CW01510370

Biomaterials and regenerative medicine in ophthalmology

Related titles:

Cellular response to biomaterials
(ISBN 978-1-84569-358-9)
The response of cells to biomaterials is critical in medical devices. It has been realised that specific cell responses may be beneficial – encouraging adhesion, healing or cell multiplication. *Cellular response to biomaterials* will discuss the response of cells to a wide range of materials, targeted at specific medical applications. Chapters in the first section review cellular response to polymers and ceramics. A second group of chapters discuss cell responses and regenerative medicine for nerves, muscles and orthopaedic materials. The final set of chapters analyse the effect surface chemistry and how it can be manipulated to provoke a useful cell response.

Degradation rate of bioresorbable materials: prediction and evaluation
(ISBN 978-1-84569-329-9)
Bioresorbable materials could be employed to provide significant advances in drug delivery systems and medical implants. The rate of material degradation is critical to performance of both implants and the controlled release of drugs; *Degradation rate of bioresorbable materials: prediction and evaluation* addresses the practicalities of this subject in detail. The first section provides an overview of bioresorbable materials and the biological environment. Degradation mechanisms are reviewed in the second group of chapters in the book, followed by bioresorption test methods in the third part. The fourth section discusses factors influencing bioresorption; finally clinical applications are reviewed.

Tissue engineering using ceramics and polymers
(ISBN 978-1-84569-176-9)
Tissue engineering is rapidly developing as a technique for the repair and regeneration of diseased tissue in the body. This authoritative and wide-ranging book reviews how ceramic and polymeric biomaterials are being used in tissue engineering. The first part of the book reviews the nature of ceramics and polymers as biomaterials together with techniques for using them such as building tissue scaffolds, transplantation techniques, surface modification and ways of combining tissue engineering with drug delivery and biosensor systems. The second part of the book discusses the regeneration of particular types of tissue from bone, cardiac and intervertebral disc tissue to skin, liver, kidney and lung tissue.

Details of these and other Woodhead Publishing materials books can be obtained by:

- visiting our web site at www.woodheadpublishing.com
- contacting Customer Services (e-mail: sales@woodheadpublishing.com; fax: +44 (0) 1223 893694; tel.: +44 (0) 1223 891358 ext. 130; address: Woodhead Publishing Limited, Abington Hall, Granta Park, Great Abington, Cambridge CB21 6AH, UK)

If you would like to receive information on forthcoming titles, please send your address details to: Francis Dodds (address, tel. and fax as above; e-mail: francis.dodds@woodhead publishing.com). Please confirm which subject areas you are interested in.

Biomaterials and regenerative medicine in ophthalmology

Edited by

Traian Chirila

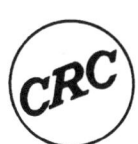

CRC Press
Boca Raton Boston New York Washington, DC

WOODHEAD PUBLISHING LIMITED
Oxford　　　Cambridge　　　New Delhi

Published by Woodhead Publishing Limited, Abington Hall, Granta Park,
Great Abington, Cambridge CB21 6AH, UK
www.woodheadpublishing.com

Woodhead Publishing India Private Limited, G-2, Vardaan House, 7/28 Ansari Road, Daryaganj,
New Delhi – 110002, India
www.woodheadpublishingindia.com

Published in North America by CRC Press LLC, 6000 Broken Sound Parkway, NW, Suite
300, Boca Raton, FL 33487, USA

First published 2010, Woodhead Publishing Limited and CRC Press LLC
© 2010, Woodhead Publishing Limited;
The authors have asserted their moral rights.

British Library Cataloguing in Publication Data
A catalogue record for this book is available from the British Library.

Library of Congress Cataloging in Publication Data
A catalog record for this book is available from the Library of Congress.

Woodhead Publishing ISBN 978-1-84569-443-2 (book)
Woodhead Publishing ISBN 978-1-84569-743-3 (e-book)
CRC Press ISBN 978-1-4398-0215-1
CRC Press order number: N10052

The publishers' policy is to use permanent paper from mills that operate a sustainable forestry
policy, and which has been manufactured from pulp which is processed using acid-free and
elemental chlorine-free practices. Furthermore, the publishers ensure that the text paper and
cover board used have met acceptable environmental accreditation standards.

Typeset by Replika Press Pvt Ltd, India
Printed by TJ International Limited, Padstow, Cornwall, UK

Contents

Part III Other applications

Contributor contact details

(*= main contact)

Chapter 1

T. V. Chirila
Queensland Eye Institute
41 Annerley Road
South Brisbane
Queensland 4101
Australia

E-mail: traian.chirila@qei.org.au

Chapter 2

D. Morrison, B. Klenkler,
    D. Morarescu and H.
    Sheardown*
School of Biomedical Engineering
    and Department of Chemical
    Engineering
McMaster University
1280 Main St West
Hamilton
ON
Canada
L8S 4L7

E-mail: sheardow@mcmaster.ca

Chapter 3

L. Werner
Intermountain Ocular Research
    Center
John A. Moran Eye Center
University of Utah
65 Mario Capecchi Drive
Salt Lake City
UT 84132
USA

E-mail: liliana.werner@hsc.utah.edu

Chapter 4

M. D. M. Evans*
Biomedical Materials and
    Regenerative Medicine Group
CSIRO Molecular and Health
    Technologies
11 Julius Avenue
North Ryde
Sydney
New South Wales 2113
Australia

E-mail: meg.evans@csiro.au

D. F. Sweeney
Vision CRC and Institute for Eye
  Research
Rupert Myers Building
Sydney
New South Wales 2052
Australia

Chapter 5

M. A. Princz and H. Sheardown*
Department of Chemical
  Engineering
McMaster University
1280 Main St West.
Hamilton ON
Canada
L8S 4L7

E-mail: sheardow@mcmaster.ca

M. Griffith
University of Ottawa
550 Cumberland Street
Ottawa ON
Canada
K1N 6NS

Chapter 6

S. Proulx, M. Guillemette, P.
  Carrier, F. A. Auger and
  L. Germain*
Departments of Oto-Rhino-
  Laryngology and Ophthalmology,
  Surgery, Laboratoire
  d'Organogénèse Expérimentale
  (LOEX), Centre de recherche
  FRSQ du CHA universitaire de
  Québec
Laval University
QC
Canada
GIS 4L8

E-mail lucie.germain@chg.ulaval.ca

C. J. Giasson
School of Optometry
Research Unit in Ophthalmology
Montréal University
Montréal QC
Canada
H3T IJ4

M. Gaudreault and S. L. Guérin
Unité de recherche en
  neurosciences, Centre de
  recherche du CHUQ, Pavillon
  CHUL
Departments of Oto-
  Rhino-Laryngology and
  Ophthalmology, Anatomy and
  Physiology
Laval University
QC
Canada
G1V OA6

Chapter 7

J. T. Jacob
Department of Ophthalmology and
    Neuroscience
Louisiana State University Health
    Sciences Center
2020 Gravier St, Suite B
New Orleans
LA 70112
USA

E-mail: jjacob@lsuhsc.edu

Chapter 8

T. V. Chirila*, L. W. Hirst,
    Z. Barnard and Zainuddin
Queensland Eye Institute
41 Annerley Road
South Brisbane
Queensland 4101
Australia

E-mail: traian.chirila@qei.org.au

D. G. Harkin
Queensland University of
    Technology
2 George St
Brisbane
Queensland 4000
Australia

I. R. Schwab
University of California, Davis
One Shields Avenue
Davis
CA 95616
USA

Chapter 9

A. Gwon
University of California, Irvine
1401 Avocado Avenue
Suite 903
Newport Beach
CA 92660
USA

E-mail: agwon@uci.edu

Chapter 10

T. Goda, T. Shimizu and
    K. Ishihara*
Departments of Materials
    Engineering and Bioengineering
Center for NanoBio Integration
The University of Tokyo
7-3-1 Hongo, Bunkyo-ku
Tokyo 113-8656
Japan

E-mail: ishihara@mpc.t.u-tokyo.ac.jp

Chapter 11

N. Efron*
Institute of Health and Biomedical
    Innovation
Queensland University of
    Technology
60 Musk Avenue, Kelvin Grove
Queensland 4059
Australia

E-mail: n.efron@qut.edu.au

P. B. Morgan and C. Maldonado-
  Codina
The University of Manchester
Moffat Building
Sackville Street
Manchester M60 1QD
UK

N. A. Brennan
Brennan Consultants Pty Ltd
110 Auburn Rd
Auburn Village
Melbourne 3122
Australia

Chapter 12

B. J. Tighe
Biomaterials Research Unit
School of Engineering and Applied
  Science
Aston University
Birmingham
B4 7ET
UK

E-mail: b.j.tighe@eggconnect.net

Chapter 13

K. E. Swindle-Reilly*
Department of Energy,
  Environmental, and Chemical
  Engineering
Washington University in St Louis
3507 Lindell Blvd
St Louis
MO 63103
USA

E-mail: kswindle@wustl.edu

N. Ravi
Veterans Affairs Medical Center
Departments of Ophthalmology and
  Visual Sciences and of Energy,
  Environmental, and Chemical
  Engineering
Washington University in St Louis
Campus Box 8096
St Louis
MO 63110
USA

E-mail: nathan.ravi@med.va.gov

Chapter 14

G. A. Limb* and J. S. Ellis
UCL Institute of Ophthalmology
Division of Ocular Biology and
  Therapeutics 11–43 Bath Street
London
ECIV 9EL
UK

E-mail g.limb@ucl.ac.uk

Chapter 15

A. S. L. Kwan*, T. V. Chirila and
  S. Cheng
Queensland Eye Institute
41 Annerley Road
South Brisbane
Queensland 4101
Australia

E-mail: tony.kwan@qei.org.au

Chapter 16

M. Wathier and M. W. Grinstaff*
Departments of Biomedical
  Engineering and Chemistry
Metcalf Center for Science and
  Engineering
Boston University
Boston
MA 02215
USA

E-mail: mgrin@bu.edu

Chapter 17

D. A. Sami
Pediatric Ophthalmology and
  Strabismus
Children's Hospital of Orange
  County (CHOC)
455 South Main Street
Orange
CA 92868
USA

E-mail: DSami@CHOC.org

S. R. Young
California Pacific Medical Center
Residency Program in
  Ophthalmology
San Francisco, California
USA

Chapter 18

E. Wentrup-Byrne* and K. George
Tissue Repair and Regeneration
  Program & School of Physical
  and Chemical Sciences
Queensland University of
  Technology
2 George St
GPO Box 2434
Brisbane
Queensland 4001
Australia

E-mail: e.wentrupbyrne@qut.edu.au

Chapter 19

B. J. Tighe
Biomaterials Research Unit
School of Engineering and Applied
  Science
Aston University
Birmingham
B4 7ET
UK

E-mail: b.j.tighe@eggconnect.net

Foreword

Biomaterials can be synthetic or biological polymers, metals, ceramics or glasses. In ophthalmology, biomaterials are mostly synthetic polymers and some biopolymers. Nevertheless, ceramics and glasses have been used in prosthetic eyeballs. A metal, titanium and a glass-ceramic have been used in keratoprostheses. Silicon, a metalloid, is used in retinal prostheses. This metalloid is also used in organosilicon polymers such as the silicones, i.e. polysiloxane backbone $(O-Si-O-Si-O-)$, and acrylic or vinyl polymers, i.e. carbon–carbon backbone, with side branches comprising tri-siloxane moieties. Biomaterials are selected from commercial materials or specially made materials, according to the physicochemical, biological and physiological properties suitable for the specific ophthalmic application.

Nearly half a century ago, when I, a chemist without experience in medical research, joined The Ophthalmic Plastics Laboratory at the Massachusetts Eye & Ear Infirmary, affiliated to Harvard Medical School, in Boston, USA, the polymer mainly used in ophthalmology was a medical-grade poly(methyl methacrylate) (PMMA), used in corneal or scleral contact lenses, intraocular lenses and keratoprostheses. Silicone rubber was used for glaucoma implants and in scleral buckling implants for retinal reattachment surgery. At that time, there were a relatively small number of scientists, engineers and medical doctors, working in academic or in industrial environments in a field that has expanded with the passage of time into the present interdisciplinary field of 'biomaterials', with numerous subspecialties, including, of course, ophthalmic biomaterials. Nowadays, there are Societies for Biomaterials in several countries, with numerous members, and several journals dealing with biomedical materials and the relatively new field of tissue engineering. Biomaterials have contributed and continue to contribute to the growth of numerous industries dealing with medical and surgical devices and, most importantly, to advances in medical procedures with devices that give patients a better quality of life, and in some cases prolong their life. The importance of biomaterials in the advances of ophthalmology and optometry is remarkable, as the reader will find in this book. The chapters by its editor, Traian Chirila, and his collaborators, and those of the outstanding group of contributors to the book, deal with the present status of ophthalmic biomaterials and their physicochemical and biological properties. This book also includes the more recent areas of biomedical investigation, tissue engineering and regenerative medicine, which aim to make or reproduce living tissues by combining materials science and cell biology.

Among the early investigators who made fundamental contributions to biomaterials, especially in ophthalmology, were Wichterle and Lim, in what was then Czechoslovakia, with their work in acrylic hydrogels, and in particularly with their invention of the hydrogel (soft) contact lenses, made of poly(2-hydroxyethyl methacrylate) (PHEMA) incorporating 38% water, an invention that was eventually refined in the USA and in other countries with great clinical and commercial success. The PHEMA hydrogel contact lens was the beginning of a series of hydrogel lenses, mostly made of HEMA copolymers, but also of hydrogels from copolymers of other hydrophilic monomers, with improved physiological properties due to improved oxygen transmissibility to the cornea, mainly a result of the higher water content and/ or lower lens thickness, compared with the original PHEMA lenses. At about the same time, several companies in the USA, France and Japan, introduced the silicone rubber contact lenses that provided optimal oxygen transmissibility to the cornea. Nevertheless, as a result of some unfavorable physical and mechanical properties of the silicone lenses, even after hydrophilic surface treatments and despite changes in lens design, their use was essentially terminated because they were too uncomfortable.

Another fundamental contribution to contact lens materials, in this case in order to improve the original oxygen-impermeable rigid PMMA lenses, was that of Gaylord and Seidner, in the USA; they developed the first rigid oxygen-permeable contact lens, made from a copolymer of MMA and methacryloxypropyl-tris(trimethylsiloxy) silane (TRIS). This material was followed by a series of rigid contact lens materials based on the same idea. The rigid gas-permeable lenses are very good as far as oxygen permeability and optical correction are concerned, but they are less comfortable, at least initially, than the hydrogel lenses. The last important development in contact lens materials has been the siloxane–hydrogel lenses that aim to have the comfort of the conventional hydrogel lenses and the oxygen permeability of the silicone- and/or TRIS-containing lenses. The priority of the invention of the siloxane–hydrogel family of contact lens materials is contentious. Nevertheless, a patent with such a claim, one of the two first generation siloxane–hydrogel contact lenses approved by the US Food and Drug Administration (FDA), is credited to 18 inventors from 3 continents. As far as nomenclature is concerned, in my opinion, silicone–hydrogel is correct when the material contains polysiloxane (silicone) moieties. However, if the hydrogel contains only TRIS or TRIS-like moieties, instead of silicone, the siloxane–hydrogel nomenclature is the correct one. Furthermore, the name siloxane–hydrogel is correct for both kinds of hydrogels, with silicone and/ or TRIS moieties.

In this book, there are chapters dealing with aspects of contact lens materials. Although corneal contact lenses are not surgical devices, but medical devices used on the ocular surface for optical correction or for therapeutic or cosmetic use, they must be approved, as must all medical devices, by the proper governmental agencies, such as the FDA in the USA. Some biomaterial devices are implanted into transparent corneas for optical correction. On the other hand, artificial corneas (keratoprostheses) are implanted in opaque corneas to restore vision to eyes that would not tolerate corneal tissue transplanted from donor eyes.

Eyes with cataract recover vision after the surgical extraction of the opaque crystalline lens, vision that is highly improved after the implantation of an intraocular lens (IOL) made of biomaterials. The original IOLs were made of PMMA, and were implanted in the eye through the relative large incision required for the extraction of the crystalline lens. However, a new cataract surgical procedure (phacoemulsification) was conceived in the late 1960s by Kelman, an ophthalmologist in New York, a procedure that emulsifies and removes the cataractous lens through a small incision. Then, new IOLs were developed made of hydrogels, silicone rubber or novel acrylic polymers that can be folded in such a way that they can be introduced into the eye through a small incision, and then unfold into the eye. In special cases of phakic eyes in need of a special optical correction, IOLs are implanted in eyes without removing the transparent crystalline lens. IOLs, as well as contact lenses, are among the biomedical devices most frequently used all over the world, and their present status and related research activities are dealt with in this book.

Other applications of polymeric biomaterials in the eye are as glaucoma implants that are used to lower the intraocular pressure by draining aqueous humor from the anterior chamber of the eye into the tissues of the external periphery of the eyeball where the aqueous is reabsorbed.

Biomaterials are used for the reattachment of detached retinas, by means of scleral buckling implants that restore the contact between the retina and the subretinal tissues, by neutralizing the traction of the shrinking vitreous on the retina. For some complicated cases of giant retinal detachment, a vitreous substitute is the only alternative to restore some degree of vision to such blind eyes. The objective in this procedure is to inject intravitreously a substance that will push the detached retina into its normal position, over the choroid, and retain it there. This procedure is currently performed with injections of gases or low viscosity perfluorocarbon liquids that are reabsorbed or removed from the eye in a relatively short postoperative time. These gases or liquids are exchanged in most cases by a vitreous substitute that will maintain the retina in its normal place for a longer time. Despite many attempts with biological polymers, such as the viscoelastic gel hyaluronan, and diverse viscous solutions of other biopolymers or synthetic hydrophilic polymers, and high water content hydrogels, the only long-lasting vitreous substitute actually in use is the hydrophobic silicone oil, with a viscosity that is 1000–2000 times higher than water. Silicone oils act as a good tamponade against the effusion of subretinal fluid in to the vitreous cavity and support the detached retina onto the choroid. Nevertheless, silicone oil is far from an ideal vitreous substitute, and new directions of research are presented in this book.

Surgical adhesives, such as the monomer butyl cyanoacrylate that polymerizes *in situ* in the presence of moisture, have been used in ophthalmology, mainly for closing corneal leaking wounds or ulcers while they heal. Other synthetic or biological polymeric adhesives for ophthalmic use have been investigated or are under investigation, as shown in this book. Polymeric biomaterials, biodegradable or non-biodegradable, are used also in devices for sustained delivery of drugs on and into the eye.

Up to this point, my comments have dealt essentially with the past and present of ophthalmic biomedical materials and devices that are most familiar to me. A number of chapters in the book deal with relatively new fields of research, tissue engineering and regenerative medicine, which are, somewhat, related to biomaterials, and aim to create a fantastic future for ophthalmology. I do not have personal experience in these fields of research, but I am aware of the excellent work of some of the authors, and I expect that the interested reader will find this portion of the book very enlightening.

In my opinion, this book can be highly recommeneded to scientists, engineers, ophthalmologists and optometrists, in academia or industry, in laboratory or clinic, who are interested in any aspect of biomaterials and regenerative medicine as applied to ophthalmology.

Miguel F. Refojo, D.Sc.
Senior Scientist Emeritus, Schepens Eye Research Institute
Associate Professor of Ophthalmology (Ret.), Harvard Medical School
Boston, MA, USA

Preface

This is the first book dedicated to ophthalmic biomaterials and ophthalmic tissue engineering and regenerative medicine. Strictly speaking, about a decade ago there was an attempt to publish such a book, following an invitation that I received from the editors of the journal *Progress in Polymer Science* to guest-edit a special issue. The result appeared in 1998 as issue number 3 of volume 23, having the additional title *'Polymer Science and the Eye'* on the title page (but not on the cover). It contained eight contributions covering not only ocular biomaterials but also the macromolecular structure of ocular tissues. I was fortunate in securing the participation of some high-calibre contributors such as Miguel Refojo, Jorge Heller, Simon Ross-Murphy, Robert Gurny, Robert Augusteyn and Vickery Trinkaus-Randall. However, a subscription-restricted circulation (it was not marketed as a book) and a rather small number of chapters dedicated specifically to biomaterials could not make that journal issue into a representative multi-author textbook in the field of ophthalmic biomaterials. I hope that the present book will be regarded and employed in such a capacity, providing a comprehensive coverage of these materials and their use for the repair and regeneration of eye structures through the techniques of tissue engineering and regenerative medicine. To this end, a collection of chapters was assembled that focuses on the materials used in ophthalmic surgery, with emphasis on certain applications and advanced methodologies for the reconstruction of ocular elements. We did not intend to have a collection of unrelated chapters, and have made efforts to achieve, at least in part, a coordinated general outlook.

I feel privileged to propose this book as a tribute to Miguel Refojo. Although I have not asked them, I am sure that the other contributors will give their consent. Miguel is the scientist who established the macromolecular basis of ophthalmic biomaterials. He did this at a time when most of the few clinicians who manifested any interest for ocular prosthetic materials were using the word 'plastic' in their reports to denote PMMA exclusively, as they were not aware that other polymers may also exist.

Miguel was born in 1928 in Santiago de Compostela, Spain. He studied at the University of Santiago where he obtained a doctorate in organic chemistry in 1956. After a 3-year postdoctoral stint at Yale University and a few years as a senior research chemist at DuPont Canada in Ontario, Miguel became a researcher at the Retina Foundation (now Schepens Eye Research Institute, SERI) in Boston, Massachusetts, where he stayed for the next 35 years. He retired in 1998 as the head of the Biomedical Polymers Laboratory at SERI and an associate professor at Harvard Medical School. Between 1965 and 1968, Miguel published a series of about ten articles regarding the synthesis, structure, properties and characterization of acrylic hydrogels and their applications in ophthalmology. These papers stood the test of time. They contributed essentially to the progress of hydrogels research, while also providing a scientific foundation for the emerging field of ophthalmic biomaterials. Subsequently, Miguel's interests expanded, and during his career he investigated almost all aspects of ophthalmic biomaterials, including: vitreous substitutes (*c*. 30 papers); materials for episcleral buckling in the treatment of retinal detachment (*c*. 20 papers); contact lens materials (*c*. 50 papers); controlled release of ocular drugs (*c*. 20 papers); ocular adhesives; corneal implants; IOLs; ocular pharmacology; and tear film physiology. He also wrote five general reviews on ophthalmic biomaterials and 32 book chapters, most of them regarded as standard references in our field, and obtained ten US patents for his inventions. Miguel's achievements were recognized through many awards and honours, and I shall mention here the prestigious Ruben Medal from the International Society for Contact Lens Research (1997), the Clemson Award from the Society for Biomaterials (2000) and the Wichterle Medal from the Czech Contactology Society (2002). Miguel accepted the invitation to write a foreword to this book with grace, and I cannot think of anyone more appropriate to do so.

I am grateful for the confidence and support from Woodhead Publishing Limited who invited me to edit this book. Special thanks are due to Laura Overend (née Bunney), the Commissioning Editor, who first approached me on behalf of the publisher – we worked together to select and recruit potential contributors; and to Lucy Cornwell, Publications Co-ordinator, who ensured that the processing of submissions became a pleasant activity. I am enormously indebted to those who agreed to contribute and write the chapters that form this book. Finally, I thank the management of the Queensland Eye Institute in Brisbane, Australia, for allowing me to carry out much of my editorial work during working hours.

1

An introduction to ophthalmic biomaterials and their application through tissue engineering and regenerative medicine

T. V. CHIRILA, Queensland Eye Institute, Australia

Abstract: This chapter presents a brief history of the development of ophthalmic biomaterials. Particularities in the development of ophthalmic biomaterials are discussed and some of their historic priorities within the general field of biomaterials are revealed or emphasized. The chapter then discusses the role and integration of ophthalmic biomaterials in tissue engineering and regenerative medicine applications.

Key words: ophthalmic biomaterials, polymers, tissue engineering, repair, regenerative medicine.

1.1 Introduction

The ultimate goal of the research and development of materials (other than drugs) for applications in medicine, which we call biomaterials, has always been to emulate natural materials. Since the natural target for biomaterials, i.e. our body's tissues and organs, is exceedingly complex, it is not surprising that in many instances the laboratory-made materials cannot match in their performance the natural entities they are meant to augment or replace. This is obviously different from the development of materials for industrial applications, which usually perform better than their natural counterparts (if the latter exist), and also evolve relatively fast, unhindered by biological constraints. For too long, an acceptable end-performance in the short term was the main requirement from a biomaterial, with little attention paid to changing its bulk and/or surface properties through the manipulation of composition and/or structure, in order to maximize the clinical outcome. Over the past six decades or so, however, the progress in bringing the properties and functionality of biomaterials close to those of their biological targets has been remarkable. While the above statements are also valid for ophthalmic biomaterials, their development has shown some particular features. The general developments in the field of biomaterials have customarily been gauged through the achievements in the branches of orthopaedic biomaterials and – to a lesser extent – biomaterials for cardiology while the progress of ophthalmic biomaterials has usually been ignored or seldom presented.

There are many definitions of the concept of 'biomaterials', all conveying essentially the same message (Ratner *et al.*, 2004). Nevertheless, the term can also be used for 'biological materials', and attempts have been made to reconcile such dual meaning (Nerem and Sambanis, 1995). I shall not delve further into terminological aspects except for warning against some unacceptable inconsistencies such as: the use of 'biopolymer' instead of 'biomaterial'; using the term 'biomaterials' exclusively for natural biological materials or, worse, to describe specifically biological matter deposited on non-biological substrata; and the more recent use of the qualifier 'biosynthetic' to designate a biomaterial resulting from the combination of a biopolymer with a synthetic polymer. In my role as an editor, I devoted much attention to avoiding such ambiguities throughout this book.

During the last two centuries, a large variety of biomaterials have been reported including metals, minerals, ceramics, wood, biopolymers and synthetic polymers. Most materials to be placed in the eye must be transparent, and this prerequisite is indeed unique to the ophthalmic biomaterials. Consequently, the focus of this book will be synthetic polymers, biopolymers (as such or modified), and combinations of the two, as the other materials are not normally transparent. Although no longer in use today, glass and quartz were the biomaterials of choice for ophthalmic applications before polymers became available, for instance in artificial corneas (Chirila *et al.*, 1998; Chirila and Hicks, 1999; Chirila *et al.*, 2005) and contact lenses (Feinbloom, 1932; Dallos, 1936; Heitz, 1984; Barr and Bailey, 1991). Opaque materials, such as ceramics, may still have minor uses in the eye, but only at locations outside the vision pathway.

1.2   Development of ophthalmic biomaterials: a brief history

In discussing here the evolution of ophthalmic biomaterials I will avoid the rather disconcerting trend of regarding, and even formally citing, biblical stories and anecdotal sources involving saints or other mythical characters, as scientific literature allegedly documenting some sort of respectable antiquity of the disciplines of biomaterials and tissue engineering. With all due respect to anyone's personal beliefs, these sources clearly do not constitute scientific evidence.

The eye is an organ of great complexity, yet it is more accessible to medical observation and surgical manipulation than most of our organs. This probably explains why the eye was the organ in which the first transplantation of donor tissue was successfully performed in humans (Zirm, 1906). Rather inexplicably, Zirm's transplantation of a donor cornea is still not recognized as being the first organ transplantation from a human donor to a human recipient. This accolade is usually reserved for the kidney transplantation reported much later (Murray *et al.*, 1955), even though the latter was performed in identical twins, while the former involved non-related human subjects. However, prior to the episode of corneal transplantation, the eye was also the organ where foreign materials were implanted for the first time with the purpose of fulfilling, in today's terms, a role as biomaterials. In 1862, Onofrio Abbate, an Italian ophthalmologist practising in Cairo (Hirschberg, 1991), presented his experiments with an artificial cornea at the Periodical International Congress of Ophthalmology in Paris. This report was published in the following year in the congress proceedings, a publication that is virtually impossible to obtain nowadays. Fortunately, details of Abbate's work are available in one of the early reviews on artificial cornea (Forster, 1923). His keratoprosthesis was made from a glass disk encased within a skirt of two successive rings, the first made of gutta-percha and the second of casein. Both are natural polymers: gutta-percha is the *trans*-isomer of natural rubber isolated from trees of the genera *Palaquium* and *Payena* (Malaya), and casein is a mixture of phosphoproteins precipitated from milk or cheese. The concept of this device illustrates Abbate's remarkable anticipation of the need for a skirt made from a material different from that used in the central zone (in this case, glass), in order to promote biointegration. His choice of the skirt materials was, however, not the most appropriate, as casein is brittle and gutta-percha becomes so on exposure to air and light. The device was maintained in animal corneas for no longer than one week. At the end of the same century, Lang implanted spheres fabricated from an artificial material (celluloid) as replacements for the enucleated eye globes (Lang, 1887). Strictly speaking, the socket implant is a cosmetic prosthesis. Soon afterwards, however, the first attempt ever to use a man-made material as a functional prosthesis took place in Germany, when – unaware of Lang's work – Dimmer made an artificial cornea (or keratoprosthesis) from celluloid and implanted it in four human patients (Dimmer, 1889; Dimmer, 1891). Celluloid, the first commercial plastic developed in the world, is a blend of nitrocellulose (a modified biopolymer), camphor, and certain stabilizing agents, therefore not actually a fully synthetic polymer. Regardless, this material was not a fortunate choice, as Dimmer's keratoprostheses were rejected within a few months.

The use of fully synthetic polymers as implantable ophthalmic biomaterials eventually occurred about half a century later, starting with poly(vinyl alcohol) gels inserted as socket implants (Thiel, 1939; Beyer, 1941), followed by the first artificial corneas made of poly(methyl methacrylate) (PMMA) (Wünsche, 1947; Franceschetti, 1949; Kuwahara, 1950; Györffy, 1951), a landmark not exempted from some controversy regarding priority (Chirila and Crawford, 1996), and culminating with the much better known and undisputed development of Ridley's PMMA intraocular lens (IOL) (Ridley, 1951; Ridley, 1952a; Ridley, 1952b). A few years later, poly(1-vinyl-2-pyrrolidinone) became the first synthetic polymer to be implanted in the vitreous cavity as a vitreous substitute (Scuderi, 1954; Hayano and Yoshino, 1959). In parallel developments, synthetic polymers also aroused the interest of the contact lens manufacturers. Feinbloom was the first to use glass (central part) in combination with commercially available synthetic polymers (peripheral part) in scleral contact lenses, and PMMA was among the polymers he proposed (Feinbloom, 1937; Feinbloom, 1940). It is not known with certainty who introduced the first scleral contact lenses made entirely from PMMA, as the unfolding of the subsequent events becomes blurred, an unfortunate result of the fact that the contact lens was perceived from the very beginning as a fast-profit-generating device. As a consequence, the research and development activities were generally carried out in the laboratories of the manufacturers, and the field became contaminated with an excessive amount of patents and litigations between competing manufacturers, while being depleted of valid scientific publications in peer-reviewed journals due to exaggerated trade secret policies. It is believed that Mullen, Obrig or Györffy were perhaps among the first to make scleral contact lenses totally from PMMA (Barr and Bailey, 1991). It is also generally accepted that around 1947, Tuohy made the first corneal contact lenses from PMMA (Barr and Bailey, 1991; Goodlaw, 2000), although he did not report it in a scientific journal. His famous patent (Tuohy, 1950) is notoriously ambiguous about what polymers are claimed for manufacture. The contact lens has a rather particular position among ophthalmic biomaterials. The device involves intimate contact with some components of the ocular surface, especially the corneal epithelium, a circumstance that is essentially different from the situation of implanting polymer devices into the eye. However, biocompatibility remains the fundamental issue for both ocular implants and contact lens materials. The latter should be, and usually are, treated as ophthalmic biomaterials – as is the case in this book. We should, however, acknowledge that the research and development of contact lenses is a discipline on its own.

The range of ophthalmic biomaterials has subsequently expanded significantly, particularly after the introduction of synthetic hydrogels (i.e. polymers that absorb and retain water without dissolving in aqueous media) by Otto Wichterle's group in Czechoslovakia (Dreifus *et al.*, 1960; Wichterle, 1960; Wichterle and Lím, 1960; Wichterle *et al.*, 1961).

Through the remarkable activity of Miguel Refojo at the Retina Foundation (now Schepens Eye Research Institute) in Boston, Massachusetts, by the mid 1970s the field of ophthalmic biomaterials became an established discipline. Brian Tighe at Aston University in Birmingham, UK, further contributed to the development of this field through fundamental studies on hydrogels and contact lens materials. The number of scientists involved in ophthalmic biomaterials worldwide increased steadily, although not to the same extent as in other branches of biomaterials. Research groups or departments dedicated to ophthalmic biomaterials and established by non-profit institutions and universities are still relatively few in number.

1.3 Tissue engineering and regenerative medicine in ophthalmology

Tissue engineering should be regarded as the next evolutionary step in the development of biomaterials. Going beyond prostheses or devices, tissue engineering aims at developing truly functional substitutes able to compensate for tissue loss or to restore failed organs. Basically, this is achievable through the *ex-vivo* manipulation of cells and tissues, and employing growth factors, angiogenic or anti-angiogenic agents, signalling molecules or other bioactive agents, and their combination with the biomaterial scaffolds. This was ideally expressed by David Williams when he defined tissue engineering as 'the persuasion of the body to heal itself, through the delivery to the appropriate sites of molecular signals, cells and supporting structures' (Williams, 1999). As cogently stated later by Linda Griffith, 'coaxing cells to form tissue is inherently an engineering process as they need physical support [...] as well as chemical and mechanical signals [...] to form the intricate hierarchical structures that characterize native tissue' (Griffith, 2002). Clearly, the field of tissue engineering involves methodologies and techniques that are much more complex than the placement of a contact lens on to the cornea or the insertion of an IOL in the anterior segment of the eye.

This multidisciplinary field probably has more definitions* than the biomaterials field has, but most are variations of the definition that appeared in the preface of the proceedings book of a tissue engineering workshop held at Granlibakken, Lake Tahoe, California in February 1988 (Skalak *et al.*, 1988), sponsored by the National Science Foundation (NSF) (USA). This definition revealed the essence of tissue engineering as 'the development of biological substitutes to restore, maintain, or improve tissue functions', and the accompanying commentary unambiguously identifies the field as it is understood today. This definition was adopted by leading researchers in the field (Nerem and Sambanis, 1995; Godbey and Atala, 2002). A popular opinion is, however, that tissue engineering was born in the late 1980s in the laboratories of Robert Langer, Joseph Vacanti, Charles Vacanti and their colleagues at Massachusetts Institute of Technology (MIT) and Harvard Medical School. In a much-cited paper from this group (Langer and Vacanti, 1993), the definition of tissue engineering was a modification of that mentioned above, a fact acknowledged by the authors.

---

* It has recently come to my attention that other investigators have been more thorough than me in searching for the origins of the term 'tissue engineering'. In an editorial (Lysaght and Crager, 2009) published in July 2009 in *Tissue Engineering Part A*, it is asserted that the very first use of the term was actually in two press releases distributed in 1982 and 1983 by a commercial information service known as *PR Newswire*. The releases, obviously not peer-reviewed publications, heralded the funding by two US medical companies of research undertaken at MIT by the late Eugene Bell, a pioneer in the field.

The origin of the term 'tissue engineering' as such is controversial. It is worth discussing the issue here, not only because it involves the activity of an ophthalmologist, but also considering that Charles Vacanti has recently dismissed as invalid any recorded use of the term tissue engineering prior to that in one of his articles published in 1991 in a surgical magazine (Vacanti and Vacanti, 1991), because – in his opinion – these earlier uses of the term do not reflect the meaning of the discipline 'as it is currently understood' (Vacanti, 2006). This statement not only disregards the fact that the term was already in correct use in 1987, as there is evidence that NSF was running at that time a 'Panel on Tissue Engineering', but also ignores the Lake Tahoe meeting and the communications presented there (Skalak *et al.*, 1988). Furthermore, as shown below, there is documented evidence that an ophthalmologist was in fact the first to use this term in a publication pre-dating these events.

J. Reimer Wolter (1924–2003) was a highly respected ophthalmologist, both as an educator and clinician, and an outstanding histologist and pathologist. He was educated in Germany but spent most of his career at the University of Michigan. He was the first to show in scientific detail how the eye tissue responds to implanted IOLs (Wolter, 1985) and other foreign materials, and he is regarded as the founder of modern ophthalmic cytopathology. Wolter was also an expert in retinal and orbital surgery, a pioneer of laser ophthalmic surgery, and he made contributions to paediatric ophthalmology and ophthalmic neuropathology. In 1984, he reported in detail the cytopathological findings of a keratoprosthesis explanted from a patient almost 20 years after implantation (Wolter and Meyer, 1984), an extraordinarily long retention for an artificial cornea, by any standard. The prosthesis was of the 'through-and-through' type, with a fenestrated skirt of Teflon and an optical zone made (probably) from PMMA. Wolter's analysis demonstrated that the skirt was embedded in the corneal stroma without inflammatory reaction. He also detected two transparent membranes: an acellular membrane formed on the anterior prosthetic surface and a cellular membrane on the posterior surface generated by macrophages that differentiated into fibroblasts. Remarkably, both membranes were transparent. Wolter hypothesized that the eye was able to produce membranes to separate the implant from the anterior chamber, and interpreted the formation of the retroprosthetic membrane as a cellular response to prevent light scattering induced by the abnormal presence of the foreign material; in other words, as if the presence of the keratoprosthesis 'engineered' the formation of the membranes. As a concluding remark, the paper contains (Wolter and Meyer, 1984, p. 198) the following statements.

This membrane took the place of the endothelium and it remained clear for 20 years. Nature impresses us with a great variety of reactive possibilities in the adaptation of its tissues to new conditions and substances. Sound progress in medicine is easiest when we work along with the physiological currents of beneficial reaction and adaptation. To understand the direction and the limits of nature's reactions is always the first step toward progress in tissue engineering.

The term 'tissue engineering' was used again on the same page, in the summary section of the article, where it was emphasized that the study revealed the 'significance of the successful adaptation of the plastic materials of the prosthesis to the tissues of the cornea and the fluids of the inner eye for the future of tissue engineering in the region of the eye [...]' (Wolter and Meyer, 1984). There is no doubt in my mind that – considering Wolter's erudition and integrity, as well as the diversity of his research interests – he used the term precisely to describe a field as he comprehended it, and there is no reason to doubt that his understanding of the term coincided with, or at least was very close to, the current meaning. Whether this will be accepted or not by the tissue engineering community is irrelevant, but it is reassuring that some leading investigators have acknowledged Wolter's first use of the term (Godbey and Atala, 2002).

In a thought-provoking essay (Williams, 2006), which perhaps should be read by all those working in the field, David Williams made a critical analysis of the current central tissue engineering paradigm. He concluded that a reason why tissue engineering has yet to deliver the expected clinical outcomes is that not only the paradigm, but also some concepts and the definition itself, might be wrong, and suggested that a combination of systems engineering and systems biology approaches will provide the conditions for cells to generate the required tissue in circumstances that are not normal. He went further and proposed a more adequate definition of tissue engineering (Williams, 2006): 'Tissue engineering is the creation of new tissue for the therapeutic reconstruction of the human body, by the deliberate and controlled stimulation of selected target cells, through a systematic combination of molecular and mechanical signals.'

Tissue engineering should be regarded as 'a major part of regenerative medicine' (Atala, 2007). The term 'regenerative medicine' is currently described by even more definitions than the terms 'biomaterials' and 'tissue engineering' put together, which is obviously suggestive of the variety of interpretations resulting from different opinions on both the aim of this discipline and the contributing disciplines. Consequently, many prominent investigators, including William Haseltine, who introduced the term (Haseltine, 2001), have made commendable efforts to formulate a consensus definition that would adequately and correctly incorporate the whole diversity of this emerging medical field (Haseltine, 2003; Mironov *et al.*, 2004; Greenwood *et al.*, 2006; Daar and Greenwood, 2007; Ingber and Levin, 2007; Mason and Dunnill, 2008). In the most thorough analysis to date, Daar and Greenwood critically and objectively discussed a range of existing definitions, and proposed a definition that captures the essence of regenerative medicine (Daar and Greenwood, 2007), a part of which is reproduced below.

> Regenerative medicine is an interdisciplinary field of research and clinical applications focused on the repair, replacement or regeneration of cells, tissues or organs to restore impaired function resulting from any cause, including congenital defects, diseases, trauma and ageing. It uses a combination of several converging technological approaches, both existing and newly emerging, that moves it beyond traditional transplantation and replacement therapies.

The definition is actually longer, further disclosing that the main role of these approaches is to trigger self-healing processes, for which bioactive molecules, stem/progenitor cell therapy, gene therapy and tissue engineering can be used (Daar and Greenwood, 2007). Aiming at formulating a more convenient definition for communications between scientists and public, other researchers processed the above definition and provided a much abbreviated version (Mason and Dunnill, 2008): 'Regenerative medicine replaces or regenerates human cells, tissue or organs, to restore or establish normal function'.

Prosthetics and transplantation are not generally regarded as valid approaches in regenerative medicine, since 'replacement' is fundamentally different from 'regeneration'. Essential to regenerative medicine is also the distinction between 'repair' and 'regeneration' (Yannas, 2001; Yannas, 2005; Mason and Dunnill, 2008), in other words the response of adult mammals to any injury that causes loss of tissue or organs. While the spontaneous repair process can accomplish the healing of a wound through contraction and formation of scar tissue, but cannot restore the original integrity and function, the process of regeneration performs full healing by synthesizing the missing tissue or organs and recovering normal structure and function. There is, however, an insurmountable problem: true regeneration never occurs in adult mammalian organisms. In humans, it only occurs in the foetus during the first 6 months of gestation. In adults, the only alternative to replacement or repair is 'induced regeneration', a process defined by Yannas as 'the synthesis of non-regenerative tissues in a severely injured adult organ that leads to, at least partial, recovery of physiological structure and function' (Yannas, 2005). To achieve induced regeneration is the cornerstone of regenerative medicine. In attempting this process, the investigators frequently use scaffolds, which in most cases have a biomaterial component, and cellular therapies. Episodes of induced regeneration have been reported so far in skin, peripheral nerves, bone, heart valves, articular cartilage, urological organs and spinal cord. It is important to note, in the context of this book, that induced regeneration has been also reported in conjunctiva (Hatton and Rubin, 2005) and cornea (Kinoshita and Nakamura, 2005).

Haseltine predicted an ongoing role for biomaterials in regenerative medicine, but he emphasized that they should fully integrate with the living cells (Haseltine, 2001). He also included the use of electronic devices to replace sensory functions (Haseltine, 2003); at least formally, the materials of such devices should be regarded as biomaterials. It is accepted (Mironov *et al.*, 2004; Daar and Greenwood, 2007) that biomaterials can be involved in regenerative medicine in a variety of ways, for instance as components of delivery systems for bioactive molecules, as nanostructured materials developed to provide new regenerative strategies, or as constituents of tissue-engineered constructs involved in certain approaches to induced regeneration.

The translation from the laboratory to the clinical setting of tissue engineering and regenerative medicine procedures has begun in respect to many specific organs (Atala, 2007; Furth and Atala, 2008; Tubo, 2008). However, in spite of occasional sensationalization in the press of laboratory-scale achievements, only a few products are commercially available and approved for clinical use; and these are almost entirely limited to the regeneration of skin (Mansbridge, 2006; Russell and Bertram, 2007; Tubo, 2008) or cartilage (Russell and Bertram, 2007; Tubo, 2008). In the eye, examples of tissue engineering applications have been reported mainly in the anterior segment (cornea, conjunctiva). As it is accepted that the scaffolds can be either biodegradable or non-biodegradable (Langer and Vacanti, 1993; Williams, 2008), the 'core-and-skirt' keratoprostheses with a porous skirt (Chirila, 1994; Chirila, 1997; Chirila *et al.*, 1998; Chirila, 2001; Duan *et al.*, 2006; Sheardown and Griffith, 2008) may be legitimately regarded as an early example of ophthalmic tissue engineering. One such artificial cornea (Chirila *et al.*, 1994; Crawford *et al.*, 2002; Hicks *et al.*, 2003), available commercially as AlphaCor™, is in routine clinical use in humans in a number of countries. Current tissue engineering and regenerative medicine applications in the ocular field include constructs to replace damaged full-thickness cornea (tissue-engineered corneal equivalents) (Germain *et al.*, 2004; Duan *et al.*, 2006; Ruberti *et al.*, 2007), which will obviate the need for keratoprostheses, and constructs for the restoration of ocular surfaces that have been damaged as a result of pathological disorders or trauma leading to the loss of epithelial stem cells (Nishida, 2003; Selvam *et al.*, 2006; Boulton *et al.*, 2007). Significant advances have been made in cellular therapies for treating retinal degenerative conditions (Lund *et al.*, 2001; Klassen, 2006; Lamba and Reh, 2008). Some progress has been made in the field of visual prostheses for restoration of vision in retina-blind people (Maynard, 2001; Weiland and Humayun, 2003; Dagnelie, 2007); although these developments involve biomaterials and elements of tissue engineering, they are essentially based on electronic engineering and neurostimulation techniques. In recent years, some efforts have been made to understand the mechanism of regeneration of the eye's crystalline lens and to investigate the possibility of creating such lenses by tissue engineering/regenerative medicine approaches (Sommer *et al.*, 2006; Tsonis, 2006). Some preliminary investigations of the regeneration of the retina have also been reported (Sommer *et al.*, 2006).

1.4   References

Atala A (2007), 'Engineering tissues, organs and cells', *J Tissue Eng Regen Med*, **1**, 83–96.

Barr J T and Bailey N J (1991), 'History and development of contact lenses', in Bennett E S and Weissman B A eds, *Clinical Contact Lens Practice*, London, J B Lippincott Co. Ch. 11, pp. 1–8.

Beyer W (1941), 'Über die Einheilung und den Erfolg der Polyviolplomben nach Thiel', *Klin Monatsbl Augenheilk*, **106**, 272–279.

Boulton M E, Albon J and Grant M B (2007), 'Stem cells in the eye', in Lanza R, Langer R and Vacanti J eds, *Principles of Tissue Engineering*, 3rd edn, Amsterdam, Elsevier, pp. 1011–1023.

Chirila T V (1994), 'Modern artificial corneas: the use of porous polymers', *Trends Polym Sci*, **2**, 296–300.

Chirila T V (1997), 'Artificial cornea with a porous polymeric skirt', *Trends Polym Sci*, **5**, 346–348.

Chirila T V (2001), 'An overview of the development of artificial corneas with porous skirts and the use of PHEMA for such an application', *Biomaterials*, **22**, 3311–3317.

Chirila T V, Vijayasekaran S, Horne R, Chen Y-C, Dalton P D, Constable I J and Crawford G J (1994), 'Interpenetrating polymer network (IPN) as a permanent joint between the elements of a new type of artificial cornea', *J Biomed Mater Res*, **28**, 745–753.

Chirila T V and Crawford G J (1996), 'A controversial episode in the history of artificial cornea: the first use of poly(methyl methacrylate)', *Gesnerus*, **53**, 236–242.

Chirila T V, Hicks C R, Dalton P D, Vijayasekaran S, Lou X, Hong Y, Clayton A B, Ziegelaar B W, Fitton J H, Platten S, Crawford G J and Constable I J (1998), 'Artificial cornea', *Prog Polym Sci*, **23**, 447–473.

Chirila T V and Hicks C R (1999), 'The origins of the artificial cornea: Pellier de Quengsy and his contribution to the modern concept of keratoprosthesis', *Gesnerus*, **56**, 96–106.

Chirila T V, Chirila M, Ikada Y, Eguchi H and Shiota H (2005), 'A historical review of artificial cornea research in Japan', *Jpn J Ophthalmol*, **49**, S1–S13.

Crawford G J, Hicks C R, Lou X, Vijayasekaran S, Tan D, Mulholland B, Chirila T V and Constable I J (2002), 'The Chirila keratoprosthesis: phase I human clinical trial', *Ophthalmology*, **109**, 883–889.

Daar A S and Greenwood H L (2007), 'A proposed definition of regenerative medicine', *J Tissue Eng Regen Med*, **1**, 179–184.

Dagnelie G (2007), 'Vision enhancement systems', in Lanza R, Langer R and Vacanti J eds, *Principles of Tissue Engineering*, 3rd edn, Amsterdam, Elsevier, pp 1049–1063.

Dallos J (1936), 'Contact glasses, the "invisible" spectacles', *Arch Ophthalmol*, **15**, 617–623.

Dimmer F (1889), 'Zur operativen Behandlung totaler Hornhautnarben mit vorderer Synechie', *Ber Versamml Ophthalmol Ges Heidelberg*, **20**, 148–163.

Dimmer F (1891), 'Notiz über Cornea arteficialis', *Klin Monatsbl Augenheilk*, **29**, 104–105.

Dreifus M, Lím D and Wichterle O (1960), 'Intracameral lenses made of hydrocolloid acylates' (Czech), *Čsl Oftal*, **16**, 154–159.

Duan D, Klenkler B J and Sheardown H (2006), 'Progress in the development of a corneal replacement: keratoprostheses and tissue-engineered corneas', *Expert Rev Med Devices*, **3**, 59–72.

Feinbloom W (1932), 'Contact lenses', *Am J Optom*, **9**, 78–111.

Feinbloom W (1937), 'A plastic contact lens', *Am J Optom*, **14**, 41–49.

Feinbloom W (1940), 'Contact lens', US Patent 2,196,066.

Forster A E (1923), 'A review of keratoplastic surgery and some experiments in keratoplasty', *Am J Ophthalmol*, **6**, 366–375.

Franceschetti A (1949), 'Corneal grafting', *Trans Ophthalmol Soc UK*, **69**, 17–35.

Furth M E and Atala A (2008), 'Current and future perspectives of regenerative medicine', in Atala A, Lanza R, Thomson J A and Nerem R M eds, *Principles of Regenerative Medicine*, Amsterdam, Elsevier, pp. 2–15.

Germain L, Giasson C J, Carrier P, Guérin S L, Salesse C and Auger F A (2004), 'Tissue engineering of the cornea', in Wnek G E and Bowlin G L eds, *Encyclopedia of Biomaterials and Biomedical Engineering*, New York, Marcel Dekker Inc., pp. 1534–1544.

Godbey W T and Atala A (2002), 'In vitro systems for tissue engineering', *Ann N Y Acad Sci*, **961**, 10–26.

Goodlaw E (2000), 'A personal perspective on the history of contact lenses', *Int Contact Lens Clin*, **27**, 139–145.

Greenwood H L, Thorsteinsdóttir H, Perry G, Renihan J, Singer P A and Daar A S (2006), 'Regenerative medicine: new opportunities for developing countries', *Int J Biotechnol*, **8**, 60–77.

Griffith L G (2002), 'Emerging design principles in biomaterials and scaffolds for tissue engineering', *Ann N Y Acad Sci*, **961**, 83–95.

Györffy I (1951), 'Acrylic corneal implant in keratoplasty', *Am J Ophthalmol*, **34**, 757–758.

Haseltine W A (2001), 'The emergence of regenerative medicine: a new field and a new society', *J Regen Med*, **2**, 17–23.

Haseltine W A (2003), 'Regenerative medicine 2003: an overview', *J Regen Med*, **4**, 15–18.

Hatton M P and Rubin P A D (2005), 'Conjunctival regeneration', *Adv Biochem Eng Biotechnol*, **94**, 125–140.

Hayano S and Yoshino T (1959), 'Local application of polyvinylpyrrolidone (PVP) for some ocular diseases' (Jpn), *Rinsho Ganka [J Clin Ophthalmol]*, **13**, 449–453.

Heitz R F (1984), 'The invention of contact lenses by August Müller (1887)', *Contact Lens Assoc Ophthalmol J*, **10**, 88–95.

Hicks C R, Crawford G J, Lou X, Tan D T, Snibson G R, Sutton G, Downie N, Werner L, Chirila T V and Constable I J (2003), 'Corneal replacement using a synthetic hydrogel cornea, AlphaCor™: device, preliminary outcomes and complications', *Eye*, **17**, 385–392.

Hirschberg J (1991), *The History of Ophthalmology*, vol. 10 (transl. Blodi F C), Bonn, J P Wayenborgh Verlag, p 342.

Ingber D E and Levin M (2007), 'What lies at the interface of regenerative medicine and developmental biology?', *Development*, **134**, 2541–2547.

Kinoshita S and Nakamura T (2005), 'Corneal cells for regeneration', in Morser J and Nishikawa S I eds, *The Promises and Challenges of Regenerative Medicine*, Berlin, Springer-Verlag, pp. 63–83.

Klassen H (2006), 'Transplantation of cultured progenitor cells to the mammalian retina', *Expert Opin Biol Ther*, **6**, 443–451.

Kuwahara Y (1950), 'Research on implantation of artificial cornea, part I' (Jpn), *Nippon Ganka Gakkai Zasshi [Acta Soc Ophthalmol Jpn]*, **54**, 400–402.

Lamba D and Reh T A (2008), 'Regenerative medicine for diseases of the retina', in Atala A, Lanza R, Thomson J A and Nerem R M eds, *Principles of Regenerative Medicine*, Amsterdam, Elsevier, pp. 418–436.

Lang W (1887), 'On the insertion of artificial globes into Tenon's capsule after excising the eye', *Trans Ophthalmol Soc UK*, **7**, 286–291.

Langer R and Vacanti J P (1993), 'Tissue engineering', *Science*, **260**, 920–926.

Lund R D, Kwan A S L, Keegan D J, Sauvé Y, Coffey P J and Lawrence J M (2001), 'Cell transplantation as a treatment for retinal disease', *Prog Ret Eye Res*, **20**, 415–449.

Lysaght M J and Crager J (2009), 'Editorial: Origins', *Tissue Eng A*, **15**, 1449–1450.

Mansbridge J (2006), 'Commercial considerations in tissue engineering', *J Anat*, **209**, 527–532.

Mason C and Dunnill P (2008), 'A brief definition of regenerative medicine', *Regen Med*, **3**, 1–5.

Maynard E M (2001), 'Visual prostheses', *Annu Rev Biomed Eng*, **3**, 145–168.

Mironov V, Visconti R P and Markwald R R (2004), 'What is regenerative medicine? Emergence of applied stem cell and developmental biology', *Expert Opin Biol Ther*, **4**, 773–781.

Murray J E, Merrill J P and Harrison J H (1955), 'Renal homotransplantation in identical twins', *Surg Forum*, **6**, 432–436.

Nerem R M and Sambanis A (1995), 'Tissue engineering: from biology to biological substitutes', *Tissue Eng*, **1**, 3–13.

Nishida K (2003), 'Tissue engineering of the cornea', *Cornea*, **22** (Suppl. 1), 28–34.

Ratner B D, Hoffman A S, Schoen F J and Lemons J E (2004), 'Biomaterials science: a multidisciplinary endeavor', in Ratner B D, Hoffman A S, Schoen F J and Lemons J E eds, *Biomaterials Science*, 2nd edn, Amsterdam, Elsevier, pp. 1–9.

Ridley H (1951), 'Intra-ocular acrylic lenses', *Trans Ophthalmol Soc UK*, **71**, 617–621.

Ridley H (1952a), 'Intra-ocular acrylic lenses after cataract extraction', *Lancet*, **1**, 118–121.

Ridley H (1952b), 'Intra-ocular acrylic lenses. A recent development in the surgery of cataract', *Br J Ophthalmol*, **36**, 113–122.

Ruberti J W, Zieske J D and Trinkaus-Randall V (2007), 'Corneal-tissue replacement', in Lanza R, Langer R and Vacanti J eds, *Principles of Tissue Engineering*, 3rd edn, Amsterdam, Elsevier, pp. 1025–1047.

Russell A J and Bertram T (2007), 'Moving into the clinic', in Lanza R, Langer R and Vacanti J eds, *Principles of Tissue Engineering*, 3rd edn, Amsterdam, Elsevier, pp. 15–31.

Scuderi G (1954), 'Ricerche sperimentali sul trapianto del vitreo (tentative di sostituzione parziale con vitreo omologo, con liquor eterologo, con soluzioni di polivinilpirrolidone)', *Ann Ottalmol Clin Ocul*, **80**, 213–220.

Selvam S, Thomas P B and Yiu S C (2006), 'Tissue engineering: current and future approaches to ocular surface reconstruction', *Ocul Surf*, **4**, 120–136.

Sheardown H and Griffith M (2008), 'Regenerative medicine in the cornea', in Atala A, Lanza R, Thomson J A and Nerem R M eds, *Principles of Regenerative Medicine*, Amsterdam, Elsevier, pp. 1060–1071.

Skalak R, Fox C F and Fung B (1988), 'Preface', in Skalak R and Fox C F eds, *Tissue Engineering*, New York, Alan R Liss Inc., pp. xix–xxi.

Sommer F, Brandl F and Göpferich A (2006), 'Ocular tissue engineering', in Fisher J P ed., *Tissue Engineering*, New York, Springer, pp. 413–429.

Thiel R (1939), 'Polyviolplomben zur plastischen Stumpfbildung nach Enucleatio bulbi', *Klin Monatsbl Augenheilk*, **103**, 530–541.

Tsonis P A (2006), 'How to build and rebuild a lens', *J Anat*, **209**, 433–437.

Tubo R (2008), 'Fundamentals of cell-based therapies', in Atala A, Lanza R, Thomson J A and Nerem R M eds, *Principles of Regenerative Medicine*, Amsterdam, Elsevier, pp. 16–26.

Tuohy K M (1950), 'Contact lens', US Patent 2,510,438.

Vacanti C A (2006), 'History of tissue engineering and a glimpse into its future', *Tissue Eng*, **12**, 1137–1142.

Vacanti C A and Vacanti J P (1991), 'Functional organ replacement. The new technology of tissue engineering', *Surgical Technol Int*, 43–49.

Weiland J D and Humayun M S (2003), 'Past, present, and future of artificial vision', *Artif Org*, **27**, 961–962.

Wichterle O (1960), 'Shaped hydrophilic articles and method of manufacturing same', British Patent 829565.

Wichterle O and Lím D (1960), 'Hydrophilic gels for biological use', *Nature*, **185**, 117–118.

Wichterle O, Lím D and Dreifus M (1961), 'A contribution to the problem of contact lens' (Czech), *Čsl Oftal*, **17**, 70–75.

Williams D F (1999), *The Williams Dictionary of Biomaterials*, Liverpool, Liverpool University Press, p. 318.

Williams D F (2006), 'To engineer is to create: the link between engineering and regeneration', *Trends Biotechnol.*, **24**, 4–8.

Williams D F (2008), 'On the mechanism of biocompatibility', *Biomaterials*, **29**, 2941–2953.

Wolter J R (1985), 'Interaction between intraocular lenses and surrounding tissues', *Contact Lens Assoc Ophthalmol J*, **11**, 300–306.

Wolter J R and Meyer R F (1984), 'Sessile macrophages forming clear endothelium-like membrane on inside of successful keratoprosthesis', *Trans Am Ophthalmol Soc*, **82**, 187–202.

Wünsche G (1947), 'Versuche zur totalen Keratoplastik und zur Cornea arteficialis', *Ärztliche Forsch*, **1**, 345–348.

Yannas I V (2001), *Tissue and Organ Regeneration in Adults*, New York, Springer, 1–25.

Yannas I V (2005), 'Similarities and differences between induced organ regeneration in adults and early foetal regeneration', *J R Soc Interface*, **2**, 403–417.

Zirm E (1906), 'Eine erfolgreiche totale Keratoplastik', *Graefes Arch Ophthalmol*, **64**, 580–593.

Part I

Applications in the anterior segment

2
Advances in intraocular lens development

D. MORRISON, B. KLENKLER, D. MORARESCU
and H. SHEARDOWN, McMaster University, Canada

Abstract: While cataracts are relatively easily treated by removal of the existing lens and its replacement with a synthetic lens, problems remain. These lenses are subject to a high incidence of secondary complications including the formation of secondary cataracts in as many as 40% of patients. Furthermore, the majority of existing intraocular lenses are unable to accommodate for vision. However, there have been a number of improvements to the materials and the lens design which have been demonstrated to and which have the potential to decrease the incidence of secondary cataracts. Additionally, new developments in the field of lens design have led to lenses that show some degree of accommodation. These are discussed in the current chapter. The chapter also highlights the results of research that may lead to truly accommodating systems in the future.

Key words: intraocular lens, posterior capsule opacification, silicone, acrylic, accommodation.

2.1   Introduction

Cataracts, responsible for the majority of blindness worldwide, and an evitable consequence of the ageing process, lead to changes in the structure of the lens resulting in the formation of opacities. However, cataracts are relatively easily treated, particularly in the developed world, by the replacement of the diseased lens with a synthetic replacement. These intraocular lenses (IOLs) have been highly successful at restoring the vision of millions of patients worldwide. However, the formation of secondary cataracts or posterior capsule opacification (PCO) remains a significant problem, occurring in as many as 40% of adult patients and a considerably greater fraction of paediatric patients. These secondary cataracts require subsequent treatment, are a burden to the healthcare system and an inconvenience to the patient. However, significant materials and manufacturing developments have resulted in a decrease in the incidence of PCO. Furthermore, current IOLs are unable to provide accommodative vision. Ongoing work aimed at further improving the success of IOL materials, including surface modifications and new materials, are highlighted in this chapter.

2.2   Native lens structure

The lens, a biconvex crystalline structure located behind the iris, is responsible for approximately 30% of the refractive power of the eye (Andley, 2007). It is generally considered to be composed of three layers: the nucleus, cortex and epithelium (Fig. 2.1); these layers are housed within the lens capsule, a bag-like structure approximately 10 mm in diameter with an axial length of 4 mm. The lens is suspended within the eye by zonular fibres which act to attach the lens capsule to the ciliary body.

The lens epithelium consists of cuboidal cells that differentiate into the cortical fibres that constitute the bulk of the lens. These lens fibres are tightly packed and contain no organelles or nuclei; they do contain proteins called lens crystallins. Lens fibres are continually added throughout life, thereby causing the lens to increase in size, eventually becoming denser, and more convex and less elastic, all of which contribute to an eventual decrease in the ability to focus light adequately.

2.3   Cataracts

Lens transparency is regulated *in vivo* by physical and chemical processes that, when disturbed, result in lens damage and opacification. The term 'cataract' has been traditionally used in a broad sense to mean any opacity or loss of transparency of the lens. Typically, cataracts are defined as lens opacities that cause some degree of visual impairment. Age-related cataracts are the most common type of cataracts; however, cataracts result from several different promoting factors including direct trauma to the eye, diabetes mellitus, heavy smoking and exposure to ultraviolet (UV) radiation. Regardless, the physiological factor leading to cataract formation appears to be the insufficient supply of nutrients to deep lens fibres (Marieb, 2001). This lack of nutrients promotes the clumping of crystalline proteins within the lens fibres. Cataracts are the leading cause of blindness worldwide, accounting for nearly 48%

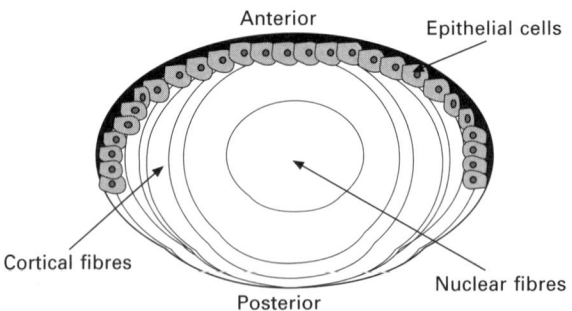

2.1 Diagram of the three layers of the native IOL.

of all blindness (Resnikoff *et al.*, 2004). As a result, cataract formation is a substantial economic and public health burden.

2.4   Cataract surgery and intraocular lens materials

Treatment of cataracts by extraction of the natural opacified lens and implantation of a polymeric IOL is currently the most common ophthalmic procedure, with approximately 6 million surgeries performed worldwide each year (Werner, 2007). Over the past 50 years, the route of surgical implantation and the nature of the materials implanted have evolved greatly. The observation by Harold Ridley that both glass and acrylic, under certain conditions, appeared to be inert within body tissues (Apple and Sims, 1996), coupled with their optical qualities and the fact that these materials were relatively inexpensive and easy to fashion into shapes, has led to the development of the materials currently used today. An appropriate biological host response to the implanted lens material is critical for maintenance of IOL transparency and visual acuity, particularly as IOLs are progressively being implanted in earlier stages of life (Werner, 2008). Developments in lens materials and designs have resulted in marked improvements in this respect.

IOL materials in current clinical use are grouped into two major categories: acrylic and silicone. Among the acrylics, the most commonly used material for IOLs since their development in 1949 is poly(methyl methacrylate) (PMMA), a rigid polymer that is well established, particularly in developing countries, owing to its cheapness and long-term reliability (Yuan, 2003). Newer, foldable lenses are now preferentially used as they require smaller incisions for implant insertion. These are made from either hydrophobic or hydrophilic (i.e. hydrogel) acrylic materials such as poly(2-hydroxyethyl methacrylate), and vary in refractive index, mechanical properties and water content based on the copolymer composition (Werner, 2008). Foldable silicone-based IOLs are also highly elastic, oxygen permeable and chemically stable, and their lower refractive index (~1.41 compared with ~1.47) results in reduced glare compared with acrylic versions (Yao *et al.*, 2006). Because they fill the entire lens capsule, the need for fixation of these lenses by polymeric haptic loops is avoided and the implant more closely mimics the natural lens (Hettlich 1991; *et al.*, Werner, 2008). In addition to differences in refractive index, the major differentiating property between foldable acrylic and silicone IOL materials is the glass transition temperature which leads to differences in unfolding time between the different materials.

2.5   Biological responses to intraocular lens materials

Upon extraction of an opacified lens and implantation of an IOL in the remaining lens capsular bag, a breakdown of the blood–aqueous barrier

(BAB) occurs with immediate release of proteins and cells into the anterior eye chamber. Numerous biological interactions to the foreign IOL material ensue; these initially include nonspecific protein deposition and complement activation, and subsequent inflammation, foreign-body response, and cellular adhesion, transformation, migration and proliferation (Yuan, 2003; Werner, 2008). Several different aspects of the host response must be assessed for an IOL material, including both capsular biocompatibility (the relationship of the IOL with the epithelial cells remaining in the lens capsule) and uveal biocompatibility (the inflammatory foreign-body reaction upon contact with the vascularized tissue of the iris, ciliary body and choroid) (Amon, 2001; Werner, 2008). The biocompatibility of a specific material in both of these respects is the subject of significant recent research, and depends on the nature of the cell–material interaction as dictated in turn by the underlying material surface properties and chemical structure.

2.5.1   Capsular biocompatibility

In most cases, the IOL comes only into direct contact with the capsular bag tissue, and resulting complications may include development of opacities in the anterior (ACO) or posterior (PCO) capsule, and capsular contraction. PCO remains the most significant late postoperative problem following cataract surgery. Because the capsule membrane is an integral part of the lens structure, it remains a platform for cellular adhesion and migration after surgery. Residual lens epithelial cells (LECs) under the anterior capsule can migrate along the posterior capsule, and upon aggregation into multilayer islets and transformation into mesenchymal cells in a process known as EMT (epithelial to mesenchymal transition), result in opacification of the central region behind the IOL and ultimately reduced vision (Yuen et al., 2006). These LECs aggregates swell and excrete extracellular matrix components including cytokines and matrix metalloproteinases which further induce proliferation and transformation of the LECs. The transformed cells become more fibroblastic and contractile in phenotype, leading to contraction and wrinkling of the capsule and to eventual decentring of the IOL (Yuen et al., 2006). While PCO is typically treated by opening the opacified capsule with a neodymium: yttrium–aluminium–garnet (Nd:YAG) laser, risks associated with this procedure include IOL damage, intraocular pressure elevation, cystoid macular oedema and retinal detachment; additionally, such laser technology is not readily available in the developing world (Yuen et al., 2006; Cheng et al., 2007).

2.5.2   Uveal biocompatibility

An IOL material may additionally invoke an inflammatory reaction upon implantation. As a result of surgical trauma causing disruption of the BAB, and in some instances direct contact of the IOL with vascularized uveal tissue, the IOL is exposed to an influx of proteins and inflammatory cells (Amon, 2001). Following initial adsorption of proteins to the surface, monocytes, macrophages and small fibroblast-like cells may then adhere through this protein layer and, upon activation, secrete cytokines to further intensify the course of the inflammation. These cells later fuse into epithelioid and foreign-body giant cells, resulting in chronic inflammation or deposition of an acellular proteinaceous membrane that is commonly detected up to 1 year after surgery (Amon, 2001; Werner, 2008). It has been suggested that PCO itself may be a late form of postoperative inflammation, as inflammatory mediators derived after BAB damage or synthesized by macrophages can also stimulate LEC proliferation and migration (Tognetto *et al.*, 2003b; Yuen *et al.*, 2006). Inflammation may result in decreased contrast sensitivity in the patient, damage to the corneal endothelial layer and other implications that are not yet understood (Werner *et al.*, 1999; Yamakawa *et al.*, 2003).

2.5.3   Lens design and material effects

While some degree of inflammation and foreign-body reaction occurs in all eyes following IOL implantation, the severity is dependent on the lens design and material factors such as surface chemistry, stability and mechanical properties. In a study by Yamakawa and coworkers, adhesion of inflammatory cells to PMMA IOLs decreased with increasing polishing time and smoothness of the IOL, possibly owing to reduced adsorption of cell-adhesive matrix proteins on smoother surfaces (Yamakawa *et al.*, 2003). Hydrophobic acrylic IOLs with intermediate values of wettability, such as PMMA, are generally associated with stronger uveal cell adhesion and growth compared with other materials (Werner *et al.*, 1999; Tognetto *et al.*, 2003a); however the increased inflammation caused by PMMA IOLs versus other types has been shown in some but not all studies (Ozdal *et al.*, 2005). High small-cell counts and membranous deposition have also been detected on silicone IOLs (Ozdal *et al.*, 2005; Yao *et al.*, 2006).

Similarly, changes in surgical technique and the design of IOLs have been instrumental in reducing PCO rates although no clinical- or material-based factor has eliminated this complication all together. In particular, the use of a square rather than a rounded edge is thought to act as a barrier to the ingrowth of LECs migrating from the lens equator along the posterior capsule, an effect that is observed among different IOL materials (Wejde *et al.*, 2003; Cheng *et al.*, 2007). The effect of the IOL material itself on PCO development is less clear, although this has been demonstrated to be significant in various clinical studies. It is noted that the effect of IOL design, surgical technique and patient-related factors is often difficult to separate from that of the material alone in these studies, and a combination of these factors probably dictates the overall outcome (Heatley *et al.*, 2005).

It was observed (Wedje *et al.*, 2003) that less PCO formation occurred after 2 years on hydrophobic acrylic versus silicone IOLs. However, other studies (Findl *et al.*, 2005; Hayashi and Hayashi, 2007) have shown that both silicone and hydrophobic acrylic IOLs had low rates of PCO when a square-edge design was introduced. Heatley *et al.* measured significantly lower PCO levels in hydrophobic versus hydrophilic acrylic lenses (Heatley *et al.*, 2005). In a meta-analysis of 23 clinical trials (Cheng *et al.*, 2007), it was determined that silicone and hydrophobic acrylic IOLs were more effective in preventing PCO than both PMMA and hydrogel IOLs.

The reasons for these differing responses to the various IOL material types is not fully understood, and may be a result of differences in protein and subsequent cell adhesion following implantation. According to the 'sandwich theory' proposed by Linnola, faster and stronger adhesion of the IOL material to the capsular bag, either directly or through a uniform monolayer of LECs, will prevent further LEC growth between the IOL surface and capsule implicated in PCO (Linnola *et al.*, 2000a; Linnola *et al.*, 2003). As such, adsorption of certain extracellular matrix proteins including fibronectin and vitronectin, which are present in plasma or synthesized by LECs themselves, can mediate the subsequent adhesion of the LEC and/or the collagenous lens capsule to the IOL material and may result in reduced PCO rates. Hydrophobic materials may be more conducive to such protein and cell binding, although the high incidence of PCO on both hydrophobic silicone and hydrophilic hydrogel IOLs indicates that a simple correlation between polymer wettability and biocompatibility does not exist (Linnola *et al.*, 2003; Okajima *et al.*, 2006). Higher levels of fibronectin and associated lens capsular adhesion were measured on hydrophobic versus hydrophilic acrylic, PMMA and silicone lens materials (Linnola *et al.*, 2000a; Linnola *et al.*, 2000b; Linnola *et al.*, 2003), in accordance with the lower PCO rates observed clinically (Wejde *et al.*, 2003). Vitronectin, which was detected on hydrophobic acrylic IOLs may also play a role in enhancing IOL–capsular bag adhesion or healing after implantation (Linnola *et al.*, 2000a; Linnola *et al.*, 2000b). Conversely, collagen type IV is a constituent of fibrotic PCO tissue, and higher amounts of this protein were detected on silicone, hydrophilic acrylic and other hydrogel IOLs which were less stimulatory to cell growth and adhesion (Linnola *et al.*, 2000a; Linnola *et al.*, 2003).

2.5.4   Surface modification for reducing complications

Various surface modifications have been investigated for minimizing the inflammatory reaction to IOL implants. One clinically proven example is the binding of heparin, which, owing to its highly hydrophilic nature diminishes the interactions of the lens surface with the cellular membranes of macrophages (Tognetto *et al.*, 2003a). The mobile surface structure of heparin-surface-modified (HSM) IOLs appears normal to the host immunological system, thus preventing a foreign-body reaction against the IOL (Werner *et al.*, 1999). HSM-PMMA IOLs showed reduced spreading and growth of fibroblasts and inflammatory cells versus those made of conventional PMMA (Larsson *et al.*, 1989; Werner *et al.*, 1999); they were, however, less biocompatible than hydrophobic AcrySof (Alcon, Inc.) and silicone IOLs in terms of inflammatory cell adhesion, ACO and PCO (Tognetto *et al.*, 2003a; Wejde *et al.*, 2003). Work continues into the use of heparin coatings to prevent cell adhesion and reduce inflammation (Schroeder *et al.*, 2008). Binding of Teflon, carbon and titanium to render PMMA IOLs more hydrophobic was also found to reduce inflammation in several studies; however, results in humans have yet to be demonstrated (Werner *et al.*, 1999; Yuan, 2003; Yuan *et al.*, 2004). Silicone IOLs have been modified by grafting of MPC, resulting in decreased adhesion of macrophages as well as LECs (Yao *et al.*, 2006).

Surface modification of IOL materials has also been investigated as a way of controlling LEC growth and adhesion to inhibit PCO development. Formation of a uniform, morphologically correct layer of LECs on the IOL surface may simulate normal optics of the human lens and adherence of the capsule according to the sandwich theory (Linnola *et al.*, 2003). The hydrophilicity or hydrophobicity of the material can affect, and in extreme cases inhibit, LEC adhesion and maintenance of normal cellular phenotype (El Khadali *et al.*, 2002). Yuen *et al.* showed that plasma treatment of IOLs increased their hydrophilicity and enhanced LEC adhesion and maintenance of normal epithelial morphology, when compared with untreated surfaces where a fibroblastic appearance was observed that could potentially promote PCO (Yuen *et al.*, 2006). Silicone IOLs, which due to their extreme hydrophobicity do not adhere to the lens capsule tissue, were modified with oxygen plasma to increase cell spreading (Hettlich *et al.*, 1991). Plasma treatment may also contribute to the low PCO rates observed clinically in AcrySof hydrophobic IOLs (Matsushima *et al.*, 2006). It was demonstrated that UV/ozone treatment, which may be less damaging to the polymer surface than plasma modification, was more effective in increasing surface wettability, and fibronectin and LEC adhesion on hydrophobic acrylic IOLs, while inhibiting LEC proliferation and PCO formation in a rabbit model (Matsushima *et al.*, 2006). An alternative approach for reducing PCO is the complete prevention of protein and subsequent cell adhesion to the IOL surface. Hydrogel IOLs were coated with poly(ethylene glycol) (PEG), which is well known to sterically inhibit the attraction of proteins and cells to surfaces, and protein deposition and LEC adhesion were reduced *in vitro* (Bozukova *et al.*, 2007). Modification of silicone IOLs with poly(2-methacryloyloxyethyl phosphorylcholine) (MPC), a biomimetic component of the cell membrane, increased hydrophilicity and inhibited LECs and fibrosis (Yao *et al.*, 2006); however, similar experiments with hydrophobic acrylic IOLs indicated that migration of LECs toward the posterior capsule may in fact be stimulated by such MPC treatment (Okajima *et al.*, 2006). Changing the chemical composition of PMMA, poly(HEMA-co-MMA) and silicone by introduction of sulfonate and carboxylate groups resulted in decreased LEC and fibroblast growth compared with the unmodified polymers, probably as a result of a conformational change in adsorbed fibronectin and vitronectin leading to altered intracellular signalling in the attached cells (Latz *et al.*, 2000; El Khadali *et al.*, 2002; Evans *et al.*, 2004; Yammine *et al.*, 2005).

2.5.5 Drug-releasing IOLs for mitigating complications

IOLs that deliver drugs that hinder LEC proliferation or reduce inflammation may have potential for reducing complications. While a choice of potent drugs is currently available, there are other limitations to designing drug-releasing IOL materials. Most importantly, the loaded material has to maintain transparency above the 1.382 refractive index limit (Lloyd *et al.*, 2001). The material should also remain foldable and easily manipulated, to avoid other surgical complications, especially in paediatric patients (Rowe *et al.*, 2004).

IOL materials, particularly acrylics and hydrogels, have been examined for the release of antibiotics, anti-inflammatory drugs and other molecules that have the potential to decrease complications such as PCO. For example, IOLs containing a drug-delivery system releasing the steroid dexamethasone or other similar molecules have been tested in rabbit eyes, and may further prevent inflammation following cataract surgery (Kleinmann *et al.*, 2006a; Kleinmann *et al.*, 2006b; Siqueira *et al.*, 2006). However, these studies have not advanced to human trials. Hydrogels releasing such drugs as diclofenac sodium, tranilast, mitomycin C, colchicines, ethylene diamine tetraacetic acid and 5-fluorouracil were tested *in vitro* (Matsushima *et al.*, 2005), and may present an alternative route for management of PCO.

Coating of IOL materials with degradable polymeric drug-delivery systems has also been used to facilitate the delivery of drugs from these materials. This method avoids direct modification of the IOL material, and therefore does not interfere with optical properties. Release duration can be modulated by coating thickness. The first report of an IOL-associated controlled drug release system came from Tetz and coworkers in 1996 (Tetz *et al.*, 1996), who used poly(DL-lactide) containing the drugs daunorubicin and indomethacin for prevention of PCO. In parallel, Nishi *et al.* used a similar degradable drug-delivery system for indomethacin, designed to be implanted as a disk sandwiched with the IOL (Nishi *et al.*, 1996). Both studies achieved controlled drug release successfully in rabbit eyes, but the drugs did not produce significant PCO reduction.

With better understanding of the biological pathways of PCO came drugs that targeted specific pathways. One very promising option seems to be the inhibition of metalloproteinase-2 (MMP-2) and MMP-9 function. These Zn^{2+}-dependent extracellular matrix (ECM)-remodelling enzymes have been shown to be necessary for both the transformation (Dwivedi *et al.*, 2006) and migration (Wong *et al.*, 2004) of remnant LECs. Two MMP inhibitors, one specific for MMP-2 and MMP-9, and a generic inhibitor, GM6001, have been identified as potent inhibitors of anterior subcataracts (Dwivedi *et al.*, 2006). Because the biological mechanisms of anterior subcataract formation and PCO formation are similar, it has been suggested that these same drugs could also mitigate PCO (Dwivedi *et al.*, 2006). The broad MMP inhibitor, GM6001, is also very efficient *in vitro* at delaying LEC migration (Wong *et al.*, 2004). Recent results suggest that it is possible to release these compounds from silicone and that the released components show significant activity in terms of reducing lens cell transformation and migration (Fig. 2.2).

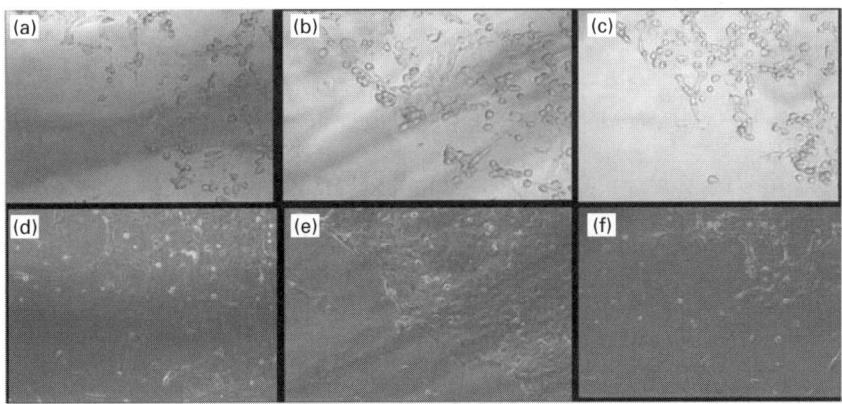

2.2 Cell migration in the presence of a drug-releasing polydimethy/siloxane (PDMS) disc was visualized at ×20 magnification, using a Zeiss Axiovert microscope. The B3 human lens epithelial cells were grown in modified Eagle's medium (MEM) F15 media, with 20% fetal bouine serum (FBS), and with 200 µM aphidicolin (a mitosis inhibitor, used to determine effects of drugs solely on migration). Photographs were taken immediately after scraping cells off one side of the dish (panels (a), (b), (c), and 3 days later (panels (d), (e) and (f). Panels (a) and (d) are untreated controls. Panels (b) and (e) are cells treated with GM6001. Calculations show a 54% ($p \leq 0.001$) reduction in migration when compared with untreated control. Panels (c) and (f) are cells treated with MMP-2-9 inhibitor II. Calculations show a 56% ($p \leq 0.001$) reduction in migration when compared with untreated control.

2.6   Multifocal intraocular lenses

Since most currently available lens materials cannot accommodate for vision, IOL recipients must wear corrective lenses to provide them with near vision. Recently, IOLs capable of providing patients with multiple focal points have begun to debut all over the world (Lane *et al.*, 2006). The Helmholtz theory of accommodation, the most accepted theory for the mechanism of accommodation of the native lens, states that vision is accommodated by the lens through the contraction and relaxation of the ciliary muscle. For near vision, the muscles contract and effectively reduce the tension on the zonule fibres and allowing the lens to become thicker, increasing the optical power of the lens. Conversely, for distance vision the ciliary muscles relax, thereby increasing the tension on the zonule fibres and decreasing the thickness and optical power of the lens.

Current multifocal IOLs provide multiple focal distances to the patient independent of ciliary body function and capsular mechanics. Once the lens is securely placed within the capsular bag, the function of these lenses will not change or deteriorate. Multifocal lenses can be designed to take advantage of many innovations in IOL technology that have led to improved outcomes (Lane *et al.*, 2006). Currently, there are two FDA-approved multifocal IOLs on the market: the ReZoom lens and the ReStor lens.

2.6.1   ReZoom lens

The ReZoom lens is a clear, foldable IOL made from a high-refractive-index acrylic material (Lane *et al.*, 2006). The second-generation refractive multifocal IOL, the first generation being the Array IOL, distributes light over five optic zones so that each lens has a distance-dominant central zone for distance vision under bright-light conditions when the pupil is constricted. In the refractive profile, the odd zones (1, 3 and 5) are adjusted for far vision and the even zones (2 and 4) are adjusted for near vision. Therefore, the optical behaviour of the IOL depends on the pupil's size. With a small pupil, light energy is sent to distance vision, but as the pupil size increases, the IOL sends light energy simultaneously to both near and distant focal points.

2.6.2   ReStor lens

The ReStor IOL is designed to provide quality near to distance vision by combining 'apodized' diffractive and refractive technologies. Apodization is defined as the gradual tapering of diffractive steps from the centre of the lens towards the outside edge to create a smooth transition of light between the distance, intermediate and near focal points (Ortiz *et al.*, 2008). On the ReStor IOL, the centre of the lens surface consists of an apodized diffractive optic with a 3.6 mm diameter for focusing light from near and distant objects. Conversely, the outer ring of the ReStor IOL surrounds the apodized diffractive region and is dedicated to focusing light for distance vision. Therefore, unlike the ReZoom lens, this IOL effectively restores near and distance vision regardless of pupil size. In bright light situations where the pupils are constricted, the lens sends light simultaneously to both near and distant focal points. In low light situations where the pupils are dilated, the apodized diffractive lens sends a greater amount of light to distance vision to minimize visual disturbances.

2.7   Accommodating intraocular lenses

Over the last several decades researchers have focused on developing a biocompatible material that is soft enough to be capable of providing truly accommodative vision. There are currently three IOLs on the market that are generally accepted as being able to provide accommodative vision: the BioComFold Ring-haptic IOL, the 1CU Accommodative IOL and the AT-45 Crystalens.

2.7.1   BioComFold ring-haptic intraocular lens

Introduced in 1996, this IOL was the first artificial accommodating IOL on the market (Menapace *et al.*, 2007). The IOL itself is constructed of a single piece of a foldable hydrophilic acrylic material with an optic size of 5.8 mm. The lens features three rigid haptics that are angled to the anterior, which is opposite to the features of most current designs. The accommodative mechanism of this lens relies on the sphincter-like ciliary muscle circumferentially compressing the haptics of the lens, which results in the forward motion of the optic and an increase in the refractive power when focusing on near objects. Similarly, there is an associated backward motion upon relaxation which is inherent in the optic owing to its elasticity.

2.7.2   1CU accommodative intraocular lens

The 1CU was first introduced on the market in 2001 and features another single-piece optic 5.5 mm in size. Like the ring-haptic IOL, the 1CU is made of a foldable hydrophilic acrylic material. The main difference between the two lies in the four delicate broad-based haptics used by the 1CU, which compress upon zonular relaxation and which move the lens forward to accommodate vision for near objects. This IOL then relies on the assumption that the capsular bag retains sufficient residual elasticity to provide backwards motion to the lens.

2.7.3   AT-45 Crystalens intraocular lens

The AT-45 Crystalens is a multipiece silicone accommodating IOL which initially received US Food and Drug Administration (FDA) approval in November 2003 to correct aphakia (Cumming *et al.*, 2006). The lens was then approved again in August 2004 to correct presbyopia following cataract extraction and to provide near, intermediate and distance vision without spectacles. Specifically, the AT-45 Crystalens is a biconvex lens with a 4.5 mm optic and flexible hinged-plate haptics that permit the forward movement of the optic during accommodation (Cumming *et al.*, 2006). The lens design incorporates grooves across the plates adjacent to the lens optic that allow for forward and backward movement of plate-haptic lenses against the vitreous face. The mechanism of accommodation is based on the working assumption of mass redistribution presumed by Coleman (Coleman and Fish, 2001), who suggested that the contraction of the ciliary muscle causes it to bulge into the incompressible vitreous body, which reacts by dislodging the anteriorly located capsule and IOL. This would then push the lens forward and increase power while accommodating for near vision.

2.8   Lens refilling

Although these multifocal IOLs are generally accepted to provide accommodative vision to patients, some researchers believe that the best way to design a solution to the problem of cataracts is to develop an artificial lens that more closely mimics the natural mechanism of accommodation of the eye. It was demonstrated that the ciliary muscle retains its function through to 80 years of age (Strenk *et al.*, 1999). Therefore, injectable materials that function as artificial lenses and which use the natural mechanism of accommodation are theoretically possible. Current work is aimed at the development of softer materials that can be stretched and compressed by the ciliary muscles of the eye through a technique known as lens refilling.

Lens refilling has been shown to be a potentially valuable alternative treatment option to the direct injection of a foldable, accommodating IOL. The technique was first explored as an IOL replacement therapy by Kessler in 1964 (Kessler, 1964). Using some of the knowledge gained during this work, Haefliger and coworkers took up the concept under the name Phaco-Ersatz (Haefliger *et al.*, 1987). In a study published in 1994, this group proved the efficacy of using lens refilling to restore visual accommodation in the senile primate eye (Haefliger and Parel, 1994). With this technique, the capsular bag was evacuated through a small capsular opening and refilled with a silicone-based elastic polymer capable of responding to changes in surface curvature according to varying zonular tension.

Hettlich and coworkers investigated the safety and efficacy of a monomer that could be polymerized under light exposure (Hettlich *et al.*, 1994). The authors conducted a histopathological study on the potential risks of lens refilling and subsequent polymerization using short-wave light, concluding that the technique did not induce any serious inflammatory reactions and that complete filling of the lens capsule resulted in reduced rates of PCO when compared with conventional IOL implantation techniques. However, they also suggested that new materials with enhanced physical properties were necessary.

More recently, Nishi and coworkers have developed a silicone-based polymeric material capable of being injected into the lens capsule for lens refilling (Nishi *et al.*, 1998). However, the study found that PCO was present in all eyes 3 days postoperatively and that lens accommodation was only a fraction of the values determined before surgery and that they decreased over time (Nishi *et al.*, 1993; Nishi and Nishi, 1998). They attributed these results to the loss of lens fibre cells within the capsule, which actively contribute to the mechanism of natural accommodation (Nishi and Nishi, 1998).

Several other slight variations to capsular bag refilling have also been presented. For example, Nishi and coworkers have also designed an inflatable balloon made of a thin silicone membrane that can be filled with a liquid silicone polymer through a delivery tube after being placed in the emptied capsule (Nishi *et al.*, 1992). The authors investigated the influence of the shape of the balloon (Nishi *et al.*, 1993) and the volume of injected silicone (Nishi *et al.*, 1997a; Nishi *et al.*, 1997b) on the accommodative amplitude. Recent work from Morrison and Sheardown suggests that hydrogel materials based on hyaluronic acid which can be photopolymerized *in situ* may also be suitable for lens refilling (Fig. 2.3).

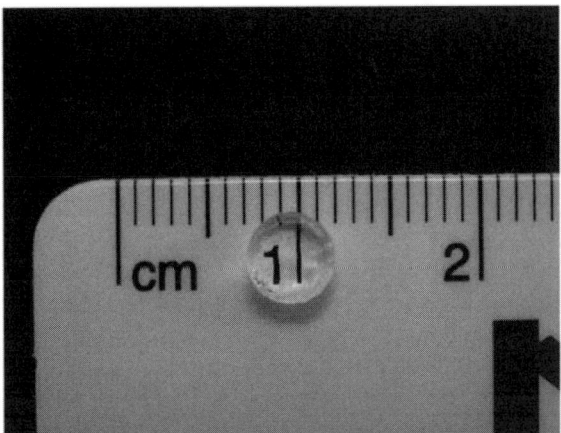

2.3 A digital photograph of a typical hyaluronic acid-based hydrogel. This hydrogel was moulded in a small, circular plastic mould of approximately the same size as the native lens capsule.

Although lens refilling holds significant potential, many problems remain to be solved. These include achieving emmetropia in the relaxed state, adequate accommodative response upon zonular relaxation, appropriate image quality throughout the full range of accommodation, and sustained functionality (Menapace *et al.*, 2007). The most significant problem, however, remains the incidence of PCO. According to Menapace and coworkers (Menapace *et al.* 2007), the ideal material for lens refilling should be cytotoxic upon direct contact with the capsule to prevent PCO but should not release toxic substances to the surroundings or leak into the anterior chamber prior to polymerization. Combination materials or materials that are capable of delivery of drugs that disrupt the pathways necessary for cellular transformations in PCO may be necessary to overcome these problems.

2.9   Conclusions

Through a better understanding of the optical and biological properties, there have been numerous advances in IOL materials since the implantation of PMMA in the eye in 1949. Through developments in lens design, lenses have a lower incidence of complications. Multifocal and even accommodative IOLs are now available. With a developing understanding of the biological processes that occur following lens implantation and the development of new materials, future generations of IOLs will have better optical properties and even fewer complications.

2.10   References

Amon M (2001), 'Biocompatibility of intraocular lenses', *J Cataract Refr Surg*, **27**, 178–179.

Andley U P (2007), 'Crystallins in the eye: function and pathology', *Prog Retin Eye Res*, **26**, 78–98.

Apple D J, Sims J (1996), 'Harold Ridley and the invention of the intraocular lens', *Surv Ophthalmol*, **40**, 279–292.

Bozukova D, Pagnoulle C, De Pauw-Gillet M C, Desbief S, Lazzaroni R, Ruth N, Jerome R, Jerome C (2007), 'Improved performances of intraocular lenses by poly(ethylene glycol) chemical coatings', *Biomacromolecules*, **8**, 2379–2387.

Cheng J W, Wei R L, Cai J P, Xi G L, Zhu H, Li Y, Ma X Y (2007), 'Efficacy of different intraocular lens materials and optic edge designs in preventing posterior capsular opacification: a meta-analysis', *Am J Ophthalmol*, **143**, 428–436.

Coleman D J, Fish S K (2001), 'Presbyopia, accommodation and the mature catentary', *Ophthalmology*, **108**, 1544–1551.

Cumming J S, Colvard D M, Dell S J, Doane J, Fine I H, Hoffman R S, Packer M, Slade S G (2006), 'Clinical evaluation of the Crystalens AT-45 accommodating intraocular lens: results of the US Food and Drug Administration clinical trial', *J Cataract Refract Surg*, **32**, 812–825.

Dwivedi D J, Pino G, Banh A, Nathu Z, Howchin D, Margetts P, Sivak J G, West-Mays

J A (2006), 'Matrix metalloproteinase inhibitors suppress transforming growth factor-beta-induced subcapsular cataract formation', *Am J Pathol*, **168**, 69–79.

El Khadali F, Helary G, Pavon-Djavid G, Migonney V (2002), 'Modulating fibroblast cell proliferation with functionalized poly(methyl methacrylate) based copolymers: chemical composition and monomer distribution effect', *Biomacromolecules*, **3**, 51–56.

Evans M D, Pavon-Djavid G, Helary G, Legeais J M, Migonney V (2004), 'Vitronectin is significant in the adhesion of lens epithelial cells to PMMA polymers', *J Biomed Mater Res*, **69**, 469–476.

Findl O, Menapace R, Sacu S, Buehl W, Rainer G (2005), 'Effect of optic material on posterior capsule opacification in intraocular lenses with sharp-edge optics: randomized clinical trial', *Ophthalmology*, **112**, 67–72.

Haefliger E, Parel J M (1994), 'Accommodation of an endocapsular silicone lens (Phaco-Ersatz) in the aging rhesus monkey', *J Refract Corneal Surg*, **10**, 550–555.

Haefliger E, Parel J M, Fantes F, Norton E W, Anderson D R, Forster R K, Hernandez E, Feuer W J (1987), 'Accommodation of an endocapsular silicone lens (Phaco-Ersatz) in the nonhuman primate', *Ophthalmology*, **94**, 471–477.

Hayashi K, Hayashi H (2007), 'Influence on posterior capsule opacification and visual function of intraocular lens optic material', *Am J Ophthalmol*, **144**, 195–202.

Heatley C J, Spalton D J, Kumar A, Jose R, Boyce J, Bender L E (2005), 'Comparison of posterior capsule opacification rates between hydrophilic and hydrophobic single-piece acrylic intraocular lenses', *J Cataract Refract Surg*, **31**, 718–724.

Hettlich H J, Lucke K, Asiyo-Vogel M N, Schulte M, Vogel A (1994), 'Lens refilling and endocapsular polymerization of an injectable intraocular lens: in vitro and in vivo study of potential risks and benefits', *J Cataract Refract Surg*, **20**, 115–123.

Hettlich H J, Otterbach F, Mittermayer C, Kaufmann R, Klee D (1991), 'Plasma-induced surface modifications on silicone intraocular lenses: chemical analysis and in vitro characterization', *Biomaterials*, **12**, 521–524.

Kessler J (1964), 'Experiments in refilling the lens', *Arch Ophthalmol*, **71**, 412–417.

Kleinmann G, Apple D J, Chew J, Hunter B, Stevens S, Larson S, Mamalis N, Olson R J (2006a), 'Hydrophilic acrylic intraocular lens as a drug-delivery system for fourth-generation fluoroquinolones', *J Cataract Refract Surg*, **32**, 1717–1721.

Kleinmann G, Apple D J, Chew J, Stevens S, Hunter B, Larson S, Mamalis N, Olson R J (2006b), 'Hydrophilic acrylic intraocular lens as a drug-delivery system: Pilot study', *J Cataract Refract Surg*, **32**, 652–654.

Lane S S, Morris M, Nordan L, Packer M, Tarantino N, Wallace R B 3rd (2006), 'Multifocal intraocular lenses', *Ophthalmol Clin North Am*, **19**, 89–105.

Larsson R, Selen G, Bjordklund H, Fagerholm P (1989), 'Intraocular PMMA lenses modified with surface-immobilized heparin: evaluation of biocompatibility in vitro and in vivo', *Biomaterials*, **10**, 511–516.

Latz C, Migonney V, Pavon-Djavid G, Rieck P, Hartmann C, Renard G, Legeais J M (2000), 'Inhibition of lens epithelial cell proliferation by substituted PMMA intraocular lenses', *Graefe's Arch Clin Exp Ophthalmol*, **238**, 696–700.

Linnola R J, Sund M, Ylonen R, Pihlajaniemi T (2003), 'Adhesion of soluble fibronectin, vitronectin, and collagen type IV to intraocular lens materials', *J Cataract Refract Surg*, **29**, 146–152.

Linnola R J, Werner L, Pandey S K, Escobar-Gomez M, Znoiko S L, Apple D J (2000a), 'Adhesion of fibronectin, vitronectin, laminin, and collagen type IV to intraocular lens materials in pseudophakic human autopsy eyes. Part 1: histological sections', *J Cataract Refract Surg*, **26**, 1792–1806.

Linnola R J, Werner L, Pandey S K, Escobar-Gomez M, Znoiko S L, Apple D J (2000b), 'Adhesion of fibronectin, vitronectin, laminin, and collagen type IV to intraocular lens materials in pseudophakic human autopsy eyes. Part 2: explanted intraocular lenses', *J Cataract Refract Surg*, **26**, 1807–1818.

Lloyd A W, Faragher R G, Denyer S P (2001), 'Ocular biomaterials and implants', *Biomaterials*, **22**, 769–785.

Marieb E N ed. (2001), *Human Anatomy and Physiology*, San Francisco, Benjamin Cummings.

Matsushima H, Iwamoto H, Mukai K, Obara Y (2006), 'Active oxygen processing for acrylic intraocular lenses to prevent posterior capsule opacification', *J Cataract Refract Surg*, **32**, 1035–1040.

Matsushima H, Mukai K, Gotoo N, Yoshida S, Yoshida T, Sawano M, Senoo T, Obara Y, Clark J I (2005), 'The effects of drug delivery via hydrophilic acrylic (hydrogel) intraocular lens systems on the epithelial cells in culture', *Ophthalmic Surg Lasers Imaging*, **36**, 386–392.

Menapace R, Findl O, Kriechbaum K, Leydolt-Koeppl C (2007), 'Accommodating intraocular lenses: a critical review of present and future concepts', *Graefe's Arch Clin Exp Ophthalmol*, **245**, 473–489.

Nishi O, Hara T, Hara T, Sakka Y, Hayashi F, Nakamae K, Yamada Y (1992), 'Refilling the lens with an inflatable endocapsular balloon: surgical procedure in animal eyes', *Graefe's Arch Clin Exp Ophthalmol*, **230**, 47–55.

Nishi O, Nakai Y, Mizumoto Y, Yamada Y (1997a), 'Capsule opacification after refilling the capsule with an inflatable endocapsular balloon', *J Cataract Refract Surg*, **23**, 1548–1555.

Nishi O, Nishi K (1998), 'Accommodation amplitude after lens refilling with injectable silicone by sealing the capsule with a plug in primates', *Arch Ophthalmol*, **116**, 1358–1361.

Nishi O, Nakai Y, Yamada Y, Mizumoto Y (1993), 'Amplitudes of accommodation of primate lenses refilled with two types of inflatable endocapsular balloons', *Arch Ophthalmol*, **111**, 1677–1684.

Nishi O, Nishi K, Mano C, Ichihara M, Honda T (1997b), 'Controlling the capsular shape in lens refilling', *Arch Ophthalmol*, **115**, 507–510.

Nishi O, Nishi K, Mano C, Ichihara M, Honda T (1998), 'Lens refilling with injectable silicone in rabbit eyes', *J Cataract Refract Surg*, **24**, 975–982.

Nishi O, Nishi K, Morita T, Tada Y, Shirasawa E, Sakanishi K (1996), 'Effect of intraocular sustained release of indomethacin on postoperative inflammation and posterior capsule opacification', *J Cataract Refract Surg*, **22**, 806–810.

Okajima Y, Saika S, Sawa M (2006), 'Effect of surface coating an acrylic intraocular lens with poly(2-methacryloyloxyethyl phosphorylcholine) polymer on lens epithelial cell line behavior', *J Cataract Refract Surg*, **32**, 666–671.

Ortiz D, Alio J L, Bernabeu G, Pongo V (2008), 'Optical performance of monofocal and multifocal intraocular lenses in the human eye', *J Cataract Refract Surg*, **34**, 755–762.

Ozdal P C, Antecka E, Baines M G, Vianna R N, Rudzinski M, Deschenes J (2005), 'Chemoattraction of inflammatory cells by various intraocular lens materials', *Ocul Immunol Inflamm*, **13**, 435–438.

Resnikoff S, Pascolini D, Etya'ale D, Kocur I, Pararajasegaram R, Pokharel G P, Mariotti S P (2004), 'Global data on visual impairment in the year 2002', *Bull World Health Organ*, **82**, 844–851.

Rowe N A, Biswas S, Lloyd I C (2004), 'Primary IOL implantation in children: a risk analysis of foldable acrylic v PMMA lenses', *Br J Ophthalmol*, **88**, 481–485.

Schroeder A C, Schmidbauer J M, Sobke A, Seitz B, Ruprecht K W, Herrmann M (2008), 'Influence of fibronectin on the adherence of *Staphylococcus epidermidis* to coated and uncoated intraocular lenses', *J Cataract Refract Surg*, **34**, 497–504.

Siqueira R C, Filho E R, Fialho S L, Lucena L R, Filho A M, Haddad A, Jorge R, Scott I U, Cunha Ada S (2006), 'Pharmacokinetic and toxicity investigations of a new intraocular lens with a dexamethasone drug delivery system: a pilot study', *Ophthalmologica*, **220**, 338–342.

Strenk S A, Semmlow J L, Strenk L M, Munoz P, Gronlund-Jacob J, DeMarco J K (1999), 'Age-related changes in human ciliary muscle and lens: a magnetic resonance imaging study', *Invest Ophthalmol Vis Sci*, **40**, 1162–1169.

Tetz M R, Ries M W, Lucas C, Stricker H, Volcker H E (1996), 'Inhibition of posterior capsule opacification by an intraocular-lens-bound sustained drug delivery system: an experimental animal study and literature review', *J Cataract Refract Surg*, **22**, 1070–1078.

Tognetto D, Toto L, Minutola D, Ballone E, Di Nicola M, Di Mascio R, Ravalico G (2003a), 'Hydrophobic acrylic versus heparin surface-modified polymethylmethacrylate intraocular lens: a biocompatibility study', *Graefe's Arch Clin Exp Ophthalmol*, **241**, 625–630.

Tognetto D, Toto L, Sanguinetti G, Cecchini P, Vattovani O, Filacorda S, Ravalico G (2003b), 'Lens epithelial cell reaction after implantation of different intraocular lens materials: two-year results of a randomized prospective trial', *Ophthalmology*, **110**, 1935–1941.

Wejde G, Kugelberg M, Zetterstrom C (2003), 'Posterior capsule opacification: comparison of 3 intraocular lenses of different materials and design', *J Cataract Refract Surg*, **29**, 1556–1559.

Werner L (2007), 'Causes of intraocular lens opacification or discoloration', *J Cataract Refract Surg*, **33**, 713–726.

Werner L (2008), 'Biocompatibility of intraocular lens materials', *Curr Opin Ophthalmol*, **19**, 41–49.

Werner L, Legeais J M, Nagel M D, Renard G (1999), 'Evaluation of teflon-coated intraocular lenses in an organ culture method', *J Biomed Mater Res*, **46**, 347–354.

Wong T T, Daniels J T, Crowston J G, Khaw P T (2004), 'MMP inhibition prevents human lens epithelial cell migration and contraction of the lens capsule', *Br J Ophthalmol*, **88**, 868–872.

Yamakawa N, Tanaka T, Shigeta M, Hamano M, Usui M (2003), 'Surface roughness of intraocular lenses and inflammatory cell adhesion to lens surfaces', *J Cataract Refract Surg*, **29**, 367–370.

Yammine P, Pavon-Djavid G, Helary G, Migonney V (2005), 'Surface modification of silicone intraocular implants to inhibit cell proliferation', *Biomacromolecules*, **6**, 2630–2637.

Yao K, Huang X D, Huang X J, Xu Z K (2006), 'Improvement of the surface biocompatibility of silicone intraocular lens by the plasma-induced tethering of phospholipid moieties', *J Biomed Mater Res*, **78**, 684–692.

Yuan Z (2003), 'Physical and cytological characters of carbon, titanium surface modified intraocular lens in rabbit eyes', *Graefe's Arch Clin Exp Ophthalmol*, **241**, 840–844.

Yuan Z, Sun H, Yuan J (2004), 'A 1-year study on carbon, titanium surface-modified intraocular lens in rabbit eyes', *Graefe's Arch Clin Exp Ophthalmol*, **242**, 1008–1013.

Yuen C, Williams R, Batterbury M, Grierson I (2006), 'Modification of the surface properties of a lens material to influence posterior capsular opacification', *Clin Exp Ophthalmol*, **34**, 568–574.

3

Opacification and degradation of implanted intraocular lenses

L. WERNER, University of Utah, USA

Abstract: This chapter presents a summary of different causes of opacification/discoloration/degradation of intraocular lenses (IOLs) manufactured from different biomaterials and in different designs. The majority of the cases presented are based on the author's own analyses, but a brief review of the literature is also provided. Different processes leading to IOL opacification/discoloration/degradation were identified and may include: formation of deposits/precipitates on the IOL surface or within the IOL substance, excess influx of water in hydrophobic materials, direct discoloration of the IOL by capsular dyes or medications, IOL coating by substances such as ophthalmic ointment and silicone oil, and slowly progressing degradation of the lens biomaterial facilitated by long-term ultraviolet exposure.

Key words: intraocular lenses, poly(methyl methacrylate), silicone, hydrophilic acrylic, hydrogel, hydrophobic acrylic.

3.1   Introduction

A significant number of intraocular lens (IOL) explantations performed in this past decade were prompted by a process related to lens opacification and/ or degradation. Based on a review of the literature, as well as on our own analyses, the types of processes identified included: formation of deposits/ precipitates on the IOL surface or within the IOL substance, IOL opacification by excess influx of water in hydrophobic materials, direct discoloration of the IOL by capsular dyes or medications, IOL coating by substances such as ophthalmic ointment and silicone oil, and slowly progressing degradation of the lens biomaterial.[1] The inability to recognize a process of IOL opacification or discoloration may prompt surgeons to perform unnecessary surgical procedures, such as neodymium: yttrium–aluminum–garnet (Nd:YAG) posterior capsulotomies, or vitrectomies, in eyes where the opacification is actually in the IOL itself, and not at the level of the posterior capsule or the vitreous. This may jeopardize subsequent implantation of a new IOL in the capsular bag, among other complications. This chapter describes causes of opacification and discoloration of IOLs of different biomaterials and designs. The text is largely, but not exclusively based on analyses performed in our laboratories in Salt Lake City, Utah, USA and in Berlin, Germany. The causes of IOL opacification and discoloration are presented according to the

35

biomaterial used in the manufacture of the IOL: poly(methyl methacrylate) (PMMA), silicone, hydrophilic acrylic, and hydrophobic acrylic.

3.2   Opacification and degradation of poly(methyl methacrylate) intraocular lenses

3.2.1   Snowflake degeneration

PMMA was used as an optic biomaterial in Sir Harold Ridley's original IOL, manufactured by Rayner Intraocular Lenses Ltd, London, UK and first implanted in 1949–1950. Since that time, as surgical techniques and IOL designs have improved, the overwhelming majority of lenses manufactured from PMMA have provided stellar results for visual rehabilitation after cataract removal. Although PMMA has largely been replaced in the industrialized world by foldable IOL biomaterials intended for small incision surgery, on a worldwide basis PMMA-optic IOLs are still commonly implanted, especially in the developing world.

By the late 1980s, most surgeons and researchers had not only concluded that PMMA was a safe biomaterial, they also had confidence in the various manufacturing techniques required for lens fabrication. However, we analyzed in our laboratory different PMMA lenses explanted because of optic opacification, characterized by a gradual and sometimes progressive late-postoperative alteration of PMMA optic biomaterial. Based on both the clinical appearance as well as the macroscopic, pathologic morphology of the affected IOL optics, we termed this a 'snowflake' degeneration of the PMMA polymer. The broad constellation of clinical findings that ensues, ranging from glare and other types of visual aberration to clinically significant decrease in visual acuity represents a distinct clinical syndrome.[2,3]

The cases were generally related to three-piece posterior-chamber IOLs with rigid PMMA optical components and blue polypropylene or extruded PMMA haptics. Most had been implanted in the 1980s to early 1990s and the clinical symptoms occurred late postoperatively, sometimes more than a decade after the implantation. A correlation of the clinical, gross, and light and electron microscopic profiles of all cases showed a distinct pattern and revealed almost identical findings. The recurrent and interconnecting finding in all cases was the presence of the roughly spherical snowflake lesion, which we interpreted as foci of degenerated PMMA biomaterial. These varied only in the number and density of the lesions, which, in general, reflected also the severity and probably the duration of the opacification. Most examiners described the white-brown opacities within the IOL optics as 'crystalline deposits' (Fig. 3.1).

Views of the cut edges of the bisected optic specimens prepared for scanning electron microscopy (SEM) confirmed that the snowflake lesions

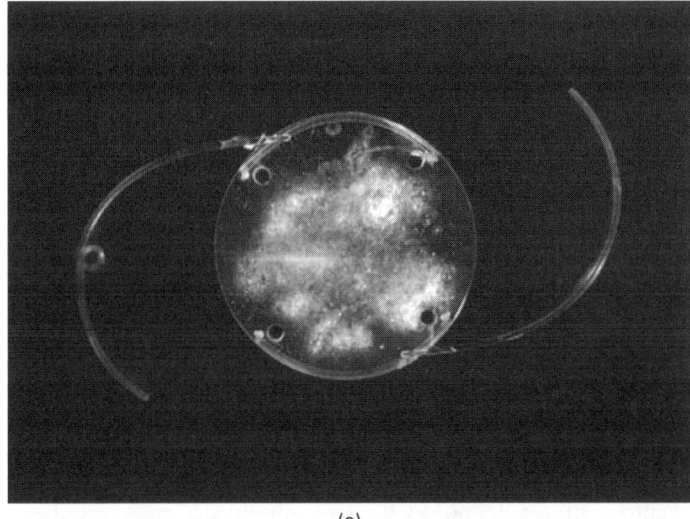

(a)

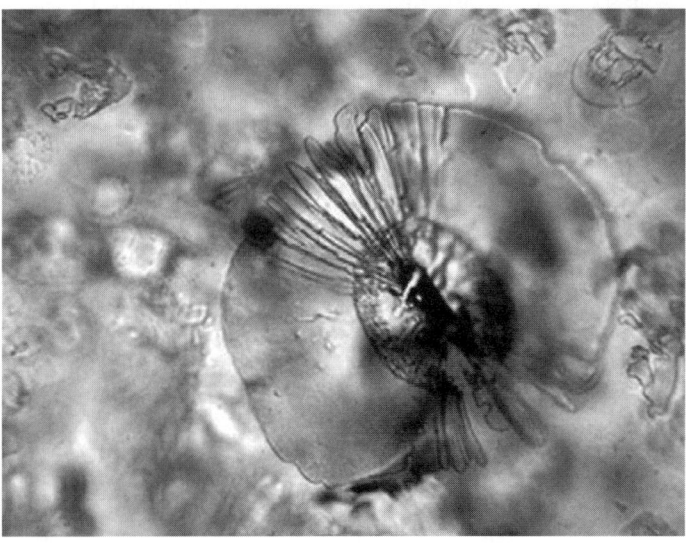

(b)

3.1 Snowflake degeneration. (a), gross photograph of a three-
piece PMMA lens explanted because of optic opacity related to
snowflake degeneration. Note that the periphery of the lens optic
is relatively free from opacities. (b), High-magnification (×400) light
photomicrograph of a snowflake lesion within the optic of the same
lens.

were not surface deposits, but rather, were all situated within the substance
of the optic. When the lenses were observed frontally, the snowflake lesions
were clustered most commonly in the central and mid-peripheral zones of
the IOL optics. The outer 0.5–1 mm peripheral rims of the lens optics were

generally less involved or free of opacification. The lesions were usually focal and discrete, with intervening clear areas, but some did appear to coalesce. Viewed in sagittal sections, the lesions generally involved the anterior third of the optic's substance. All histochemical and energy dispersive x-ray spectroscopy (EDS) analyses were negative indicating that the materials involved in the snowflake lesions are non-proteinaceous and are composed of elements common to PMMA (carbon, oxygen).

We suggested that manufacturing variations in some lenses fabricated in the 1980s to early 1990s may be responsible. It is possible that the late change in the PMMA material process is facilitated by long-term ultraviolet (UV, solar) exposure. This is supported by two pathologic observations. First, many opacities have been clustered in the central zone of the optic, extending to the mid-peripheral portion but often leaving the distal peripheral rim free of the opacities. This observation would support the hypothesis that the slow and sometimes progressive lesion formation might relate to the fact that the IOL's central optic is exposed to UV radiation over an extended period, whereas the peripheral optic may be protected by the iris. Furthermore, the opacities are present most commonly and intensely within the anterior third of the optic's substance. Since the anterior strata of the optic are the first to encounter the UV light, this might explain why the opacities are seen more frequently in this zone. The manufacturing process of PMMA utilizes many different polymerization techniques, and various components such as UV absorbers and initiators. Therefore, various impurity profiles are possible. A frequently used initiator is azo-bis-isobutyryl nitrile (AIBN). It is possible that UV radiation is a contributing factor; however, the exact pathogenesis can as of now only be hypothesized. Potential causes of a snowflake lesion include: (a) insufficient post-annealing of the cured PMMA polymer; (b) excessive thermal energy during the curing process leaving voids in the polymer matrix; (c) non-homogeneous distribution of the UV chromophore and/or thermal initiator into the polymer chain; (d) poor filtration of the pre-cured monomeric components (MMA, UV blocker, thermal initiator). Another possible pathogenic factor could be an inadvertent use of excessive initiator substance during the polymerization process that may facilitate the formation of the snowflake lesions. The $N{=}N$ bond of the AIBN initiator may be disrupted by gradual UV exposure with a release of nitrogen gas (N_2). Such gas formation can be caused by either heat or UV light exposure. Indeed the normal polymerization process for PMMA synthesis consists in part of a heat-induced N_2 formation as a byproduct. During normal polymerization the N_2 escapes from the mixture. However, in cases where there is excessive initiator, more than the fractional amount required, unwanted initiator may be entrapped in the PMMA substance. Slow release of gaseous N_2 within the PMMA substance trigged by long-term UV exposure would explain the formation of the cavitations within the snowflake lesions. Additional experimentation is necessary to determine if any of these proposed mechanisms for the formation of a snowflake lesion are probable.

Our initial belief when first looking at the spherical lesions was that fluid permeates into the cavitated lesions, forming vacuoles or 'glistenings'. Further examination of the lesions however, suggested that they are dry, rather than fluid-filled lesions. We have recently analyzed a PMMA lens explanted because of snowflake degeneration in the dry and hydrated states.[4] The lesions characteristic of the condition were restricted to the central 2 mm of the lens optic in the dry state. This is the smallest area ever observed, and may be related to the fact that the patient's pupils were relatively constricted as noted on the exam before and after dilation. Upon hydration of the explanted lens, an unusual amount of water was collected within the central 4 mm of the lens optic, where multiple linear cracks were present. These cracks were not evident under light microscopy in the dry state. They may represent the initial injury before the typical snowflake lesions are seen, or they may be secondary to the initial presence of the more central snowflake lesions. In any case, the clinical significance of snowflake degeneration may depend on the amount of water collected within the area of cracks. The emergence of this complication could have represented a more significant problem, except for the fact that many of the patients implanted with these IOLs are now deceased. However, surgeons must be aware that there are probably still a number of patients living with varying stages of snowflake degeneration.

3.3   Opacification and degradation of silicone intraocular lenses

3.3.1   Early opacification

We reported on the laboratory analyses of six IOLs explanted from patients who had visual disturbances caused by early postoperative opacification of the lens optic.[5,6] Six patients with three-piece silicone lenses presented with optic cloudiness, as early as a few hours after implantation. The lenses were implanted in four different locations in Brazil, and in France. The lenses in Brazil were stored at the same location before implantation. Gross and microscopic analyses were performed (dry and hydrated states). One-half of each specimen underwent gas chromatography–mass spectrometry (GC–MS) analysis and/or extraction by isopropyl alcohol or acetonitrile. One lens also underwent SEM with EDS. The IOLs were examined for the presence of contaminants and/or deposits that could cause fast optic opacification. The lenses showed whitish optic discoloration in the hydrated state, but became transparent upon complete dehydration (Fig. 3.2). Suspect exogenous chemical compounds were identified in GC–MS analyses; general classes included terpenes and ketones, typically found in industrial cleaning agents and

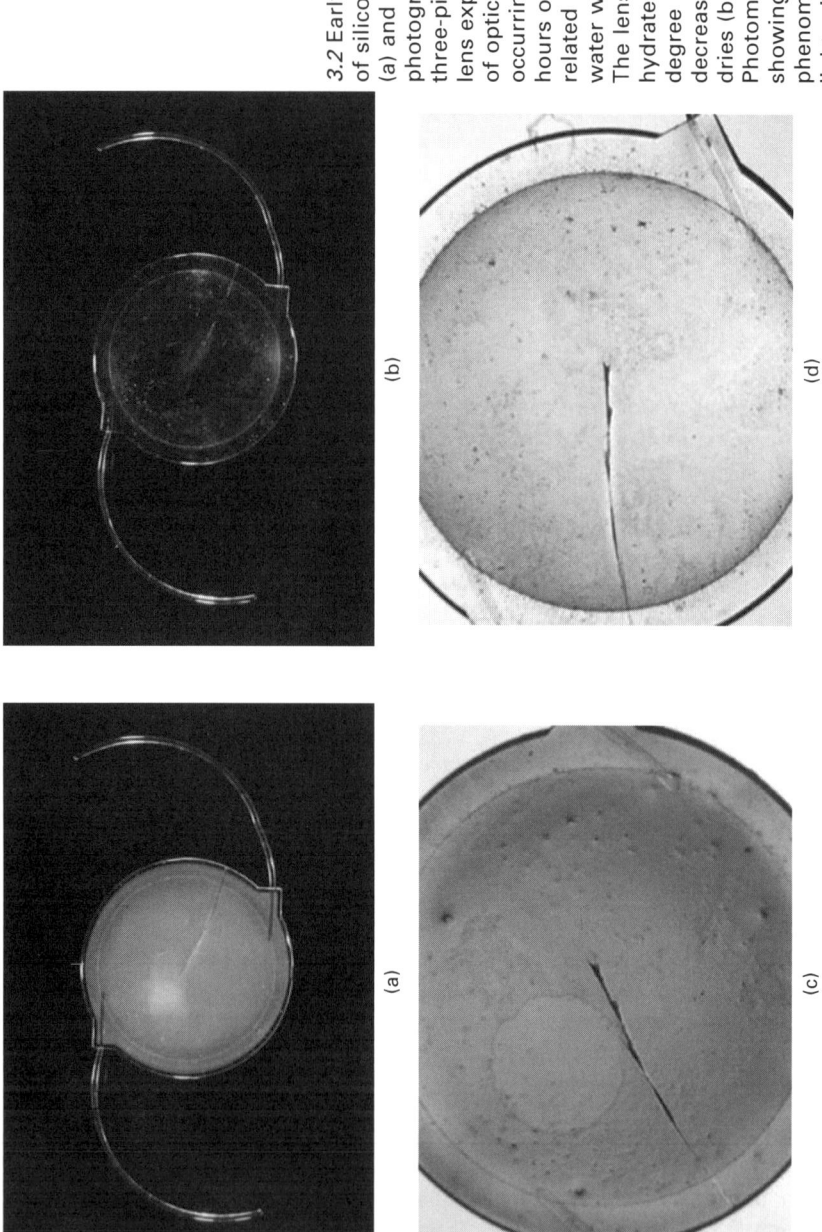

3.2 Early opacification of silicone lenses. (a) and (b) Gross photographs of a three-piece silicone lens explanted because of optic opacification occurring within 24 hours of implantation, related to influx of water within the optic. The lens is white while hydrated (a) and the degree of opacity decreases as the lens dries (b). (c) and (d) Photomicrographs showing the same phenomenon under light microscopy.

(a)

(b)

(c)

(d)

fumigants. Surface analyses (SEM and EDS) did not show any significant deposits on the external surfaces and sagittal cut of one of the specimens. Later, we reported on two other similar cases, from the United Kingdom and Hong Kong.[7]

Tanaka et al.[8] observed a phenomenon similar to our eight cases, in an 83-year-old Japanese patient implanted with an SI40 NB. In his report, the IOL presented with a 'brown haze' on the first postoperative day. The haze did not decrease until day 15 postoperatively, when the IOL was then explanted. Light microscopic evaluation of the explanted lens showed the presence of numerous spheroid structures in the central region of the optic, similar to glistenings. The authors suggested that the haze was secondary to influx of water within the lens, but no analyses to determine possible causative factors were carried out.

A thorough review of the history of the lenses evaluated in this study was carried out by the manufacturer (AMO, Santa Ana, CA, USA), according to their serial numbers. Although all the implantations in Brazil were carried out in different locations, and the lenses were from different manufacturing lots, it was determined that they had all been stored in the same area in Brazil, preoperatively. Spraying of the storage area with cleaning and insecticide agents was reportedly performed. Taking this fact into account, as well as the presence of exogenous chemical compounds in GC-MS analyses of these lenses, we hypothesized that chemical contamination of the lenses might have occurred preoperatively. This might have caused surface changes, rendering the relatively hydrophobic silicone surfaces more hydrophilic, allowing influx of water and therefore opacification of the IOL optic. It was noteworthy that after complete lens extraction of the lenses in some cases (i.e. removal of all adsorbed molecules), re-immersion of the lenses in solution did not cause any degree of optic opacification. Of particular interest was the presence of terpenes in some cases, and cyclohexanone in one case, which are not expected to be found in an IOL as they are not used in the lens manufacturing process, but are used in the manufacture of cleaning and insecticide agents. However, no clear history of preoperative contamination could be determined in some cases.

Three-piece silicone IOLs with PMMA haptics require sterilization by techniques using low temperature and pressure. Therefore, ethylene oxide gas sterilization is used.[9] For effective sterilization with ethylene oxide, selection of packaging material is very important, and permeability is one of the most important criteria. The packaging material must be permeable enough for ethylene oxide and moisture to enter the package (and air escape) and sterilize the contents within the desired cycle time. The packaging material must also have sufficient breathability to permit release of toxic residues (e.g. ethylene oxide residual gas). At the same time, the packaging material must be impermeable to bacteria and other contaminants. If this kind of packaging allows sterilization by ethylene oxide, one must assume that other chemical vapors may also penetrate the package and contaminate the lenses.

3.3.2   Late opacification

There have been reports of brownish discoloration and central haze of silicone lenses in the early 1990s.[10–15] In 1991, Milauskas reported 15 cases of brownish discoloration with IOLs manufactured by Staar and Iolab, observed from 15 to 60 months after implantation.[12] A decrease in the contrast sensitivity of the patients affected was observed in the more severe cases. Later, Milauskas identified 9 other cases, with the same kind of lenses.[13] Watt has also reported a case of central brownish discoloration of another silicone lens (AMO SI18 NGB), observed 6 weeks after implantation.[14] Koch and Heit reported on two other similar cases, with the same lens design.[11] In general this complication was considered clinically insignificant; IOL explantation has rarely been performed. These reports have suggested that the brown haze was due to light scatter from water vapor that may diffuse into the silicone when immersed in an aqueous medium. This may be caused by some anomaly of the curing process during the manufacture of those lenses or by incomplete extraction of large polymers. UV blocking agents did not seem to be an issue with lens discoloration since the phenomenon was also observed with silicone IOL models not containing these agents. Additional filtration steps in the manufacturing process of silicone lenses seemed to solve the problem.

More recently, we reported on 12 cases of late-postoperative opacification of silicone lenses (4 weeks to 2 years); all lenses were explanted in the United States (Werner L, Mamalis N, Olson RJ. Postoperative optic opacification of silicone IOLs: Analyses of 20 explants. Best-Paper-of-Session Award, Free Papers, Cataract Session, at the American Academy of Ophthalmology – AAO meeting, New Orleans, LA, USA, November 11, 2007). The degree of optic opacification was not as marked as for the lenses that showed earlier-onset opacification. GC-MS analyses of the lenses also showed components not matching chemicals used in AMO's silicone material synthesis, or components used while manufacturing the lenses. Of particular interest, is the presence of benzophenone in 7 out of 12 lenses. Although this compound may also be used as a UV blocker, the one used by the manufacturer on the corresponding designs is a modified benzotriazole compound.

AMO have reviewed the lot of history files for all lenses with known serial numbers, and no deviations regarding procedures used at the time of their manufacture were found. These lenses and the one without a serial number but with information on implant/explant dates were all manufactured at the Pharmacia facility in Groningen, before improvements in AMO's synthesis process (refinement of raw materials used during synthesis) were introduced. To date, to the best of their knowledge, no similar cases of opacification of silicone lenses manufactured after the improvements in the synthesis process were observed. According to the manufacturer, the incidents/complaints reported in this study represent a very low fraction of the total lenses sold and no relationship to manufacturing batches and components used – among other factors considered – was found. AMO currently performs several chemical analyses on their silicone material. These include analyses of the molecular weight of extracts obtained during silicone synthesis and IOL manufacturing, as residual monomers and short polymer chains may cause opacification when lenses are kept in water for some time at 37 °C.

3.3.3   Discoloration associated with dyes

Although experimental studies demonstrated that silicone lenses do not significantly interact with commonly used capsular dyes, we reported one case of blue discoloration of a silicone IOL.[16] The patient was a 52-year-old man who underwent uneventful phacoemulsification with implantation of an SI40 NB (AMO) in the right eye. A 'blue dye' was used to enhance visualization during capsulorhexis. Postoperatively, the patient presented with corneal edema and a discolored IOL (Fig. 3.3(a). The lens was therefore explanted and exchanged. The corneal edema resolved within 1 month of the initial surgical procedure. After explantation, gross and microscopic analyses of the explanted silicone lens revealed that its surface and internal substance had been permanently stained blue. It was then determined in this case that methylene blue had been inadvertently used instead of trypan blue to stain the anterior capsule. Of course, the most significant problem in this case was not the discoloration of the IOL itself, but the use of a solution that was not appropriate for the intraocular environment, raising concerns about toxic anterior segment syndrome (TASS).[17]

3.3.4   Discoloration associated with systemic medication

Silicone IOL opacification/discoloration has also been associated with the long-term use of systemic medications. Katai *et al.* reported on a patient who was treated with amiodarone for 3 years and developed brown discoloration of the silicone lenses in both eyes.[18] Jones and Irwin described the case of a patient who developed a rose discoloration of the silicone lenses in both eyes after receiving rifabutin for 10 months.[19] Recently, there have been reports from South India of green discoloration of silicone IOLs.[20,21] The phenomenon was noted at 6 months postoperatively, but as the patients were asymptomatic, the lenses were not explanted. To date, careful scrutiny of the medical and surgical history of the patients failed to reveal factors that

3.3 Other causes of explantation of silicone lenses. (a) Light photomicrograph of a three-piece silicone lens explanted because of inadvertent use of methylene blue as a capsular dye instead of trypan blue, with blue discoloration of the lens. (b) Clinical photograph showing adhesion of silicone oil used in retinal surgery to the implanted silicone lens. (c) Light photomicrograph of a three-piece silicone lens explanted because of coating of the optic component with ophthalmic ointment used by the surgeon after the implantation procedure. (d) Gross photograph of a silicone plate lens, explanted because of optic calcification in an eye with asteroid hyalosis.

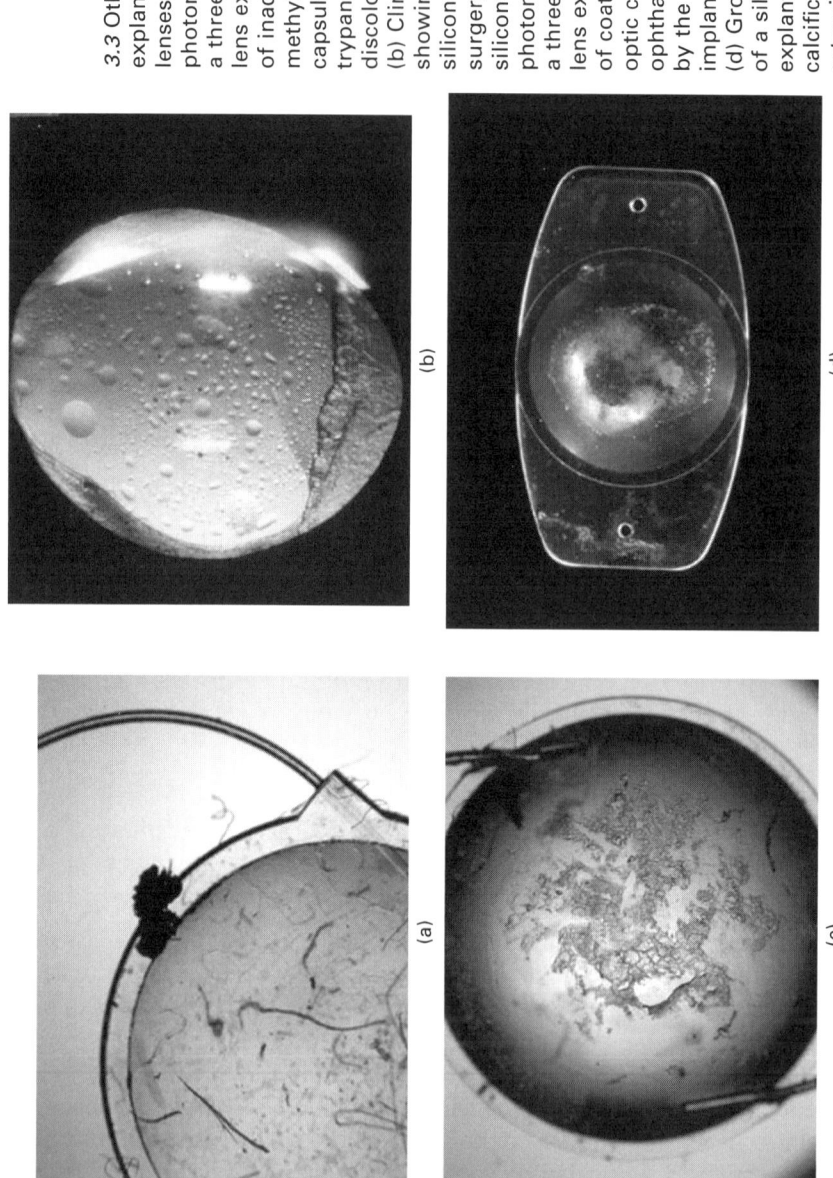

(a)

(b)

(c)

(d)

might have predisposed the IOLs to green discoloration. A previous report from Pakistan had also described a similar complication.[21]

3.3.5 Coating with silicone oil

Opacification/discoloration of silicone lenses in the late-postoperative period was also observed in relation to deposition of material on the lens surfaces. The interaction of silicone oil, used in vitreoretinal surgery, with standard silicone IOLs in a given patient is a well-documented clinical complication (Fig. 3.3(b).[22,23] Patients with vitreoretinal problems that may require use of silicone oil should not be implanted with silicone lenses, as the oil will attach to the lens surfaces, causing optical irregularities. This irreversible adherence of silicone oil to the IOL optic may lead to different sequelae, including visual disturbances and visual loss for the patient, as well as obstruction of the vitreoretinal surgeon's view into the eye. This is a complication not generally seen by the implanting cataract surgeon but, rather, at a later stage in a patient's postoperative course, by a vitreoretinal surgeon. Experimental studies showed that, although silicone IOLs show maximal adherence to silicone oil, other lens biomaterials are not immune to this complication. Silicone oil coverage was related to the dispersive energy component of the surface charge of the IOL biomaterial. Low dispersive energy materials had less silicone oil coverage, while those with higher dispersive energy had more oil coverage. Regardless of the degree of oil-induced cloudiness of the IOL, visual loss is often severe by the time most patients develop severe vitreoretinal disease that requires radical treatment with silicone oil. Therefore the clinical importance of this complication actually relates most significantly to patients who may be deemed to have a high propensity for severe vitreoretinal disease that may require silicone oil treatment at a later date. Common conditions that may fall into this category include: rhegmatogenous retinal degeneration, previous retinal tears or detachment in the same or fellow eye, family history of hereditary retinal detachment, high risk of ocular trauma, high myopia or ocular developmental abnormalities, congenital cataract and proliferative diabetic retinopathy. Patients that fall in any of the above categories should proactively receive an appropriate IOL with the future complications borne in mind.

3.3.6 Coating with ophthalmic ointment

We have recently reported eight cases of TASS related to an oily material within the anterior chamber of the patients' eyes.[24] The eight patients had undergone uneventful phacoemulsification by the same surgeon via clear corneal incisions, with implantation of three-piece silicone lens designs. Postoperative medications included antibiotic/steroid ointment, and pilocarpine gel; each eye was firmly patched at the end of the procedure. On the first postoperative day, some patients presented with diffuse corneal edema, increased intraocular pressure (IOP), and an oily, film-like material within the anterior chamber, coating the corneal endothelium. The others presented with an oily bubble floating inside the anterior chamber, which was later seen coating the IOL. Additional surgical procedures required included penetrating keratoplasty (N = 4), IOL explantation (N = 6), and trabeculectomy (N = 1). Two corneal buttons were analyzed histopathologically, two explanted IOLs underwent gross and light microscopic analyses (as well as surface analyses on one of them), and four other explanted IOLs underwent GC-MS.

Pathological examination of the corneas showed variable thinning of the epithelium, with edema. The stroma was diffusely thickened, and the endothelial cell layer was absent. Evaluation of the explanted IOLs confirmed the presence of an oily substance coating large areas of their anterior and posterior optic surfaces (Fig. 3.3(c). GC-MS of the lens extracts identified a mixed chain hydrocarbon compound, which was also found in the GC-MS analyses of the ointment used postoperatively. Therefore, the results indicated that the ointment gained access to the eye, causing the postoperative complications described. These cases highlight the importance of appropriate wound construction and integrity, as well as the risks of tight eye patching following placement of ointment. McDonnell et al. evaluated the dynamic morphology of clear corneal cataract incisions by creating clear corneal incisions in human and rabbit eyes obtained postmortem.[25] They found that, at low pressures, wound edges tended to gape, starting at the internal aspect of the wound. In a retrospective study, Shingleton et al. demonstrated that a significant percentage of eyes having clear corneal phacoemulsification had an IOP of 5 mm Hg or less 30 minutes after surgery.[26]

Intraocular penetration of ointments has already been described in the literature. In 1973, Fraunfelder and Hanna, published a report on a survey sent to 400 randomly selected ophthalmologists from the Fellows in the American Academy of Ophthalmology and Otolaryngology.[27] Of the 327 surveys returned, 65 (20%) reported having seen ointment entrapped in the anterior chamber postoperatively in a total of 95 patients. Garzozi et al. reported the case of a patient who presented with a bubble floating in the anterior chamber after radial keratotomy.[28] Aralikatti et al. reported the case of a patient who underwent uneventful phacoemulsification through an oblique, self-sealing clear corneal incision, and presented with a white lump of a substance in the anterior chamber, overlying the pupil, on the first postoperative day.[29] More recently, Riedl et al. described ointment entering the anterior chamber after cataract surgery through a temporal corneal incision.[30] Therefore, the possibility of intraocular penetration of any kind of ointment used postoperatively, not only in cataract surgery, but in different types of penetrating procedures, should therefore be anticipated.

Ophthalmic ointment may also gain intraocular access after surgery, but only coat the IOL implanted later postoperatively. We have recently evaluated the case of a patient who underwent uneventful phacoemulsification with implantation of a three-piece silicone IOL (SI30 NB, AMO) via a 3.0 mm scleral tunnel incision.[31] Postoperative medications included antibiotic/steroid drops and ointments. Eight months postoperatively, the patient started having recurrent episodes of anterior-chamber inflammatory reaction. The suspicion that lens instability was causing the reactions led to two repositioning procedures, including performance of McCannel sutures. Finally, 18 months postoperatively, the IOL presented with a 'greasy' film and it was later exchanged. GC-MS analysis of the ointment used after each surgical procedure showed several compounds that had mass spectra characteristic of hydrocarbons similar to those detected in the extract prepared from the explanted IOL. In this case, it is possible that the ointment entered the anterior chamber after the IOL repositioning procedures, perhaps through clear corneal paracentesis usually required for the placement of McCannel iris-suture fixation. The first observation of globules on the IOL was only noted 5 months after the last procedure. The reasons for this late onset remain unclear to us. Chen *et al.* have also recently reported a case where an oily-like material was only observed inside the anterior chamber in the late-postoperative period after cataract surgery.[32] The material was identified as ointment by Fourier transform infrared and confocal Raman microspectroscopies.

3.3.7   Calcification in asteroid hyalosis

Calcified deposits leading to significant opacification requiring explantation were observed on the surface of silicone IOLs in eyes with asteroid hyalosis. Four cases were initially reported in the literature, all with silicone-plate lenses in patients with unilateral asteroid hyalosis (Fig. 3.3(d)).[33,34] Whitish deposits appeared only on the posterior optic surface of the lens late postoperatively. Two out of the four reported patients had diabetes. In two of the cases, the deposits were noted before Nd:YAG laser capsulotomy was performed. Fast re-accumulation of the deposits on the posterior surface of the lenses was described after the procedure. In the other two cases, it is not clear whether or not the deposits were present before the Nd:YAG procedure. While in the three cases reported by us, the deposits were observed mostly within the area of the Nd:YAG capsulotomy,[33] in the case reported by Wackernagel *et al.*, the deposits also appeared on the periphery of the optic, covered by the posterior capsule.[34]

Later we described the first similar case related to a three-piece silicone lens, in a patient with bilateral asteroid hyalosis.[35] The 76-year-old diabetic woman underwent uneventful cataract surgery in 1994 with implantation of an SI30 NB (AMO) IOL in the left eye. An Nd:YAG laser posterior capsulotomy was performed 2 years after cataract surgery, but persistent whitish deposits were observed on the posterior optic surface of the lens. Over the next 3 years, the opacification increased in the region corresponding to the capsulotomy. The IOL was explanted/exchanged. The right eye had cataract surgery in 1995. The acrylic lens implanted in this eye developed no opacities after 6 years.

There are only a few cases in the recent literature describing the association between dystrophic calcification of silicone lenses and asteroid hyalosis. Calcification of silicone lenses in the absence of this vitreous condition has not been reported. Indeed, in the absence of asteroid hyalosis, long-term calcified deposits were previously observed only on the surface or within the substance of some hydrophilic acrylic IOL designs. There is, therefore, increasing evidence that the material opacifying the silicone lenses is derived from the asteroid bodies, or derived from a similar process that results in this vitreous condition, as its composition was found to be similar to that of hydroxyapatite (calcium and phosphate). The latter is more likely the case because the asteroid calcium is already 'out of solution'. It is, however, still unclear why only a few cases have been observed, while there have probably been many implantations of silicone lenses of various designs in patients with asteroid hyalosis. Careful clinical examination of pseudophakic patients with asteroid hyalosis will confirm if this phenomenon is more widespread, but only significant enough to require IOL explantation in a few cases. This will also confirm if the phenomenon is restricted to silicone lenses. Without such knowledge, it is difficult to proscribe silicone IOL implantation in the presence of asteroid hyalosis.

3.4 Opacification and degradation of hydrophilic acrylic intraocular lenses

3.4.1 Discoloration

Capsular dyes such as fluorescein sodium, indocyanine green (ICG), and trypan blue have been successfully used for staining the anterior capsule (injection under an air bubble or intracameral subcapsular injection), for performing capsulorhexis in advanced/white, intumescent, or hypermature cataracts. We described for the first time the occurrence of blue discoloration of an IOL by a capsular dye (Fig. 3.4).[36] The lens was an hydrophilic acrylic design (Acqua, Mediphacos). The patient was a 79-year-old Caucasian male patient, who underwent cataract surgery with implantation of this hydrophilic acrylic design. Trypan blue 0.1% was injected under an air bubble to stain the anterior capsule before capsulorhexis. Seven days after surgery, the patient presented with 'dark and double' vision (monocular diplopia). The IOL was decentered superiorly and appeared dark blue. The lens was explanted

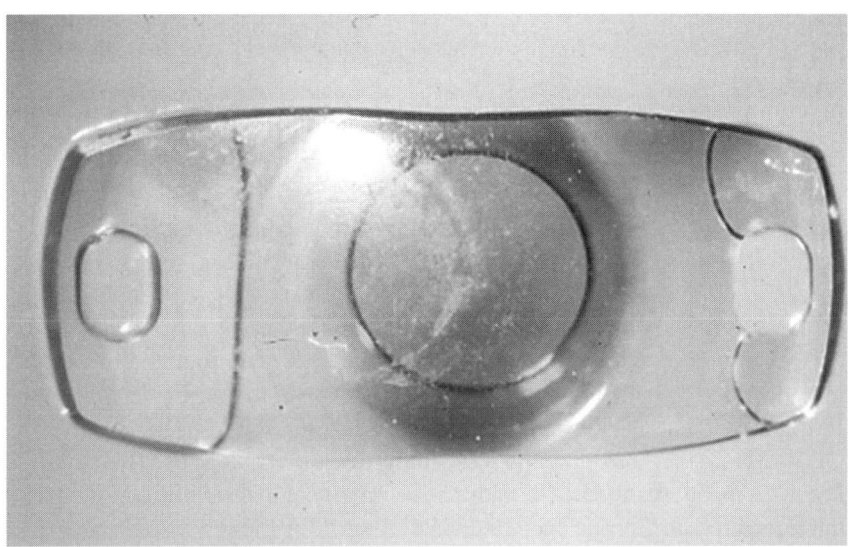

3.4 Gross photograph of a plate hydrophilic acrylic lens (Acqua) explanted because of blue discoloration related to intraoperative use of capsular dyes (trypan blue).

2 months after surgery and submitted for gross and microscopic analyses performed in a dry state and after hydration. Analyses of the lens revealed that the dark blue staining was denser within the optic component, especially in the optical periphery. The blue discoloration could not be removed after 24 hours of immersion of the lens in balanced salt solution at 37 °C. The same analyses were performed on two unused lenses of the same design, which had been immersed in diluted trypan blue solutions (0.01% and 0.001%). Permanent staining of the unused lenses was also obtained after immersion in the experimental solutions.

Most of the currently available hydrophilic acrylic lenses have water contents ranging from 18% to 28%. They are packaged in a vial containing distilled water or balanced salt solutions, thus they are implanted in the hydrated state and in their final dimensions. Hydration renders these lenses flexible, enabling the surgeons to fold and insert them through small incisions. To our knowledge, the Acqua lens is manufactured from the hydrophilic acrylic material with the highest water content (73.5%) currently used for the manufacture of IOLs. This lens is implanted in the dry state, its expansion depending on its hydration by the fluids within the capsular bag. It appears that minimal amounts of dye still present in the capsular bag during IOL implantation may be absorbed by this lens. Therefore, capsular dyes should not be used in association with the Acqua lens.

After this report, trypan blue, ICG, and fluorescein sodium have been tested in laboratory settings to evaluate their interaction with various IOL materials. These tests showed that only the hydrophilic acrylic lenses could significantly absorb commonly used capsular dyes.

3.4.2 Calcification

Postoperative optic opacification of modern hydrophilic acrylic IOL designs has been a significant complication leading to IOL explantation since 1999.[1,37] Different studies using histopathological, histochemical, electron microscopic, as well as elemental or molecular surface analytical techniques demonstrated that the opacification was related to calcium/phosphate precipitation on (Fig. 3.5) and/or within (Fig. 3.6) the lenses.[38–47] The four major designs manufactured in the United States that were involved in the problem were the Hydroview (Bausch & Lomb), the MemoryLens (Ciba Vision), the SC60B-OUV (Medical Developmental Research), and the Aqua-Sense (Ophthalmic Innovations International). Sporadic cases involving hydrophilic acrylic lenses manufactured in Europe were also described.[37] Although in many cases it was difficult to determine the time that optic opacification was first observed, the lenses involved in the problem were on average explanted during the second year after implantation. The opacification was not associated with anterior segment inflammatory reaction and Nd:YAG laser was ineffective in removing the calcified deposits from the lenses.

Different experimental methods have been used in an attempt to elucidate the factors involved in the calcification of hydrophilic acrylic lenses. In the case of the Hydroview, the silicone gasket sealing the SureFold cap came under suspicion early, as the lenses in the previous packaging did not calcify. Guan et al. evaluated the role of silicone compounds interacting with long-chain saturated fatty acids present in the aqueous humor (myristic, palmitic, stearic, arachidic, and behenic) on the calcification process.[40] The IOLs were exposed to cyclic silicone compounds, and treated with one of the above-mentioned fatty acids, at different concentrations. Then, they were rinsed and placed in supersaturated solutions of calcium chloride and potassium dihydrogen phosphate. The authors demonstrated that hydrophobic cyclic silicone compounds adsorbed at the IOL surfaces interacted strongly with the hydrophobic carbon chains of the fatty acids, to create a layer of fatty acids oriented with polar, functional hydrophilic groups exposed to the aqueous solution, providing nucleation sites for calcium/phosphate. Interestingly, in a retrospective study of 949 cases of Hydroview IOL implantations carried out between 1998 and 2000, a phosphate-buffered ophthalmic viscosurgical device (OVD) preparation had been used intraoperatively in all of the cases of calcification requiring explantation ($N = 20$).[44] Ohrstrom et al. had already demonstrated that the amount of silicone oil within the syringes of the same OVD was one of the highest among five different brands.[48]

Dorey et al. analyzed 17 explanted Hydroview lenses and demonstrated

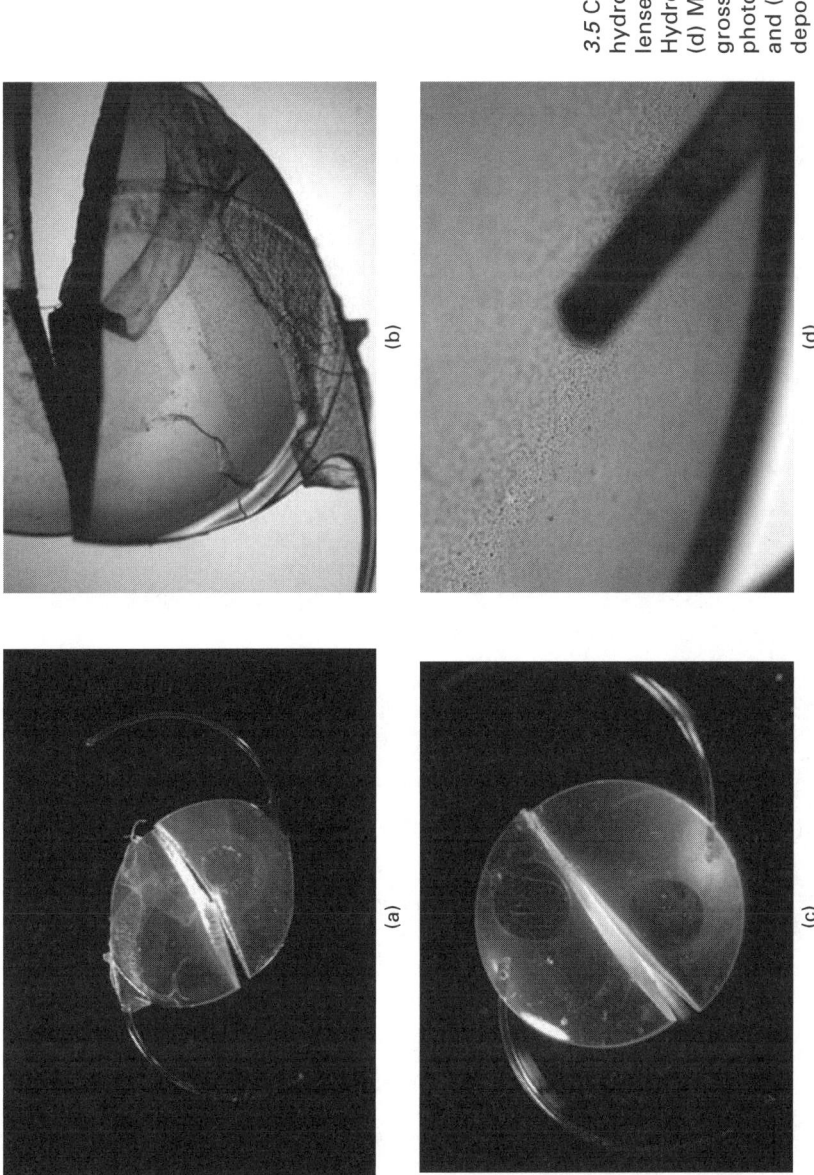

3.5 Calcification of hydrophilic acrylic lenses. (a) and (b) Hydroview lens. (c) and (d) MemoryLens. The gross (a) and (c) and light photomicrographs (b) and (d) show the calcified deposits mostly on the surfaces of the lenses.

(a)

(b)

(c)

(d)

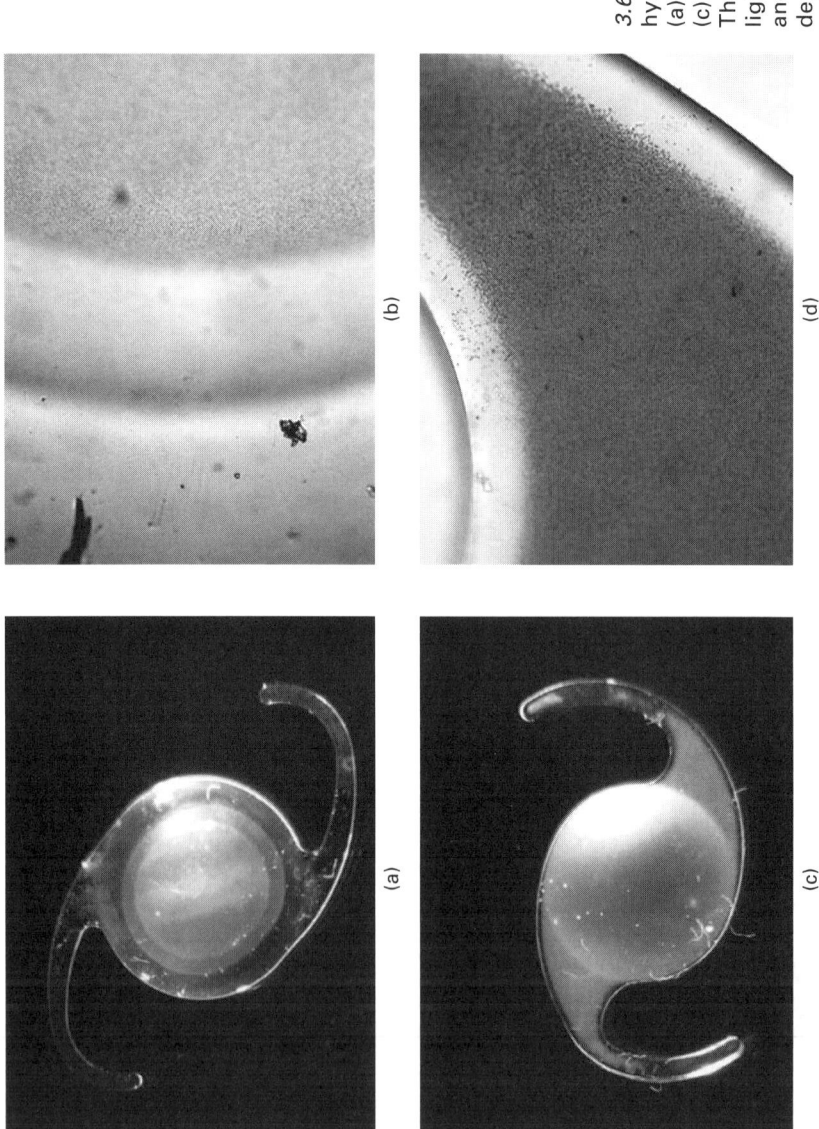

3.6 Calcification of hydrophilic acrylic lenses. (a) and (b) SC60B-OUV lens. (c) and (d) Aqua-Sense lens. The gross (a) and (c) and light photomicrographs (b) and (d) show the calcified deposits mostly within the substance of the lenses.

(a)

(b)

(c)

(d)

the presence of the element silicon mainly at the center of the calcified deposits, in surface analyses using EDS coupled with transmission electron microscopy.[38] Later, we demonstrated the presence of the element silicon in relation to calcified deposits with the three other major hydrophilic acrylic designs that have been associated with calcification, by using an EDS system attached to an environmental scanning electron microscope.[47] Ophthalmic Innovations International also confirmed the presence of siloxane silicone elastomers in the packaging components used at that time. As a result of the above-mentioned research the packaging of the Hydroview and Aqua-Sense lenses was significantly changed. When comparing different studies on surface analyses of explanted calcified lenses, one should be aware of the differences between the techniques used. The analyses carried out by the manufacturers of the Hydroview and Aqua-Sense designs give information at the molecular level. According to them, the contamination with those designs was in the form of low molecular weight silicone compounds forming a thin fluid film (although it is referred to as 'particles' in some publications). Therefore, further investigation is necessary regarding the relationship between our results and those of Dorey and the silicone compounds found on the Hydroview and Aqua-Sense by analyses performed at the molecular level.

Gartaganis et al. provided further contribution to the understanding of the IOL calcification process.[39] They described their three-part study involving morphological analyses of explants (24 Hydroview, two SC60B-OUV, two MemoryLens, and two Aqua-Sense), chemical analyses of aqueous humor collected from cases of explanted calcified IOLs, and in vitro experiments using PMMA and poly(2-hydroxyethyl methacrylate) (PHEMA) polymer powder suspended in solutions supersaturated with calcium and phosphate. They concluded that a key factor in the development of crystalline phosphate salts is represented by local conditions of supersaturation either in the vicinity of the surface of the IOLs, or within their substance, where salts develop by diffusion of calcium/phosphate ions. The authors, as well as others before them,[49] recognized that calcium/phosphate may be derived from residual cataractous lens material. Perhaps differences in surgical technique, including the extent of cortical clean up may explain, at least in part, why patients bilaterally implanted with hydrophilic acrylic IOLs from the same lot sometimes develop calcification in only one of the lenses.

Similar studies have also been performed by Nakanome et al.[42] These authors measured the concentration of calcium, phosphate, and albumin in the aqueous humor collected from ten eyes with calcified IOLs (all diabetic patients; nine with diabetic retinopathy and five from patients on hemodialysis). High concentrations of the three parameters measured were found, believed to be associated with chronic breakdown of the blood–aqueous barrier. The authors also placed Hydroview lenses in calcium/phosphate solutions with 25 mg/dL albumin. One group of lenses was subjected to large fluctuations in the concentrations of calcium and phosphate in the solutions (simulating hemodialysis conditions), while the other group was kept under constant calcium/phosphate concentrations. Calcified deposits were observed on the surface of the lenses in the first group within 7 days, while no significant calcification was observed on the lenses in the second group.

Regarding the MemoryLens design, the manufacturer (Ciba Vision) correlated the opacification problem with a change in the polishing process in 1999.[43] The modified manufacturing method used a phosphate buffer in the tumbling process, which would attract more protein. The process would then continue to progress with the deposition of minerals, most likely calcium, on top of the protein film. According to the manufacturer, a worldwide recall of this lens in April 2000 (associated with cases of sterile hypopyon) also included all MemoryLens IOLs manufactured using the modified tumbling process. Ciba Vision then changed the polishing process and re-introduced the MemoryLens in October 2000 with the models U940S and CV232, the latter featuring a square optic-edge design.

More recently, we described for the first time the case of a MemoryLens IOL model CV232 that was explanted 18 months postoperatively.[50] The patient had decreased visual acuity with the presence of a well-circumscribed, centrally/paracentrally located opacification of the optic. The area had the aspect of a small 'lens within the lens' or a regular, round bubble. The opacification observed within the CV232 lens remained well localized, without notable changes in its aspect since it was first noted 1 year after the surgery, until the lens was explanted 6 months later. It was actually difficult to determine the clinical significance of the IOL opacity precisely in that case. The postoperative decrease in visual acuity could eventually be, at least partially, related to posterior capsule opacification (PCO) formation, and eventually to retinal and glaucoma problems. The analyses of the explanted CV232 lens revealed that within the localized round area of opacification there were deposits (large crystals) distributed within an optic 'void', seen as a linear breach in sagittal cuts. We hypothesized that the precipitation of calcium in this case was a process secondary to the optic defect. The origin of the optic defect remains speculative at this point. We are aware of other similar cases with the new CV232 design, including asymptomatic cases where explantation was not necessary, and cases where the localized area within the optic has the aspect of a clear bubble (Fig. 3.7), without significant opacification. Whether or not secondary calcification will occur within the optic void in these cases at some point in the postoperative period is still unknown.

Calcification of hydrophilic acrylic lenses appears to be a multifactorial problem, and factors related to IOL manufacture, IOL packaging, surgical techniques and adjuvants, as well as patient metabolic conditions, among others, may be implicated. As the exact combination of factors and sequence

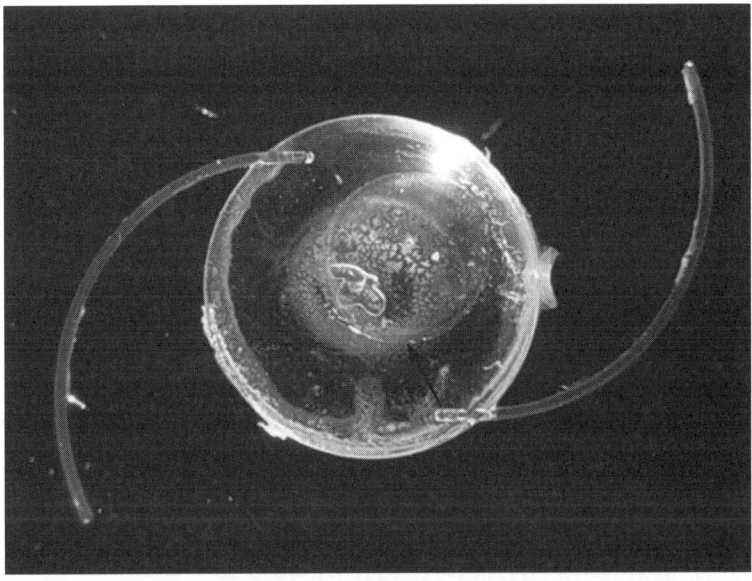

(a)

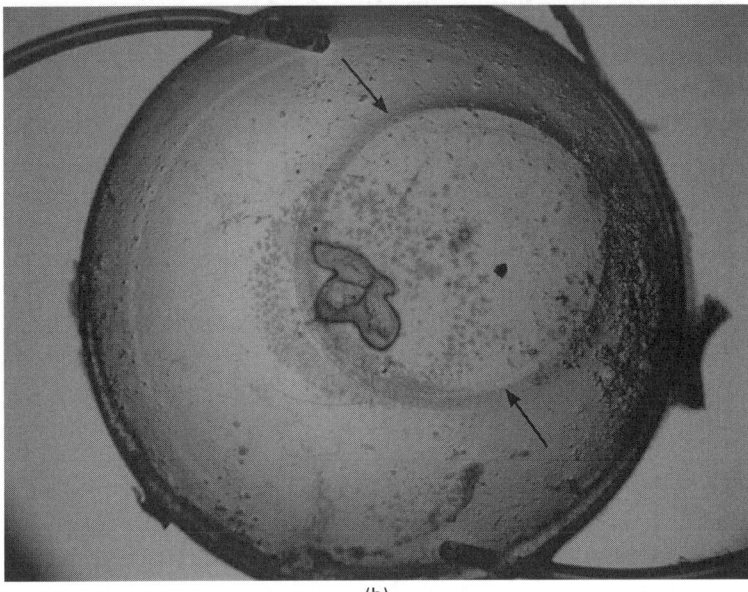

(b)

3.7 Gross photograph (a) and light photomicrograph (b) of a three-piece hydrophilic acrylic lens, which was explanted because of the presence of a localized optic void, with the aspect of a relatively clear bubble (arrows). Unspecific surface deposits (crystallized viscoelastic solution, etc.) can be observed on the optic surface.

of events ultimately leading to calcification of the lenses is still unknown, continuous research on this complication is warranted. This requires a multidisciplinary approach, which is further complicated by the fact that detailed manufacturing procedures are considered proprietary information, and some IOL designs are distributed in different countries with different commercial names. In the meantime, surgeons must be able to recognize this condition during clinical examination, to avoid performance of unnecessary procedures, such as Nd:YAG laser posterior capsulotomy (after a misdiagnosis of PCO), or vitrectomy (after a misdiagnosis of some form of vitreous opacity). We have recently described eight cases where calcification of the implanted MemoryLens IOLs was not recognized, with unnecessary procedures and repeated interventions ultimately leading to complications such as retinal detachment and endophthalmitis.[41] Explantation/exchange of the opacified/calcified IOL is to date the only possible treatment.

3.5   Opacification and degradation of hydrophobic acrylic intraocular lenses

3.5.1   Interlenticular opacification

Although not representing a cause of opacification of the IOL itself, the problem of interlenticular opacification (ILO) has only been significantly related to hydrophobic acrylic IOLs. ILO is the opacification of the opposing surfaces of IOLs implanted in a piggyback manner. The purpose of implanting two or more posterior-chamber IOLs (polypseudophakia or piggyback IOLs) is to (a) provide adequate pseudophakic optical correction for patients requiring high IOL power or (b) provide secondary correction of an undesirable optical result following cataract–IOL surgery.[51,52] To date, all cases analyzed in our laboratory seemed to be related to two posterior-chamber IOLs being implanted in the capsular bag through a small capsulorhexis, with its margins overlapping the optic edge of the anterior IOL for 360° (Fig. 3.8).[51–54] In addition, all of the explanted lenses we received were three-piece AcrySof IOLs (Alcon, Inc.). The adhesive nature of the acrylic material of this lens may play a role in the outcome of this complication, rendering removal of any opacity within the interlenticular space surgically difficult. Laboratory analyses allowed us to conclude that the opacification within the interlenticular space is derived from retained/regenerative cortex and pearls, which is similar to the pathogenesis of the pearl form of PCO. The aspect of the opacifying material varies according to the space available in the interlenticular interface.[53]

One should be aware that careful cortical clean up is mandatory in piggyback implantation. Also, based on the common features of different cases of ILO, some surgical methods were proposed for its prevention. The

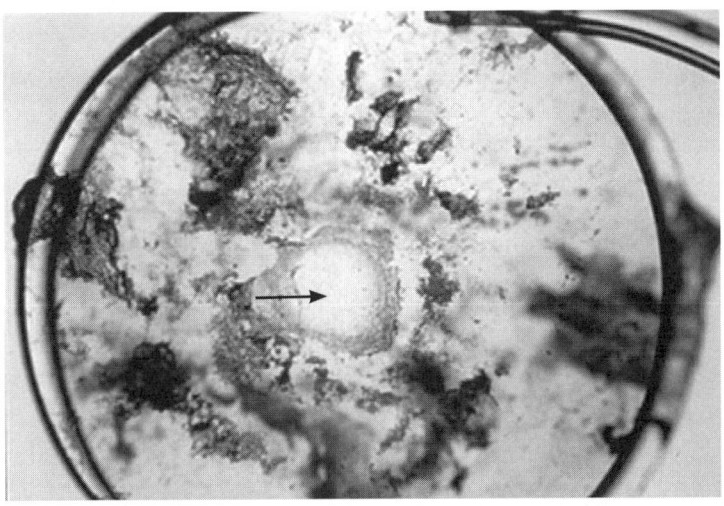

3.8 Light photomicrograph of a pair of three-piece hydrophobic acrylic lenses, which were implanted in the capsular bag, and were explanted because of interlenticular opacification. The arrow shows the central contact area between the optic components of the lenses, where no opacification is present.

first option would be to implant both IOLs in the capsular bag but with a relatively larger diameter capsulorhexis. The other possibility is to implant the anterior IOL in the sulcus and the posterior IOL in the bag with a small rhexis. In both scenarios, the lens epithelial cells within the equatorial fornix will be sequestered.

To the best of our knowledge, ILO is not a common occurrence in association with silicone lenses. We performed an animal study to evaluate and compare the incidence of capsular bag opacification, focusing on ILO in rabbit eyes implanted with a dual-optic silicone IOL or piggyback lenses.[54] Ten dual-optic study IOLs (Synchrony, Visiogen), ten control pairs of piggyback silicone-plate lenses, and ten control pairs of piggyback single-piece hydrophobic acrylic lenses were implanted in the bag following phacoemulsification. After a follow-up of 6 weeks, the rabbits were killed; their eyes were enucleated and underwent gross and microscopic evaluation after histopathological processing. In this study, ILO formation was statistically different among the three groups of lenses, but the differences between the study IOL group and the pair of silicone-plate lens group were not significant. ILO comparisons between the hydrophobic acrylic lenses and the study lens, or the silicone-plate lenses were significant. Histopathological examination showed extension of the proliferating cortical material from the peripheral Soemmering's ring into the interlenticular space, causing ILO, especially with the pairs of hydrophobic acrylic lenses.

3.5.2   Glistenings

Glistenings are fluid-filled microvacuoles (1–20 microns in diameter) that form within the IOL optic when the lens is in an aqueous environment.[55] Although they are largely described in association with hydrophobic acrylic IOLs (Fig. 3.9),[56] they can actually be observed with different IOL materials, including PMMA.[57–59] The majority of peer-reviewed articles on glistenings available in the literature describe them in relation to the AcrySof material. Earlier *in vitro* studies demonstrated that glistenings were confined to IOLs packaged in AcryPak folders maintained at constant body temperature.[55] Glistenings were noted in the Wagon Wheel-packaged IOLs only under fluctuating temperature conditions. Other studies demonstrated *in vitro* glistening formation after incubating different types of hydrophobic acrylic lenses in salt solution, and subjecting them to changes in temperature. The change in the equilibrium water content caused by temperature changes between 30 and 40 °C was found to be an important factor in glistening formation, and IOL materials featuring less temperature-dependent water absorption would be less likely to form glistenings.[60–62]

There is still controversy on whether or not glistenings have any impact on the visual function of the patient, and if they progress over time. Regarding clinical significance, an earlier study evaluated 17 patients implanted with a hydrophobic acrylic IOL (three-piece AcrySof in AcryPak folders), 10 of the patients having a silicone IOL in the contralateral eye.[63] All 17 eyes with the acrylic IOLs had some lenticular glistenings, ranging from trace to 2+. Statistical analysis of visual acuity, contrast sensitivity, and glare testing revealed a statistically significant difference between the acrylic and the silicone IOLs only in contrast sensitivity. A later study comparing eyes implanted with a hydrophobic acrylic IOL (Wagon Wheel-packaged three-piece AcrySof) with glistenings, and eyes with the same IOL but without glistenings, only showed a statistically significant difference in contrast sensitivity at the high spatial frequency.[64] Christiansen *et al.* graded glistenings in 42 eyes implanted with the same hydrophobic acrylic lens from trace to 4+.[65] They found a slight decrease in visual function in eyes with glistenings graded as 2+ or more, in comparison to eyes with lower grades of glistenings. However, Oshika *et al.* experimentally created 1+ to 4+ glistenings in Wagon Wheel-packaged three-piece AcrySof lenses, among which the 4+ glistenings were found to be beyond the range of clinical settings.[66] By using optical bench tests, the authors determined that only the 4+ glistenings obtained would cause mild to moderate deterioration of the optical quality of the lens.

Different studies looked at the progression of glistenings over time. In clinical and experimental settings, Miyata *et al.* found that glistenings reached their peak in number within a few months of formation in all cases, showing no further increase thereafter.[67] Experimental glistenings first appeared on

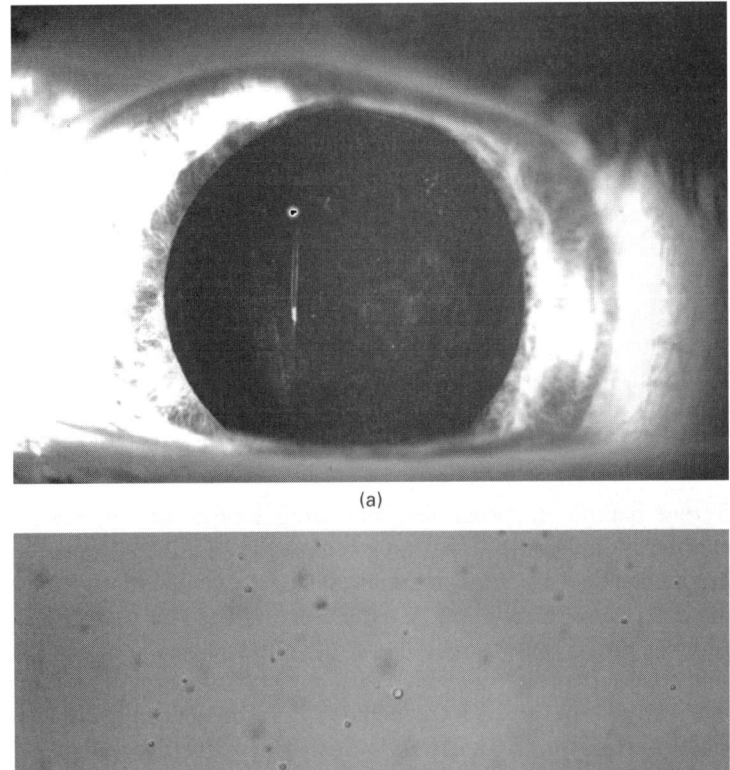

(a)

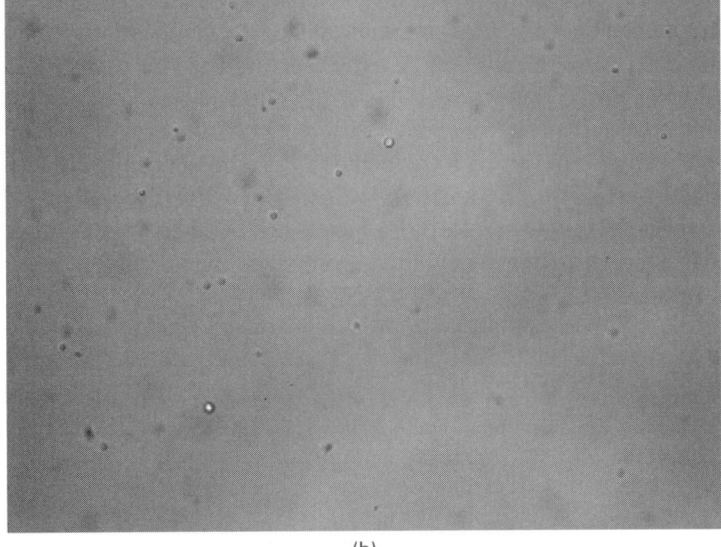

(b)

3.9 Intraoptical glistenings. (a) Clinical photograph of an eye implanted with a hydrophobic acrylic lens exhibiting glistenings. (b) High-magnification (×400) light photomicrograph of a single-piece hydrophobic acrylic lens exhibiting glistenings. The photograph was taken immediately after removing the explanted lens from balanced salt solution under a temperature of 37 °C.

the tenth day of the experiment and remained at the same level for the next 60 days without showing any increase. However, the frequency and intensity of glistenings in the Wagon Wheel-packaged three-piece AcrySof lenses was found to be related to the time between surgery and clinical evaluation, in a study on 38 eyes by Moreno-Montañés *et al.*[68] In another clinical study, the authors evaluated the occurrence of glistenings in seven different foldable IOLs, including two silicone designs (911A and SI40 NB), three hydrophilic acrylic designs (ACR6D, Hydroview, and Stabibag), and two hydrophobic acrylic designs (Sensar and 3-piece AcrySof).[58] The percentage of patients with glistenings increased over time with the AcrySof lenses. The mean grade of glistenings also increased over time in the AcrySof and 911A groups (the mean grade being significantly higher in the AcrySof group). Regarding single-piece AcrySof lenses, in an *in vitro* study they exhibited more and smaller glistenings than the three-piece IOLs. A recently published clinical study evaluating models SA60AT and SN60AT showed that glistenings were found in all IOLs studied and became worse over time.[69]

3.6   Conclusions

Different pathologic processes, including long-term degradation of the lens optic biomaterial, may lead to clinically significant opacification or discoloration of the optic component of IOLs manufactured from different biomaterials and in different designs. Factors such as patient's associated conditions, IOL manufacture, IOL storage, surgical techniques and adjuvants, among others, may be involved in different combinations. The complication may already be observed intraoperatively, or only postoperatively, from a few hours after lens implantation to many years after surgery, depending on the processes involved. With the increasing number of new lenses on the market every year, constant vigilance regarding overall IOL biocompatibility is warranted.

3.7   References

1 Werner L. Calcification of hydrophilic acrylic intraocular lenses. *Am J Ophthalmol* 2008; **146**: 341–343 (Editorial).
2 Apple DJ, Peng Q, Arthur SN, *et al.* Snowflake degeneration of polymethyl methacrylate posterior chamber intraocular lens optic material: a newly described clinical condition caused by unexpected late opacification of polymethyl methacrylate. *Ophthalmology* 2002; **109**: 1666–1675.
3 Apple DJ, Werner L. Complications of cataract and refractive surgery: A clinicopathological documentation. *Trans Am Ophthalmol Soc* 2001; **99**: 95–109.
4 Dahle N, Werner L, Fry L, Mamalis N. Localized, central optic snowflake degeneration of a PMMA intraocular lens: Clinical report with pathological correlation. *Arch Ophthalmol* 2006; **124**: 1350–1353.
5 Hilgert CR, Hilgert A, Hofling-Lima AL, Farah ME, Werner L. Early opacification of SI-40NB silicone intraocular lenses. *J Cataract Refract Surg* 2004; **30**: 2225–2229.
6 Werner L, Dornelles F, Hilgert CR, Botelho F, Conte PF, Rozot P, Andrenyak DM, Mamalis N, Olson RJ. Early opacification of silicone intraocular lenses: Laboratory analyses of six explants. *J Cataract Refract Surg* 2006; **32**: 499–509.

7 Elgohary M, Zaheer A, Werner L, Ionides A, Sheldrick J, Ahmed N. Opacification of Array SA40N silicone multifocal intraocular lens. *J Cataract Refract Surg* 2007; **33**: 342–347.

8 Tanaka T, Saika S, Hashizume N, Ohnishi Y. Brown haze in an Allergan SI-40NB silicone intraocular lens. *J Cataract Refract Surg* 2004; **30**: 250–252.

9 American National Standard, ANSI/AAMI ST27-1988, Guideline for industrial ethylene oxide sterilization of medical devices, 1988.

10 Kershner R. In reply to: Milauskas AT. Silicone intraocular lens implant discoloration in humans. *Arch Ophthalmol* 1991; **109**: 913–914.

11 Koch DD, Heit LE. Discoloration of silicone intraocular lenses. *Arch Ophthalmol* 1992; **110**: 319–320.

12 Milauskas AT. Silicone intraocular lens implant discoloration in humans. *Arch Ophthalmol* 1991; **109**: 913.

13 Milauskas AT. In reply to: Watt RH. Discoloration of a silicone intraocular lens 6 weeks after surgery. *Arch Ophthalmol* 1991; **109**: 1495.

14 Watt RH. Discoloration of a silicone intraocular lens 6 weeks after surgery. *Arch Ophthalmol* 1991; **109**: 1494–1495.

15 Ziemba S. In reply to: Milauskas AT. Silicone intraocular lens implant discoloration in humans. *Arch Ophthalmol* 1991; **109**: 914–915.

16 Stevens S, Werner L, Mamalis N. Corneal edema and permanent blue discoloration of a silicone intraocular lens by methylene blue. *Ophthalmic Surg Lasers Imaging* 2007; **38**: 136–141.

17 Mamalis N, Edelhauser HF, Dawson DG, Chew J, LeBoyer RM, Werner L. Toxic anterior segment syndrome (TASS). *J Cataract Refract Surg* 2006; **32**: 324–333.

18 Katai N, Yokoyama R, Yoshimura N. Progressive brown discoloration of silicone intraocular lenses after vitrectomy in a patient on amiodarone. *J Cataract Refract Surg* 1999; **25**: 451–452.

19 Jones DF, Irwin AE. Discoloration of intraocular lens subsequent to rifabutin use. *Arch Ophthalmol* 2002; **120**: 1211–1212.

20 Sathyan P, Myint K, Singh G, *et al.* Late green discoloration of Allergan SI-40NB silicone intraocular lens. *J Cataract Refract Surg* 2006; **32**: 1584–1585.

21 Siddique M, Ashraf KM, Qazi ZA. Greenish discoloration of a CeeOn 911A silicone intraocular lens. *Eye* 2005; **19**: 1349–1350.

22 Apple DJ, Federman JL, Krolicki TJ, *et al.* Irreversible silicone oil adhesion to silicone intraocular lenses. A clinicopathologic analysis. *Ophthalmology* 1996; **103**: 1555–1561.

23 Apple DJ, Isaacs RT, Kent DG, *et al.* Silicone oil adhesion to intraocular lenses: an experimental study comparing various biomaterials. *J Cataract Refract Surg* 1997; **23**: 536–544.

24 Werner L, Sher JH, Taylor JR, *et al.* Toxic anterior segment syndrome and possible association with ointment in the anterior chamber following cataract surgery. *J Cataract Refract Surg* 2006; **32**: 227–235.

25 McDonnell PJ, Taban M, Sarayba M, *et al.* Dynamic morphology of clear corneal cataract incisions. *Ophthalmology* 2003; **110**: 2342–2348.

26 Shingleton BJ, Wadhwani RA, O'Donoghue MW, *et al.* Evaluation of intraocular pressure in the immediate period after phacoemulsification. *J Cataract Refract Surg* 2001; **27**: 524–527.

27 Fraunfelder FT, Hanna C. Ophthalmic ointment. *Trans Am Acad Ophthalmol Otolaryngol* 1973; **77**: 467–475.

28 Garzozi HJ, Muallem M, Harris A. Recurrent anterior uveitis and glaucoma associated with inadvertent entry of ointment into the anterior chamber after radial keratotomy. *J Cataract Refract Surg* 1999; **25**: 1685–1687.

29 Aralikatti AK, Needham AD, Lee MW, Prasad S. Entry of antibiotic ointment into the anterior chamber after uneventful phacoemulsification. *J Cataract Refract Surg* 2003; **29**: 595–597.

30 Reidl M, Maca S, Amon M, *et al.* Intraocular ointment after small-incision cataract surgery causing chronic uveitis and secondary glaucoma. *J Cataract Refract Surg* 2003; **29**: 1022–1025.

31 Chew JJL, Werner L, Mackman G, Mamalis N. Late opacification of a silicone intraocular lens caused by ophthalmic ointment. *J Cataract Refract Surg* 2006; **32**: 341–346.

32 Chen KH, Lin SY, Li MJ, Cheng WT. Retained antibiotic ophthalmic ointment on an intraocular lens 34 months after sutureless cataract surgery. *Am J Ophthalmol* 2005; **139**: 743–745.

33 Foot L, Werner L, Gills JP, *et al.* Surface calcification of silicone plate intraocular lenses in patients with asteroid hyalosis. *Am J Ophthalmol* 2004; **137**: 979–987.

34 Wackernagel W, Ettinger K, Weitgasser U, *et al.* Opacification of a silicone intraocular lens caused by calcium deposits on the optic. *J Cataract Refract Surg* 2004; **30**: 517–520.

35 Werner L, Kollarits CR, Mamalis N, Olson RJ. Surface calcification of a three-piece silicone intraocular lens in a patient with asteroid hyalosis: A clinicopathologic case report. *Ophthalmology* 2005; **112**: 447–452.

36 Werner L, Apple DJ, Crema AS, *et al.* Permanent blue discoloration of a hydrogel intraocular lens caused by intraoperative use of trypan blue. *J Cataract Refract Surg* 2002; **28**: 1279–1286.

37 Werner L. Causes of intraocular lens opacification or discoloration. *J Cataract Refract Surg* 2007; **33**: 713–726 (Review).

38 Dorey MW, Brownstein S, Hill VE, *et al.* Proposed pathogenesis for the delayed postoperative opacification of the hydroview hydrogel intraocular lens. *Am J Ophthalmol* 2003; **135**: 591–598.

39 Gartaganis SP, Kanellopoulou DG, Mela EK, *et al.* Opacification of hydrophilic acrylic intraocular lens attributable to calcification: Investigation on mechanism. *Am J Ophthalmol* 2008; **146**: 395–403.

40 Guan X, Tang R, Nancollas GH. The potential calcification of octacalcium phosphate on intraocular lens surfaces. *J Biomed Mater Res* 2004; **71A**: 488–496.

41 Haymore J, Zaidman G, Werner L, *et al.* Misdiagnosis of hydrophilic acrylic intraocular lens optic opacification: report of 8 cases with the MemoryLens. *Ophthalmology* 2007; **114**: 1689–1695.

42 Nakanome S, Watanabe H, Tanaka K, Tochikubo T. Calcification of Hydroview H60M intraocular lenses: aqueous humor analysis and comparisons with other intraocular lens materials. *J Cataract Refract Surg* 2008; **34**: 80–86.

43 Neuhann IM, Werner L, Izak AM, *et al.* Late postoperative opacification of a hydrophilic acrylic (hydrogel) intraocular lens: A clinicopathological analysis of 106 explants. *Ophthalmology* 2004; **111**: 2094–2101.

44 Sher JH, Gooi P, Dubinski W, *et al.* Comparison of the incidence of opacification of Hydroview hydrogel intraocular lenses with the ophthalmic viscosurgical device used during surgery. *J Cataract Refract Surg* 2008; **34**: 459–464.

45 Werner L, Apple DJ, Escobar-Gomez M, *et al.* Postoperative deposition of calcium

on the surfaces of a hydrogel intraocular lens. *Ophthalmology* 2000; **107**: 2179–2185.

46   Werner L, Apple DJ, Kaskaloglu M, Pandey SK. Dense opacification of the optical component of a hydrophilic acrylic intraocular lens: a clinicopathological analysis of 9 explanted lenses. *J Cataract Refract Surg* 2001; **27**: 1485–1492.

47   Werner L, Hunter B, Stevens S, Chew JJL, Mamalis N. Role of silicon contamination on calcification of hydrophilic acrylic intraocular lenses. *Am J Ophthalmol* 2006; **141**: 35–43.

48   Ohrstrom A, Svensson B, Tegenfeldt S, Celiker C, Lignell B. Silicone oil content in ophthalmic viscosurgical devices. *J Cataract Refract Surg* 2004; **30**: 1278–1280.

49   Bucher PJM, Buchi ER, Daicker BC. Dystrophic calcification of an implanted hydroxyethylmethacrylate intraocular lens. *Arch Ophthalmol* 1995; **113**: 1431–1435.

50   Hunter B, Werner L, Memmen JE, Mamalis N. Postoperative localized opacification of the new MemoryLens design: Analyses of an explant. *J Cataract Refract Surg* 2005; **31**: 1836–1840.

51   Gayton JL, Apple DJ, Peng Q, *et al*. Interlenticular opacification: A clinicopathological correlation of a new complication of piggyback posterior chamber intraocular lenses. *J Cataract Refract Surg* 2000; **26**: 330–336.

52   Werner L, Shugar JK, Apple DJ, *et al*. Opacification of piggyback IOLs associated with an amorphous material attached to interlenticular surfaces. *J Cataract Refract Surg* 2000; **26**: 1612–1619.

53   Werner L, Apple DJ, Pandey SK, *et al*. Analysis of elements of interlenticular opacification. *Am J Ophthalmol* 2002; **133**: 320–326.

54   Werner L, Mamalis N, Stevens S, Hunter B, Chew JL, Vargas LG. Interlenticular opacification: Dual-optic versus piggyback intraocular lenses. *J Cataract Refract Surg* 2006; **32**: 656–662.

55   Omar O, Pirayesh A, Mamalis N, Olson RJ. In vitro analysis of AcrySof intraocular lens glistenings in AcryPak and Wagon Wheel packaging. *J Cataract Refract Surg* 1998; **24**: 107–113.

56   Werner L, Storsberg J, Mauger O, *et al*. Unusual pattern of glistening formation on a 3-piece hydrophobic acrylic intraocular lens. *J Cataract Refract Surg* 2008; **34**: 1604–1609.

57   Cisneros-Lanuza A, Hurtado-Sarrió M, Duch-Samper A, *et al*. Glistenings in the Artiflex phakic intraocular lens. *J Cataract Refract Surg* 2007; **33**: 1405–1408.

58   Tognetto D, Toto L, Sanguinetti G, Ravalico G. Glistenings in foldable intraocular lenses. *J Cataract Refract Surg* 2002; **28**: 1211–1216.

59   Wilkins E, Olson RJ. Glistenings with long-term follow-up of the Surgidev B20/20 polymethylmethacrylate intraocular lens. *Am J Ophthalmol* 2001; **132**: 783–785.

60   Gregori NZ, Spencer TS, Mamalis N, Olson RJ. *In vitro* comparison of glistening formation among hydrophobic acrylic intraocular lenses. *J Cataract Refract Surg* 2002; **28**: 1262–1268.

61   Kato K, Nishida M, Yamane H, *et al*. Glistening formation in an AcrySof lens initiated by spinodal decomposition of the polymer network by temperature change. *J Cataract Refract Surg* 2001; **27**: 1493–1498.

62   Miyata A, Yaguchi S. Equilibrium water content and glistenings in acrylic intraocular lenses. *J Cataract Refract Surg* 2004; **30**: 1768–1772.

63   Dhaliwal DK, Mamalis N, Olson RJ, *et al*. Visual significance of glistenings seen in the AcrySof intraocular lens. *J Cataract Refract Surg* 1996; **22**: 452–457.

64 Gunenc U, Oner FH, Tongal S, Ferliel M. Effects on visual function of glistenings and folding marks in AcrySof intraocular lenses. *J Cataract Refract Surg* 2001; **27**: 1611–1614.

65 Christiansen G, Durcan FJ, Olson RJ, Christiansen K. Glistenings in the AcrySof intraocular lens: pilot study. *J Cataract Refract Surg* 2001; **27**: 728–733.

66 Oshika T, Shiokawa Y, Amano S, Mitomo K. Influence of glistenings on the optical quality of acrylic foldable intraocular lens. *Br J Ophthalmol* 2001; **85**: 1034–1037.

67 Miyata A, Uchida N, Nakajima K, Yaguchi S. Clinical and experimental observation of glistening in acrylic intraocular lenses. *Jpn J Ophthalmol* 2001; **45**: 564–569.

68 Moreno-Montañés J, Alvarez A, Rodríguez-Conde R, Fernández-Hortelano A. Clinical factors related to the frequency and intensity of glistenings in AcrySof intraocular lenses. *J Cataract Refract Surg* 2003; **29**: 1980–1984.

69 Waite A, Faulkner N, Olson RJ. Glistenings in the single-piece, hydrophobic, acrylic intraocular lenses. *Am J Ophthalmol* 2007; **144**: 143–144.

4

Synthetic corneal implants

M. D. M. EVANS, CSIRO Molecular and Health Technologies
and Vision CRC, Australia; D. F. SWEENEY, Vision CRC
and Institute for Eye Research, Australia

Abstract: The cornea is the transparent tissue at the front of the eye that refracts light on to the retina. Devices can be implanted into the cornea to correct refractive errors (corneal inlay, corneal onlay, intracorneal rings) or to replace damaged and diseased corneal tissue to restore vision (keratoprosthesis, shields). Synthetic materials used in these devices present a challenging set of requirements necessitating an understanding of the tissue, impact of surgery and wound-healing processes, material science and optical design. This chapter considers the history of corneal implants, currently available technologies and future developments using synthetic materials as implantable devices and scaffolds in the cornea to improve vision.

Key words: cornea, corneal implant, synthetic material, inlay, onlay, keratoprosthesis.

4.1 The function and structure of the cornea

4.1.1 Function of the cornea

The cornea is the transparent tissue at the front of the eye; it is approximately 12 mm in diameter and covers an area of 123 mm^2 in humans (Dua *et al.*, 1994). Human corneal tissue is approximately 500–550 μm thick centrally and is composed of several layers of specialised tissue, as seen in Fig. 4.1. The cornea has dual functions of protection and refraction of light on to the retina. Protection is afforded by the corneal tissue, tear film and eyelids working together as a barrier to the entry of pathogens. Light refraction is due to the relatively smooth anterior corneal surface and its associated tear film which together are responsible for approximately 70% of the refractive power of the eye (Cotlier, 1975).

4.1.2 Epithelium

The outermost layer of the corneal tissue is a stratified epithelium, approximately 50 μm thick and made up of five to seven layers of regularly arranged epithelial cells, as seen in Fig. 4.2. The anterior layers of the corneal epithelium are formed by terminally differentiated squamous cells

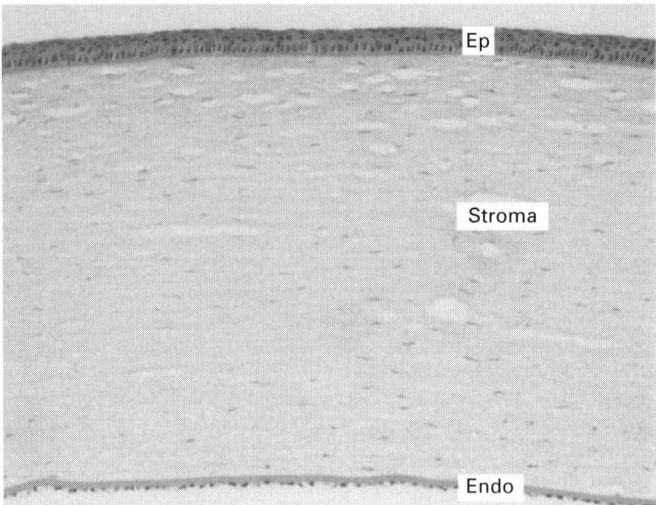

4.1 Light micrograph of section through the central cornea of the rabbit showing the stratified epithelium (Ep) on the anterior surface, the stroma (Stroma) and the single layer of endothelial cells (Endo) bounding the anterior chamber (original magnification ×100).

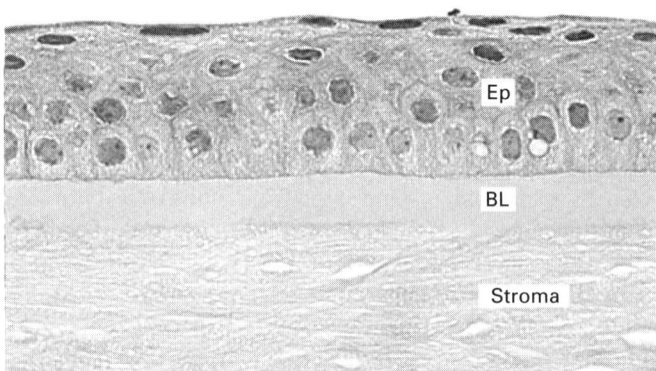

4.2 Light micrograph of section through the anterior portion of the central human cornea showing the arrangement of the squamous, wing and basal cells that constitute the stratified epithelium (Ep) and Bowman's layer (BL) in the anterior portion of the stroma (original magnification ×400).

which have small projections (microvilli and microplicae) to support the tear film that keeps the non-keratinised epithelium moist and contribute to the refractile properties of the cornea (Pfister, 1973; Andrews, 1976). These superficial cells are connected by tight junctions that form an occlusive barrier that is constantly reformed as the superficial cells are lost from the anterior corneal surface into the tear film. This layer is replenished from beneath by the intermediate cell layers formed by polygonal wing cells with highly interdigitated cell membranes and cell–cell junctions known as desmosomes which bind them together (Beuerman and Pedroza, 1996). Beneath the wing cells is the layer of basal cells of the corneal epithelium which is in direct contact with their basement membrane on the posterior aspect. Basal cells are typically 18–20 μm high and 10 μm in diameter and are attached on their lateral aspects by specialised cell–cell junctions, the zonula adherens and gap junctions. The basal cells are anchored on their posterior aspect by a series of specialised cell–matrix junctions known as adhesion complexes. These comprise an intracellular adhesive plaque (hemidesmosome) linking through the basement membrane to anchoring fibrils formed by collagen type VII which are located in the anterior portion of the underlying stroma (Buck, 1983; Gipson *et al.*, 1987; Burgeson *et al.*, 1990; Binder *et al.*, 1991; Green and Jones, 1996; Borrodori and Sonnenberg, 1999), as seen in Fig. 4.3. The corneal epithelial basement membrane is approximately 120 nm thick and composed of laminin, collagen IV, nidogen/entactin and heparan sulphate proteoglycan (Yurchenco and Schittny, 1990; Aumailley, 1995) with some of these components showing regional heterogeneity of expression across the cornea (Ljubimov *et al.*, 1995).

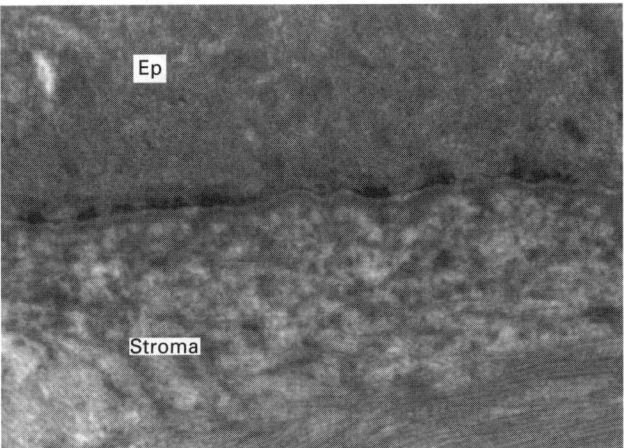

4.3 Transmission electron micrograph of the interface of a basal epithelial cell (Ep) with the anterior stroma (Stroma) in the normal rabbit cornea showing ultrastructural details of the basement membrane zone with adhesion complexes formed by electron-dense hemidesmosomal plaques along the posterior face of the epithelial plasma membrane and anchoring fibrils in the anterior stroma (original magnification ×10 500).

4.1.3   Bowman's layer, corneal stroma and keratocytes

The corneal stroma lies posterior to the epithelium and accounts for 90% of the total corneal volume. The bulk of the stromal tissue (substantia propria or stroma proper) is composed of aligned arrays of hydrated heterotypic fibrils of collagen types I and V with collagen VI filaments running between and some isolated collagen III fibrils (Newsome *et al.*, 1981; Birk *et al.*, 1986; Beuerman and Pedroza, 1996; Linsenmayer *et al.*, 1998). The fibrillar collagens are embedded in a hydrated matrix made up of non-fibrillar collagen types (type VI, XII, XIV and XVIII), glycoproteins (such as fibronectin and laminin) and proteoglycans including dermatan sulphate proteoglycan (decorin) and keratan sulphate proteoglycans (lumican, mimecan and keratocan) (Linsenmayer *et al.*, 1998). The collagen fibrils have a uniform diameter of 32 ± 0.7 nm with regular interfibrillar spacing and are arranged into parallel arrays forming 300–500 orthogonally packed lamellae, as seen in Fig. 4.4. This arrangement, together with the nature of the ground substance in which they are embedded, provides the transparency that is so critical to corneal function (Maurice, 1984; Birk *et al.*, 1986; Meek and Fullwood, 2001). A new model for the three-dimensional organisation of collagen fibrils and proteoglycans in the human corneal stroma (Müller *et al.*, 2004) updates the original thinking of corneal transparency and also adds to the explanation of the resistance of the cornea to stretching and compression. The ultrastructural data describe a hexagonal arrangement of collagen fibrils interconnected to neighbouring fibrils at regular intervals by groups of six

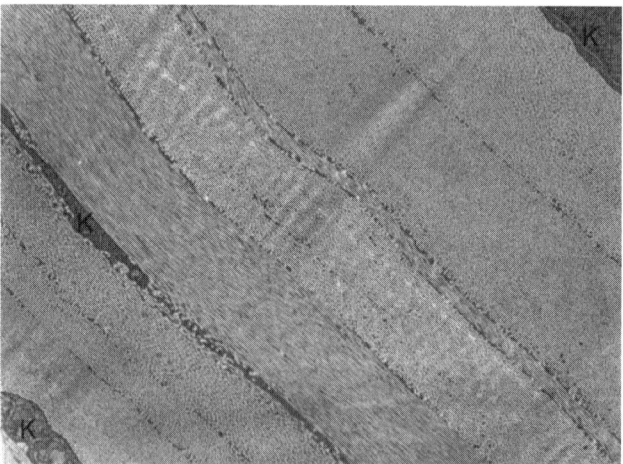

4.4 Transmission electron micrograph of the stroma in the central bovine cornea showing ultrastructural details of the arrangement of keratocytes (K) between the orthogonally packed lamellae formed by bundles of collagen fibrils arranged in layers (original magnification ×15 000).

proteoglycans that are attached orthogonal to the fibril circumference. While the most predominant collagen in the normal corneal stroma is collagen type I, constituting 71% of its dry weight, a change in the ratio of corneal collagens is found in some disease states. This is also the case after wounding, with an increased amount of collagen type III found to be associated with scars (Newsome *et al.*, 1981).

In the anterior stroma of primates and birds an acellular band approximately 8–10 µm thick can be distinguished immediately subjacent to the epithelial basement membrane (Bergmanson, 2008). This is known as Bowman's layer (or the anterior limiting lamina) as seen in Fig. 4.2. The collagen fibrils in Bowman's layer are of similar types to the stroma proper but differ in their diameter (narrower) and arrangement (random orientation) with irregular interweaving (Komai and Ushiki, 1991; Jacobsen *et al.*, 1984; Linsenmayer *et al.*, 1998; Wilson and Hong, 2000). Bowman's layer is generally regarded as separating the epithelium and stroma (Obata and Tsuru, 2007) and being a visible indicator of ongoing stromal–epithelial interactions (Wilson and Hong, 2000). It is also thought to have a role in the mechanical integrity and curvature of the cornea (Müller *et al.*, 2001), although one study reported that the mechanical properties of the cornea were unchanged after its removal (Seiler *et al.*, 1992). The interface of Bowman's layer with the underlying stromal tissue has been the subject of several studies; which support a role for Bowman's layer in corneal biomechanics yet question the concept that the collagen lamellae of the stroma extend from limbus- to- limbus. An early electron microscopy study of this region showed that some of the fibres do run parallel to the corneal surface while others run at angles into Bowman's layer (Kayes and Holmberg, 1960). Second harmonic imaging microscopy showed that the anterior lamellae interweave and confirmed that some project into Bowman's layer with a transverse orientation in normal cornea (Morishige *et al.*, 2007). This differed in keratoconic corneas with weakened corneal biomechanics which have shown less lamellar interweaving and fewer projections (Morishige *et al.*, 2007). High-magnification transmission electron microscopy has confirmed that collagen fibrils link the anterior limiting layer to the anterior stroma (Mathew *et al.*, 2008). A functional biomechanical role for Bowman's layer and the anterior stroma is supported if one considers the cases where Bowman's layer has been disrupted leading to a condition affecting vision, such as sub-epithelial fibrosis (corneal dystrophy and bullous keratopathy) or ectasia (keratoconus) (Obata and Tsuru, 2007).

Keratocytes are the cellular elements of the corneal stroma and account for at least 3–5% (Beuerman and Pedroza, 1996) and possibly up to 10% (Müller *et al.*, 1995) of the total stromal mass. Although they are generally regarded as quiescent cells, they are actively involved in the routine maintenance of stromal extracellular matrix and also in its repair after injury. The majority of keratocytes are characterised by flattened triangulate cell bodies with clearly defined cell processes (Poole *et al.*, 1993), which appear as long, slender tapering profiles in cross-sections of the corneal stroma (Müller *et al.*, 1995). The relatively sparse distribution of keratocytes in the stroma is thought to retain transparency of the corneal tissue, yet these cells interconnect through the stromal lamellae to form a three-dimensional network allowing for communication at the tips of the cell processes via gap junctions (Poole *et al.*, 2003). A three-dimensional reconstruction of the central corneal stroma showed the keratocytes were arranged in a corkscrew pattern with the highest density in the anterior stroma near Bowman's layer (Müller *et al.*, 1995). This change in density has since been confirmed by confocal microscopy (Poole *et al.*, 2003; Tervo and Moilanen, 2003; Moilanen *et al.*, 2008). There appear to be different types of keratocytes present in the stroma, with those in the anterior portion possessing twice the number of mitochondria, indicative of a higher metabolic state, which may be associated with oxygen gradients in the stromal tissue and/or the synthesis of different substances (Müller *et al.*, 1995). It is generally accepted that there are few actively proliferating keratocytes in the normal corneal stroma (Zieske, 2004), although data based on stem-cell-specific markers have identified a population of keratocyte progenitor cells near the limbus of the adult cornea (Du *et al.*, 2005).

4.1.4   Descemet's membrane and corneal endothelium

The posterior stroma is separated from the underlying endothelium by a thickened basement membrane known as Descemet's membrane, which is 2–3 μm thick at birth increasing to 7–10 μm in adults (Binder *et al.*, 1991; Joyce, 2003). A single layer of endothelial cells, characteristically 5 μm in height and 15–20 μm in width, binds the anterior chamber (Binder *et al.*, 1991). Both Descemet's membrane and the endothelium can be seen in Fig. 4.1. The number of corneal endothelial cells decreases with age with approximately 400 000 cells/mm^2 of hexagonal shape in young children and 2000 cells/mm^2 of less regular shape in adults (Joyce, 2003). The hexagonal morphology is thought to maximise the surface area exposed to neighbouring cells which are linked by specialised cell–cell junctions, including leaky tight junctions, to facilitate the movement of fluid and solutes. This is in keeping with the major function of the corneal endothelium which is to regulate stromal hydration to maintain corneal transparency. The generally accepted 'pump-leak' mechanism by which the corneal endothelium maintains corneal hydration was first proposed by David Maurice (Maurice, 1972) and accounts for the leaking of fluids and solutes across the endothelium into the stroma that is balanced by the pumping of solutes and passive fluid transfer back across the endothelium and into the aqueous humour. Injury and disease can upset this balance and this can directly impact on corneal thickness and transparency, diminishing vision. Significant to this, endothelial cells lack a robust proliferative response and, with the number and density of endothelial cells decreasing with age, it is possible for injury or disease to cause a reduction in density below a critical point causing the corneal stroma to imbibe fluid and become oedematous and opaque (Joyce, 2003; Bourne and McLaren, 2004). Healing of endothelial wounds occurs by the sliding and enlargement of adjacent cells rather than by mitosis which adds to the changed cell density and shape (Joyce, 2003). The impact of such changes on vision is exemplified in disease states such as Fuch's endothelial dystrophy, where inherited morphological and functional abnormalities of the endothelium cause a progressive loss of pump function leading to stromal oedema and diminished visual acuity, which can lead to blindness (Wilson and Bourne, 1988; Bourne and McLaren, 2004). Since the endothelium has a limited regenerative capacity, and relies mostly on cell movement and shape changes within the existing cell population to repair wounds, it is particularly vulnerable to insult and injury such as may occur during surgical procedures related to the cornea or lens.

4.1.5   Nutrient supply to the cornea

The transparent nature of the cornea is absolutely critical to its optical properties. Transparency is maintained by a highly organised tissue structure and a complete lack of blood vessels in the central cornea. Metabolites (e.g. oxygen and glucose) and waste products (e.g. carbon dioxide and lactate) diffuse in and out of the cornea via the tear film, the abundant blood vessels in the scleral tissue peripheral to the cornea and also from the aqueous humour contained in the anterior chamber. Oxygen in the open eye is supplied by atmospheric oxygen dissolved in the tear film and from the aqueous humour (Friend, 1979). In the closed eye oxygen comes from the blood vessels in the sclera, limbus and the palpebral vessels of the eyelids (Friend, 1979). Glucose is principally provided by the aqueous humour and is distributed forwards towards the epithelium in the stromal fluid, with smaller contributions diffusing from the tears and limbus (Friend, 1979; McCarey and Schmidt, 1990). Glycogen stores in the epithelium are utilised if there is insufficient free glucose available as a result of anaerobic conditions or trauma (Friend, 1979).

4.1.6   Nerve supply to the cornea

Despite its avascular nature, the cornea is well-innervated tissue and has a high density of sensory free nerve endings which make it one of the body's most sensitive tissues (Rozsa and Beuerman, 1982). The cornea is innervated by the ophthalmic and maxillary branches of the fifth cranial (trigeminal) nerve and sympathetic nerves, which enter the stroma from the periphery and fan in a radial pattern parallel to the corneal surface. The majority of these nerve fibre trunks are located in the anterior third of the stroma, where they turn at right angles to penetrate Bowman's layer and then fan out along the base of the epithelium as epithelial leashes, which are partially interconnected and form a sub-basal nerve plexus (Müller *et al.*, 2003). The diameter of these fibres varies between 1 and 5 µm as measured by confocal microscopy (Stachs *et al.*, 2007). Single nerves or nerve fibres arising from this network protrude between adjacent basal cells of the epithelium (Müller *et al.*, 2003). Equal numbers of nerves penetrate the stroma in all quadrants of the cornea (Müller *et al.*, 2003), although previously it was thought that the majority were located in the nasal and temporal quadrants (Müller *et al.*, 1997). Communication via soluble messengers between the nerve cells, epithelial cells, keratocytes and possibly the endothelial cells is an essential part of normal corneal function and homeostasis (Wilson *et al.*, 2003). One such soluble mediator is Substance P, which is released by the nerve endings and bound by receptors on the epithelial cells promoting cellular activities including proliferation and migration (Garcia-Hirschfeld *et al.*, 1994). It is interesting to note that neural disease states of the cornea, such as neurotrophic keratopathy, are characterised by decreased corneal sensitivity and poor corneal healing and, in these corneas, a breakdown of the epithelium may result in ulceration, infection and degradation (melting) of the underlying stroma (Nishida *et al.*, 2007). Denervation of the cornea results in decreased cell metabolism, increased corneal permeability, with decreased levels of neurotransmitters and decreased cell proliferation, which can lead to an erosion of the epithelium even in the absence of injury as a result of the continuous turnover of corneal epithelial cells.

4.1.7   Immune cells in the cornea

The cornea has long been regarded as a site of immune privilege since it was avascular and was thought to lack resident immune cells. Since then, populations of bone marrow-derived leukocytes, which are distinct from stromal keratocytes and include bone marrow-derived cells and macrophages, have been identified in the cornea (Hamrah *et al.*, 2003; Sosnová *et al.*, 2005). Dendritic cells, which are capable of initiating an immune response, including epithelial Langerhans cells and anterior stromal dendritic cells, are not restricted to the peripheral cornea but have been identified in the central portion of healthy corneal tissue, indicating that the entire cornea is able to participate actively in the immune response to foreign antigens and autoantigens (Hamrah and Dana, 2007). While much of this immune activity may remain muted during normal corneal homeostasis, it can be activated by infections or trauma such as that caused by injury or surgery, and epithelial cells and keratocytes respond by chemokine production which attracts inflammatory cells to the damaged area (Wilson *et al.*, 2003). Indeed, communication between the corneal epithelial cells and stromal keratocytes (and possibly endothelial cells as well) via cell-mediated substances such as cytokines is recognised to be of great importance in the regulation of corneal tissue metabolism (Wilson and Kim, 1998).

4.1.8   Corneal renewal and wound healing

Despite its avascular nature, the regenerative capacity of the corneal epithelium is considerable and occurs continuously in normal cornea to maintain the epithelium in good health (Lemp and Mathers, 1991). The corneal epithelial replacement process was originally shown to take 5–7 days to complete in the rat cornea (Hanna and O'Brien, 1960), although more recent cell-labelling studies have shown it to take 2 weeks for complete turnover of the epithelium (Cenedella and Fleschner, 1990). Regeneration is primarily achieved by the migration of the epithelial cells from the periphery of the cornea inwards along the basement membrane and upwards to the superficial layers where they are continuously shed from the corneal surface into the tear film. This was proposed by Thoft and Friend (1983) in their X, Y, Z hypothesis of corneal epithelial cell replacement; where X represented proliferation in the basal cells, Y was the proliferation and migration of the limbal cells, and Z was the loss of epithelial cells from the ocular surface. Equilibrium in regular corneal epithelial cell replacement is maintained if $X + Y = Z$. The driving force for the centripetal migration of corneal epithelial cells is not fully understood, but is believed to involve desquamation of the central corneal epithelium in a preferential exfoliative process driven at least partly by the shearing force of the upper eyelid (Lavker *et al.*, 1991; Lemp and Mathers, 1991; Mathers and Lemp, 1992). Davanger and Evensen (1971) first proposed that the regenerative capacity of the corneal epithelium resided in the papillary structure of the limbus at the corneal periphery, which is richly supplied with blood. Corneal epithelial stem cells were later identified in this location using monoclonal antibodies (Schermer *et al.*, 1986; Zieske, 1992) and their slow-cycling nature while in the limbal microenvironment was demonstrated by thymidine labelling (Cotsarelis *et al.*, 1989). Studies in skin (Watt, 1984; Jones and Watt, 1993) and then in cornea lead to the proposal that the pluripotent corneal epithelial stem cells from the limbus gave rise to semi-differentiated, multipotent 'transient amplifying cells' that migrated on to the cornea proper to divide and replenish the stratified epithelial layers of the central cornea as non-proliferative 'terminally differentiated cells' (Schermer *et al.*, 1986).

Superficial wounding to the epithelium activates a rapid wound-healing response to quickly restore epithelial barrier function and normal vision. Epithelial cells around the wound periphery disassemble their hemidesmosomes and rearrange themselves, flattening and migrating inwards as a tissue front, which contracts in a 'purse-string' fashion to cover the defect (Buschke, 1949; Crosson *et al.*, 1986; Gipson, 1989; Beuerman and Thompson, 1992; Dua *et al.*, 1994). Once the wound is covered, the cells proliferate and stratify to restore normal epithelial thickness and hemidesmosomes reform in a wound-healing process that takes only days to complete (Hanna, 1966; Gipson, 1989; Dua *et al.*, 1994). During this wound-healing phase, the undifferentiated epithelial stem cells located in the limbus and slightly differentiated 'transient amplifying cells' in the basal cell layer are stimulated to proliferate, providing additional cells to complete the restratification process (Dua and Azuara-Blanco, 2000). A direct linkage between differentiation status and proliferative capacity of corneal epithelial cells has been questioned in a study that showed that the daughter cells arising from cell division in the basal layer did not all differentiate synchronously to become wing cells, but rather, some remained in the basal layer with potential to undergo additional rounds of cell division (Beebe and Masters, 1996). Consistent with this are recent findings based on a human organotypic model where donut epithelial wounds were made to the central cornea, with dimensions 7 mm outer diameter and 3 mm inner diameter, and where the limbus was left intact or ablated. Data from the ablated limbus group showed that epithelial cells in the central corneal epithelium had the capacity to undergo sufficient cell division and migration to heal the epithelial wounds in the initial 12 hours post-surgery without recruiting cells from the limbus (Chang *et al.*, 2008).

A substantially longer healing process of weeks to months is involved if the wound has penetrated both the epithelium and the stromal tissue (Stock *et al.*, 1992; Jester *et al.*, 1999). Wound repair in the corneal stroma is undertaken by the stromal keratocytes in a complex process modulated by soluble signalling molecules such as cytokines and growth factors such as platelet-derived growth factor (PDGF), keratocyte growth factor (KGF) and transforming growth factor-beta (TGF-β) that are produced by the injured epithelial cells above. It is not clear whether soluble signalling molecules derived from the epithelium penetrate the full thickness of the stroma or involve the interconnected keratocyte network in transmitting messages (Wilson *et al.*, 2003). The response of the keratocytes to wounding is rapid and causes the keratocytes in the wounded stroma beneath to enter into programmed cell death known as 'apoptosis' (Wilson *et al.*, 2003). Keratocytes in the stroma adjacent to the wound are activated to proliferate within hours of wounding and they transform into a fibroblastic phenotype and migrate into the affected area to repair damage (Fini, 1999; Jester *et al.*, 1999; Wilson *et al.*, 2003; West-Mays and Dwivedi, 2006). Repair fibroblasts may develop into a contractile phenotype known as myofibroblast during the wound-healing process and this is strongly mediated by the presence of TGF-β released from epithelial cells (Mohan *et al.*, 2003). Activated fibroblasts and myofibroblasts synthesise and assemble new extracellular matrix, which has different components and properties to the normal uninjured stromal tissue (Funderburgh *et al.*, 2003; Guo *et al.*, 2007). Notable among these is hyaluronan, which is absent in the stroma of normal cornea but present in abundance in wounded corneas and those with chronic pathology and is regarded as a fibrotic matrix component (Guo *et al.*, 2007).

Stromal–epithelial interactions are recognised to be a core part of the wound-healing processes that take place in response to corneal stromal injury (Melles *et al.*, 1995). Significant to these interactions are the integrity of the epithelium and the exposure of keratocytes to epithelial-derived factors during wounding which determine whether corneal repair will be regenerative or fibrotic in nature (West-Mays and Dwivedi, 2006). Myofibroblasts and other cell types, such as bone marrow-derived cells, may be present in the stroma during the repair process depending on the nature and severity of the wound and their presence at the repair site causes haze (Dupps and Wilson, 2006). As the wound-healing response continues, stromal cells – such as keratocytes, fibroblasts, myofibroblasts and inflammatory cells – die by necrosis (Mohan *et al.*, 2003). Damaged cells release pro-inflammatory chemokines which attract great numbers of bone-marrow-derived cells to clean up degenerative cells by engulfing debris into their cytoplasm in a process of phagocytosis (Dupps and Wilson, 2006). A study of myofibroblasts in tissues other than cornea (Dupps and Wilson, 2006) has suggested that myofibroblasts may originate in the bone marrow. These cells tend to be present in the stroma near the epithelium or sites of epithelial ingrowth into the stroma, implying that cytokines produced by epithelial cells are linked to their presence. Myofibroblasts are found where abnormalities of the stromal surface or regenerated basement membrane occur, as seen following refractive surgical procedures, such as surface laser ablation (Netto *et al.*, 2006). Adult human corneal stromal wounds heal slowly and incompletely and may result in abnormalities such as scar tissue and reduplicated basement membrane (Melles *et al.*, 1995; Dawson *et al.*, 2008). These findings are consistent with the idea that the structural integrity of the epithelial basement membrane is significant in minimising the fibrotic response of the keratocytes and any subsequent scarring and loss of corneal clarity (West-Mays and Dwivedi, 2006).

4.2   Using the cornea to correct refractive error

4.2.1   Refractive error

Light rays pass through the cornea and lens and then focus on the retina. The retina receives the light rays and converts them to neural signals that are transmitted by the optic nerve to the brain, where the signals are translated into images. The cornea is responsible for 70% of the refractive power of the eye. Vision is blurred if light does not bend or refract correctly and focus directly on the retina. Blurred vision is a refractive error, which is the most common disorder of the eye. Myopia (short-sightedness) occurs when the eyeball is too long in relation to the refractive power of the eye and light rays focus in front of the retina making distant objects appear blurry. Myopia is the leading cause of vision loss in the Asia–Pacific region and affects approximately one-third of people in the world. Hyperopia (long-sightedness) occurs when the image is focused on a point beyond the retina because the eyeball is too short in relation to the refractive power of the eye. Approximately one-quarter of the world's population is hyperopic. Many people with myopia or hyperopia also have some astigmatism which is caused by the shape of the cornea. A normal cornea is spherically shaped and astigmatism occurs if the curvature of the cornea is irregular/unequal causing light rays to have more than one focal point, which results in blur and distortion to both distant and near objects. Presbyopia is an age-related condition where the flexibility of the natural lens is gradually reduced and is accompanied by a reduction in the ability of the muscles to change the shape of the lens to focus light on the retina when observing near objects (accommodation). The global increase in life expectancy translates to an increased number of people over the age of 45 years with presbyopia.

4.2.2 Alternative approaches in using the cornea to correct refractive error

There is a need for more permanent and convenient solutions for the correction of refractive error as an alternative to spectacles or contact lenses (rigid gas-permeable, soft and orthokeratology lenses). Currently, there are alternative technologies available to treat all types of refractive errors and this section deals with those that involve the cornea. Technologies that address this demand can be categorised broadly into two groups: those that remove corneal tissue to correct refractive error (subtractive) and those technologies that add to corneal tissue to achieve a correction (additive). Subtractive solutions, such as the laser-based procedures, are non-reversible in the sense that tissue is permanently removed. The excimer laser is used to flatten the cornea in the treatment of myopia, to steepen the cornea to correct hyperopia, and to reshape the corneal topography in the treatment of astigmatism. Depending on the type of laser used, the corneal epithelium may need removal or lifting and replacement to expose the stroma for the laser ablation and this has given rise to the development of a range of associated surgical techniques. Newer laser technologies such as the femtosecond laser are able to pass through the tissue to the target area with apparently minimal damage and therefore leave the epithelium intact. Additive solutions embrace a range of intracorneal devices made from either biological or synthetic materials or a combination of both, which are technically removable and are therefore reversible procedures. There is some cross-over between these groups, since all devices require some form of surgical procedure to implant them. Frequently, surgical techniques that have been developed to enable laser procedures are used for implanting intracorneal devices. Sections 4.3 and 4.4 examine different approaches taken in the correction of refractive errors involving the cornea. Optical and biological outcomes of the technologies that have been developed are considered along with the knowledge gained from those endeavours.

4.3   Subtractive approaches to correct refractive error: refractive surgery

4.3.1   Incisional refractive surgery techniques

The demand for solutions to the correction of refractive error that offer convenience and cosmesis has driven the development of a range of refractive surgical techniques that have been well reviewed in the literature (Kaufman, 1989; Waring, 1992; Aquavella, 1994; Tervo and Moilanen, 2003; Sakimoto et al., 2006). Initially, ophthalmic surgeons addressed this need with incisional refractive procedures such as radial keratotomy (RK), where the cornea was flattened by a series of radial incisions to treat myopia (Sato et al., 1953). Regression in many patients following this type of surgery cast doubt on its predictability and this problem was attributed to contraction of the wound bed during healing. Studies of incisional gape wounds in animals, such as used in RK, showed healing involved the rapid migration of the corneal epithelium to cover the wounded surface and fill the wound site with an epithelial plug (over the first few days) that was gradually replaced by stromal fibroblasts which produced new extracellular matrix material (by 2 weeks), which eventually contracted (by 4 weeks) (Garana et al., 1992). The wound-healing process was biphasic and strongly linked to the presence of epithelium in the wound bed (pre-contractile phase), with contraction occurring once this was replaced by fibroblastic tissue (contractile phase) (Jester et al., 1992). Further animal studies identified that the tension responsible for the contraction was generated by actin stress fibres formed in myofibroblasts interacting with fibronectin in the local extracellular matrix (Garana et al., 1992). Animal data showing the initiation of wound contraction by myofibroblasts and re-steepening of the cornea observed 2 weeks post-operatively were found to correlate temporally with the progressive hyperopic shift observed in 30% of patients following incisional refractive surgery (Waring et al., 1994; Jester et al., 1999).

4.3.2   Ablative refractive surgery techniques

The transition from incisional to ablative refractive surgery occurred with the advent of excimer laser technology in the 1980s. Photorefractive keratectomy (PRK) used the excimer laser in a surface ablation technique to change the curvature of the central cornea after debridement of the epithelium, which healed afterwards (Trokel *et al.*, 1983; McDonald *et al.*, 1990). While clinically this procedure has successfully corrected refractive errors, it has been associated with complications including post-surgical pain, regression of the refractive effect and post-surgical sub-epithelial haze (Azar *et al.*, 1998; Azar *et al.*, 2001). Histological analyses of corneas have shown reduced keratocyte densities, undulations in Bowman's layer, incomplete stromal wound healing and scar formation months to years after PRK (Hanna *et al.*, 1990; SundarRaj *et al.*, 1990; Linna and Tervo, 1997). Studies in animals and humans have linked the regression and haze issues to the presence of myofibroblasts in the healing wound bed and the deposition of new collagen above the photoablated stromal surface (Møller-Pedersen *et al.*, 1998; Møller-Pedersen *et al.*, 2000). In recent years, problems relating to cutting a flap and wound-healing issues with laser *in situ* keratomileusis (LASIK) procedures have revived the use of PRK. Alternative methods of epithelial removal in the PRK procedure have been investigated to address the issues of post-operative pain and re-epithelialisation of the wound bed following surface ablation. The aim of the new approaches was to make a superficial corneal flap minimising damage to the underlying stromal tissue. Instruments for blunt dissection are used to cleave the epithelium through the basement membrane zone creating a flap of epithelial tissue, which is repositioned after the stromal surface has been ablated. The techniques vary in the method of removal of the epithelial sheet (Pallikaris *et al.*, 2003).

In laser-assisted sub-epithelial keratomileusis (LASEK), diluted alcohol is used to loosen the epithelial sheet which is freed with a spatula (Azar *et al.*, 2001). Brief periods (25–30 seconds) of exposure to diluted alcohol (15–20%) allow the creation of a reproducible flap with a smooth cleavage plane through the basement membrane zone (Browning *et al.*, 2003; Espana *et al.*, 2003), with low levels of cell death found in epithelium and underlying stromal keratocytes (Lee *et al.*, 2002). *In vitro* studies on the effect of various alcohol dilutions on cultured epithelial monolayers resulted in increasing cell death in a dose- and time-dependent manner (Chen *et al.*, 2002). Nerve damage is also caused by the LASEK procedure and persists for some time after the procedure. A confocal microscopy study of 35 patients reported that the sub-basal nerves were not recovered 6 months after the LASEK procedure although corneal sensitivity, evaluated using aesthesiometry, was restored after 3 months (Darwish *et al.*, 2007). Overall, LASEK may be useful for patients unable to have LASIK but they would have to accept the disadvantages of the LASEK procedure, which include post-operative discomfort and delayed visual recovery resulting from the 4–7 day epithelial closure time (Taneri *et al.*, 2004).

In epi-LASIK, the epithelial sheet is removed mechanically using an epikeratome with a blade to avoid the use of alcohol. The cleavage plane and the viability of the epithelial sheet after epi-LASIK procedures have been examined by a range of techniques (Tanioka *et al.*, 2007; Chen *et al.*, 2008; Choi *et al.*, 2008a; Choi *et al.*, 2008b). Immunohistochemistry of the epithelial flap has shown that the cleavage plane in epi-LASIK procedures depends on the type of epikeratome used in human eyes (Choi *et al.*, 2008b). A comparison of different commercially available epikeratomes using immunohistochemistry and electron microscopy has shown that each epikeratome tested had successfully cleaved through the basement membrane zone without damage to the stromal surface in the pig and human corneas used (Herrmann *et al.*, 2008). Trypan Blue staining of the epithelial flaps created in the abattoir-sourced pig eyes in this study revealed minimal damage to the cells of the central portion of the flaps (with <12% damaged) but this outcome might be different in the corneas of live subjects where the epithelium is more difficult to cleave. *In vivo* confocal microscopy used to monitor wound healing in patients following epi-LASIK treatment for myopia showed that cells in most of the epithelial flaps were damaged during the first few days and were rapidly replaced by new cells during the healing process (Chen *et al.*, 2008). The possibility that the presence of the flap of epithelium, whether vital or not, might confer any benefit – such as reduction in post-operative pain, promotion of epithelial healing and/or impact on apoptosis of keratocytes in the underlying stroma – is the subject of current discussion. The role of the epithelial flap in epi-LASIK was the subject of a recent study in 56 human subjects being treated for myopia where the flap was replaced in one eye and removed in the contralateral eye (Kalyvianaki *et al.*, 2008). Both techniques revealed similar epithelial wound-healing responses with equivalent haze scores, and visual and refractive outcomes but lower subjective pain scores were noted at the 2 hours post-operative time point in the eyes without flaps, indicating that retention of the flap may not offer benefit in this respect. This is consistent with earlier studies that compared various epithelial removal techniques for PRK and showed that post-operative pain, sub-epithelial opacity and visual acuity were similar regardless of the epithelial removal procedure (Lee *et al.*, 2005; Sakimoto *et al.*, 2006). It has been suggested that combining these techniques of LASEK and epi-LASIK, using alcohol with an epikeratome, may improve the quality of the epithelial flap and hinge (Camellin and Wyler, 2008).

Butterfly LASEK is another method of epithelial removal for surface ablation; the method was introduced to try and improve the viability of the epithelial flap tissue to facilitate wound healing and post-operative recovery.

This technique involves making two epithelial pockets created on either side of a central corneal epithelial incision where the epithelium has been eased back using alcohol to expose the stromal surface for laser ablation (Vinciguerra and Camesasca, 2002; Vinciguerra *et al.*, 2003). Interestingly, re-epithelialisation of the stromal surface occurs more rapidly after PRK without the use of alcohol, than with butterfly LASEK where alcohol is used, and PRK also showed lower post-operative pain scores (Ghanem *et al.*, 2008).

LASIK arose in the 1990s and combined photoablation using the excimer laser with a lamellar cut to create a hinged corneal flap aimed at preserving the integrity of the central anterior cornea including an intact epithelium (Pallikaris *et al.*, 1990). The procedure involved use of the microkeratome to cut through the central cornea creating a corneal flap approximately 120–180 microns thick and 8–10 mm in diameter. The flap was lifted to expose the underlying stroma for ablation with the laser to achieve the desired change of shape and the flap was repositioned without sutures. LASIK is currently the most frequently performed refractive surgical procedure; reports indicate that 700 000 procedures are performed annually and over 15 million people are treated using LASIK worldwide, with 6 million of those in the USA (AAO, 2008). The popularity of this laser-based refractive procedure is related to the perceived advantages for the patient – including rapid visual rehabilitation, reduced post-operative discomfort and a reduced wound-healing scenario that is likely to provide a more stable outcome (Ambrósio *et al.*, 2008). Problems with LASIK are associated with the creation of a hinged flap in the anterior one-third of the cornea and include dry eye, glare, epithelial ingrowth, corneal haze and diffuse lamellar keratitis (Kramer *et al.*, 2005; Sandoval *et al.*, 2005). LASIK-associated dry eye is the most commonly reported problem affecting approximately 50% (Ambrósio *et al.*, 2008) to 95% (Sandoval *et al.*, 2005) of LASIK patients. The fact that not all LASIK patients suffer from dry eye is curious and may be related to factors such as the size and thickness of the corneal flap, the depth of ablation with the laser, underlying sub-clinical conditions and/or the questions asked in surveys. Dry eye symptoms are caused by a combination of transection of corneal nerve axons with the microkeratome changing the function of the lacrimal gland–ocular surface unit and an altered distribution of the tear film due to the changed corneal curvature (Ambrósio *et al.*, 2008). Inflammation caused by LASIK may also contribute to dry eye and would explain the reported efficacy of treatment with topical anti-inflammatory drugs such as cyclosporine A for up to 6 months after surgery (Ambrósio *et al.*, 2008). This timing correlates with studies that showed that the return of corneal sensation, substantially diminished immediately after LASIK, was restored over the 6–12 months that it took the sub-epithelial and sub-basal nerve plexus to regrow. However, some studies report that the total length and morphology of nerve fibres after LASIK is never completely restored to pre-operative levels (Vesaluoma *et al.*, 2000; Lee *et al.*, 2002; Dawson *et al.*, 2005; Moilanen *et al.*, 2008). Confocal microscopy of post-LASIK corneas out to 12 months has revealed decreased keratocyte numbers on both sides of the lamellar cut (Vesaluoma *et al.*, 2000; Mitooka *et al.*, 2002), increased numbers of activated keratocytes compared with PRK (Mitooka *et al.*, 2002) and undulations in Bowman's layer (Vesaluoma *et al.*, 2000; Mitooka *et al.*, 2002). Histology of post-LASIK corneal tissue has shown incomplete stromal wound healing and scar formation months to years after procedures (Anderson *et al.*, 2002; Dawson *et al.*, 2005; Schmack *et al.*, 2005). Issues with flap thickness related to the difficulties of cutting of the cornea with a mechanical microkeratome underlie many of the problems observed with LASIK (Binder, 2006). Additionally, biomechanical issues are of concern with LASIK (and PRK) procedures, as chronic interlamellar and interfibrillar slippage akin to keratoconus may result in biomechanical failure and ectasia (Pallikaris *et al.*, 2001; Dawson *et al.*, 2008).

Some of these issues may be reduced by the development of new instruments such as the femtosecond laser introduced in 2002 (e.g. the IntraLase FS laser from IntraLase Corp, USA), which allows the surgeon greater precision and consistency in cutting predictable and uniform flaps in the cornea (Binder, 2006). The use of lower raster energy levels with femtosecond LASIK procedures reduces keratocyte activation and post-LASIK haze (Petroll *et al.*, 2006; Netto *et al.*, 2007). Newer versions of the femtosecond laser that require less energy to make flaps combined with laser software updates may improve flap accuracy and outcomes in the future. Thin-flap-assisted-*in-situ*-keratomileusis uses the femtosecond laser to make a much thinner customised corneal flap just beneath Bowman's layer in a procedure named 'sub-Bowman's keratomileusis' (SBK). This is aimed at reducing the flap thickness, thereby leaving more residual stromal tissue which enables safer/greater ablation of stromal tissue in high myopes. SBK also reduces the corneal biomechanical stability effects reported with conventional LASIK procedures and reduces the pain associated with PRK techniques (Azar *et al.*, 2008; Slade, 2008). Some regard this technique as the new generation of corneal surgery. Femtosecond lenticule extraction (FLE or FLEX) is a new approach for myopia that uses the femtosecond laser to create a flap and carve a stromal lenticule, which is manually removed from the cornea to give the desired correction (Sekundo *et al.*, 2008). Overall, there is still a need for alternative or parallel approaches that offer the cosmesis and convenience of the refractive surgeries, but which are more predictable and reversible with no permanent damage to the corneal structure and tissue.

4.4   Additive approaches to correct refractive error: corneal implants

An alternative approach is to correct refractive errors by inserting an implant made from synthetic and/or biological materials into the corneal tissue. Changed corneal power can be achieved by altering the curvature of the anterior corneal surface by using a pre-shaped implant made from an iso-refractive material, or by inserting a lens made from a material with a different refractive index than the corneal tissue, or by a combination of these approaches. Additive technologies have the potential to correct hyperopia, myopia, astigmatism and presbyopia. The implant may be placed within the stromal tissue (keratophakia, intracorneal rings, intracorneal lens, corneal inlay) or immediately beneath the epithelium (epikeratophakia, sub-epithelial, corneal onlay). Additive technologies offer several advantages over currently used subtractive refractive surgical techniques, paramount of which is the fact that the implant may be removed, making the procedures adjustable and reversible.

4.4.1   Early use of materials for corneal implants

The original work on corneal implants was performed to explore new treatments for clinical problems and to correct refractive error. The choice of materials was based on what was available at the time that offered good optical properties and might be tolerated by corneal tissue. Barraquer (1949) first demonstrated that it was possible to alter corneal curvature, with the potential to correct refractive errors, by surgically implanting lenses of biconvex flint glass and Plexiglas into the corneal stroma of rabbits using a freehand lamellar pocket. Both materials were solid and, while tissue posterior to the implant remained clear, tissue forward of the lenses developed necrosis and resulted in extrusion of the implants. Despite the clinical failure, the outcome was instructive as Barraquer recognised that lenses made of impermeable materials blocked a metabolic exchange that occurred from the posterior to anterior cornea, which was essential to the health of corneal tissue forward of the implanted lens. During this time, Krwawicz (1960) implanted impermeable plastic lenses in rabbits, which eventually eroded out, but they demonstrated that corneal curvature could be altered by an intracorneal implant. These outcomes with impermeable materials informed clinicians such as Choyce, Brown and Dohlman of the opportunity to use membranes to reduce the fluid flow from the aqueous humour through the cornea, which would enable treatment of conditions such as endothelial dystrophies, which resulted in stromal and epithelial oedema (Brown and Dohlman, 1965; Choyce, 1968; Choyce, 1982). Silicone membranes implanted in rabbits to test this idea did result in dehydration of the stromal tissue anterior to the implant (Brown and

Dohlman, 1965). These investigators also noted that the material had good qualities as it was transparent, flexible and able to be sterilised. In order to address the issue of permeability in intracorneal implants for the correction of refractive error, Barraquer implanted a 'large size interlamellar inclusion with a large central perforation' to allow for metabolic exchange that was aimed at modifying the corneal curvature to alter its power (Barraquer, 1966). The clinical failure of these implants was attributed to their large size and to the fact that they were a different shape to the cornea and had exerted compression on the corneal tissue. A greater understanding of the causes of failure of impermeable materials implanted in the cornea came later from modelling work presented originally by Maurice (1969) and refined by McCarey and Schmidt (1990), which considered the movement of glucose through the corneal tissue in the presence of an intracorneal implant made from a non-permeable material. Modelling showed that an impermeable material could only allow glucose into the stromal tissue anterior to the implant via lateral flow if the intracorneal lens was implanted deep in the stroma (McCarey and Schmidt, 1990).

4.4.2   Corneal implants made from biological tissue

Barraquer concluded in his article that the best material to be included in the cornea was 'the corneal parenchyma itself' (Barraquer, 1966) and we note that this is a permeable material. Barraquer went on to question issues of maintaining corneal transparency if a tissue lenticule was used, the possibility of the lenticule being reabsorbed, the cells of the recipient invading the lenticule, the size of the 'inclusion' and the possibility that the cornea might modify its form. These ideas were tested by implanting lenticules of corneal tissue in interlamellar pockets in the stroma of rabbits which were maintained for up to one year (Barraquer, 1966). Clinical data from this trial showed changed curvature of the anterior face of the cornea which was 'in perfect relation to the curve of the lenticule included in the thickness of the cornea' (Barraquer, 1966). Histological evaluation showed that donor cells had died and the lenticule was slowly repopulated with cells of the host. Problems with the lathing of the tissue lenticules were noted and it was suggested that lenticules should be of minimal thickness and be implanted as superficially as possible (Barraquer, 1966). Later, lenticules were cut from the patient's own tissue, which was frozen and lathed to the desired shape, then sutured back into the patient's cornea, giving that cornea new refractive power in a procedure named 'keratomileusis'. Some patients were implanted with desiccated positive lenticules cut from human corneal stroma using a superficial interlamellar pocket and were maintained for up to 11 months (Barraquer, 1966). The outcomes of the human trial were similar to the rabbit trial except for the presence of some opacities that formed at the lenticule interface and a less marked change in corneal curvature, which was attributed to the 'lesser elasticity' of the rabbit tissue due to the absence of Bowman's layer present in the human cornea. Barraquer named this procedure of implanting tissue lenticules into the cornea 'keratophakia' (Barraquer, 1966). Significantly, he suggested that it should be possible to manufacture lenticules 'with a foreign substance', possibly with a high refractive index, which would allow for diminished thickness of the intracorneal implant (Barraquer, 1966).

In the early 1980s, Kaufman and Werblin modified the keratophakia technique to a more superficial procedure named 'epikeratophakia', aimed at correcting refractive error associated with aphakia by placing a lenticule of donor stromal tissue lathed to a specified dioptric power on to the debrided surface of the recipient's cornea to be incorporated into the cornea by the regrowth of the epithelium (Kaufman, 1980; Werblin and Kaufman, 1981; Werblin and Klyce, 1981). This technique offered several advantages over keratophakia including a simple surgical technique, minimal damage to the central optical zone, maintaining central Bowman's intact and the possibility of reversibility (Kaufman, 1980; McDonald and Dingeldein, 1988). An early study sutured shaped donor lenticules on to debrided primate corneas with an annular keratectomy groove, which were maintained for up to 25 months (Yamaguchi et al., 1984a; Yamaguchi et al., 1984b). Histology showed that the host epithelium covered the donor lenticules with hemidesmosomes formed at the epithelial–lenticule interface. Interestingly, they also found that the host keratocytes repopulated the donor lenticule through surgical breaches of Bowman's layer in the host. Clinical data from later epikeratophakia studies by McDonald et al. (McDonald et al., 1987; McDonald and Dingeldein, 1988) showed that a predictable optical correction was not achieved because of inaccuracies with stromal tissue cryolathing associated with the effect of freezing and thawing of allograft tissue, remodelling of the implanted lens tissue, graft haze and difficulties in maintaining epithelial cover. Other studies – which tested the potential of epikeratoplasty in the treatment of aphakia, myopia and/or keratoconus – revealed stromal scarring (Lass et al., 1987) and difficulties in maintaining epithelial growth over the surface of the tissue lenticule (Lass et al., 1987; Rao et al., 1987) that were attributed to the possibility of corneal hypesthesia (diminished nerve response) (Rao et al., 1987). The main reason for clinical failure of epikeratophakia was imperfect re-epithelisation of the implanted tissue lenticule (Young et al., 1994). Failed human epikeratoplasty lenticules were histologically examined and structural abnormalities were identified at all levels of the donor lenticules including irregular epithelium, changes in the basement membrane, focal breaks and undulations in Bowman's layer, changes in keratocyte population and stromal collagens (Binder and Zavala, 1987). Another histological study on failed epikeratoplasty tissue removed from patients treated for keratoconus and aphakia revealed corneal scarring and accumulation of electron-dense material associated with the keratocytes around the implanted stromal tissue (Grossniklaus *et al.*, 1989). This outcome was similar to that reported on explanted tissue from epikeratoplasty used in the treatment of keratoconus, which showed problems with epithelial irregularity and sub-epithelial fibrosis as well as folds in Descemet's membrane and stromal scars (Rodrigues *et al.*, 1992).

Biological materials other than corneal stroma have also been considered as intracorneal implants to correct refractive error. In one study, human placental collagen IV stabilised by aldehyde treatment was implanted in the corneas of dogs for 2 years and showed good clinical biocompatibility with clear corneas and no inflammatory response (Dupont *et al.*, 1989). Histology conducted on implanted corneas showed thinned epithelium forward of the implants, degenerated keratocytes near the implant and foreign material at interfaces. Alternative materials were also considered including collagen types I, III, or IV, collagen–hydrogel copolymers, bioactive synthetics, and coated hydrogels, such as poly(2-hydroxyethyl methacrylate) (PHEMA) (Thompson *et al.*, 1991). It was recognised that a suitable material should offer optical clarity, support of epithelial migration and adhesion, be permeable to glucose and other solutes and not be degraded (Thompson *et al.*, 1991). In addition, it was also suggested that attachment strategies to fix the synthetic implants to the cornea without cutting Bowman's layer (such as adhesives) might improve the efficacy of the procedure, named 'synthetic epikeratoplasty' (Thompson *et al.*, 1991). A study of human placental collagen IV discs, stabilised by aldehyde treatment, implanted in the corneas of rhesus monkeys using the epikeratoplasty technique ensued (Thompson *et al.*, 1993). These implants remained clear and maintained epithelial cover for up to 30 months with some formation of cell–matrix junctions at the epithelial–lenticule interface during that time, but all showed degradation of the lenticule with time that involved neutral protease activity which degraded the collagen. As with the use of tissue lenticules, the stability of the collagen material in the corneal environment was recognised as an issue that needed to be addressed. Problems with the use of tissue lenticules in keratophakia and epikeratophakia procedures focused attention on alternative materials such as those of synthetic origin, and alternative designs and surgical procedures in the intracorneal implant area.

4.4.3   Corneal implants made from impermeable synthetic materials

Barraquer concluded from his early work that synthetic materials would be ideal as intracorneal inclusions since they could offer a refractive index higher than native corneal tissue (1.376) and could be produced as thin lenses (Barraquer, 1966). Researchers at the time recognised polysulphone as a candidate material as it had a high refractive index (1.633) permitting the creation of thin lenses to give refractive correction without altering the shape of the corneal surface. In addition, polysulphone had excellent optical properties, could be easily moulded or lathed, absorbed ultraviolet and infrared light, and was already known to be biocompatible for biomedical applications, including intraocular lenses (McCarey *et al.*, 1988). On this basis, lenses made of polysulphone and other materials, such as poly(methyl methacrylate) (PMMA) (refractive index of 1.49), were implanted intrastromally in animals and humans (Choyce, 1982; Kirkness *et al.*, 1985; Lane *et al.*, 1986; Climenhaga *et al.*, 1988; Deg and Binder, 1988; McCarey *et al.*, 1988; Rodrigues *et al.*, 1990). Some implants were tolerated for months to years with few reports of inflammation being a problem (Choyce, 1982; Deg and Binder, 1988; Rodrigues *et al.*, 1990). The impermeable nature of the materials tested may have overwhelmed any subtlety in response that might have been noted among the different materials tested; these included glass (Barraquer, 1949), polysulphone (Choyce, 1982; Choyce, 1985; Kirkness *et al.*, 1985; Lane *et al.*, 1986; Climenhaga *et al.*, 1988; Deg and Binder, 1988; McCarey *et al.*, 1988; Rodrigues *et al.*, 1990) and PMMA (Choyce, 1982; Rodrigues *et al.*, 1990). The influence of the type of material used in the tissue response was considered by some authors (Choyce, 1982; Kirkness *et al.*, 1985; Deg and Binder, 1988; Rodrigues *et al.*, 1990), although it was difficult to distinguish any real evidence that one material offered any benefit over another. Typical complications included interface opacities, epithelial thinning and stromal necrosis which resulted in lens extrusion. Concern about the chemical stability of the material and its effect on the corneal tissue during the period of implantation were also noted (Barraquer, 1966; Kirkness *et al.*, 1985; Deg and Binder, 1988). Opacities associated with the implant interface, particularly lipid or crystalline deposits, were a frequently reported occurrence (Choyce, 1982; Choyce, 1985; Lane *et al.*, 1986; Climenhaga *et al.*, 1988; Deg and Binder, 1988; McCarey *et al.*, 1988; Rodrigues *et al.*, 1990). While some consideration was given to the inappropriate stiffness of the material used (Barraquer, 1966; Deg and Binder, 1988), failures were, in general, attributed to inadequate nutrition of the tissue anterior to the lens owing to the solid nature of the material used (Barraquer, 1949; Choyce, 1982; Choyce, 1985; Kirkness *et al.*, 1985; Lane *et al.*, 1986; Deg and Binder, 1988; McCarey *et al.*, 1988; Rodrigues *et al.*, 1990). Attempts to improve the permeability of polysulphone, such as the addition of large holes (Barraquer, 1966; Choyce, 1982) or small fenestrations (McCarey *et al.*, 1988), offered some benefit in reducing opacification of corneal tissue forward of the implant and in improved retention time of the devices in the cornea, but failed to completely resolve these problems. Implanting the lens deeper in the stromal tissue close to Descemet's membrane enabled some implants to be retained for longer but resulted in other problems such as tearing of Descemet's membrane and protrusion of the inlays into the anterior chamber (Choyce, 1985; McCarey et al., 1988; Rodrigues et al., 1990).

4.4.4   Corneal implants made from permeable synthetic materials

The difficulties encountered with intracorneal lenses made from solid materials and the growing significance of material permeability and modulus gave rise to concurrent activity with alternative materials such as hydrogels. Hydrogels are three-dimensional hydrophilic polymer networks capable of swelling in water and retaining large amounts of fluid between the polymer chains, which impart solute permeability to this class of materials. The water content is generally accepted to reflect the permeability of the material and hydrogels can be manufactured with a range of water contents, although those with a great deal of water have a low modulus and can be difficult to handle. The permeability and optical properties of hydrogels were already understood in the 1960s from their use as materials for the manufacture of contact lenses. Hydrogels could also be made with a refractive index matching that of the cornea (1.376), offering the potential to be shaped to change the corneal curvature and achieve the desired refractive outcome. Dohlman et al. (1967) used a hydrogel material, poly(glycerol methacrylate) (PGMA; refractive index 1.353) with 88% water content, as an intracorneal implant; this was well tolerated by the corneal tissue (no inflammation), but implants were extruded in a response that was attributed to insufficient permeability and mechanical issues due to their flat form. Mester et al. (1972) demonstrated that corneal curvature and the dioptric power of the cornea could be changed using implants made from hydrogels, mostly PHEMA (refractive index 1.44). Following those initial trials, various hydrogel materials with a range of water contents, originally developed as contact lens materials, were tested as intracorneal implants in animal and human trials. Included in these trials were Perfilcon A, Lidofilcon A, Lidofilcon B, Surfilcon A and Etafilcon A (see Table 4.1 for details).

Generally, each of these hydrogel implants was reported to have been well tolerated by the corneal tissue for extended periods of time (Mester et al., 1972; McCarey and Andrews, 1981; Werblin et al., 1983; Koenig et al., 1984; Samples et al., 1984; Yamaguchi et al., 1984b; Beekhuis et al., 1986; McCarey et al., 1990; McCarey, 1991; Parks and McCarey, 1991; Werblin et al., 1992a; Werblin et al., 1992b; McDonald et al., 1993). Early work with hydrogels concentrated on testing the significance of the water content of the materials on the biological and optical outcomes. Biocompatibility was linked to the water content of the implanted material following work in rabbits where implants of a low water content material (glycerol methacrylate;

Table 4.1 Chemical components and typical water contents of hydrogel contact lens materials commonly used as intracorneal implants

Name (trade name)	Principal components	Typical water content (%)	Reference to testing as an intracorneal implant
Perfilcon A (Permalens)	HEMA, VP, MA	70–71	Binder *et al.*, 1981/82; McCarey and Andrews, 1981; Sendele *et al.*, 1983; Werblin *et al.*, 1983; Samples *et al.*, 1984; McCarey, 1991; Parks and McCarey, 1991; Werblin *et al.*, 1992a; Werblin *et al.*, 1992b
Lidofilcon A (Sauflon 70)	MMA, VP	68–70	Binder *et al.*, 1981/82; Werblin *et al.*, 1983; Samples *et al.*, 1984; McCarey *et al.*, 1990; McCarey, 1991; Parks *et al.*, 1993; McDonald *et al.*, 1993
Surfilcon A (Permaflex)	AMA, VP	70–74	Koenig *et al.*, 1984; Yamaguchi *et al.*, 1984b
Etafilcon A	HEMA, MA	58–72	Beekhuis *et al.*, 1986; Beekhuis *et al.*, 1987
Lidofilcon B	MMA, VP	79	Beekhuis *et al.*, 1987; McDonald *et al.*, 1993

HEMA, 2-hydroxyethyl methacrylate; VP, *N*-vinyl pyrrolidone; MA, methacrylic acid; MMA, methyl methacrylate; AMA, alkyl methacrylate.

GMA) failed quickly because of non-inflammatory ulceration while implants of a high water content hydrogel, Perfilcon A (70%), were tolerated for 12 months (Sendele *et al.*, 1983). Longer-term testing of two high water content materials, Lidofilcon A (70%) and Lidofilcon B (79%), implanted in lamellar pockets in monkey eyes, showed that both materials were equally well tolerated by the cornea for up to 5 years (McDonald *et al.*, 1993). During this period, McCarey and Schmidt (1990) modelled glucose distribution in the cornea in the presence of intracorneal lenses of varying diameter, depth, permeability and thickness. They identified that the glucose permeability of the material was more significant in maintaining corneal health than the diameter or depth of the implanted lens.

Refractive data from many of the studies suggested that the type of hydrogel material was perhaps less significant than the species used to test it and the depth at which the implant was placed in the cornea. Optical data from studies that compared lenses made of hydrogels with different water contents (various hydrogels ranging between 38 and 79% water content) (Binder *et al.*, 1981/82) and also similar water contents (Lidofilcon A and Perfilcon A, both with 70% water content) (Werblin *et al.*, 1983) that were implanted in primate eyes, reported no difference in the optical outcomes among the materials tested. The curvature change achieved when hydrogels were tested in primates (which have a Bowman's layer present in the anterior stroma) were encouraging over considerable periods from months to years (Mester *et al.*, 1972; Binder *et al.*, 1981/82; Werblin *et al.*, 1983; Beekhuis *et al.*, 1986; Beekhuis *et al.*, 1987; McCarey *et al.*, 1990; McDonald *et al.*, 1993; Parks *et al.*, 1993). In another study, refractive changes that had been observed in rabbits (without Bowman's layer) did not occur in the first human patient (with Bowman's layer present) and it was suggested that moving the lens more anteriorly might help (Sendele *et al.*, 1983). The depth at which the lenses of differing water contents were implanted was also considered and tested. Etafilcon A lenses with a range of water contents (58%, 68% and 72%) were implanted at different depths in the monkey stroma and data showed that the higher water content materials did not necessarily give the best refractive data when implanted at 60% depth (Beekhuis *et al.*, 1986). Deeper implants of Lidofilcon A placed at >79% corneal depth, were found to give little, or less predictable, refractive outcomes than those mid-depth or shallower in the cornea (Koenig *et al.*, 1984; McCarey *et al.*, 1990). However, deeper implants were generally well tolerated by corneal tissue, as demonstrated with lenses made of Lidofilcon A and Perfilcon A (McCarey, 1991; Parks *et al.*, 1993) and Surfilcon A (Koenig *et al.*, 1984). It is likely that a contributing factor to this outcome was the availability of glucose to the tissue forward of the implant being increased if the lens was deep (McCarey and Schmidt, 1990), rather than the type of hydrogel material that was used. Often these deep stromal implants were associated with bulging of the posterior stroma and endothelium into the anterior chamber (Koenig *et al.*, 1984; McCarey, 1991; Parks *et al.*, 1993). In addition, the stability of the refractive outcomes with deeper hydrogel implants was not always assured and the contraction of stromal tissue that occurs during wound healing was implicated in at least one study (McCarey *et al.*, 1990).

Factors such as the design and size of the implant, inconsistent microkeratome cuts and decentration caused by migration of the implants were reported to have caused poor outcomes in some cases (Beekhuis *et al.*, 1987; McCarey *et al.*, 1990; McDonald *et al.*, 1993), as did contaminants associated with materials used for implants (Beekhuis *et al.*, 1987; Werblin *et al.*, 1992b). Overall, clinical complications that developed with hydrogel intracorneal lenses included oedema and inflammation, crystalline deposits, accumulation of extracellular matrix around the implant, epithelial ingrowth, fibrosis around implant and ulceration of tissue forward of the implant (McCarey and Andrews, 1981; Sendele *et al.*, 1983; Samples *et al.*, 1984; Yamaguchi *et al.*, 1984b; Beekhuis *et al.*, 1987; McCarey *et al.*, 1990; Parks *et al.*, 1993). Variation in the biological response to the same material was also evident (Parks *et al.*, 1993). While many implants were well tolerated, thinning of the epithelium forward of the implant and the presence of keratocytes and debris at the stromal–lens interface were commonly reported in cases where histology was conducted (Sendele *et al.*, 1983; Samples *et al.*, 1984; Yamaguchi *et al.*, 1984b; Beekhuis *et al.*, 1987; McCarey, 1991; Werblin *et al.*, 1992b; McDonald *et al.*, 1993). Data arising from these studies with hydrogels showed notable similarities to those that tested the biocompatibility of acellular biological tissue for intracorneal implants.

Guiding principles arose from this work with hydrogels, with these studies flagging the significance of high permeability and biocompatibility as essential to the success of synthetic materials as intracorneal implants. The possibility of slow stromal alterations occurring in response to hydrogel intracorneal implants, either by remodelling or by encapsulation of non-biological hydrogel, material, was raised (McCarey and Andrews, 1981). Later, it was noted that the need for biocompatibility of hydrogels depended on the toxicity, stability and solute–solvent permeability of materials and, based on this, it was recommended that materials be free of residual monomers, cleaning agents and debris that could stimulate inflammation (McCarey *et al.*, 1988). Further work lead to the identification of requirements for the use of hydrogels for intracorneal implants to correct refractive error that included: minimising the thickness of the implant to reduce hypoplasia of the overlying epithelium; provision of the refractive power correction should come from the optics of the implant; simplification of the surgical procedure; the permeability of the implant should be retained in the long term to provide for nutritional biocompatibility (McCarey, 1991). Implant thickness was acknowledged to be an issue for glucose transport and recommendations were made that lens thickness be minimised (McDonald *et al.*, 1993). Given that hydrogel thickness could be a limiting factor in intracorneal lens design, it was clear that developments in surgical techniques, materials and lens designs were required to address these issues.

New microkeratome technology allowed the creation of hinged corneal flaps for use in LASIK surgery. Concurrently, new materials were developed for use as intracorneal implants. The combination offered the opportunity to place the lens under the corneal flap in a sutureless synthetic keratoplasty procedure which was potentially reversible (corneal inlay). Hyperopic correction was the target of the new technology since the optical designs were relatively simple and myopia was being treated using LASIK as it was easier to flatten the cornea effectively than to steepen it at that time (Esquenazi *et al.*, 2006). Nutrapore, described as a microporous hydrogel material with 70% water content and a refractive index close to corneal tissue, was made into a thin hyperopic design lens to correct up to +6D (PermaVision from Anamed Inc., Lake Forest, California, USA). Confocal microscopy on PermaVision implants placed under a 150 μm corneal flap in rabbits showed a minimal tissue response over 6 months to the presence of implant in an outcome that was attributed to the thin design of the inlay made from what was regarded to be a highly permeable material (Ismail, 2002). Refractive data on PermaVision implants came from another study (Michieletto *et al.*, 2004), where hyperopic implants made from a 78% water content version of the hydrogel with a central thickness ranging from 25 to 60 μm were maintained in the corneas of patients with promising optical outcomes and relatively few complications over the 6 month period. A third study (Alio *et al.*, 2004) on PermaVision Nutrapore implants in 11 eyes reported early, and serious, complications during the 6-month period including patient discomfort and loss of best-corrected visual acuity (BCVA), combined with edge opacities that did not respond to steroids and were attributed to the presence of epithelial cells under the inlay. In another study (Knorz, 2005), stable refractive outcomes were shown after 'first-generation' PermaVision inlays were implanted in 21 eyes of 12 patients, but the majority developed corneal haze which started around the implant edge at 3 months and gradually covered the lens in up to 3 years. A follow-up study with PermaVision lenses implanted in 23 eyes of 20 patients over 2 years reported relative refractive predictability with 70% ±0.5D but with many complications such as decentration, induced astigmatism, stromal opacification, night halos and glare (Ismail, 2006). Confocal microscopy was used to compare hyperopic PermaVision inlays with LASIK performed using a femtosecond laser (IntraLase) and identified interface particles and activated keratocytes in both groups with chronic central corneal epithelial thinning in the inlay group (Petroll *et al.*, 2006). It is possible that the permeability of hydrogel materials such as these is not maintained in the long term due to fouling or other reasons. Only recently, Larrea *et al.* (2007) developed a three-dimensional model of solute transport in the cornea which simultaneously addressed the axisymmetric oxygen and glucose diffusion for different lens permeabilities and positions of the implant in the cornea. Simulations using inlay with 3 mm diameter and 20 μm thick with a range of permeabilities (supplied by BioVision AG) showed the mid-posterior stroma (75% depth) to be the optimal position for the inlay to be implanted to enhance the supply of oxygen and glucose to the cornea. This publication (Larrea *et al.*, 2007) also reminds us that transport of other solutes through the cornea, such as lactate, is significant and may be affected by the presence of an implanted lens. Lactic acid is a product of cell metabolism that increases in concentration under hypoxic conditions and can lead to accumulation of lactate which causes stromal oedema.

4.4.5   Current corneal implant technologies

Previous work with intracorneal inclusions for the correction of refractive error has clearly shown that permeability of the implant is critical to a good outcome and that this can be addressed by decreasing the diameter of the implant, increasing the permeability of the material or decreasing the thickness of the implant, or a combination of all these approaches. Additionally, placing the implant superficially is less damaging to the corneal tissue and offers reversibility. The currently available technologies in the synthetic intracorneal implant area reflect a good understanding of the knowledge gained from this research. A range of materials and designs have been tested as corneal inlays and onlays and these are well documented in review articles (Hughes and Chan, 2001; Xie *et al.*, 2001; Sweeney *et al.*, 2008). Currently, the majority of technologies emerging in this area are corneal inlays aimed at presbyopia to provide an alternative to reading glasses for the growing market arising from the ageing 'baby-boomer' generation (Pieper, 2006). These presbyopic implants make use of synthetic materials in small-diameter, thin designs and are generally being implanted intracorneally in the non-dominant eye of subjects with no other refractive error (emmetropes), some of whom may have had previous or concurrent refractive surgery (Alio, 2007; Dalton, 2008). In each case, the inlays and accompanying surgical procedures are directed toward a solution that is convenient, minimally invasive, preserving of distance visual acuity and reversible.

ReVision Optics has manufactured the PermaVision hydrogel into small, thin, plano-presbyopic lenses to treat presbyopia (Presbylens from ReVision Optics, Lake Forest, California, USA). The material is iso-refractive with corneal tissue and works by changing the anterior curvature of the cornea with a central near-add and an additional draping effect that improves intermediate vision. This 'refractively neutral' approach is expected to reduce the incidence of halos and glare (Bethke, 2007). The small 1.5–2 mm diameter inlays are implanted into the central cornea using either a microkeratome flap or delivered using an applicator into a tunnel pocket made with a femtosecond laser. General reports suggest that these inlays show predictable and stable visual outcomes in a procedure that is reversible and exchangeable (Slade, 2006; Dalton, 2008; Lang *et al.*, 2008). ReVision Optics is working towards a combination 'one-visit' therapy where LASIK and an inlay are used concurrently in a presby-LASIK approach (Bethke, 2007).

BioVision AG has also designed a small, thin lens to improve near vision for emmetropic presbyopes using a monovision approach (Invue from BioVision AG, Brüggs, Switzerland). The 3 mm diameter inlay is made of a permeable acrylic hydrogel material that is implanted in the patient's non-dominant eye. The donut-shaped bifocal lens has a central neutral zone of 1.8 mm and a peripheral zone with refractive power to correct near vision. The implant has a small hole centrally that provides for corneal nutrition without interfering with the optics. The lens is implanted mid-depth in the central cornea in a tunnel made using a microkeratome dissector (Visitome from BioVision AG) or femtosecond laser. The Invue inlay potentially offers a multifocal cornea to emmetropic presbyopes with no astigmatism, allowing them to read. Some reports suggest that this can be achieved in the majority of cases (Sanchez Leon, 2006; Kymionis *et al.*, 2007a; Sanchez Leon, 2008), but there are several disadvantages reported with this technology, including slow visual rehabilitation, a small loss of contrast sensitivity or quality of distance vision, some night-vision problems such as halo, and complications requiring the removal of the inlay in a small number of patients (Lindstrom, 2005; Bethke, 2007; Dalton, 2008).

AcuFocus has addressed the correction of presbyopia using a small-diameter device (ACI-7000 intracorneal inlay from AcuFocus, Inc., Irvine, California, USA) with a central pinhole 1.6 mm in diameter to increase the depth of field based on the principle of small-aperture optics (Yilmaz *et al.*, 2008). The current version of this inlay is a made from poly(vinylidene fluoride) (PVDF; refractive index 1.42) with carbon nanoparticles to make it opaque. The lens is very thin (approximately 10 µm thick) with a 3.6 mm area around the central hole that incorporates a random arrangement of 160 pores (25 µm) to provide for nutritional flow (Yilmaz *et al.*, 2008). The inlay is placed on the non-dominant eye beneath a conventional corneal flap (approximately 160 µm deep) cut with a microkeratome or a femtosecond laser. ACI-7000 inlays are being implanted in naturally emmetropic patients and previously ametropic patients who have had LASIK surgery (Yilmaz *et al.*, 2008). The depth of the implant appears to be significant in minimising flap complications and preventing a change in shape of the corneal curvature (Yilmaz *et al.*, 2008). Centration of the inlay over the pupil is essential to a good outcome as the opaque ACI-7000 inlay is placed over the pupil to create a fixed aperture setting of 1.6 mm to increase the depth of field, improving intermediate and near vision in presbyopic patients without significantly reducing distance vision (Yilmaz *et al.*, 2008). Clinical testing has shown improved near vision (of about +1.5D) without marked loss of distance vision over a period of 1 year (Dalton, 2008; Yilmaz *et al.*, 2008). In some patients there were problems with glare caused by high light transmission from the pinholes, which also reduced contrast sensitivity. The manufacturers have addressed this by design modifications that resulted in an even thinner implant (5 µm thick), with lower light transmission through the pinholes (Bethke, 2007). Disadvantages of this technology include the appearance of the inlay (black) and some loss of night vision because of reduced light entering the eye (Dalton, 2008). Data from a Phase III trial of 200 eyes implanted with the ACI-7000 were presented to the US Food and Drug Administration (FDA) in 2007. In the future, the company plans to implant inlays in ametropic patients who are undergoing LASIK with the intention of correcting refractive error and treating presbyopia in a single visit (Bethke, 2007).

Vision CRC (Vision Cooperative Research Centre, Sydney, Australia) has developed a non-hydrogel material with broad potential in the additive refractive keratoplasty area. The higher permeability nature of this material does not restrict its use to the correction of presbyopia but offers the potential for broader corrections – including myopia, hyperopia, presbyopia and astigmatism – since thickness is not a limiting factor in the implant design. The group has drawn on the considerable experience gained from their own research and that of others in the field to produce a non-hydrogel material family with characteristics defined as ideal for an intracorneal application. Implants made of the perfluoropolyether (PFPE) -based material create a stable change in corneal curvature when implanted and could be used to treat presbyopia, myopia or hyperopia. This material offers many advantages for corneal augmentation as it is iso-refractive (refractive index of 1.34 (Rice and Ihlenfeld, 1989)), inert, transparent, flexible and chemically and thermally stable. Biostability of the PFPE material has been demonstrated in samples implanted subcutaneously in sheep over 2 years (G. F. Meijs, K. Schindhelm, R. Odell and H. Chen, unpublished data). PFPE is inherently hydrophobic and some hydrophilicity has been introduced by co-polymerisation with monomers containing a zwitterion, which has also enhanced its anti-fouling properties. Permeability has been chemically induced into the PFPE material (Chaouk et al., 2001) to meet requirements established by implanting model polymer membranes with a calculated range of permeabilities into the feline cornea and monitoring clinical outcomes (Sweeney et al., 1998). Porous PFPE membranes have demonstrated permeability to appropriate corneal metabolites such as glucose and model proteins such as albumin and inulin (Evans et al., 2000; Hughes and Chan, 2001).

The Vision CRC polymer has been tested as an inlay in both animal and human trials. PFPE inlays, 4.3 mm diameter and 80 μm thick centrally, in a hyperopic-shaped design with tapered sides, were well tolerated by corneal tissue over the long term when placed under a microkeratome corneal flap in rabbit corneas (Xie et al., 2006) and in unsighted human subjects (Sweeney et al., 2005; Sweeney et al., 2006; Prakasam et al., 2007a; Sweeney et al., 2008; Sweeney et al., 2009). In both cases, clinical data have shown that corneas remained clear without inflammation, neo-vascularisation or increased redness compared with accompanying sham-operated corneas for 2 years in rabbits (Xie et al., 2006) and over 4 years in humans (Sweeney et al., 2009), as seen in Fig. 4.5. Confocal microscopy of the implanted human eyes showed the presence of activated keratocytes immediately around the lens at 6 months, which was accompanied by reflective deposits on inlay surfaces in a low-grade response that had stabilised by 12 months (Vaddavalli et al., 2007; Sweeney et al., 2009). Histology and electron microscopy on the implanted rabbit corneas showed a similar overall response with activated and degenerative keratocytes, with some accompanying cell debris along the surfaces of the inlay noted at 6 months, which showed no increase at 12 or 24 months (Xie et al., 2006), as seen in Fig. 4.6. Despite the overall good biocompatibility, PFPE inlays in both human and rabbit eyes have shown a

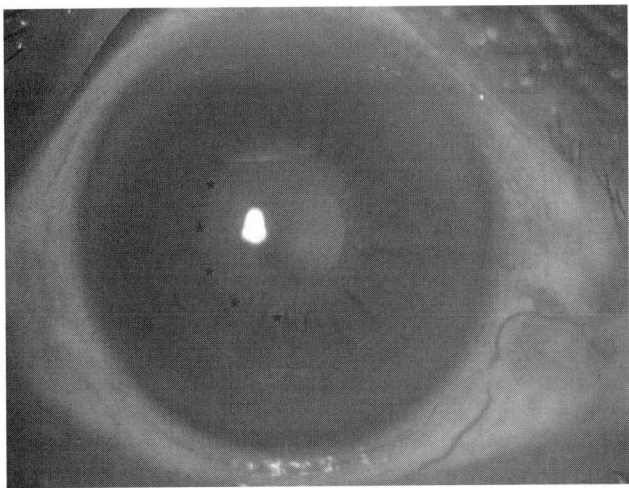

4.5 Diffuse light image of a Vision CRC PFPE inlay implanted in the human cornea at 39 month timepoint (asterisks mark a portion of the outer edge of the inlay).

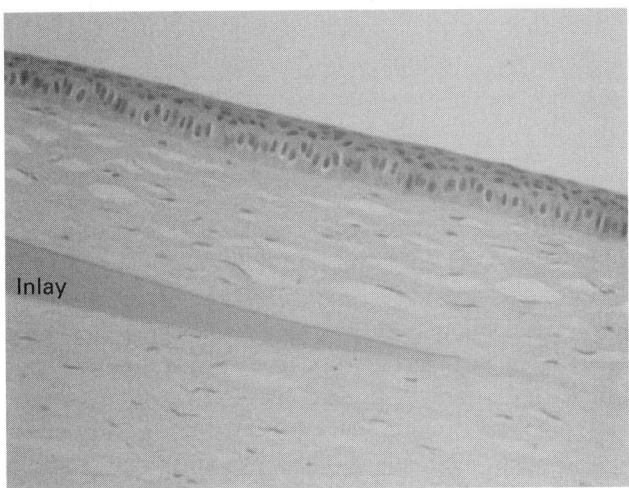

Inlay

4.6 Light micrograph of a transverse histological section of rabbit cornea showing a Vision CRC PFPE inlay 24 months after it was implanted under a corneal flap (nasal side of inlay at original magnification ×20).

low level of reduction in clarity with time. Ultrastructural data from the 2-year rabbit trial showed that the presence of extracellular matrix components and debris from degenerated cells along the inlay surfaces is likely to be involved in this loss of clarity (Evans *et al.*, 2002). Keratometry data from the human trial showed a relatively stable change in corneal dioptric power in the implanted eyes of average 6.5D (range 4–14D) at 48 months with fluctuations related to the patients' poor fixation in their unsighted eyes as well as to the patients' age (Sweeney *et al.*, 2008; Sweeney *et al.*, 2009). Reversibility has also been demonstrated when some inlays were removed and the corneal flap replaced (Sweeney *et al.*, 2008; Sweeney *et al.*, 2009). Interestingly, the changed corneal curvature in implanted human eyes caused the formation of iron rings in the peripheral cornea, which were similar to Fleisher's ring that occurs in keratoconus (Prakasam *et al.*, 2007b). Iron rings are non-pathological and result from iron deposition in the basal layer of the corneal epithelium, usually in response to sudden changes in corneal contour.

The Vision CRC polymer has also been tested as a synthetic corneal onlay. Onlays are placed superficially under the corneal epithelium without disturbing Bowman's layer and are incorporated into the cornea by epithelial tissue covering the anterior surface of the lens. Refractive correction is obtained by a change in corneal curvature. This is a challenging application for any synthetic material since, in addition to being inert, biostable, nutrient permeable, transparent and mechanically compliant, it must also allow for the growth and stable adhesion of a stratified epithelium on its anterior surface (Evans *et al.*, 2001a; Hughes and Chan, 2001; Xie *et al.*, 2001). The surface chemistry and topography of the polymer are known to be significant in achieving this outcome and have been carefully examined by this group using in vitro modelling systems (Evans and Steele, 1997; Evans and Steele, 1998; Fitton *et al.*, 1998; Dalton *et al.*, 1999; Evans *et al.*, 1999; Dalton *et al.*, 2001; Evans *et al.*, 2001b; Evans *et al.*, 2003). Initial *in vivo* work by Vision CRC determined that covalently immobilised collagen type I promoted epithelial growth across the surface of a model synthetic polymer implanted in feline eyes (Sweeney *et al.*, 1997; Sweeney *et al.*, 2003). This coating strategy was applied to PFPE lenses, which supported the growth of epithelial tissue implanted in an open pocket made in feline corneas (Evans *et al.*, 2000). Longer-term trials in feline corneas showed that collagen-coated PFPE lens not only supported epithelial growth but also the formation of recognisable basement membrane and components of cell–matrix junctions (hemidesmosomes and anchoring fibrils) along the epithelial–lens interface (Evans *et al.*, 2002). *In vivo* studies have demonstrated that a PFPE lens with a collagen I coat could be glued on to a debrided feline cornea and be incorporated into the cornea by the migration and adhesion of stratified corneal epithelial tissue, as seen in Fig. 4.7.

4.4.6   Intracorneal rings

Non-permeable synthetic materials have been used to make intracorneal rings, which were originally designed to treat myopia but are now used mostly in

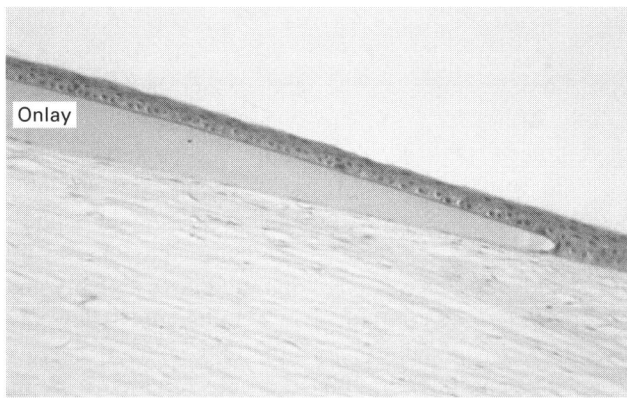

4.7 Light micrograph of a transverse histological section showing a Vision CRC PFPE onlay that had been fully covered with epithelial tissue for 3 months after placement on a debrided feline cornea (inferior side of onlay at original magnification ×200).

the treatment of disorders involving corneal ectasia and keratoconus. Intacs (Addition Technology Inc., previously KeraVision, Fremont, California, USA) originally developed a one-piece PMMA intracorneal ring, which was implanted in a tunnel made in the peripheral cornea to flatten the central area and reduce myopia. Subsequent designs produced two half-ring segments made from impermeable PMMA, which were easier to implant. This technology offered the advantage of leaving the central cornea undisturbed (Linebarger *et al.*, 2000; Ruckhofer *et al.*, 2001a) but has failed to provide reliable optical outcomes except in the case of very low myopes (Ruckhofer *et al.*, 2001b). Complications reported with intracorneal rings include corneal dehydration, crystal formation, lipid deposits, opacities and difficulties with implant edges which have caused thinning, fibrosis and ulceration of the stroma, keratitis and corneal vascularisation, with some of these difficulties likely to be associated with the stretching of the corneal tissue. This would be consistent with recent histological evaluation of failed cases of intracorneal rings used in the treatment of keratoconus and post-LASIK keratectasia that showed an abnormal accumulation of fibrotic extracellular matrix components and proteases near the rings, suggesting ongoing lysis and remodelling of corneal stroma (Maguen *et al.*, 2008). Currently, intracorneal rings are being used in the treatment of keratoconus where they may offer some benefit (Kymionis *et al.*, 2007b). Recent figures show that intracorneal rings have been used to treat 50 000 keratoconus cases worldwide since the first implantation 10 years ago, with stable correction provided for most of those cases (Colin, 2008). Outcomes may be improved with use of the femtosecond laser instead of mechanical methods to create the channels used to implant the rings (Carrasquillo *et al.*, 2007). The KeraRing (Mediphacos,

Belo Horizonte, Brazil) consists of two semi-circular ring segments made of PMMA that were specifically designed for the treatment of corneal ectasia. This technology now uses the femtosecond laser to create a tunnel for implantation with some reasonable outcomes at 12 months reported for patients with keratoconus (Coskunseven *et al.*, 2008). Ferrara rings (Ferrara Ophthalmics, Belo Horizonte, Brazil) are two semi-circular ring segments made of Perspex CQ Acrylic (PMMA), a material known to be tolerated by ocular tissue from its previous use as an ophthalmic biomaterial. Originally, the rings were intended for the treatment of moderate to high myopia, myopic astigmatism and irregular astigmatism in keratoconus. They have shown benefit for keratoconus patients unable to wear contact lenses (Miranda *et al.*, 2003; Kwitko and Severo, 2004) and are reported to reinforce and stabilise the cornea and possibly delay or prevent progression of keratoconus and improve vision acuity. Another intracorneal ring technology, Myoring (Dioptix, Linz, Austria), is a solid, but flexible, one-piece PMMA ring that is implanted in a closed intrastromal pocket made in the peripheral cornea using a pocketmaker microkeratome (Corneal Intrastromal Implantation System, also from Dioptix) (Daxer, 2008). The dimensions of the ring are determined by the refractive power needed, with the presence of the implant changing the shape of the cornea, flattening the central area. Myoring is reported to achieve this change in cornea shape without alteration to the biomechanics (Daxer, 2008). The technique is described by the inventor as being a quick and minimally invasive way to treat patients with moderate and high myopia and is reported to offer a safe and effective alternative to LASIK and phakic intraocular lens implantation (Daxer, 2008). At this time, there are no data from long-term trials from which to evaluate the safety and efficacy of this PMMA-based corneal implant system (Daxer, 2008).

4.4.7   Overall outcomes of using the cornea to correct refractive error

Additive approaches offer advantages over subtractive approaches in using the cornea to correct refractive errors. Paramount among these is the possibility of being able to remove the intracorneal implant if necessary. Design principles for ideal intracorneal implants to correct refractive error can be drawn from the outcomes of research and clinical trials in this area, as summarised in Table 4.2. Clearly, the material and the implant design, as well as the surgical procedure, have a significant impact on the outcome. The material for such an intracorneal implant must be transparent, highly nutrient permeable, chemically stable, biostable, biocompatible and mechanically compliant with corneal tissue. The optical design should result in an implant as small and as thin as needed to achieve the desired refractive outcome. Surgical procedures used for the implant should be minimised and the implant placed

Table 4.2 Characteristics of an ideal intracorneal implant system to correct refractive error

- Transparent material
- Design should be aimed at a small, thin and flexible lens
- Optical design should be optimised to be as thin as possible with good edges
- Permeable material to allow for nutrient flux and nerve regrowth
- Refractive index of material could match or be different from that of corneal tissue
- Modulus of material should match that of central corneal tissue
- Material chemically inactive with low residual extractables and no contaminants
- Low-fouling material needed to reduce accumulation of proteins, lipids, etc.
- Biocompatible material should not initiate an inflammatory or immune response
- Anterior surface treatment to support stable corneal epithelium (onlay)
- Lens surfaces designed to minimise fibrosis
- Posterior lens surface treated with adhesive (onlay)
- Lens design to prevent epithelial undergrowth
- Lens design to minimise mechanical stresses on cornea
- Surgical procedure should be quick, minimal and superficial (sub-epithelial if possible)
- Lens should be easily handled by surgeon
- Lens should be easy for surgeon to orient right side up
- Centration of implant should be easy for surgeon

as superficially as possible leaving Bowman's layer intact to preserve nerves and maintain optimal corneal biomechanics and, most importantly, to confine the wound-healing events to those associated with an epithelial abrasion. This appears to a very significant factor since penetrating the stroma by any means such as scalpel, microkeratome or laser initiates a stromal wound-healing process that is complicated and prolonged, and is likely to result in opacity or interface haze caused by incomplete healing. Ideally, a synthetic implant placed beneath the epithelium as an onlay is most likely to succeed since an epithelial wound can heal quickly to incorporate the device, offering rapid visual rehabilitation and the opportunity of reversibility. Correction of hyperopia, myopia and presbyopia with this type of approach would deliver breakthrough products to the ophthalmic marketplace.

4.5   Corneal repair and replacement

4.5.1   The need for materials to repair and replace the cornea

Diseases, infection or damage to the cornea may result in corneal opacity and blindness. Corneal disease is the second most common cause of blindness in the world and is frequently associated with severe damage to the ocular surface. Corneal blindness is particularly prevalent in less-developed nations where diseases and infections may progress untreated (Garg *et al.*, 2005). Diseased and damaged corneas can be surgically removed and replaced with a button of corneal tissue sourced from cadavers (allografts) in a penetrating keratoplasty procedure. Corneal allografts may be successful and remain clear and provide a successful solution for some, but this is not always the case and recipients may require a second graft or an alternative option. The insufficient number of cadaveric corneas available for transplant is a serious issue and results from the unsuitability of some donated eyes for transplant, the low levels of organ donation due to religious and cultural factors, a lack of general education and the absence of eye-banking facilities, particularly in developing countries. Some ocular surface disorders can now be treated effectively by newer procedures involving the transplantation of biological entities such as autologus limbal stem cells (Tseng, 1989; Kenyon and Tseng, 1989; Dua and Azuara-Blanco, 2000) and/or amniotic membrane (Kim and Tseng, 1995; Park *et al.*, 2008). However, there are many ocular conditions that are recognised as having a 'high risk of failure' for the transplant of either corneal grafts or limbal stem cell/amnion approaches and these require an alternative option.

Together, these severe cases have left an unmet clinical need that has driven the development of synthetic corneal replacements. Synthetic devices that replace corneal tissue are known as 'keratoprostheses' (KPros) and are used to restore functional visual acuity (and, less commonly, alleviate pain in conditions such as keratopathy) in eyes with severe corneal disease and opacity that carry a poor prognosis for standard corneal transplantation. The ideal keratoprosthesis would be inert and not rejected by the patient's immune system, it would also be inexpensive and able to maintain long-term clarity. In addition, it would be quick to implant, easy to examine and allow an excellent view of the retina. Section 4.5 examines the history of design approaches to KPros and draws on the knowledge gained from those experiences, noting that each approach has a considerable device history which has been built on in the creation of newer iterations of KPro technologies.

4.5.2   Early use of materials as keratoprostheses

The material requirements and design of KPro devices are extremely challenging and have a substantial developmental lineage, which has been well reviewed in several articles (Hicks *et al.*, 1997; Chirila *et al.*, 1998). Pellier de Quengsy first proposed replacing the cornea with a device made of glass in the eighteenth century and also suggested that the artificial corneal device should have a porous skirt (Chirila *et al.*, 1998; Chirila and Hicks, 1999). In the mid-nineteenth century, this idea was tested when glass was implanted into the eyes of rabbits by Von Nussbaum and Neptuk. Heusser later implanted glass into human eyes that was retained for 3 months (Chirila *et al.*, 1998). In both cases, the implants were extruded, but these early efforts demonstrated that it was practically possible to replace the cornea with a synthetic material to let light into the eye, even if only for a short period. Interest in KPro development waned after the first successful human-to-human corneal tissue graft was performed in 1906 (Barnham and Roper-Hall, 1983). That interest was revived when it became evident that penetrating keratoplasty procedures were ineffective in cases of severe corneal disease and damage. Various reports of PMMA showing a relatively inert response when implanted or lodged in the corneas of animals and humans (Chirila and Crawford, 1996; Chirila *et al.*, 1998) served to increase awareness of new materials that might be used to replace the cornea.

Since that time, there have been many attempts at developing KPros with a variety of designs, such as fully penetrating and anterior or posterior perforating lamellar implants; the latter had a lower rate of extrusion but visual results were often compromised because of the presence of the residual stroma. These KPro devices utilised a range of materials and material treatments, implanted using various surgical techniques, and have been well reviewed by others (Barber, 1988; Hicks *et al.*, 1997; Chirila *et al.*, 1998; Chirila and Hicks, 1999; Khan *et al.*, 2001; Aquavella *et al.*, 2006; Liu *et al.*, 2008a; Myung *et al.*, 2008a). While KPro technologies vary in their approaches and design, all are aimed at replacing the central cornea with an optical core made from a transparent material (optic) that is anchored in the surrounding stromal tissue by a support or skirt (haptic). For the purposes of this chapter, a different classification of devices will be considered, namely those incorporating a biological support and those that are fully synthetic and without a biological support.

4.5.3   Keratoprostheses with a synthetic core with a biological support

Some of the working KPro designs have used PMMA for the optic and attached that to a biological material as a haptic to increase the likelihood of anchorage of the device in the cornea. The Cardona 'bolt and nut' two-piece penetrating KPro had retrocorneal fixation that required removal of the corneal epithelium, conjunctiva, tarsus plate, lid margin, inner outer rectus muscles, lens, vitreous and iris. A teflon supporting plate with dacron mesh was placed over the cornea and covered with autologous tissue, usually periosteum (Polack, 1976). The device was then covered by the upper lid, which was permanently sutured to the lower lid. The soft lid tissue was trephined to allow the PMMA optical cylinder to be threaded on to the retention plate and passed through the cornea into the globe. This KPro was designed to reduce the rate of extrusion seen with penetrating types of

KPros. A relatively recent histological evaluation of an eye implanted with a Cardona device showed that PMMA was a suitable material for an optic and had provided good post-operative visual acuity for the 14-year implantation period (Vijayasekaran *et al.*, 2005). The complex skirt area was considered to be predisposed to long-term inflammation. Less complicated surgery and a simple inert device with a flange with good mechanical and biological integration were recommended to reduce post-operative complications (Vijayasekaran *et al.*, 2005).

A slightly different approach was taken in the osteo-odonto-keratoprosthesis (OOKP) type of KPro originally developed by Strampelli in the 1960s and refined by Falcinelli in the 1970s (Falcinelli *et al.*, 2005; Hille *et al.*, 2005). Like the Cardona and other devices, the OOKP uses PMMA for the transparent optical cylinder and has undergone several design modifications over time. The OOKP has the PMMA optic mounted in a biological support consisting of a longitudinal section of an autologus tooth including some surrounding alveolar bone and ligament with periosteum (Falcinelli *et al.*, 2005; Liu *et al.*, 2005). In the absence of usable teeth, other tissues and matrices of biological origin have been tested such as cartilage (Casey, 1966), tibial bone in the osteo-KPro or Temprano-KPro (Michael *et al.*, 2008) or hydroxyapatite/coral (León *et al.*, 1997). OOKP and osteo-KPro devices are stabilised in the recipient's cornea by placing autologus buccal mucosa over the top which is opened some time later in a second procedure. These and other penetrating KPros are used to treat end-stage corneal blindness not amenable to penetrating keratoplasty, such as dry keratinised eye resulting from severe Stevens–Johnson syndrome, ocular cicatricial pemphigoid, trachoma and chemical injury resulting in severe corneal scarring leaving the ocular surface keratinised. Falcinelli and co-workers reported good long-term prognosis with the OOKP when they reviewed data from 181 patients implanted between 1973 and 1999 (Falcinelli *et al.*, 2005). Functional and anatomical analysis of the osteo-KPro and OOKP devices showed that both had similar functional results, with the OOKP having slightly better anatomical outcomes; the analysis showed that the difference was influenced more by the status of the retina rather than the actual procedure (Michael *et al.*, 2008). Complications include glaucoma, vitreo-retinal complications, inflammation, epithelial downgrowth and extrusion of the device which is frequently associated with resorption of the biological support (Stoiber *et al.*, 2002). Nonetheless, OOKP is particularly resilient to a hostile environment such as the severely dry eye and is regarded by many as 'the keratoprosthesis of choice for end-stage corneal blindness not amenable to penetrating keratoplasty' (Liu *et al.*, 2005; Liu *et al.*, 2008a). Liu has identified the interpentetrating pore network of the alveolar bone used for the biological support to be a key feature in the success of OOKP devices (Liu *et al.*, 2005). Interestingly, coral skeletons that have also shown good outcomes when tested as biological supports in this type of KPro are reported to have possess a similar pore geometry to dental bone (León *et al.*, 1997).

Dohlman and colleagues used PMMA for the optic of a 'collar button'-type KPro implanted in patients in 1974. The device, known as the Boston KPro, has involved a series of design iterations over 30 years, leading to the development of the two currently available versions aimed at full-thickness replacement of the cornea. Both designs require the patient's crystalline lens to be removed to allow implantation of the KPro. The Boston Type I device is designed for patients with sufficient tear production (wet eyes) and the Boston Type II is a device for people with ocular pemphigoid and very dry eyes, and is implanted through a closed eyelid (Dohlman and Doane, 1994). The Boston Type 1 KPro was approved by the FDA in 1992 and is the most effective and widely used of these designs. The current version incorporates a rim of donor corneal tissue that is placed over the stem of the front PMMA plate which is clamped and locked with a titanium ring. The periphery of the donor graft tissue is then sutured into the recipient's cornea, as it would be in a standard corneal graft procedure, and the corneal surface is covered with a soft contact lens. This KPro has shown good outcomes for many patients with non-autoimmune disease and those with previous graft failures who have no other ocular problems. Complications such as inflammation, endophthalmitis, vitritis, glaucoma and retroprosthetic membrane formation do occur and may respond to treatment. Analysis of device failures correlates to pre-operative diagnosis and patients with immune-related disease of the corneal surface are reported to develop inflammation leading to necrosis and melting of the corneal tissue and epithelial downgrowth around the front plate of the device that results in extrusion (Dudenhoefer *et al.*, 2003). Continual modifications to the design in response to problems and new understandings have improved the clinical outcomes for this device over the years of its development (Dohlman and Doane, 1994). The use of biological tissue with the device, in the form of a remnant rim of donor corneal tissue grafted with the device, encourages tissue integration to anchor the device in the cornea. The addition of holes to the PMMA back plate, previously solid, to improve the flow of nutrients from the aqueous humour forward to the grafted corneal tissue has increased the health of the graft and reduced the amount of tissue melt associated with the device (Harissi-Dagher *et al.*, 2007). The application of a soft contact lens to cover the anterior surface of the device and graft tissue post-operatively and continued in the long term has reduced the problem of corneal dehydration and tissue melting around the neck of the device (Harissi-Dagher *et al.*, 2008). Analysis of data from a multicentre study on 210 eyes fitted with the modified Boston Type 1 KPro between 2003 and 2007 showed graft retention rates up to 96% at 8–10 months post-operative, accompanied by vision improvements for 63% of recipients (Zerbe *et al.*, 2006; Belin, 2007). Other problems – such as advanced glaucoma, macular degeneration or retinal detachment – were found to be the primary cause of failures (Belin, 2007). The modified Boston Type I KPro may have better outcomes with patients who have had repeated graft failure rather than Stevens–Johnsons syndrome, cicatricial pemphigoid and chemical burns.

4.5.4   Keratoprostheses with a synthetic core and skirt

Concurrent activity involving a different KPro design approach utilised a fully synthetic 'core and skirt' device made possible by the development of microporous materials. These aimed to reduce the complication rates seen with the use of biological supports by replacing the biological tissue with skirts/haptics made from soft, microporous polymers to assist in the stable integration of the device into the host cornea. Several KPros have been developed on this design principle, some using optical cores made of PMMA which were attached to porous skirts, and other versions using soft hydrogels to create optics and skirts that were fused together to form one-piece devices.

The Seoul-type KPro (S-KPro) used PMMA for the optic in a double-fixed device with a porous flange of polyurethane or polypropylene material for stromal fixation and polypropylene haptics that were sutured to the sclera posterior to the iris to improve device stability. Initial studies (Lee *et al.*, 2000) conducted on the S-KPro involved implantation of the device into 25 rabbit eyes with histology showing that stromal fibroblasts colonised a polyurethane version of the flange/skirt material with a 40 μm pore size over the 2–4 month period of implantation. No retroprosthetic membrane formation was noted during that time, although retinal detachment was a problem and was thought to have been caused by the scleral haptics. Two human subjects, one with chemical burns and one with Stevens–Johnson syndrome, were also implanted with the S-KPro and both devices gave improved vision for the period of retention, which was 8 and 18 months respectively (Lee *et al.*, 2000). These preliminary studies suggested that a porous skirt material could allow biological integration with corneal tissue. Several different porous materials were then compared in rabbits with the best outcomes reported using a polypropylene skirt material (Kim *et al.*, 2002). More recent data from a small group of patients showed that S-KPro devices were retained for an average of 31.6 months, although all suffered from retinal detachments (Kim *et al.*, 2007).

The Pintucci KPro also used a PMMA optic, in this case secured to a soft, pliable skirt made from Dacron (polyethylene terephthalate; PET) fibres, which had an already established track record of use in cardiovascular devices. The porous skirt was designed to encourage integration of new collagen fibres and thus aid integration of the keratoprosthesis into the surrounding ocular tissue. The Pintucci KPro was colonised in the lower lid for 2 months to allow the porous skirt to populate with autologous fibroblasts; it was then removed and implanted in the cornea and covered with buccal mucosa until stable, and then exposed. Trials of this device in bilaterally blind patients who were unsuitable for corneal transplant showed a range of complications over several years including necrosis of the oral mucosa before exposure of the device, formation of retro-implant membranes, deposit formation, retinal and choroidal detachment, and device extrusion (Pintucci *et al.*, 1995). Some optimisation of the Dacron used in the haptic occurred to further encourage ingrowth of stromal fibroblasts (Pintucci *et al.*, 2001) and developments in the surgical technique used to implant the device have improved the clinical outcomes in patients with vascularised corneas (Pintucci *et al.*, 1996). More recent data from 31 patients blinded with corneal burns, vascularised corneas and dry eye have shown some retention of these devices in patients for up to 6–7 years but not without complications (Maskati and Maskati, 2006). Dacron has been reported to degrade significantly following implantation and this degradation may have contributed to the complications seen in long-term follow-up (Coury *et al.*, 1996). An 85% complication rate after 10 years' follow-up was reported with the Girard nut and bolt style KPro using a similar Dacron skirt with a PMMA optic (Girard, 1983).

Concurrently, a French group led by Legeais were developing a new KPro device with dimensions similar to the normal cornea which was initially based on a PMMA optic joined to a microporous fluorocarbon skirt made from expanded polytetrafluoroethylene (ePFTE). The haptic was inserted into a stromal lamellar pocket, then a PMMA optic was positioned in a hole made in the central cornea and clipped to the haptic with a PMMA clip and sealing ring which was covered with buccal mucosa for 2 months and then exposed. Implantation of this device did not require the removal of the iris or lens. Trials of this device in a small group of young bilaterally blind patients showed that the microporous skirt was colonised by stromal fibroblasts but the devices were not retained in the long term leading the group to conclude that the biocompatible, inert microporous polymer did not eliminate all of the mechanical complications associated with a KPro (Legeais *et al.*, 1995). The group continued to optimise the ePFTE used as the skirt to encourage stromal integration of the device (Drubaix *et al.*, 1996; Legeais *et al.*, 1997) and the material was also pre-seeded with corneal fibroblasts using a range of chemo-attractants to encourage their ingrowth prior to implantation (Dupuy *et al.*, 2001). The mechanical issues were also addressed by replacement of the rigid PMMA optical core by polydimethylsiloxane (PDMS) coated with polyvinylpyrrolidone and this was fused to the ePTFE skirt in a new one-piece design known as the BioKPro II (Legeais and Renard, 1998). This second-generation device was tested in human eyes with some acceptable optical outcomes but resulted in some anatomical failures that involved extrusions, retroprosthetic membranes and endophthalmitis (Legeais and Renard, 1998).

Legeais recognised that epithelial growth over the anterior surface of the device was essential for the long-term stability of the implant.

A synthetic cornea was also being developed at Boston University (Trinkaus-Randall group) using a transparent, flexible polyvinylalcohol (PVA) hydrogel with a refractive index of 1.42 which was bonded to a fibrous skirt of blown microfibre polybutylene and polypropylene (Tsuk *et al.*, 1997). The design of this KPro was strongly driven by an understanding of corneal biology, with the surface of the PVA optic plasma modified to encourage the growth of epithelial tissue, which occurred without any added biological coating when tested in an organ culture system (Latkany *et al.*, 1997). Devices were pre-seeded with stromal fibroblasts and epithelial cells to create a three-dimensional construct. Various iterations of these devices were implanted into rabbit corneas using different surgical procedures which resulted in partial epithelialisation of the surfaces at 3 weeks post-operative (Trinkaus-Randall *et al.*, 1997). Controlled release technology was also incorporated into the skirt to deliver growth factors aimed at promoting anchorage by increasing fibroplasia (Trinkaus-Randall and Nugent, 1998) and alternative materials were tested to improve the function of the skirt (Wu *et al.*, 1998). This work acknowledged the need for fibrous ingrowth for anchorage and also identified the need for epithelialisation of the anterior surface of a synthetic cornea but overall it failed to provide a long-term solution as a synthetic cornea.

Concurrent activity at the Lions Eye Institute and Centre for Ophthalmology and Visual Science in Perth in Western Australia (Chirila group) gave rise to a new design concept and material approach that involved a one-part, fused 'core-and-skirt' KPro. Both the core and skirt were made of the same soft, hydrogel material, PHEMA, that was prepared slightly differently to produce a transparent optical core that was fused to an opaque, macroporous peripheral skirt intended to promote anchorage of the device in the stromal tissue (Chirila *et al.*, 1993; Chirila *et al.*, 1994). Originally known as the Chirila KPro, this device was eventually marketed as the AlphaCor KPro (first by Argus Biomedical in Perth Australia, then by CooperVision in the USA, and now by Addition Technologies Inc., Des Plaines, Illinois, USA). It offered several advantages over competitive technologies at the time. It was a one-part device that could be sutured in place in a relatively simple procedure and in this sense was truly a synthetic corneal graft. The initial design version was sutured in place and covered with conjuctival tissue which was opened in a second procedure some months later. The later version was slightly smaller than the original and was implanted into a lamellar pocket with its posterior face removed and the anterior surface of the device covered by a corneal tissue and a conjunctival flap, which again was opened some months later. Early data arising from devices implanted in rabbit and human corneas demonstrated the potential of the AlphaCor technology (Hicks *et al.*, 1998; Hicks *et al.*, 2000; Hicks *et al.*, 2003). Later trials with 337 carefully selected patients showing retention rates of 80% at 1 year and 62% at 2 years (Hicks *et al.*, 2006). Over 300 AlphaCor devices have been implanted to date and followed for up to 7 years (Liu *et al.*, 2008a). The retention rates may be attributed to the porous nature of the KPro skirt, optimised during the design phase for fibroblastic ingrowth to anchor the device (Vijayasekaran *et al.*, 1998), which showed the presence of stromal fibroblasts and new collagen formation within the porous pHEMA material when explanted and examined histologically (Hicks *et al.*, 2005). Complications of the AlphaCor KPro include stromal melting and white deposits within the optical core (Hicks *et al.*, 2006), with topical medications used in conjunction with the AlphaCor KPro found to have contributed to the white calcium deposits (Vijayasekaran *et al.*, 2000; Hicks *et al.*, 2004). Cigarette smoke was identified as the cause of brown pigmentation noted in other AlphaCor implants (Hicks *et al.*, 2004) revealing the unexpected impact that environmental factors might have on KPro devices. Stromal melting has historically been recognised as a major problem with all KPro devices and is mediated by matrix metalloproteases that digest corneal stromal collagens. Melting associated with the AlphaCor KPro was addressed using topical treatment with medroxyprogesterone in some patients and data compared against those who were not treated. Outcomes showed the incidence of melting increased if medroxyprogesterone was used, but its use delayed the onset of the melting process (Hicks and Crawford, 2003). A more recent study of three patients implanted with AlphaCor devices which failed owing to stromal melting, used immunohistochemistry to show that fibroblasts that colonised the skirt to achieve biointegration were activated and transformed into a contractile, myofibroblast phenotype that was identified as a likely source of pro-inflammatory cytokines associated with stromal melting (Coassin *et al.*, 2007). These outcomes suggest that there might be an inadequate flux through the material causing tissue necrosis by nutritional deprivation of tissue forward of the implant. It is possible that the material used in the AlphaCor device may be slowly fouling, causing a progressive reduction of permeability with time. PHEMA hydrogels are recognised to be prone to calcification and, although the causes of this are not fully understood, their porous nature inherently creates surface defects which have been shown to increase the tendency for calcification (Lou *et al.*, 2005). Different techniques that simplified the surgical procedure used to implant the AlphaCor device, with the aim of reducing the surgical trauma, appear to have failed to improve the outcomes of this KPro device.

4.5.5   Overall outcomes on materials and devices for corneal repair and replacement

The health burden associated with corneal blindness, particularly in developing countries, will continue to drive research into improved KPro and corneal replacement technologies. The outcomes described with penetrating KPros demonstrate the degree of difficulty and the immense challenge presented in the retention of these devices which are the last choice of visual recovery for patients. The experience and efforts of previous researchers and clinicians provide guiding design principles for corneal replacement devices, as summarised in Table 4.3. Current information suggests that the best outcomes for KPro surgery are associated with careful pre-operative patient selection and lifelong post-operative care (Khan *et al.*, 2001; Liu *et al.*, 2008a). The AlphaCor PHEMA hydrogel device, which showed considerable promise initially, may be unable to meet the long-term challenge unless patients

Table 4.3 Characteristics of an ideal corneal replacement system

- Material(s) should be biocompatible with corneal tissue, i.e. non-inflammatory
- Material(s) for the central core should be transparent and have a refractive index close to corneal tissue
- Central core should be short and soft
- Central core should have a large enough diameter to maximise the field of view
- Good integration of the central core and peripheral skirt is essential, ideally a strong flexible union
- Material(s) for the peripheral skirt should allow ingrowth of stromal tissue and deposition of extracellular matrix in an ordered way to regenerate stromal tissue
- Materials for the skirt should be able to hold sutures or have a self-adhesive strategy
- Device should be tightly anchored in the cornea to retain the device and prevent leakage, infection and epithelial downgrowth
- Material(s) for the device should have a modulus that provides resistance to intraocular pressure but is flexible like corneal tissue to minimise mechanical stress
- Material(s) for the device should not impede the flow of nutrients through corneal tissue
- Anterior surface of device should be colonised with corneal epithelial cells in patients with a normal ocular environment, with a modified design and surgical procedure for others
- Downgrowth of epithelial cells around the internal components of the device should be prevented by the design and treatment of materials
- Posterior surface of the device should not support the formation of a retroprosthetic membrane but encourage the regrowth of an endothelial layer if possible
- Surgical procedure used to implant device should be minimised according to the needs of the patient with endothelium preserved wherever possible
- Patients should be carefully evaluated prior to surgery
- Patients should be closely monitored post-operatively for inflammation, glaucoma, infection, etc.
- Devices should be presented in various iterations specifically designed and tuned to treat the individual conditions that have made corneal replacement surgery necessary

are selected with great care. The Boston and OOKP devices, with their biological supports and PMMA cores, can achieve functional and anatomical outcomes for years in some patients. PMMA offers many good properties, such as transparency and chemical stability, but it is a very stiff material and while providing acceptable functional outcomes it may account for some of the anatomical failures. This issue may have been reduced by the soft modulus and porous nature of the PHEMA material used in the AlphaCor one-piece device. The development of posterior segment complications such as retroprosthetic membranes and retinal detachments may be addressed by improved KPro designs and new surgical techniques. Removal of opacified tissue in preparation for the implantation of KPro devices is traumatic to the corneal tissue. Less aggressive surgical techniques using new technological advances in equipment may help to achieve better outcomes in full-thickness corneal replacement. Infection with KPro devices is an issue that plagues this type of surgery and, although endophthalmitis can be treated with antibiotics, devices with anti-microbial strategies incorporated into/on to the materials could assist in reducing this problem. Epithelial growth over the anterior surface of the device would be ideal in protecting against necrosis and in assisting to retain the device in the cornea but the epithelium would need to be stable and multilayered to be beneficial (Hicks *et al.*, 1997; Allan, 1999). Rigid polymers like PMMA would not support epithelial growth nor would many hydrogels. Clearly, epithelial growth would not be a possibility in patients with compromised epithelial status (very dry eye or limbal damage) unless concurrent transplant therapies were used in combination, such as cleverly modified surfaces pre-colonised with stem cells.

4.6   Future trends

Much has been studied and attempted in the field of synthetic implants in the cornea but there is still a need for safe and effective long-term solutions. The successes and failures of previous work are instructive and provide a foundation for future approaches. Clearly, there is a need for systems that bring together innovations in materials, device design and surgical instrumentation combined with a knowledge and understanding of corneal biology, anatomy, physiology, neurobiology and wound healing.

4.6.1   Corneal implants to treat refractive errors

Intracorneal implants aimed at changing the refractive power of the eye should be manufactured from materials that are biostable in the corneal environment. These materials should also be transparent and highly permeable with low-fouling surfaces to address issues of loss of long-term clarity. Better optical designs that provide stable and predictable outcomes from the smallest and thinnest lens possible are most likely to succeed. Materials should also offer high levels of dimensional stability to provide stable optical outcomes. Improved manufacturing processes that enable porous materials to be made to specification are needed to address issues such as permeability and nerve regeneration. Pores should be small enough to not interfere with the scatter of light, numerous enough to provide adequate nutritional flux and ideally should provide for the regeneration of some nerves. Material treatments should reflect an understanding of corneal biology and, for onlays, be bi-functional, promoting epithelial growth and the sustained adhesion of a stratified epithelium on the anterior surface with anti-fibrotic treatments to reduce keratocyte activation on the posterior face. Micro- and nano-patterning may be used to encourage tissue adhesion on the anterior lens surface to compliment or even reduce the need for the addition of biological signals such as extracellular matrix molecules, peptides or growth factors to the polymer surface. Alternatively, layer-by-layer technology could be used to deliver signals in a specific temporal sequence. Patterning on the posterior surface could be used to reduce the chronic responses of the stromal tissue and minimise epithelial undergrowth. Minimally invasive surgical procedures, ideally above Bowman's layer, using instrumentation designed to reduce trauma to corneal tissue and allow centration of the implant would contribute to more predictable and stable refractive outcomes. New adhesive strategies based on chemistry rather than on physical glues or sutures could be used to attach a lens to a debrided stromal surface or beneath an epithelial pocket and assist in centration and prevention of device expulsion caused by epithelial undergrowth. Whatever the approaches, they need to be well integrated and involve multidisciplinary teams to achieve a synthetic intracorneal implant that offers rapid visual rehabilitation with a predictable refractive outcome in a fully reversible procedure.

4.6.2   Corneal replacement and repair: tissue regeneration

The challenge of corneal replacement and repair also requires new approaches, as the benefit of currently available technologies is limited to carefully selected patients and, even then, outcomes are not optimal. Solutions should be safe and effective in the long term. For the most part, emerging technologies in this area are being directed at scaffolds for *corneal regeneration* and may be used alone or pre-colonised with cells in tissue culture prior to implantation. Many involve new treatments and fabrication techniques for fully synthetic materials. Other strategies employ a tissue engineering approach using biologically based materials stabilised by chemical cross-linking or co-polymerisation with synthetic polymers to optimise the characteristics of the material. These scaffolds are likely to have great potential in corneal regeneration and may be used in the replacement of specific layers of the cornea providing an alternative to the trauma of penetrating keratoplasty where the full thickness of corneal tissue is removed and replaced with either transplanted cadaver corneal tissue or KPro devices. Target areas for the partial-thickness replacement of the cornea are the endothelial layer in cases of endothelial decompensation (e.g. endothelial dystrophies) or corneal stoma where it has been damaged by disease or trauma.

Stanford University's Bio-X initiative has enabled a cross-disciplinary group to design and fabricate a photolithographically patterned hydrogel construct (Duoptix™ arising from Stanford University in California, USA) based on an optic made from a double network of high water content polyethylene glycol/polyacrylic acid (PEG/PAA), with an interpenetrating skirt made of a microperforated hydrogel poly(hydroxyethyl acrylate) (PHEA) (Myung *et al.*, 2007; Myung *et al.*, 2008a). The design principles of this KPro reflect knowledge gained from all precedent devices and recognise many aspects of corneal biology. The skirt material is porous with microperforations created using photolithographic techniques to allow stromal ingrowth to anchor the device (Myung *et al.*, 2007). The optic component is permeable to the glucose flux that occurs from the aqueous humour to the epithelium to promote epithelialisation of the anterior surface of the device (Myung *et al.*, 2008b). The necessity of cell adhesion to the core and skirt material has been recognised and a coating of collagen I is provided to both to facilitate this process (Myung *et al.*, 2007). Recent data have shown that the PEG/PAA materials used in the optic support epithelial closure in an *in vitro* organ culture system when coated with collagen I (Myung *et al.*, 2009). This bioengineered cornea arising from the cross-disciplinary initiative has the potential to be used as a corneal replacement and possibly also as a material for a corneal implant (inlay or onlay) to correct refractive error.

The University of Ottawa Eye Institute (Griffith group) has developed a biosynthetic corneal matrix replacement that is intended to stabilise damaged tissue and allow for regeneration. Initial testing was conducted on hydrated collagen and *N*-isopropylacrylamide copolymers which formed a transparent, permeable biosynthetic material that supported cell and nerve growth *in vitro* (Li *et al.*, 2003). Since then, various collagen types have been stabilised by cross-linking with water-soluble carbodiimide chemistry and tested in animal corneas using lamellar keratectomy procedures. Stabilised porcine collagen type I implants showed evidence of stable integration in the stroma with some nerve regeneration at 6 months (Liu *et al.*, 2006). Mechanical testing of these implants at 12 months demonstrated 'seamless integration' in the host cornea which was attributed to the gradual turnover of the implanted matrix during the natural remodelling process (McLaughlin *et al.*, 2008). Stabilised human recombinant collagen types I and III have also been compared over 12 months with similar outcomes, including maintenance of optical clarity, stable integration in the corneal stroma and regeneration of the tear film, corneal cells and nerves (Liu et al., 2008b; Merrett et al., 2008). The cross-linked human recombinant collagen III was shown to be superior to a human amniotic membrane as a scaffold for the transplantation of limbal stem cells when tested in vitro (Dravida et al., 2008). The ability of this co-polymeric extracellular matrix replacement material to support nerve regeneration and the growth of corneal epithelial, stromal and stem cells in vitro shows great promise (Griffith et al., 2009). Recent reports on clinical testing of these corneal substitutes in patients with keratoconus and corneal scarring using a deep lamellar procedure reveal that keratocyte ingrowth occurred with these bioengineered implants, which also supported nerve ingrowth and re-surfacing by host epithelium for 9 months (Fagerholm et al., 2009).

McMaster University in Toronto (Sheardown group) has identified significant biological issues that were problematical to the success of KPro devices and has endeavoured to solve these issues using surface immobilisation strategies applied to PDMS. This material was selected as it possesses many of the target properties needed for a corneal replacement, including transparency, oxygen permeability and appropriate mechanical properties. The inherently hydrophobic surface of the PDMS was altered using gas plasma polymerisation techniques which enabled the linkage of various growth factors aimed at controlling cell adhesion. A 'growth factor therapy' approach was directed at the problems identified with existing KPro devices. One such problem was the downgrowth of corneal epithelial tissue, which contributes to the extrusion of KPro devices in vivo. TGF-β-modified surfaces, intended to increase stromal cell adhesion (needed for device anchorage) and decrease epithelial cell adhesion (the cause of downgrowth), were tested in vitro but this surface strategy failed to satisfy either requirement fully (Merrett et al., 2003). Another issue tackled with this approach was to improve the retention time of artificial corneal devices by promoting epithelial tissue adhesion to the anterior surface. To address this issue, epidermal growth factor (EGF) was covalently tethered to plasma-modified PDMS substrates and in vitro assays showed that this growth factor did increase the growth and proliferation of epithelial cells (Klenkler et al., 2005). More recently, slow release of growth factors has been achieved in vitro using cross-linked collagen matrices modified with heparin to deliver basic fibroblast growth factor (FGF-2) (Princz and Sheardown, 2008). Cell-adhesion peptides have also been incorporated into stabilised collagen scaffolds using similar dendrimer methodology and these have been shown to support corneal epithelial cell stratification using in vitro systems (Duan and Sheardown, 2007). The long-term stability and efficacy of these types of surfaces in vivo remains to be tested.

Biomimetic approaches to corneal replacement and/or repair are demonstrating the impact of combining new materials with fabrication technologies. The University of Wisconsin (Murphy and Nealey group) have considered the surface on which corneal epithelial cells would be migrating and growing if a synthetic material were implanted below the epithelium. Initial work used a range of microscopy techniques to characterise the topographical and morphological features of the corneal epithelial basement membrane in rhesus monkeys (Abrams *et al.*, 2000a) and humans (Abrams *et al.*, 2000b). This information was used to create replicates of basement membrane topography on culture substrates using lithographic techniques which were tested with corneal epithelial cells *in vitro*. Data showed that the cells were extremely sensitive to the defined surface features for their alignment and spreading behaviour (Teixeira *et al.*, 2003), strength of adhesion to the surface (Karuri *et al.*, 2004), migration over the surface (Diehl *et al.*, 2005), proliferation and differentiation (Liliensiek *et al.*, 2006) and protein adsorbed to the test surfaces (Fraser *et al.*, 2008). A collaborative approach in Europe (coordinated by David Hulmes) has produced a three-dimensional scaffold made from collagen fibrils aligned using horizontal magnetic fields in combination with a series of gelation–rotation–gelation cycles to produce orthogonal packing that resembles the lamellae of the corneal stroma (Torbet *et al.*, 2007). The California Institute of Technology (Tirrell group) is developing regenerative scaffolds for corneal repair using genetically engineered protein hydrogels with specified macromolecular architectures tuned to match the mechanical and erosion characteristics of the target tissue (Maskarinec and Tirrell, 2005; Shen *et al.*, 2006). The University of Sheffield (MacNeil/Rimmer collaboration) has developed a biocompatible, non-degradable material treatment for use in corneal replacement. This involves the chemical modification of the surface of low-adhesive hydrogel materials with plasma techniques to allow the attachment, migration and growth of corneal epithelial cells, which has shown promising outcomes when tested over the short term in co-culture with stromal cells *in vitro* (Rimmer *et al.*, 2007). The technology has been commercialised (CellTran Ltd) for a range of applications including corneal repair where corneal epithelial cells isolated from a healthy contra-lateral eye are expanded on the modified substrates under culture conditions and then transferred to help heal the damaged eye.

Research in the fields of biology, biochemistry and protein chemistry is also being directed at the challenge of corneal repair and replacement. At the University of Aarhus in Denmark (Enghild group), proteomics is being directed at the development of new therapies for treating corneal diseases by comparing proteins in normal corneas to those in disease states such as granular and lattice dystrophies that would usually require a transplant (Karring *et al.*, 2005). Various groups in the UK (Sandeman, Lloyd, Tighe) have worked together to screen materials for KPro devices by developing *in vitro* assays to model the inflammatory processes that occur following implantation of corneal replacement devices (Sandeman *et al.*, 2003). Biological studies at University College in London and the University of Auckland in New Zealand have shown that cell–cell communication through connexin 43 (Cx43) gap junction channels plays a major role in the epithelial and stromal wound-healing process following epithelial injury in cornea (Qiu *et al.*, 2003) and skin (Coutinho *et al.*, 2005; Mori *et al.*, 2006). This technology is being developed in a spin-out company (CoDa Therapeutics Inc., San Diego, California, USA) with a gel product containing Cx43 antisense that results in a transient downregulation of Cx43 protein levels and an increase in the rate of wound closure after a single topical application.

Concurrent developments in surgical techniques and instruments may reduce damage associated with surgery, speeding recovery and improving both anatomical and refractive outcomes in corneal replacement and repair. SupraDescemetic implantation is one new surgical technique which involves removal of the central corneal epithelium and stroma leaving Descemet's membrane and the endothelium intact. This potentially avoids the perforation of the anterior chamber, with its associated risks of leakage and infection, that occurs with conventional KPro surgery. Various synthetic materials have been tested in rabbit corneas to test this supraDescemetic synthetic cornea (sDSC) procedure (Stoiber *et al.*, 2004; Stoiber *et al.*, 2005) and have demonstrated that it is possible to implant a KPro device into the cornea without perforating Descemet's membrane, but progress has been thwarted by complications such as the formation of neovascularised tissue at the device–Descemet's membrane interface, which may prevent the long-term utility of this type of surgery. Descemet-stripping endothelial keratoplasty (DSEK) is a relatively new surgical procedure that is being used to replace the corneal endothelium in patients with endothelial dysfunction as an alternative to penetrating keratoplasty (Ham *et al.*, 2009). While the technique was developed to transplant donor Descemet's membrane carrying its endothelium (Ham *et al.*, 2009), other materials such as chitosan are being tested as degradable supports for the transfer of corneal endothelial cells (Gao *et al.*, 2008). The femtosecond laser is being used in a variety of surgical techniques and has allowed improved precision in making corneal incisions with laser energy focused to a particular depth minimising injury to the surrounding tissue (Donate *et al.*, 2004). At the current time, the femtosecond laser has been approved for use in a variety of refractive and corneal surgeries including LASIK flaps, and intrastromal incisions such as those used with ring implants, lamellar keratoplasty as well as penetrating keratoplasty.

4.7   Conclusions

The future relies on the outcome of innovative cross-disciplinary approaches that draw on knowledge and expertise in corneal biology, device design, materials and material treatments, surgery and surgical instrumentation. The events involved in corneal wound healing are complex and involve an interaction of all constituent cell and tissue types. Overlying corneal biology and physiology with mathematical disciplines such as biological modelling and network science may speed the understanding of the complexity of the interactions that occur between cells, tissues, nerves, proteins, functional molecules, etc. (Mete *et al.*, 2008; Winkler, 2008). Combinatorial approaches based on these and other initiatives can be expected to lead to the development of new multifunctional materials and designs offering innovative solutions for improving and restoring vision with intracorneal implants that augment, repair or replace specific parts or the entire cornea.

4.8   Acknowledgements

The authors would like to thank their colleagues Jukka Moilanen, Andrea Petznick, Tim Hughes and Keith McLean for their helpful comments during the preparation of this chapter.

4.9   References

American Academy of Ophthalmology (AAO) (2008), 'Academy testifies at FDA meeting on LASIK outcomes and satisfaction', *Medical News Today*, 28 April 2008, http://www.medicalnewstoday.com/articles/105545.php.

Abrams GA, Goodman SL, Nealey PF, Franco M and Murphy CJ (2000a), 'Nanoscale topography of the basement membrane underlying the corneal epithelium of the rhesus macaque', *Cell Tissue Res*, **299**, 39–46.

Abrams GA, Schaus SS, Goodman SL, Nealey PF and Murphy CJ (2000b), 'Nanoscale topography of the corneal epithelial basement membrane and Descemet's membrane of the human', *Cornea*, **19**, 57–64.

Alio JL, Mulet ME, Zapata LF, Vidal MT, De Rojas V and Javloy J (2004), 'Intracorneal inlay complicated by intrastromal epithelial opacification', *Arch Ophthalmol*, **122**, 1441–46.

Alio JL (2007), 'Presbyopia-correcting surgery: What, when and where to do it', *OSN SuperSite*, March 2007, http://www.osnsupersite.com/print.asp?rID=20917.

Allan B (1999), 'Artificial corneas', *BMJ*, **318**, 821–22.

Ambrósio RJ, Tervo T and Wilson SE (2008), 'LASIK-associated dry eye and neurotrophic epitheliopathy: pathophysiology and strategies for prevention and treatment', *J Refract Surg*, **24**, 396–407.

Anderson NJ, Edelhauser HF, Sharara N, Thompson KP, Rubinfeld RS, Devaney DM, L'hernault N and Grossniklaus HE (2002), 'Histologic and ultrastructural findings in human corneas after successful laser in situ keratomileusis', *Arch Ophthalmol*, **120**, 288–93.

Andrews PM (1976), 'Microplicae: characteristic ridge-like folds of the plasmalemma', *J. Cell Biol*, **68**, 420–29.

Aquavella JV (1994), 'Major refractive surgical techniques', *Ophthalmic Surg*, **25**, 573–75.

Aquavella JV, Qian Y, McCormick GJ and Palakuru JR (2006), 'Keratoprosthesis – current techniques', *Cornea*, **25**, 656–62.

Aumailley M (1995), 'Structure and supramolecular organisation of basement membranes', *Kidney Int*, **47**, S4–S7.

Azar DT, Pluznik D, Jain S and Khoury JM (1998), 'Gelatinase B and A expression after laser in situ keratomileusis and photorefractive keratectomy', *Arch Ophthalmol*, **116**, 1206–08.

Azar DT, Ang RT, Lee JB, Kato T, Chen CC, Jain S, Gabison E and Abad JC (2001), 'Laser subepithelial keratomileusis: electron microscopy and visual outcomes of flap photorefractive keratectomy', *Curr Opin Ophthalmol*, **12**, 323–28.

Azar DT, Ghanem RC, de la Cruz J, Hallak JA, Kojima T, Al-Tobaigy FM and Jain S (2008), 'Thin-flap (sub-Bowman keratomileusis) versus thick-flap laser in situ keratomileusis for moderate to high myopia: Case-control analysis', *J Cataract Refract Surg*, **34**, 2073–78.

Barber JC (1988), 'Keratoprosthesis: past and present', *Int Ophthalmol Clin*, **28**, 103–09.

Barnham JJ and Roper-Hall MJ (1983), 'Keratoprosthesis: a long-term review', *Br J Ophthalmol*, **67**, 468–74.

Barraquer JI (1949), 'Queratoplastia refractiva. estudios e informaciones oftalmologicas', **2**, 10–30.

Barraquer JI (1966), 'Modification of refraction by means of intracorneal inclusions', *Int Ophthalmol Clin*, **6**, 53–79.

Beebe DC and Masters BR (1996), 'Cell lineage and the differentiation of corneal epithelial cells', *Invest Ophthalmol Vis Sci*, **37**, 1815–25.

Beekhuis WH, McCarey BE, Waring GO and Van Rij G (1986), 'Hydrogel keratophakia: a microkeratome dissection in the monkey model', *Br J Ophthalmol*, **70**, 192–98.

Beekhuis WH, McCarey BE, Van Rij G and Waring GO (1987), 'Complications of hydrogel intracorneal lens in monkeys', *Arch Ophthalmol*, **105**, 116–22.

Belin MV (2007), 'Boston KPro collaborative study results', *Acta Ophthalmol Scand*, **85**, s240.

Bergmanson JPG (2008), *Clinical Ocular Anatomy and Physiology* (Texas Eye Research and Technology Center, Houston, Texas). ISBN-13:978-0-9800708-0-4

Bethke W (2007), 'Treating presbyopia from inside the cornea', *Rev Ophthalmolo News*, 14:09, http://www.revophth.com/index.asp?page=1_13509.htm.

Beuerman RW and Thompson HW (1992), 'Molecular and cellular responses of the corneal epithelium to wound healing', *Acta Ophthalmol Suppl*, **202**, 7–12.

Beuerman RW and Pedroza L (1996), 'Ultrastructure of the human cornea', *Micros Res Tech*, **33**, 320–35.

Binder PS, Deg JK, Zavala EY and Grossman KR (1981/82), 'Hydrogel keratophakia in non-human primates', *Curr Eye Res*, **1**, 535–42.

Binder PS and Zavala EY (1987), 'Why do some epikeratoplasties fail?', *Arch Ophthalmol*, **105**, 63–69.

Binder PS, Rock ME, Schmidt KC and Anderson JA (1991), 'High voltage electron microscopy of normal human cornea', *Invest Ophthalmol Vis Sci*, **32**, 2234–43.

Binder PS (2006), 'One thousand consecutive IntraLase laser in situ keratomileusis flaps', *J Cat Refract Surg*, **32**, 962–69.

Birk DE, Fitch JM and Linsenmayer TF (1986), 'Organisation of collagen types I and V in the embryonic chick cornea', *Invest Ophthalmol Vis Sci*, **27**, 1470–77.

Borrodori L and Sonnenberg A (1999), 'Structure and function of hemidesmosomes: more than simple adhesion complexes', *J Invest Dermatol*, **112**, 411–18.

Bourne WM and McLaren JW (2004), 'Clinical responses of the corneal endothelium', *Exp Eye Res*, **78**, 561–72.

Brown SI and Dohlman CH (1965), 'A buried corneal implant serving as a barrier to fluid', *Arch Ophthalmol*, **73**, 635–39.

Browning AC, Shah S, Dua HS, Maharajan SV, Gray T and Bragheeth MA (2003), 'Alcohol debridement of the corneal epithelium in PRK and LASEK: an electron microscopic study', *Invest Ophthalmol Vis Sci*, **44**, 510–13.

Buck RC (1983), 'Ultrastructural characteristics associated with the anchoring of the corneal epithelium in several classes of vertebrates', *J Anat*, **137**, 743–56.

Burgeson RE, Lundstrum GP, Rokosova B, Rimberg CS, Rosenbaum LM and Keene DR (1990), 'The structure and function of type VII collagen', *Ann N Y Acad Sci*, **580**, 32–43.

Buschke W (1949), 'Morphologic changes in cells of corneal epithelium in wound healing', *Arch Ophthalmol*, **41**, 306–16.

Camellin M and Wyler D (2008), 'Epi-LASIK versus epi-LASEK', *J Refract Surg*, **24**, S57–S63.

Carrasquillo KG, Rand J and Talamo JH (2007), 'Intacs for keratoconus and post-LASIK ectasia: mechanical versus femtosecond laser-assisted channel creation', *Cornea*, **26**, 956–62.

Casey TA (1966), 'Osteo-odonto-keratoprosthesis', *Proc R Soc Med*, **59**, 530–1.

Cenedella RJ and Fleschner CR (1990), 'Kinetics of corneal epithelium turnover *in vivo*. Studies of lovastatin', *Invest Ophthalmol Vis Sci*, **31**, 1957–62.

Chang CY, Green CR, McGhee CN and Sherwin T (2008), 'Acute wound healing in the human central corneal epithelium appears to be independent of limbal stem cell influence', *Invest Ophthalmol Vis Sci*, **49**, 5279–86.

Chaouk H, Wilkie JS, Meijs GF and Cheng HY (2001), 'New porous perfluoropolyether membranes', *J Appl Polym Sci*, **80**, 1756–63.

Chen CC, Chang JH, Lee JB, Javier J and Azar DT (2002), 'Human corneal epithelial cell viability and morphology after dilute alcohol exposure', *Invest Ophthalmol Vis Sci*, **43**, 2593–602.

Chen WL, Chang HW and Hu FR (2008), '*In vivo* confocal microscopic evaluation of corneal wound healing after epi-LASIK', *Invest Ophthalmol Vis Sci*, **49**, 2416–23.

Chirila TV, Constable IJ, Crawford J, Vijayasekaran S, Thompson DE, Chen Y-C, Fletcher WA and Griffin BJ (1993), 'Poly(2-hydroxyethyl methacrylate) sponges as implant materials: *in vivo* and *in vitro* evaluation of cellular invasion', *Biomaterials*, **14**, 26–38.

Chirila TV, Vijayasekaran S, Horne R, Chen Y-C, Dalton P, Constable IJ and Crawford GJ (1994), 'Interpenetrating polymer network (IPN) as a permanent joint between the elements of a new type of artificial cornea', *J Biomed Mater Res*, **28**, 745–53.

Chirila TV and Crawford GJ (1996), 'A controversial episode in the history of artificial cornea: the first use of poly(methyl methacrylate)', *Gesnerus*, **53**, 236–42.

Chirila TV, Hicks CR, Vijayasekaran S, Lou X, Hong Y, Clayton AB, Ziegelaar BW, Fitton JH, Platten S, Crawford GJ and Constable IJ (1998), 'Artificial cornea', *Prog Polym Sci*, **23**, 447–73.

Chirila TV and Hicks CR (1999), 'The origins of the artificial cornea: Pellier de Quengsy and his contribution to the modern concept of keratoprosthesis', *Gesnerus*, **56**, 96–106.

Choi CY, Kim JY, Kim MJ and Tchah H (2008a), 'Transmission electron microscopy study of corneal epithelial flaps following removal using mechanical scraping, alcohol, and epikeratome techniques', *J Refract Surg*, **24**, 667–70.

Choi SK, Kim JH, Lee D, Lee JB, Kim HM, Tchah HW, Hahn TW, Joo M and Ha CI (2008b), 'Different epithelial cleavage planes produced by various epikeratomes in epithelial laser in situ keratomileusis', *J Cataract Refract Surg*, **34**, 2079–84.

Choyce DP (1968), 'The present status of intracameral and intra-corneal implants', *Canad J Ophthalmol*, **3**, 295–311.

Choyce DP (1982) 'Semi-rigid corneal inlays in the management of albinism, aniridia and ametropia', in Henkind P (Ed.), *Proceedings of the 24th International Congress of Ophthalmology*. San Francisco, Lippincott.

Choyce DP (1985), 'The correction of refractive errors with polysulfone corneal inlays', *Trans Ophthalmol Soc UK*, **104**, 332.

Climenhaga H, Macdonald JM, McCarey BE and Waring GO (1988), 'Effect of diameter and depth on the response to solid polysulphone intracorneal lenses in cats', *Arch Ophthalmol*, **106**, 818–24.

Coassin M, Zhang C, Green WR, Aquavella JV and Akpek EK (2007), 'Histopathologic and immunologic aspects of AlphaCor artificial cornea failure', *Am J Ophthalmol*, **144**, 699–704.

Colin J (2008) 'Expert shows intracorneal rings stable over 10 years', *OSN SuperSite Top Story*, http.www.osnsupersite.com/view.aspx?rid = 31222 jump.

Coskunseven E, Kymionis GD, Tsiklis NS, Atun S, Arslan E, Jankov MR and Pallikaris IG (2008), 'One-year results of intrastromal corneal ring segment implantation (KeraRing) using femtosecond laser in patients with keratoconus', *Am J Ophthalmol*, **145**, 775–79.

Cotlier E (1975), 'The lens', in Moses RA (Ed.), *Adler's Physiology of the Eye; Clinical Applications*. Saint Louis, USA, C.V. Mosby Company, pp. 275–97.

Cotsarelis G, Cheng S-Z, Dong G, Sun T-T and Lavker RM (1989), 'Existence of slow-cycling limbal epithelial basal cells that can be preferentially stimulated to proliferate: implications on epithelial stem cells', *Cell*, **57**, 201–09.

Coury AJ, Levy RJ, McMillin CR, Pathak Y, Ratner BD, Schoen FJ, Williams DF and Williams RL (1996), 'Degradation of materials in the biological environment', in Rattner BD, Hoffman AS, Schoen FJ and Lemon JE (Eds), *Biomaterials Science: An Introduction to Materials in Medicine*. San Diego, Academic Press, pp. 243–60.

Coutinho P, Qiu C, Frank S, Wang CM, Brown T, Green CR and Becker DL (2005), 'Limiting burn extension by transient inhibition of Connexin43 expression at the site of injury', *Br J Plast Surg*, **58**, 658–67.

Crosson CE, Klyce SD and Beuerman RW (1986), 'Epithelial wound closure in the rabbit cornea: a biphasic process', *Invest Ophthalmol Vis Sci*, **27**, 464–73.

Dalton BA, Evans MDM, McFarland GA and Steele JG (1999), 'Modulation of corneal epithelial stratification by polymer surface topography', *J Biomed Mater Res*, **45**, 384–94.

Dalton BA, McFarland GA and Steele JG (2001), 'Stimulation of epithelial tissue migration by certain porous topographies is independent of fluid flux', *J Biomed Mater Res*, **56**, 83–92.

Dalton M (2008), 'Presbyopia – Corneal inlays: the next big thing?', *Eyeworld News Mag*, http.//www.eyeworld.orlarticle.php?sid = 4286.

Darwish T, Brahma A, Efron N and O'Donnell C (2007), 'Subbasal nerve regeneration after LASEK measured by confocal microscopy', *J Refract Surg*, **23**, 709–15.

Davanger M and Evensen A (1971), 'Role of pericorneal papillary structure in renewal of corneal epithelium', *Nature*, **229**, 560–61.

Dawson DG, Holley GP, Geroski DH, Waring GO 3rd, Grossniklaus HE and Edelhauser

HF (2005), 'Ex vivo confocal microscopy of human LASIK corneas with histologic and ultrastructural correlation', *Ophthalmology*, **112**, 634–44.

Dawson DG, Grossniklaus HE, McCarey BE and Edelhauser HF (2008), 'Biomechanical and wound healing characteristics of corneas after excimer laser keratorefractive surgery: is there a difference between advanced surface ablation and sub-Bowman's keratomileusis?', *J Refract Surg*, **24**, S90–S96.

Daxer A (2008), 'Corneal intrastromal implantation surgery for the treatment of moderate and high myopia', *J Cataract Refract Surg*, **34**, 194–98.

Deg JK and Binder PS (1988), 'Histopathology and clinical behavior of polysulfone intracorneal implants in the baboon model. Polysulfone lens implants', *Ophthalmology*, **95**, 506–15.

Diehl KA, Foley JD, Nealey PF and Murphy CJ (2005), 'Nanoscale topography modulates corneal epithelial cell migration', *J Biomed Mater Res A*, **75**, 603–11.

Dohlman CA, Refojo MF and Rose J (1967), 'Synthetic polymers in corneal surgery. I. Glycerol methacrylate', *Arch Ophthalmol*, **77**, 252–57.

Dohlman CH and Doane MG (1994), 'Some factors influencing outcome after keratoprosthesis surgery', *Cornea*, **13**, 214–18.

Donate D, Albert O, Colliac JP, Tubelis P, Sabatier P, Mourou G, Burillon C, Pouliquen YM and Legeais J-M (2004), 'Femtosecond laser: a micromachining system for corneal surgery', *J Fr Ophtalmol*, **27**, 783–89.

Dravida S, Gaddipati S, Griffith M, Merrett K, Lakshmi Madhira S, Sangwan VS and Vemuganti GK (2008), 'A biomimetic scaffold for culturing limbal stem cells: a promising alternative for clinical transplantation', *J Tissue Eng Regen Med*, **2**, 263–71.

Drubaix I, Legeais J-M, Malek-Chesire N, Savoldelli M, Menasche M, Robert L, Renard G and Pouliquen Y (1996), 'Collagen synthesised in fluorocarbon polymer implant in the rabbit cornea', *Exp Eye Res*, **62**, 367–76.

Du Y, Funderburgh ML, Mann MM, SundarRaj N and Funderburgh JL (2005), 'Multipotent stem cells in human corneal stroma', *Stem Cells*, **23**, 1266–75.

Dua HS, Gomes JAP and Singh A (1994), 'Corneal epithelial wound healing', *Br J Ophthalmol*, **78**, 401–08.

Dua HS and Azuara-Blanco A (2000), 'Limbal stem cells of the corneal epithelium', *Surv Ophthalmol*, **44**, 415–25.

Duan X and Sheardown H (2007), 'Incorporation of cell-adhesion peptides into collagen scaffolds promotes corneal epithelial stratification', *J Biomater Sci Polym Ed*, **18**, 701–11.

Dudenhoefer EJ, Nouri M, Gipson IK, Baratz KH, Tisdale AS, Dryja TP, Abad JC and Dohlman CH (2003), 'Histopathology of explanted collar and button keratoprostheses: a clinicopathologic correlation', *Cornea*, **22**, 424–28.

Dupont D, Gravagna P, Albinet P, Tayot J-L, Romanet J-P, Mouillon M and Eloy R (1989), 'Biocompatability of human type IV intracorneal implants', *Cornea*, **8**, 251–58.

Dupps WJJ and Wilson SE (2006), 'Biomechanics and wound healing in the cornea', *Exp Eye Res*, **83**, 709–20.

Dupuy FP, Savoldelli M, Robert AM, Robert L, Legeais J-M and Renard G (2001), 'Chemotactic penetration of keratocytes in ePTFE polymer *in vitro*', *J Biomed Mater Res*, **56**, 487–93.

Espana EM, Grueterich M, Mateo A, Romano AC, Yee SB, Yee RW and Tseng SC (2003), 'Cleavage of corneal basement membrane components by ethanol exposure in laser-assisted subepithelial keratectomy', *J Cat Refract Surg*, **26**, 1192–97.

Esquenazi S, Bui V and Bibas O (2006), 'Surgical correction of hyperopia', *Surv Ophthalmol*, **51**, 381–418.

Evans MDM and Steele JG (1997), 'Multiple attachment mechanisms of corneal epithelial cells to a polymer – cells can attach in the absence of exogenous adhesion proteins through a mechanism that requires microtubules', *Exp Cell Res*, **233**, 88–98.

Evans MDM and Steele JG (1998), 'The effect of polymer surface chemistry on cell attachment, growth and deposition of extracellular matrix components by corneal epithelial cells', *J Biomed Mater Res*, **40**, 621–30.

Evans MDM, Dalton BA and Steele JG (1999), 'Persistent adhesion of epithelial tissue is sensitive to polymer topography', *J Biomed Mater Res*, **45**, 485–93.

Evans MDM, Xie RZ, Fabbri M, Madigan MC, Chaouk H, Beumer GJ, Meijs GF, Griesser H, Steele JG and Sweeney DF (2000), 'Epithelialization of a synthetic polymer in the feline cornea – a preliminary study', *Invest Ophthalmol Vis Sci*, **41**, 1674–80.

Evans MDM, McLean KM, Hughes TC and Sweeney DF (2001a), 'A review of the development of a synthetic corneal onlay for refractive correction', *Biomaterials*, **22**, 3319–28.

Evans MDM, McFarland GA, Taylor S, Johnson G and McLean KM (2001b), 'The architecture of a collagen coating on a synthetic polymer influences epithelial adhesion', *J Biomed Mater Res*, **56**, 461–68.

Evans MDM, Xie RZ, Fabbri M, Bojarski B, Chaouk H, Wilkie JS, McLean KM, Chen HY and Sweeney DF (2002), 'Progress in the development of a synthetic corneal onlay', *Invest Ophthalmol Vis Sci*, **43**, 319–201.

Evans MDM, Taylor S, Dalton BA and Lohmann D (2003), 'Polymer design for corneal epithelial tissue adhesion: Pore density', *J Biomed Mater Res A*, **64**, 357–64.

Fagerholm P, Lagali N and Griffith M (2009) 'Biosynthetic corneas: Evaluation in humans', European Society of Cataract and Refractive Surgeons (ESCRS), 13th Winter Meeting, Rome, February 2009, http://www.escrs.org/EVENTS/09rome/free paperlisting.asp?day=07102/2009.

Falcinelli G, Falsini B, Taloni M, Colliardo P and Falcinelli G (2005), 'Modified osteo-odonto-keratoprosthesis for treatment of corneal blindness: long-term anatomical and functional outcomes in 181 cases', *Arch Ophthalmol*, **123**, 1319–29.

Fini ME (1999), 'Keratocyte and fibroblast phenotypes in the repairing cornea', *Prog Retin Eye Res*, **18**, 529–51.

Fitton HJ, Dalton BA, Beumer G, Johnson G, Griesser HJ and Steele JG (1998), 'Surface topography can interfere with epithelial tissue migration', *J Biomed Mater Res*, **42**, 245–57.

Fraser SA, Ting YH, Mallon KS, Wendt AE, Murphy CJ and Nealey PF (2008), 'Sub-micron and nanoscale feature depth modulates alignment of stromal fibroblasts and corneal epithelial cells in serum-rich and serum-free media', *Biomed Mater Res A*, **86**, 725–35.

Friend J (1979), 'Biochemistry of ocular surface epithelium', *Int Ophthalmol Clin*, **19**, 73–91.

Funderburgh JL, Mann MM and Funderburgh ML (2003), 'Keratocyte phenotype mediates proteoglycan structure: a role for fibroblasts in corneal fibrosis', *J Biol Chem*, **278**, 45629–37.

Gao X, Liu W, Han B, Wei X and Yang C (2008), 'Preparation and properties of a chitosan-based carrier of corneal endothelial cells', *J Mater Sci Mater Med*, **19**, 3611–19.

Garana RMR, Petroll WM, Chen W-T, Herman IM, Barry P, Andrews P, Cavanagh HD and Jester JV (1992), 'Radial keratectomy II. Role of the myofibroblast in corneal wound contraction', *Invest Ophthalmol Vis Sci*, **33**, 3271–82.

Garcia-Hirschfeld J, Lopez-Briones LG and Belmonte C (1994), 'Neurotrophic influences on corneal epithelial cells', *Exp Eye Res*, **59**, 597–605.

Garg P, Krishna PV, Stratis AK and Gopinathan U (2005), 'The value of corneal transplantation in reducing blindness', *Eye*, **19**, 1106–14.

Ghanem VC, Souza GC, Souza DC, Viese JM, Weber SL and Kara-José N (2008), 'PRK and butterfly LASEK: prospective, randomized, contralateral eye comparison of epithelial healing and ocular discomfort', *J Refract Surg*, **24**, 591–99.

Gipson IK, Spurr-Michaud S and Tisdale AS (1987), 'Anchoring fibrils form a complex network in human and rabbit cornea', *Invest Ophthalmol Vis Sci*, **28**, 212–20.

Gipson IK (1989) 'Epithelial response to injury', in Proceedings of *Corneal Biomechanics and Wound Healing*, pp. 161–70.

Girard LJ (1983), 'Keratoprosthesis', *Cornea*, **2**, 207–24.

Green KJ and Jones JCR (1996), 'Desmosomes and hemidesmosomes: structure and function of molecular components', *FASEB*, **10**, 871–81.

Griffith M, Jackson WB, Lagali N, Merrett K, Li F and Fagerholm P (2009), 'Artificial corneas: a regenerative medicine approach', *Eye*, advance online publication, doi: 10.1038/eye.2008,409.

Grossniklaus HE, Lass JH, Jacobs G, Margo CE and McAuliffe KM (1989), 'Light microscopic and ultrastructural findings in failed epikeratoplasty', *Refract Corneal Surg*, **5**, 296–301.

Guo N, Kanter D, Funderburgh ML, Mann MM, Du Y and Funderburgh JL (2007), 'A rapid transient increase in hyaluronan synthase-2 mRNA initiates secretion of hyaluronan by corneal keratocytes in response to transforming growth factor beta', *J Biol Chem*, **282**, 12475–83.

Ham L, Dapena I, van Luijk C, van der Wees J and Melles GR (2009), 'Descemet membrane endothelial keratoplasty (DMEK) for Fuch's endothelial dystrophy: review of the first 50 consecutive cases', *Eye*, advance online publication, doi: 10.1038/eye.2008.393.

Hamrah P, Liu Y, Zhang Q and Dana MR (2003), 'The corneal stroma is endowed with a significant number of resident dendritic cells', *Invest Ophthalmol Vis Sci*, **44**, 581–89.

Hamrah P and Dana MR (2007), 'Corneal antigen-presenting cells', *Chem Immunol Allergy*, **92**, 58–70.

Hanna C and O'Brien JE (1960), 'Cell production and migration in the epithelial layer of the cornea', *Arch Ophthalmol*, **64**, 88–91.

Hanna C (1966), 'Proliferation and migration of epithelial cells during corneal wound repair in the rabbit and rat', *Am J Ophthalmol*, **61**, 55–63.

Hanna KD, Pouliquen YM, Savoldelli M, Fantes F, Thompson KP, Waring GO 3rd and Samson J (1990), 'Corneal wound healing in monkeys 18 months after excimer laser photorefractive keratectomy', *Refract Corneal Surg*, **6**, 343–45.

Harissi-Dagher M, Khan BF, Schaumberg DA and Dohlman CH (2007), 'Importance of nutrition to corneal grafts when used as a carrier of the Boston Keratoprosthesis', *Cornea*, **26**, 564–68.

Harissi-Dagher M, Beyer J and Dohlman CH (2008), 'The role of soft contact lenses as an adjunct to the Boston keratoprosthesis', *Int Ophthalmol Clin*, **48**, 43–51.

Herrmann WA, Hillenkamp J, Hufendiek K, Prahs P, Lohmann CP, Helbig H and Kobuch K (2008), 'Epi-laser in situ keratomileusis: comparative evaluation of epithelial separation with 3 microkeratomes', *J Cataract Refract Surg*, **34**, 1761–66.

Hicks C, Crawford G, Chirila T, Wiffen S, Vijayasekaran S, Lou X, Fitton J, Maley M, Clayton A, Dalton P, Platten S, Ziegelaar B, Hong Y, Russo A and Constable I (2000), 'Development and clinical assessment of an artificial cornea', *Prog Retin Eye Res*, **19**, 149–70.

Hicks CR, Fitton JH, Chirila TV, Crawford GJ and Constable IJ (1997), 'Keratoprostheses: advancing toward a true artificial cornea', *Surv Ophthalmol*, **42**, 175–89.

Hicks CR, Chirila TV, Clayton AB, Fitton HJ, Vijayasekaran S, Dalton PD, Lou X, Platten S, Ziegelaar B, Hong Y, Crawford GJ and Constable IJ (1998), 'Clinical results of implantation of the Chirila keratoprosthesis in rabbits', *Br J Ophthalmol*, **82**, 18–25.

Hicks CR, Crawford GJ, Lou X, Tan DT, Snibson GR, Sutton G, Downie N, Werner L, Chirila TV and Constable IJ (2003), 'Corneal replacement using a synthetic hydrogel cornea', *Eye*, **17**, 385–92.

Hicks CR and Crawford GJ (2003), 'Melting after keratoprostheis implantation: the effects of medroxyprogesterone', *Cornea*, **22**, 497–500.

Hicks CR, Chirila TV, Werner L, Crawford GJ, Apple DJ and Constable IJ (2004), 'Deposits in artificial corneas: risk factors and prevention', *Clin Experiment Ophthalmol*, **32**, 185–91.

Hicks CR, Werner L, Vijayasekaran S, Mamalis N and Apple DJ (2005), 'Histology of AlphaCor skirts: evaluation of biointegration', *Cornea*, **24**, 933–40.

Hicks CR, Crawford GJ, Dart JK, Grabner G, Holland EJ, Stulting RD, Tan DT and Bulsara M (2006), 'AlphaCor: Clinical outcomes', *Cornea*, **25**, 1034–42.

Hille K, Grabner G, Liu C, Colliardo P, Falcinelli G, Taloni M and Falcinelli G (2005), 'Standards for modified osteoodontokeratoprosthesis (OOKP) surgery according to Strampelli and Falcinelli: the Rome–Vienna Protocol', *Cornea*, **24**, 895–908.

Hughes TC and Chan GYN (2001), 'Design principles of synthetic corneal inlays and onlays', *Materials Forum*, **25**, 216–45.

Ismail MM (2002), 'Correction of hyperopia with intracorneal implants', *J Cat Refract Surg*, **28**, 527–30.

Ismail MM (2006), 'Correction of hyperopia by intracorneal lenses – Two-year follow-up', *J Cataract Refract Surg*, **32**, 1657–60.

Jacobsen IE, Jensen OA and Prause JU (1984), 'Structure and composition of Bowman's membrane', *Acta Ophthalmol*, **62**, 39–53.

Jester JV, Petroll WM, Feng W, Essepian J and Cavanagh HD (1992), 'Radial keratotomy. 1. The wound healing process and measurement of incisional gape in two animal models using in vivo confocal microscopy', *Invest Ophthalmol Vis Sci*, **33**, 3255–70.

Jester JV, Petroll WM and Cavanagh HD (1999), 'Corneal stromal wound healing in refractive surgery: the role of myofibroblasts', *Prog Retin Eye Res*, **18**, 311–56.

Jones PH and Watt FM (1993), 'Separation of human epidermal cells from transient amplifying cells on the basis of differences in integrin function and expression', *Cell*, **73**, 713–24.

Joyce NC (2003), 'Proliferative capacity of the corneal endothelium', *Prog Retin Eye Res*, **22**, 359–89.

Kalyvianaki MI, Kymionis GD, Kounis GA, Panagopoulou SI, Grentzelos MA and Pallikaris IG (2008), 'Comparison of Epi-LASIK and off-flap Epi-LASIK for the treatment of low and moderate myopia', *Ophthalmology*, **115**, 2174–80.

Karring H, Thøgersen IB, Klintworth GK, Møller-Pedersen T and Enghild JJ (2005), 'A dataset of human cornea proteins identified by Peptide mass fingerprinting and tandem mass spectrometry', *Mol Cell Proteomics*, **4**, 1406–08.

Karuri NW, Liliensiek SJ, Teixeira AI, Abrams G, Campbell S, Nealey PF and Murphy CJ (2004), 'Biological length scale topography enhances cell-substratum adhesion of human corneal epithelial cells', *J Cell Sci*, **117**, 3153–64.

Kaufman HE (1980), 'The correction of aphakia', *Am J Ophthalmol*, **89**, 1–10.

Kaufman HE (1989), 'Refractive surgery: through the looking glass', *Acta Ophthalmol Suppl*, **192**, 30–37.

Kayes J and Holmberg A (1960), 'The fine structure of Bowman's layer and the basement membrane of the corneal epithelium', *Am J Ophthalmol*, **50**, 1013–21.

Kenyon KR and Tseng SCG (1989), 'Limbal autograft transplantation for ocular surface disorders', *Ophthalmology*, **96**, 709–23.

Khan BF, Dudenhoefer EJ and Dohlman CH (2001), 'Keratoprosthesis: an update', *Ophthalmology*, **12**, 288–93.

Kim JC and Tseng SC (1995), 'Transplantation of preserved human amniotic membrane for surface reconstruction in severely damaged rabbit corneas', *Cornea*, **14**, 473–84.

Kim MK, Lee JL, Wee WR and Lee JH (2002), 'Comparative experiments for in vivo fibroplasia and biological stability of four porous polymers intended for use in the Seoul-type keratoprosthesis', *Br J Ophthalmol*, **86**, 809–14.

Kim MK, Lee SM, Lee JL, Chung TY, Kim YH, Wee WR and Lee JH (2007), 'Long-term outcome in ocular intractable surface disease with Seoul-type keratoprosthesis', *Cornea*, **26**, 546–51.

Kirkness CM, Steele AD and Garner A (1985), 'Polysulphone corneal inlays. Adverse reactions: A preliminary report', *Trans Ophthalmol Soc UK*, **104**, 343–50.

Klenkler BJ, Griffith M, Becerril C, West-Mays JA and Sheardown H (2005), 'EGF-grafted PDMS surfaces in artificial cornea applications', *Biomaterials*, **26**, 7286–96.

Knorz MC (2005), 'PermaVision corneal implants show good results in phase 2 trials', reported by Schultz J, *OSN SuperSite*, March 1st 2005, http://www.osnsupersite.com/view.aspx?rid=5894.

Koenig SB, Hamano T, Yamaguchi T, Kimura T, McDonald MB and Kaufman HE (1984), 'Refractive keratoplasty with hydrogel implants in primates', *Ophthalmic Surg*, **15**, 225–29.

Komai Y and Ushiki T (1991), 'The three-dimensional organization of collagen fibrils in the human cornea and sclera', *Invest Ophthalmol Vis Sci*, **32**, 2244–58.

Kramer TR, Chuckpaiwong V, Dawson DG, L'hernault N, Grossniklaus HE and Edelhauser HF (2005), 'Pathologic findings in postmortem corneas after successful laser *in situ* keratomileusis', *Cornea*, **24**, 92–102.

Krwawicz T (1960), 'Attempted modification of corneal curvature by means of experimental plastic surgery', *Klin Oczna*, **30**, 229.

Kwitko S and Severo NS (2004), 'Ferrara intracorneal ring segments for keratoconus', *J Cataract Refract Surg*, **30**, 812–20.

Kymionis GD, Bouzoukis DI and Pallikaris IG (2007a), 'Corneal inlays: a surgical correction of presbyopia', *Cataract Refract Surg Today*, September, http://www.crstodayeurope.com/Pages/whichArticle.php?id=66.

Kymionis GD, Siganos CS, Tsiklis NS, Anastasakis A, Yoo SH, Pallikaris AI, Astyrakakis N and Pallikaris IG (2007b), 'Long-term follow-up of Intacs in keratoconus', *Am J Ophthalmol*, **143**, 236–44.

Lane SL, Lindstrom RL, Cameron JD, Thaomas RH, Mindrup EA, Waring GO 3rd, McCarey BE and Binder PS (1986), 'Polysulfone corneal lenses', *J Cataract Refract Surg*, **12**, 50–60.

Lang AJ, Icenogle T, Franz S, Vatz A, Holliday K, Schneider N, Miller T, Le A, Chayet A and Barraga E (2008), 'Clinical efficacy of the PRESBYLENS® intracorneal inlay for the correction of presbyopia', ARVO Annual Meeting, Program number 3353; Poster number A171.

Larrea X, De Courten C, Feingold V, Burger J and Büchler P (2007), 'Oxygen and glucose distribution after intracorneal lens implantation', *Optom Vis Sci*, **84**, 1074–81.

Lass JH, Stocker EG, Fritz ME and Collie DM (1987), 'Epikeratoplasty: the surgical correction of aphakia, myopia and keratoconus', *Ophthalmology*, **94**, 912–25.

Latkany R, Tsuk A, Sheu MS, Loh IH and Trinkaus-Randall V (1997), 'Plasma surface modification of artificial corneas for optimal epithelialization', *J Biomed Mater Res*, **36**, 29–37.

Lavker RM, Dong G, Cheng SZ, Kudah K, Costarelis G and Sun T-T (1991), 'Relative proliferative rates of limbal and corneal epithelia', *Invest Ophthalmol Vis Sci*, **32**, 1864–75.

Lee HK, Lee KS, Kim JK, Kim HC, Seo KR and Kim EK (2005), 'Epithelial healing and clinical outcomes in excimer laser photorefractive surgery following three epithelial removal techniques: mechanical, alcohol, and excimer laser', *Am J Ophthalmol*, **139**, 56–63.

Lee JB, Javier JA, Chang JH, Chen CC, Kato T and Azar DT (2002), 'Confocal and electron microscopic studies of laser subepithelial keratomileusis (LASEK) in the white leghorn chick eye', *Arch Ophthalmol*, **120**, 1700–06.

Lee JH, Wee WR, Chung ES, Kim HY, Park SH and Kim YH (2000), 'Development of a newly designed double-fixed Seoul-type keratoprosthesis', *Arch Ophthalmol*, **118**, 1673–78.

Legeais J-M, Renard G, Parel J-M, Ing E-G, Savoldelli M and Pouliquen Y (1995), 'Keratoprosthesis with biocolonizable microporous fluorocarbon haptic', *Arch Ophthalmol*, **113**, 757–63.

Legeais J-M, Drubaix I, Briat B, Savoldelli M, Menasche M, Robert L, Renard G and Poulinquen Y (1997), 'Influence of ePFTE polymer implant permeability on the rate and density of corneal extracellular matrix synthesis', *J Biomed Mater Res*, **36**, 49–54.

Legeais J-M and Renard G (1998), 'A second generation of artificial cornea (Biokpro II)', *Biomaterials*, **19**, 1517–22.

Lemp MA and Mathers WD (1991), 'Conrad Berens lecture. Renewal of corneal epithelium', *CLAO J*, **17**, 258–66.

León CR, Barraquer JIJ and Barraquer JIS (1997), 'Coralline hydroxyapatite keratoprosthesis in rabbits', *J Refract Surg*, **13**, 74–78.

Li F, Carlsson DJ, Lohmann C, Suuronen E, Vascotto S, Kobuch K, Sheardown H, Munger R, Nakamura M and Griffith M (2003), 'Cellular and nerve regeneration within a biosynthetic extracellular matrix for corneal transplantation', *PNAS*, **100**, 15346–51.

Liliensiek SJ, Campbell S, Nealey PF and Murphy CJ (2006), 'The scale of substratum topographic features modulates proliferation of corneal epithelial cells and corneal fibroblasts', *J Biomed Mater Res A*, **79**, 185–92.

Lindstrom RL (2005), 'Coming at presbyopia from a new direction', *Rev Ophthalmol News*, **12**, http://www.revophth.com/index.asp?page=1_795.htm.

Linebarger EJ, Song D and Ruckhofer J (2000), 'Intacs: the intrastromal corneal ring', *Int Ophthalmol Clin*, **40**, 199–208.

Linna T and Tervo T (1997), 'Real-time confocal microscopic observations on human corneal nerves and wound healing after excimer laser photorefractive keratectomy', *Curr Eye Res*, **16**, 640–49.

Linsenmayer TF, Fitch JM, Gordon MK, Cai CX, Igoe F, Marchant JK and Birk DE (1998), 'Development and roles of collagenous matrices in the embryonic avian cornea', *Prog Retin Eye Res*, **17**, 231–65.

Liu C, Paul B, Tandon R, Lee E, Fong K, Mavrikakis I, Herold J, Thorp S, Brittain P, Francis I, Ferret C, Hull C, Lloyd A, Green D, Franklin V, Tighe B, Fukuda M and Hamada S (2005), 'The osteo-odonto-keratoprosthesis', *Semin Ophthalmol*, **20**, 113–28.

Liu C, Hille K, Tan DT, Hicks CR and Herold J (2008a), 'Keratoprosthesis surgery', *Dev Ophthalmol*, **41**, 171–86.

Liu W, Merrett K, Griffith M, Fagerholm P, Dravida S, Heyne B, Scaiano JB, Watsky MA, Shinozaki N, Lagali N, Munger R and Li F (2008b), 'Recombinant human collagen for tissue engineered corneal substitutes', *Biomaterials*, **29**, 1147–58.

Liu Y, Gan L, Carlsson DJ, Fagerholm P, Lagali N, Watsky MA, Munger R, Hodge WG, Priest D and Griffith M (2006), 'A simple, cross-linked collagen tissue substitute for corneal implantation', *Invest Ophthalmol Vis Sci*, **47**, 1869–75.

Ljubimov AV, Burgeson RE, Butkowski RJ, Michael AF, Sun T-T and Kenney MC (1995), 'Human corneal basement membrane heterogeneity: Topographical differences in the expression of type IV collagen and laminin isoforms', *Lab Invest*, **72**, 461–73.

Lou X, Vijayasekaran S, Sugiharti R and Robertson T (2005), 'Morphological and topographic effects on calcification tendency of pHEMA hydrogels', *Biomaterials*, **26**, 5808–17.

Maguen E, Rabinowitz YS, Regev L, Saghizadeh M, Sasaki T and Ljubimov AV (2008), 'Alterations of extracellular matrix components and proteinases in human corneal buttons with INTACS for post-laser in situ keratomileusis keratectasia and keratoconus', *Cornea*, **27**, 565–73.

Maskarinec SA and Tirrell DA (2005), 'Protein engineering approaches to biomaterials design', *Curr Opin Biotech*, **16**, 422–26.

Maskati QB and Maskati BT (2006), 'Asian experience with the Pintucci keratoprosthesis', *Indian J Ophthalmol*, **54**, 89–94.

Mathers WD and Lemp MA (1992), 'Morphology and movement of corneal surface cells in humans', *Curr Eye Res*, **11**, 517–23.

Mathew JH, Bergmanson JPG and Doughty MJ (2008), 'Fine structure of the interface between the anterior limiting lamina and the anterior stromal fibrils of the human cornea', *Invest Ophthalmol Vis Sci*, **49**, 3914–18.

Maurice DM (1969) 'Nutritional aspects of corneal grafts and prostheses', in Rycroft PV (Ed.) *Corneo-Plastic Surgery, International* Corneo-plastic Conference, London, 1967. Oxford and New York, Pergamon Press, p. 197.

Maurice DM (1972), 'The location of the fluid pump in the cornea', *J Physiol*, **221**, 43–54.

Maurice DM (1984), *The Cornea and Sclera*. New York, Academic Press.

McCarey BE and Andrews DM (1981), 'Refractive keratoplasty with intrastromal hydrogel lenticular implants', *Invest Ophthalmol Vis Sci*, **21**, 107–15.

McCarey BE, Lane SS and Lindstrom RL (1988), 'Alloplastic corneal lenses', *Int Ophthalmol Clin*, **28**, 155–63.

McCarey BE and Schmidt FH (1990), 'Modeling glucose distribution in the cornea', *Curr Eye Res*, **9**, 1025–39.

McCarey BE, Storie BR, Van Rij G and Knight PM (1990), 'Refractive predictability of myopic hydrogel intracorneal lenses in nonhuman primate eyes', *Arch Ophthalmol*, **108**, 1310–15.

McCarey BE (1991), 'Refractive keratoplasty with synthetic lens implants', *Refract Surg*, **31**, 87–99.

McDonald MB, Kaufman HE, Aquavella JV, Durrie DS, Hiles DA, Hunkeler JD, Keates RH, Morgan KS and Sanders DR (1987), 'The nationwide study of epikeratophakia for myopia', *Am J Ophthalmol*, **103**, 375–83.

McDonald MB and Dingeldein SA (1988) 'Complications of Epikeratophakia', in Cavanagh HD (Ed.) *World Congress on the Cornea*. New York, Raven Press Ltd.

McDonald MB, Frantz JM, Klyce SD, Salmeron B, Beuerman RW, C.R. M, Clapham TN, Koons SJ and Kaufman HE (1990), 'One-year refractive results of central photorefractive keratectomy for myopia in nonhuman primate cornea', *Arch Ophthalmol*, **108**, 40–47.

McDonald MB, McCarey BE, Storie B, Beuerman RW, Salmeron B, Van Rij G and Knight PM (1993), 'Assessment of the long-term corneal response to hydrogel intrastromal lenses implanted in monkey eyes for up to five years', *J Cataract Refract Surg*, **19**, 213–22.

McLaughlin CR, Fagerholm P, Muzakare L, Lagali N, Forrester JV, Kuffova L, Rafat MA, Liu Y, Shinozaki N, Vascotto S, Munger R and Griffith M (2008), 'Regeneration of corneal cells and nerves in an implanted collagen corneal substitute', *Cornea*, **27**, 580–89.

Meek KM and Fullwood NJ (2001), 'Corneal and scleral collagens – a microscopist's perspective', *Micron*, **32**, 261–72.

Melles GR, Binder PS, Moore MN and Anderson JA (1995), 'Epithelial–stromal interactions in human keratotomy wound healing', *Arch Ophthalmol*, **113**, 1124–30.

Merrett K, Griffith CM, Deslandes Y, Pleizier G, Dube MA and Sheardown H (2003), 'Interactions of corneal cells with transforming growth factor beta 2-modified poly dimethyl siloxane surfaces', *J Biomed Mater Res*, **67A**, 981–93.

Merrett K, Fagerholm P, McLaughlin CR, Dravida S, Lagali N, Shinozaki N, Watsky MA, Munger R, Kato Y, Li F, Marmo CJ and Griffith M (2008), 'Tissue-engineered recombinant human collagen-based corneal substitutes for implantation: performance of type I versus type III collagen', *Invest Ophthalmol Vis Sci*, **49**, 3887–94.

Mester U, Roth K and Dardenne MU (1972), 'Versvchemit 2-hydroxyaethylmethycrylatlinsen als keratophakiematerial', *Ber Ophthalmol Ges*, **72**, 326.

Mete M, Tang F, Xu X and Yuruk N (2008), 'A structural approach for finding functional modules from large biological networks', *BMC Bioinformatics*, **12**, S19.

Michael R, Charoenrook V, de la Paz MF, Hitzl W, Temprano J and Barraquer RI (2008), 'Long-term functional and anatomical results of osteo- and osteoodonto-keratoprosthesis', *Graefes Arch Clin Exp Ophthalmol*, **246**, 1133–37.

Michieletto P, Ligabue E, Balestrazzi A, Balestrazzi A and Giglio S (2004), 'PermaVision intracorneal lens for the correction of hyperopia', *J Cat Refract Surg*, **30**, 2152–57.

Miranda D, Sartori M, Francesconi C, Allemann N, Ferrara P and Campos M (2003), 'Ferrara intrastromal corneal ring segments for severe keratoconus', *J Refract Surg*, **19**, 645–53.

Mitooka K, Ramirez M, Maguire LJ, Erie JC, Patel SC, McLaren JW, Hodge DO and Bourne WM (2002), 'Keratocyte density of central human cornea after laser *in situ* keratomileusis', *Am J Ophthalmol*, **133**, 307–14.

Mohan RR, Hutcheson AEK, Choi R, Hong J-W, Lee J-S, Mohan RR, Ambrosio R, Zieske JD and Wilson SE (2003), 'Apoptosis, necrosis, proliferation and myofibroblast generation in the stroma following LASIK and PRK', *Exp Eye Res*, **76**, 71–87.

Moilanen JA, Holopainen JM, Vesaluoma MH and Tervo TM (2008), 'Corneal recovery after lasik for high myopia: a 2-year prospective confocal microscopic study', *Br J Ophthalmol*, **92**, 1397–402.

Møller-Pedersen T, Li HF, Petroll WM, Cavanagh HD and Jester JV (1998), 'Confocal microscopic characterization of wound repair after photorefractive keratectomy', *Invest Ophthalmol Vis Sci*, **39**, 487–501.

Møller-Pedersen T, Cavanagh HD, Petroll WM and Jester JV (2000), 'Stromal wound healing explains refractive instability and haze development after photorefractive keratectomy: a 1-year confocal microscopic study', *Ophthalmology*, **107**, 1235–45.

Mori R, Power KT, Wang CM, Martin P and Becker DL (2006), 'Acute downregulation of connexin43 at wound sites leads to a reduced inflammatory response, enhanced keratinocyte proliferation and wound fibroblast migration', *J Cell Sci*, **119**, 5193–203.

Morishige N, Wahlert AJ, Kenney MC, Brown DJ, Kawamoto K, Chikama T, Nishida T and Jester JV (2007), 'Second-harmonic imaging microscopy of normal human and keratoconus cornea', *Invest Ophthalmol Vis Sci*, **48**, 1087–94.

Müller LJ, Pels L and Vrensen GFJM (1995), 'Novel aspects of ultrastructural organization of human corneal keratocytes', *Invest Ophthalmol Vis Sci*, **36**, 2557–67.

Müller LJ, Vrensen GFJM, Pels L, Cardoza BN and Willekens B (1997), 'Architecture of human corneal nerves', *Invest Ophthalmol Vis Sci*, **38**, 985–94.

Müller LJ, Pels E and Vrensen GF (2001), 'The specific architecture of the anterior stroma accounts for maintenance of corneal curvature', *Br J Opthalmol*, **85**, 437–43.

Müller LJ, Marfurt CF, Kruse F and Tervo TMT (2003), 'Corneal nerves: structure, contents and function', *Exp Eye Res*, **76**, 521–42.

Müller LJ, Pels E, Schurmans LR and Vrensen GF (2004), 'A new three-dimensional model of the organization of proteoglycans and collagen fibrils in the human corneal stroma', *Exp Eye Res*, **78**, 493–501.

Myung D, Koh W, Bakri A, Zhang F, Marshall A, Ko J, Noolandi J, Carrasco M, Cochran JR, Frank CW and Ta CN (2007), 'Design and fabrication of an artificial cornea based on a photolithographically patterned hydrogel construct', *Biomed Microdevices*, **9**, 911–22.

Myung D, Duhamel P-E, Cochran JR, Noolandi J, Ta CN and Frank CW (2008a), 'Development of hydrogel-based keratoprosthesis: a materials perspective', *Biotechnol Prog*, **24**, 735–41.

Myung D, Farooqui N, Waters D, Schaber S, Koh W, Carrasco M, Noolandi J, Frank CW and Ta CN (2008b), 'Glucose-permeable interpenetrating polymer network hydrogels for corneal implant applications: a pilot study', *Curr Eye Res*, **33**, 29–43.

Myung D, Farooqui N, Zheng LL, Koh W, Gupta S, Bakri A, Noolandi J, Cochran JR, Frank CW and Ta CN (2009), 'Bioactive interpenetrating polymer network hydrogels that support corneal epithelial wound healing', *J Biomed Mater Res A*, **90**, 70–81.

Netto MV, Mohan RR, Sinha S, Sharma A, Dupps WJJ and Wilson SE (2006), 'Stromal haze, myofibroblasts, and surface irregularity after PRK', *Exp Eye Res*, **82**, 788–97.

Netto MV, Mohan RR, Medeiros FW, Dupps WJJ, Sinha S, Krueger RR, Stapleton WM, Rayborn M, Suto C and Wilson SE (2007), 'Femtosecond laser and microkeratome corneal flaps: comparison of stromal wound healing and inflammation', *J Refract Surg*, **23**, 667–76.

Newsome DA, Foidart J-M, Hassell JR, Krachmer JH, Rodrigues MM and Katz SI (1981), 'Detection of specific collagen types in normal and keratoconus corneas', *Invest Ophthalmol Vis Sci*, **20**, 738–50.

Nishida T, Chikama T, Morishige N, Yanai R, Yamada N and Saito J (2007), 'Persistent epithelial defects due to neurotrophic keratopathy treated with a substance p-derived peptide and insulin-like growth factor 1', *Jpn J Ophthalmol*, **51**, 442–47.

Obata H and Tsuru T (2007), 'Corneal wound healing from the perspective of keratoplasty specimens with special reference to the function of the Bowman layer and Descemet membrane', *Cornea*, **26**, S82–89.

Pallikaris IG, Papatzanaki ME, Stathi EZ, Frenschock O and Georgiadis A (1990), 'Laser *in situ* keratomileusis', *Lasers Surg Med*, **10**, 463–68.

Pallikaris IG, Kymionis GD and Astyrakakis NI (2001), 'Corneal ectasia induced by laser *in situ* keratomileusis', *J Cataract Refract Surg*, **27**, 1803–11.

Pallikaris IG, Naoumidi II, Kalyvianaki MI and Katsanevaki VJ (2003), 'Epi-LASIK: comparative histological evaluation of mechanical and alcohol-assisted separation', *J Cataract Refract Surg*, **29**, 1496–501.

Park JH, Jeoung JW, Wee WR, Lee JH, Kim MK and Lee JL (2008), 'Clinical efficacy of amniotic membrane transplantation in the treatment of various ocular surface diseases', *Cont Lens Anterior Eye*, **31**, 73–80.

Parks RA and McCarey BE (1991), 'Hydrogel keratophakia: Long term morphology in the monkey model', *CLAO J*, **17**, 216–22.

Parks RA, McCarey BE, Knight PM and Storie BR (1993), 'Intrastromal crystalline deposits following hydrogel keratophakia in monkeys', *Cornea*, **12**, 29–34.

Petroll WM, Goldberg D, Lindsey SS, Kelley PS, Cavanagh HD, Bowman RW, Parmar DN, Verity SM and McCulley JP (2006), 'Confocal assessment of the corneal response to intracorneal lens insertion and laser *in situ* keratomileusis with flap creation using IntraLase', *J Cataract Refract Surg*, **32**, 1119–28.

Pfister RR (1973), 'The normal surface of the corneal epithelium: a scanning electron microscopic study', *Invest Ophthalmol*, **12**, 654–68.

Pieper B (2006), 'Reaching baby boomers: 2020 and beyond', *Optometry*, **77**, 141–44.

Pintucci S, Pintucci F, Cecconi M and Caiazza S (1995), 'New dacron tissue colonisable keratoprosthesis: clinical experience', *Br J Ophthalmol*, **79**, 825–29.

Pintucci S, Pintucci F, Caiazza S and Cecconi M (1996), 'The Dacron felt colonizable keratoprosthesis: after 15 years', *Eur J Ophthalmol*, **6**, 125–30.

Pintucci S, Perilli R, Formisano G and Caiazza S (2001), 'Influence of dacron tissue thickness on the performance of the Pintucci biointegrable keratoprosthesis: an in vitro and in vivo study', *Cornea*, **20**, 647–50.

Polack FM (1976), 'Editorial: Keratoprosthesis', *Invest Ophthalmol*, **15**, 593–95.

Poole CA, Brookes NH and Clover GM (1993), 'Keratocyte networks visualised in the living cornea using vital dyes', *J Cell Sci*, **106**, 685–92.

Poole CA, Brookes NH and Clover GM (2003), 'Confocal imaging of the human keratocyte network using the vital dye 5-chloromethylfluorescein diacetate', *Clin Exp Ophthalmol*, **31**, 147–54.

Prakasam RK, Sweeney DF, Vaddavalli PK, Evans MDM, Hughes TC, Xie R-Z, McLean KM, Vannas A and Sridhar MS (2007a), 'Corneal inlay is a reversible refractive procedure', Asia ARVO, Singapore, Poster 342(703) B142.

Prakasam RK, Sweeney DF, Vaddavalli PK, Evans MDM, Hughes TC, Xie R-Z, McLean KM, Vannas A and Sridhar MS (2007b), 'Corneal pigment ring deposits after corneal inlay', Asia ARVO, Singapore, Poster 343(711) B143.

Princz MA and Sheardown H (2008), 'Heparin-modified dendrimer cross-linked collagen matrices for the delivery of basic fibroblast growth factor (FGF-2)', *J Biomater Sci Polym Ed*, **19**, 1201–18.

Qiu C, Coutinho P, Frank S, Franke S, Law LY, Martin P, Green CR and Becker DL (2003), 'Targeting connexin43 expression accelerates the rate of wound repair', *Curr Biol*, **13**, 1697–703.

Rao GN, Ganti S and Aquavella JV (1987), 'Specular microscopy of corneal epithelium after epikeratophakia', *Am J Ophthalmol*, **103**, 392–96.

Rice DE and Ihlenfeld JV (1989), 'Ophthalmic device comprising a polymer of telechelic perfluoropolyether', US Patent 4,818,801; File date April 4, 1989, Affiliation of inventors: Minnesota Mining and Manufacturing Company (St Paul, Minnesota USA).

Rimmer S, Johnson C, Zhao B, Collier J, Gilmore L, Sabnis S, Wyman P, Sammon C, Fullwood NJ and MacNeil S (2007), 'Epithelialization of hydrogels achieved by amine functionalization and co-culture with stromal cells', *Biomaterials*, **28**, 5319–31.

Rodrigues M, Nirankari V, Rajagopalan S, Jones K and Funderburgh J (1992), 'Clinical and histopathologic changes in the host cornea after epikeratophakia for keratoconus', *Am J Ophthalmol*, **114**, 161–70.

Rodrigues MM, McCarey BE, Waring GO, Hidayat AA and Kruth H (1990), 'Lipid deposits posterior to impermeable intracorneal lenses in rhesus monkeys: clinical, histochemical and ultrastructural studies', *Refract Corneal Surg*, **6**, 32–37.

Rozsa AJ and Beuerman RW (1982), 'Density and organisation of free nerve endings in the corneal epithelium of the rabbit', *Pain*, **14**, 105–20.

Ruckhofer J, Stoiber J, Alzner E and Grabner G (2001a), 'One year results of European multicenter study of intrastromal corneal ring segments. Part 1: Refractive outcomes', *J Cataract Refract Surg*, **27**, 287–96.

Ruckhofer J, Stoiber J, Alzner E and Grabner G (2001b), 'One year results of European multicenter study of intrastromal corneal ring segments. Part 2: Complications, visual symptoms and patient satisfaction', *J Cataract Refract Surg*, **27**, 287–96.

Sakimoto T, Rosenblatt MI and Azar DT (2006), 'Laser eye surgery for refractive errors', *Lancet*, **367**(9520), 1432–47.

Samples JR, Binder PS, Zavala EY, Baumgartner SD and Deg JK (1984), 'Morphology of hydrogel implants used for refractive keratoplasty', *Invest Ophthalmol Vis Sci*, **25**, 843–50.

Sanchez Leon F (2006), 'Small study shows immediate benefit from intracorneal presbyopia implant', *OSN SuperSite*, August 9th 2006, http://www.osnsupersite.com/view.aspx?rid=17974.

Sanchez Leon F (2008), 'Corneal inlay shows promise for presbyopic correction', *OSN SuperSite*, 2/21/2008, http://www.osnsupersite.com/view.asp?rID=26548.

Sandeman SR, Lloyd AW, Tighe BJ, Franklin V, Li J, Lydon F, Liu CS, Mann DJ, James SE and Martin R (2003), 'A model for the preliminary biological screening of potential keratoprosthetic biomaterials', *Biomaterials*, **24**, 4729–39.

Sandoval HP, de Castro LE, Vroman DT and Solomon KD (2005), 'Refractive Surgery Survey 2004', *J Cataract Refract Surg*, **31**, 221–33.

Sato T, Akiyama K and Shibata H (1953), 'A new surgical approach to myopia', *Am J Ophthalmol*, **36**, 823–29.

Schermer A, Galvin S and Sun T-T (1986), 'Differentiation-related expression of a major 64K corneal keratin in vivo and in culture suggests limbal location of corneal epithelial stem cells', *J Cell Biology*, **103**, 49–62.

Schmack I, Dawson DG, McCarey BE, Waring GOr, Grossniklaus HE and Edelhauser HF (2005), 'Cohesive tensile strength of human LASIK wounds with histologic, ultrastructural, and clinical correlations', *J Refract Surg*, **21**, 433–45.

Seiler T, Matallana M, Sendler S and Bende T (1992), 'Does Bowman's layer determine the biomechanical properties of the cornea?', *Refract Corneal Surg*, **8**, 139–42.

Sekundo W, Kunert K, Russmann C, Gille A, Bissmann W, Stobrawa G, Sticker M, Bischoff M and Blum M (2008), 'First efficacy and safety study of femtosecond lenticule extraction for the correction of myopia: six-month results', *J Cataract Refract Surg*, **34**, 1513–20.

Sendele DD, Abelson MB, Kenyon KR and Hannimen LA (1983), 'Intracorneal lens implantation', *Arch Ophthalmol*, **101**, 940.

Shen W, Zhang K, Kornfield JA and Tirrell DA (2006), 'Tuning the erosion rate of artificial protein hydrogels through control of network topology', *Nature Mater*, **5**, 153–58.

Slade SG (2006), 'Intracorneal lens with femtosecond laser promising as hyperopia treatment', reported by Altersitz K, *OSN SuperSite*, 9/15/06, http.//www.osnsupersite. com view.aspx?rid = 18416.

Slade SG (2008), 'Thin-flap laser-assised *in situ* keratomileusis', *Curr Opin Ophthalmol*, **19**, 325–29.

Sosnová M, Bradl M and Forrester JV (2005), 'CD34+ corneal stromal cells are bone marrow-derived and express hemopoietic stem cell markers', *Stem Cells*, **23**, 507–15.

Stachs O, Zhivov A, Kraak R, Stave J and Guthoff R (2007), '*In vivo* three-dimensional confocal laser scanning microscopy of the epithelial nerve structure in the human cornea', *Graefes Arch Clin Exp Ophthalmol*, **245**, 569–75.

Stock EL, Kurpakus MA, Sambol B and Jones JCR (1992), 'Adhesion complex formation after small keratectomy wounds in the cornea', *Invest Ophthalmol Vis Sci*, **33**, 304–13.

Stoiber J, Csaky D, Schedle A, Ruckhofer J and Grabner G (2002), 'Histopathologic findings in explanted osteoodontokeratoprosthesis', *Cornea*, **21**, 400–4.

Stoiber J, Fernandez V, Kaminski S, Lamar PD, Dubovy SR, Alfonso E and Parel JM (2004), 'Biological response to a supraDescemetic synthetic cornea in rabbits', *Arch Ophthalmol*, **122**, 1850–55.

Stoiber J, Fernandez V, Lamar PD, Kaminski S, Acosta AC, Dubovy SR, Alfonso E and Parel JM (2005), 'Biocompatibility of a nonpenetrating synthetic cornea in vascularized rabbit corneas', *Cornea*, **24**, 467–73.

SundarRaj N, Geiss MJ, Fantes F, Hanna K, Anderson SC, Thompson KP, Thoft RA and Waring GO (1990), 'Healing of excimer laser ablated monkey corneas', *Arch Ophthalmol*, **108**, 1604–10.

Sweeney DF, Xie RZ, Tout SD, Steele JG, Holden BA, Beumer GJ and Griesser HJ (1997), 'Effects of biologically modified surface of synthetic lenticules on corneal epithelialization in vivo', *Invest Ophthalmol Vis Sci*, **38**(4), (ARVO) Abstract 1903.

Sweeney DF, Xie RZ, O'Leary DJ, Vannas A, O'Dell R, Schindhelm K, Cheng H, Steele JG and Holden BA (1998), 'Nutritional requirements of the corneal epithelium and anterior stroma: Clinical findings', *Invest Ophthalmol Vis Sci*, **39**, 284–91.

Sweeney DF, Xie R-Z, Evans MDM, Vannas A, Tout SD, Griesser HJ, Johnson G and Steele JG (2003), 'A comparison of biological coatings for the promotion of corneal epithelialization of synthetic surface *in vivo*', *Invest Ophthalmol Vis Sci*, **44**, 3301–09.

Sweeney DF, Sridhar MS, Vannas A, Pravin VK, Prakasam RK, Hughes TC, Evans MDM, McLean KM, Xie R-Z, Chan GY, Nguyen X, McFarland GA, Johnson G, Knower WS and Wilkie JS (2005), 'Corneal inlays: results of a 6 month phase 1 clinical trial', Annual Meeting of The Association for Research in Vision and Ophthalmology (ARVO), Florida, USA, May 2005, Abstract 4372, p. 188.

Sweeney DF, Pravin VK, Prakasam RK, Sridhar MS, Vannas A, Hughes TC, Evans MDM, McLean KM and Xie R-Z (2006), 'Corneal inlays: results of an 18 month phase 1 clinical trial', Annual Meeting of The Association for Research in Vision and Ophthalmology (ARVO), Florida, USA, May 2006, p. 204, Abstract 4335.

Sweeney DF, Vannas A, Hughes TC, Evans MDM, McLean KM, Xie R-Z, Pravin VK and Prakasam RK (2008), 'Synthetic corneal inlays', *Clin Exp Optom*, **91**, 56–66.

Sweeney DF, Prakasam RK, Vaddavalli PK, Vannas A, Hughes TC, Sridhar MS, Evans MDM, McLean KM, Moilanen J and Xie R-Z (2009), 'Clnical performance of a perfluoropolyether corneal inlay', *Invest Ophthalmol Vis Sci*, submitted.

Taneri S, Zieske JD and Azar DT (2004), 'Evolution, techniques, clinical outcomes, and pathophysiology of LASEK: review of the literature', *Surv Ophthalmol*, **49**, 576–602.

Tanioka H, Hieda O, Kawasaki S, Nakai Y and Kinoshita S (2007), 'Assessment of epithelial integrity and cell viability in epithelial flaps prepared with the epi-LASIK procedure', *J Catarack Refract Surg*, **33**, 1195–220.

Teixeira AI, Abrams GA, Bertics PJ, Murphy CJ and Nealey PF (2003), 'Epithelial contact guidance on well-defined micro- and nanostructured substrates', *J Cell Sci*, **116**, 1881–92.

Tervo T and Moilanen J (2003), 'In vivo confocal microscopy for evaluation of wound healing following corneal refractive surgery', *Prog Retin Eye Res*, **22**, 339–58.

Thoft RA and Friend J (1983), 'The X, Y, Z hypothesis of corneal epithelial maintenance', *Invest Ophthalmol Vis Sci*, **24**, 1442–43.

Thompson KP, Hanna K, Waring GO, Gipson IK, Liu Y, Gailitis RP, Johnson-Witt B and Green K (1991), 'Current status of synthetic epikeratoplasty', *J Refract Surg*, **7**, 240–48.

Thompson KP, Hanna KD, Gipson IK, Gravagna P, Waring GO and Johnson-Wint B (1993), 'Synthetic epikeratoplasty in rhesus monkeys with human type IV collagen', *Cornea*, **12**, 35–45.

Torbet J, Malbouyres M, Builles N, Justin V, Roulet M, Damour O, Oldberg A, Ruggiero F and Hulmes DJ (2007), 'Orthogonal scaffold of magnetically aligned collagen lamellae for corneal stroma reconstruction', *Biomaterials*, **28**, 4268–76.

Trinkaus-Randall V, Wu XY, Tablante R and Tsuk A (1997), 'Implantation of a synthetic cornea: design, development and biological response', *Artif Organs*, **21**, 1185–91.

Trinkaus-Randall V and Nugent MA (1998), 'Biological response to a synthetic cornea', *J Controlled Release*, **53**, 205–14.

Trokel S, Srinivasan R and Braren B (1983), 'Excimer laser surgery of the cornea', *Am J Ophthalmol*, **96**, 710–15.

Tseng SCG (1989), 'Concept and application of limbal stem cells', *Eye*, **3**, 141–57.

Tsuk AG, Trinkaus-Randall V and Leibowitz HM (1997), 'Advances in polyvinyl alcohol hydrogel keratoprostheses: Protection against ultraviolet light and fabrication by a molding process', *J Biomed Mater Res*, **34**, 299–304.

Vaddavalli PK, Moilanen J, Prakasam RK, Sweeney DF, Evans MDM, Hughes TC, Xie R-Z, McLean KM and Vannas A (2007) 'Confocal microscopy in corneal inlays', Annual Meeting of the International Society for Contact Lens Research, Whistler, Canada.

Vesaluoma MH, Pérez-Santonja J, Petroll WM, Linna T, Alió J and Tervo T (2000), 'Corneal stromal changes induced by myopic LASIK', *Invest Ophthalmol Vis Sci*, **41**, 369–76.

Vijayasekaran S, Fitton JH, Hicks CR, Chirila TV, Crawford GJ and Constable IJ (1998), 'Cell viability and inflammatory response in hydrogel sponges implanted in the rabbit cornea', *Biomaterials*, **19**, 2255–67.

Vijayasekaran S, Chirila TV, Robertson TA, Lou X, Fitton JH, Hicks CR and Constable IJ (2000), 'Calcification of poly(2-hydroxyethyl methacrylate) hydrogel sponges implanted in the rabbit cornea: a 3-month study', *J Biomater Sci Polym Ed*, **11**, 599–615.

Vijayasekaran S, Robertson T, Hicks C and Hirst L (2005), 'Histopathology of long-term Cardona keratoprosthesis: a case report', *Cornea*, **24**, 233–37.

Vinciguerra P and Camesasca FI (2002), 'Butterfly laser epithelial keratomileusis for myopia', *J Refract Surg*, **18**, S371–73.

Vinciguerra P, Camesasca FI and Randazzo A (2003), 'One-year results of butterfly laser epithelial keratomileusis', *J Refract Surg*, **19**, S223–6.

Waring GO (1992), 'Making sense of keratospeak IV', *Arch Ophthalmol*, **110**, 1385–92.

Waring GO 3rd, Lynn MJ and McDonnell PJ (1994), 'Results of the prospective evaluation of radial keratotomy (PERK) study 10 years after surgery', *Arch Ophthalmol*, **112**, 1298–308.

Watt FM (1984), 'Selective migration of terminally differentiating cells from the basal layer of cultured human epidermis', *J Cell Biol*, **98**, 16–21.

Werblin TP and Kaufman HE (1981), 'Epikeratophakia: the surgical correction of aphakia. II Preliminary results in a non-human primate model', *Curr Eye Res*, **1**, 131–37.

Werblin TP and Klyce SD (1981), 'Epikeratophakia: the surgical correction of aphakia. I. Lathing of corneal tissue', *Curr Eye Res*, **1**, 123–29.

Werblin TP, Blaydes JE, Fryezkowski A and Peiffer RL (1983), 'Stability of hydrogel intracorneal implants in non-human primates', *CLAO J*, **9**, 157–61.

Werblin TP, Patel AS and Barraquer JI (1992a), 'Initial human experience with Permalens myopic hydrogel intracorneal lens implants', *Refract Corneal Surg*, **8**, 23–32.

Werblin TP, Peiffer RL, Binder PS, McCarey BE and Patel AS (1992b), 'Eight years experience with Permalens intracorneal lenses in nonhuman primates', *Refract Corneal Surg*, **8**, 12–22.

West-Mays JA and Dwivedi DJ (2006), 'The keratocyte: Corneal stromal cell with variable repair phenotypes', *Int J Biochem Cell Biol*, **38**, 1625–31.

Wilson SE and Bourne WM (1988), 'Fuchs' dystrophy', *Cornea*, **7**, 2–18.

Wilson SE and Kim W-J (1998), 'Keratocyte apoptosis: implications on corneal wound healing, tissue organization and disease', *Invest Ophthalmol Vis Sci*, **39**, 220–26.

Wilson SE and Hong J-W (2000), 'Bowman's layer structure and funtion', *Cornea*, **19**, 417–20.

Wilson SE, Netto M and Ambrósio RJ (2003), 'Corneal cells: chatty in development, homeostasis, wound healing, and disease', *Am J Ophthalmol*, **136**, 530–36.

Winkler DA (2008), 'Network models in drug discovery and regenerative medicine', *Biotechnol Annu Rev*, **14**, 143–70.

Wu XY, Tsuk A, Leibowitz HM and Trinkaus-Randall V (1998), 'In vivo comparison of three different porous materials intended for use in a keratoprosthesis', *Br J Ophthalmol*, **82**, 569–76.

Xie R-Z, Stretton S and Sweeney DF (2001), 'Artificial cornea: towards a synthetic onlay for correction of refractive error', *Biosci Rep*, **21**, 513–36.

Xie R-Z, Evans MDM, Bojarski B, Hughes TC, Chan GY, Nguyen X, Wilkie JS, McLean KM, Vannas A and Sweeney DF (2006), 'Two-year preclinical testing of perfluoropolyether as a corneal inlay', *Invest Ophthalmol Vis Sci*, **47**, 574–81.

Yamaguchi T, Koenig SB, Kimura T, Werblin TP, McDonald MB and Kaufman HE (1984a), 'Histological study of epikeratophakia in primates', *Ophthal Surg*, **15**, 230–35.

Yamaguchi T, Koenig SB, Hamano T, Kimura T, Santana E, McDonald MB and Kanfman HE (1984b), 'Electron microscopic study of intrastromal hydrogel implants in primates', *Ophthalmology*, **91**, 1170–75.

Yilmaz OF, Bayraktar S, Agca A, Yilmaz B, McDonald MB and van de Pol C (2008), 'Intracorneal inlay for the surgical correction of presbyopia', *J Cataract Refract Surg*, **34**, 1921–27.

Young RD, Armitage WJ, Bowerman P, Cook SD and Easty DL (1994), 'Improved preservation of human corneal basement membrane following freezing of donor tissue for epikeratophakia', *Br J Ophthalmol*, **78**, 863–70.

Yurchenco PD and Schittny JC (1990), 'Molecular architecture of basement membranes', *FASEB J*, **4**, 1577–90.

Zerbe BL, Belin MW, Ciolino JB and Study BTK (2006), 'Results from the multicenter Boston type 1 Keratoprosthesis Study', *Ophthalmology*, **113**, 1779–84.

Zieske JD (1992), 'Characterisation of a potential marker of corneal epithelial stem cells', *Invest Ophthalmol Vis Sci*, **33**, 143–52.

Zieske JD (2004), 'Corneal development associated with eyelid opening', *Int J Dev Biol*, **48**, 903–11.

5

Corneal tissue engineering versus synthetic artificial corneas

M. A. PRINCZ and H. SHEARDOWN, McMaster University, Canada; M. GRIFFITH, University of Ottawa, Canada

Abstract: With corneal blindness as the second leading cause of blindness worldwide, there have been significant efforts toward understanding how corneal cells interact with artificial materials and toward developing a corneal substitute. Two approaches have been taken. In the first, synthetic materials have been used to develop a scaffold with which the native tissue interacts. In the second, corneal tissue engineering has been used to develop material–cell combinations that mimic the structure of the native tissue. The state of the art in both cases is discussed and summarized. Promising future directions for research are outlined.

Key words: artificial cornea, corneal tissue engineering, collagen, corneal cells, synthetic polymers.

5.1   The cornea

The cornea is a transparent tissue, acting not only as the eye's main refractive constituent, but also as a physical barrier to protect the interior ocular elements.[1] It consists of three cellular layers – the epithelium, the stroma and the endothelium – which are in turn separated by discrete layers, namely Bowman's layer and Descemet's membrane. The epithelium mainly contains three cell types that are tightly organized into five to seven layers, providing much of the cornea's protective barrier functions. The stroma is the thickest and strongest part of the cornea, consisting mostly of water and collagen fibrils, with keratocyte cells found within the fibril network. The endothelium is a single layer of cells, organized hexagonally, and regulates corneal hydration. As the cornea reflects light on to the retina, any damage or opacification of the organ will result in vision impairment or blindness.[2]

5.2   The need for an artificial cornea

According to the World Health Organization, vision loss due to corneal disease, trauma, scarring or ulceration constitutes to the second leading cause of blindness,[3] roughly affecting 10 million people worldwide[4]. In fact, 1.5–2 million new cases of corneal blindness occur annually as a result of corneal trauma or ulceration.[4]

The most successful and accepted treatment for corneal blindness is corneal allograft surgery, also known as penetrating keratoplasty, whereby donor tissue is implanted into the host cornea. Although 80% success rates are achieved within the first 2 years,[4] this rate falls to 65% 5 years post-surgery,[5] and is further complicated by underlying corneal damage or disease.[1] There are also disease transmission risks associated with allograph surgeries, primarily HIV and hepatitis.[6] Furthermore, there is a shortage of donor tissue, with surgery wait times averaging 2 years in North America; these wait times are only expected to lengthen due to an ageing population[4] and the increased popularity of laser *in situ* keratomileusis (LASIK) surgery, which renders the cornea unsuitable for transplantation.[6] An attractive alternative is therefore artificial replacement of the cornea, either with a keratoprosthesis or a tissue -engineered corneal equivalent (TECE).[2]

5.3   Artificial cornea

The artificial cornea must be non-toxic and able to interact well with surrounding corneal cells and tissue, transparent with a refractive index similar to the native cornea, be strong enough to withstand intraocular pressure, and allow for oxygen and nutrient diffusion to keep remaining corneal cells viable.[1,2,6,7] Current artificial corneal devices can be considered as keratoprostheses, which are made from synthetic polymers, or as tissue-engineered corneal equivalents, which are typically made from natural polymers combined with a biological component.[7]

5.4   Keratoprostheses

Keratoprostheses (KPros) are typically designed as a collar button device, also referred to as the optical stem with skirt implant, or as a core and skirt device.[8] The former design has two plates joined by an optical core, while the latter design has an optical core surrounded by a skirt used to anchor the device into the stroma. The optical core in both designs should be transparent and as a short as possible to avoid anterior chamber penetration,[9] while device segments intended for anchorage must be flexible but durable to withstand placement and suturing.[8] In many designs, the skirt is porous to allow for nutrient and oxygen diffusion and for device integration with the host's tissue,[4] with pore sizes being able to accommodate cell–cell interactions and extracellular matrix deposition.[6] The anterior surface of the KPro should encourage epithelialization to promote tear interactions, but avoid epithelial downgrowth to avoid device extrusion.[7] Furthermore, the posterior should inhibit cell integration to maintain device clarity on the optical core.

Early KPros fabricated from gold, quartz, and glass were met with a high incidence of device extrusion.[9,10] In the late 1940s, the second generation of

KPros were fabricated from synthetic polymers, the first being composed of poly(methyl methacrylate) (PMMA).[10] However, a variety of polymer materials have been examined in this application including polytetrafluoroethylene (PTFE), polybutylene:polypropylene, polyurethane, Dacron, poly(2-hydroxyethyl methacylate) (PHEMA) and poly(dimethyl siloxane) (PDMS).[2,10]

Synthetic KPro devices are advantageous owing to their potential for off-the-shelf availability, their durability in the prevention of postoperative remodeling, and a reduction in the risk of disease transmission that is associated with allograft surgeries.[2] However, KPros often fail to interact sufficiently with host tissue which results in device extrusion, tissue rejection (in the form of stromal melting and epithelial thinning), aqueous humour leakage, infection, retroprosthetic membrane formation, retinal detachment and glaucoma.[6,7,11]

5.4.1   Dohlman–Doane Keratoprosthesis

The Dohlman–Doane KPro (D-KPro) is a PMMA collar button device that sandwiches the corneal tissue between 2 plates.[12,13] It has been approved by the United States Food and Drug Administration and has been implanted in over 190 eyes since the 1990s.[12,13] There are 2 PMMA prototypes: type I is utilized for patients with good ocular surface hydration, while type II is intended for patients with ocular surface disease – such as dry eye, ocular mucous membrane pemphigoid, or Stevens–Johnson syndrome – who thus can not support the type I device.[12,13] A third prototype has been created with a titanium ring to enhance mechanical stability.[12]

Following implantation in 63 eyes between 1990 and 1997, 6 devices required replacement, while 10 devices were permanently removed.[14] Complications associated with the D-KPro were glaucoma (46%), retroprosthetic membrane (37%), tissue melting (29%), retinal detachment (19%) and endophthalmitis (8%). Although visual acuities between 20/20 and 20/200 were initially achieved, 42% of patients lost vision improvements because of device complications. Preoperative conditions were attributed to complications, with non-cicatrizing conditions, such as graft failure, having the best outcomes, while the Stevens–Johnson syndrome group had the worst outcomes. Elsewhere, histological analysis revealed epithelial downgrowth.[13]

Further development of both the design and surgical and postoperative techniques (anti-inflammatory agents, contact lens bandages, antibiotics, shunts, etc.) resulted in no device extrusion and improved visual acuity.[15,16] Furthermore, no occurrences of endophthalmitis, reoperations, dislocations or extrusions of 25 implanted D-KPros have been reported as of 2005.[17]

5.4.2   Osteo-odonto keratoprosthesis

The osteo-odonto KPro (OOKP) has a PMMA optic, which is secured to a haptic made from a tooth root, containing its alveolar ligament, belonging to the patient or a compatible donor.[18] Long-term studies of 224 eyes beween 1973 and 1999 demonstrated 85% retention over 18 years with fewer instances of complications;[18] however, there are concerns regarding increased intraocular pressure and resorption of the bone, owing to chronic inflammation, which loosens and leads to the eventual failure of the device.[19,20] Synthetic OOKP devices have been fabricated from aluminum oxide, hydroxyapatite (HA) ceramic and glass ceramic.[20] However, degradation of corals, HA-based materials, tooth and bone was rapid and may not be suitable for the ocular environment; hence more chemically stable materials are necessary.[20]

5.4.3   Seoul-type keratoprosthesis

The Seoul-type KPro (S-KPro) consists of a PMMA optic, of the collar button design, surrounded by a polyurethane or polypropylene skirt, which is secured to the cornea, with monofilament polypropylene haptics that are secured to the sclera for enhanced mechanical stability.[21] Preliminary animal *in vivo* studies with both prototypes demonstrated fibroblast integration, collagen deposition and corneal neovascularization, and only mild tissue necrosis and inflammation, with the polypropylene device performing best.[22] However, short-term human trials using the polypropylene prototype demonstrated tissue melting around the skirt, which may have been related to preoperative conditions.[21] Other complications included retroprosthetic membrane formation, retinal detachment, glaucoma and endophthalmitis.[21] Long-term usage of S-KPro, resulted in visual rehabilitation for about 32 months; however, instances of tissue melting and exposure of the skirt after approximately 13 months and retinal detachment following S-KPro exchange, which was attributable to poor vitrectomy techniques, were also evident.[23] Further *in vivo* animal research to improve vitrectomy techniques following device exchange resulted in a decrease in retinal detachment and may enhance the long-term success of the S-KPro.[24]

5.4.4   AlphaCor keratoprosthesis

Previously referred to as the Chirila KPro, the AlphaCor KPro, is a core and porous skirt design, all composed of PHEMA.[9] Initially there were two prototypes: type I is intended for patients with an intact conjuctival flap and is no longer available; type II, which has a smaller diameter, is less invasive, does not require a healthy conjuctiva and can be reversed if required.

As of February 2006, 322 AlphaCor KPro devices have been implanted in the United States, Europe and Australia with 416 patient years of experience.[25] Retention of this device after 1 year is high, approximately 80%, as a result of stromal fibroblast integration into the porous skirt; however, tissue melting, retroprosthetic membrane formation, optic damage and in some cases opacification due to calcification of the KPro can occur.[25,26] Extracted devices have provided evidence of stromal cell integration, along with chronic inflammation.[27–29] Omitting the second-stage surgical procedure, whereby the implant is exposed to the external surface of the eye, resulted in improved KPro outcomes, including longer device (14–38 months) tolerance, despite having a non-functioning endothelium; however, it is unknown how this will affect corneal hydration.[30]

5.4.5   BIOKPro device

There are three prototypes of the BIOKPro device: type I has a PMMA optic core while types II and III are composed of silicone with a polyvinylpyrrolidone coating; all have porous PTFE haptics.[31] Following implantation, the BIOKPro I demonstrated tissue integration through keratocyte migration and collagen production.[32] Clinical trials with 11 devices implanted for 5 years were less successful, with evidence of glaucoma, tissue necrosis, device extrusion, endophthalmitis, lens dislocation and retroprosthetic membrane formation.[33] Only 36% were retained, with 8 cases of melting, 10 cases of retroprosthetic membrane formation, 5 cases of endophthalmitis and 4 cases of device extrusion[33]. BIOKPro II had increased short-term clinical success with increased keratocyte integration and few corneal complications[34]. Although long-term studies with this KPro were more successful than those for type I (38% failure), there were still instances of skirt exposure, retroprosthetic membrane formation, endophthalmitis and device extrusion.[31] Further design led to the development of the BIOKPro III, which has a smaller optic and larger skirt, in comparison with BIOKPro II.[35] However, long-term human implantation results were disappointing, with only 1 of 7 devices remaining intact.

5.4.6   SupraDescemetic keratoprosthesis

The SupraDescemetic KPro (SDKP) can be fabricated from PMMA, or copolymers of PHEMA with MMA (PHEMA-MMA) or N-vinylpyrrolidinone (PHEMA-NVP).[36] Following implantation into seven rabbit corneas, these KPros were well tolerated after 8 weeks, and there was no evidence of inflammation in five eyes, with mild inflammation in the remaining two eyes, and no cases of retinal detachment.[36] Subsequent long-term studies in rabbits revealed 100% of the PHEMA-MMA, 80% of the PMMA and 60% of the PHEMA-NVP devices retained transparency.[37] Furthermore, deposited collagen was observed in the device skirt.[37] Implantation was also performed in feline corneas, which resulted in device extrusion between 15 and 150 days, but these results may not be representative of human wound healing as felines demonstrated complete cornea regeneration which is not possible in humans.[38]

5.4.7   Aachen keratoprosthesis

The Aachen KPro is made of silicone rubber, and the design boasts easy surgical handling and flexibility.[39] Following short-term implantation into ten patients, there were no occurrences of retinal detachment, clear visual acuity in four eyes, and edema in three eyes.[39] The type II Aachen KPro, with immobilized fibronectin for increased cellular attachment, was implanted as a temporary implant prior to retinal surgery or corneal grafting.[40,41] It also allows for intraocular pressure measurements in porcine eyes.[42]

5.4.8   Other keratoprostheses in development

An interpenetrating polymer network of PDMS and poly(*N*-isopropylacrylamide) (PNIPAAM) has been fabricated to combine the mechanical strength, transparency, wettability and glucose permeability of these two materials for ophthalmic applications.[43]

Elsewhere, three porous materials, polybutylene:polypropylene (80:20), poly(ethylene terephthalate) and PTFE, intended for application as a KPro, were evaluated in rabbit corneal stroma over 12 weeks.[44] PTFE demonstrated decreased inflammation and stromal cell migration, while edema and neovascularization were similar among the implants.[44]

A poly(ethylene glycol)–poly(acrylic acid) (PEG–PAA) interpenetrating polymer network hydrogel, with glucose permeability comparable with the human cornea, was evaluated over 2 weeks in rabbit stromas and was well tolerated in nine out of ten eyes.[45,46] Further development in fabrication lead to the usage of photolithography to form a patterned skirt of poly(2-hydroxyethyl acrylate) (PHEA) around the PEG–PAA core.[47]

5.4.9   Biological keratoprostheses

KPro devices have been fabricated using biological components – such as extracellular matrix components including collagen, fibronectin and laminin, or oligopeptides – to render the device more able to interact with host cells and tissue.[6,7] To aid with epithelialization and tissue integration, collagen type I was tethered to a PEG–PAA hydrogel; however, corneal epithelial migration and wound healing rates were decreased from 2–3 days to 14 days.[46] This was attributed by the authors to antimicrobials leaching from the hydrogel, improper surgical technique and the choice of collagen that did not properly mimic the corneal basement membrane.[48] Elsewhere, a poly(vinyl alcohol) (PVA) hydrogel with tethered collagen demonstrated enhanced epithelialization *in vitro*,[48] but required modification with an amniotic membrane (PVA-AM) to result in epithelialization, reduced inflammation and opacification *in vivo*.[49]

Corneal onlays fabricated from porous perfluoropolyether (PFPE) coated with collagen type I enhanced epithelialization in four feline corneas for 39 days.[50] In another study, porous polycarbonate membranes coated with collagen type I, collagen type IV, or laminin enhanced corneal epithelial cell migration and adhesion *in vivo*, while fibronectin, endothelial extracellular matrix, hyaluronic acid or chondroitin sulfate did not support epithelialization.[51]

PHEMA–MAA–PEG hydrogels were fabricated with extracellular matrix components (fibronectin, laminin, substance P and insulin-like growth factor) or peptide sequences such as arginine–glycine–aspartic acid (RGD) or fibronectin adhesion-promoting (FAP); FAP enhanced epithelialization significantly.[52] Previous work showed that tethered FAP and laminin had better epithelial adhesion compared with fibronectin.[53] Furthermore, cornea epithelial cell adhesion was increased *in vitro* on PHEMA hydrogels through tethering of RGDS (arginin–glycine–asparticacid–serine) and YIGSR (tyrosine–isoleucine–glycine–serine–arginine) cell adhesion peptides.[54]

Incorporation of growth factors, including epidermal growth factor (EGF) and transforming growth factor beta (TGF-β), has been utilized to manipulate epithelialization.[7] Specifically, EGF was tethered to PDMS through a PEG spacer to improve epithelialization of the surface, which was found to rely heavily on the underlying surface chemistry.[55–57] Tethered TGF-β2 was also demonstrated to enhance epithelialization and to hinder stromal cell adhesion.[58]

5.5   Tissue-engineered corneal equivalents

TECEs combine natural polymers or biological components – including but not restricted to proteins, polysaccharides, nucleic acids or polyphenols – and corneal cells to fabricate a device that could mimic one or more native corneal tissue layers for seamless integration into the host.[2] There are generally three approaches to TECE devices: seeding cells directly on a surface or gel that can be reorganized by the cells; seeding cells on to a substrate where they secrete their own extracellular matrix scaffold;[59] and using a preformed substrate or scaffold that allows integration of either pre-seeded progenitor cells or in-growing host cells. Many TECEs are based on collagen, as the cornea is mainly type I collagen.[7] TECEs with cellular components include cells from immortalized cell lines[60] or from primary/low-passage limbal or central corneal cells.[61–63]

5.5.1 Cell-based tissue-engineered corneal equivalent (Okano laboratory, Japan)

Corneal or oral mucosal epithelial stem cell sheets are grown on a temperature-sensitive layer of PNIPAAM, which allows cell growth and cell sheet detachment at 37 °C and below 32 °C, respectively.[64,65] Cells are removed from the PNIPAAM coating without digestive enzymes – retaining cell–cell junctions, cellular proteins and their extracellular matrix – and multiple sheets can be layered to form three-dimensional matrices.[64] During surgery, cell sheets are transplanted to the host using a donut-shaped support that can be removed following attachment of the cell sheets; cell sheets do not need to be sutured in place.[64] In order to aid availability, a device was fabricated for transportation of the cell sheets at 37 °C for 8 hours.[66] A regenerated epithelium and improved visual acuity 1 year postoperatively has been achieved with this technique.[64]

5.5.2 Collagen sponge-based tissue-engineered corneal equivalent (Hubel laboratory, USA)

A collagen sponge, fabricated through dehydrothermal crosslinking and lyophilization, supported epithelial, keratocyte and endothelial cell proliferation and migration, and extracellular matrix production *in vitro*.[63] Further studies investigated the development of a corneal stromal equivalent, whereby stromal cells cultured on these collagen sponges demonstrated a myofibroblast phenotype, evident via alpha smooth muscle actin staining, matrix contraction and matrix remodelin.[67,68] Transparency was further enhanced with the addition of chondroitin sulphate, while matrix contraction decreased.[67] Recently, collagen matrices were created with glucose-mediated ultraviolet (UV) crosslinking, with improved mechanical strength and transparency.[69] Microgroove patterning (2 μm) resulted in stromal cell alignment along the grooves after 1 week in culture.[69]

5.5.3 Chemically crosslinked collagen and cell-based tissue-engineered corneal equivalent (Griffith and Fagerholm laboratories, Canada and Sweden)

The Griffith group has developed various porcine and recombinant human collagen-based corneal substitutes that have been implanted successfully into mice, rabbits, guinea pigs, dogs and pigs as either deep lamellar grafts or full-thickness implants that aim to promote regeneration of corneal tissue by mobilizing endogenous progenitor cells. The hydrogels were fabricated by moulding to the appropriate dimensions and curvatures, which allow for transmission of 90% or higher of white light. Crosslinking, co-polymerization and development of interpenetrating networks have been used to enhance the mechanical properties of the gels to allow suturing and resist biodegradation. They demonstrated that a simple type I collagen-based corneal stroma mimic (fabricated by crosslinking porcine or recombinant collagen with 1-ethyl-3-(3-dimethylaminopropyl) carbodiimide hydrochloride (EDC) and N-hydroxysuccinimide (NHS)) could be successfully implanted into mini-pigs with stable host–graft integration.[70,71] At 12 months post-implantation, the implants had regenerated an epithelium, the stroma and corneal nerves. Results of recent Phase I human clinical trials in Sweden of corneal transplantation with the EDC crosslinked recombinant human collagen corneas as deep lamellar grafts are shown in Fig. 5.1. Early postoperative results show regeneration of corneal epithelium, stroma and early signs of nerve regeneration.[72] These implants, which are completely synthetic, using a synthethically produced recombinant human collagen did not cause adverse reactions and therefore are suitable as temporary grafts or patches. However, longer-term monitoring is needed to determine whether or not they will be useful as substitutes for donor tissue. In addition, further modifications are probably needed in order to be useful in a wider range of clinical indications.

The group has also shown that synthetic materials can be combined with collagen to enhance interaction with the host cornea, e.g. by grafting of laminin-derived pentapeptide, YIGSR, on to a synthetic crosslinker of poly(N-isopropylacrylamide-coacrylic acid-coacryloxysuccinimide),[73] enhanced nerve regeneration and restoration of corneal touch sensitivity was achieved in pigs within a 6 week period, compared with still insensitive allografts. Constructs could also be stabilized against enzymatic or UV degradation by fabrication of collagen–phosphorylcholine interpenetrating networks.[74] Where the patients are lacking endogenous progenitors, these collagen-based constructs have been shown *in vitro* to support expansion of corneal progenitor cells, e.g. limbal cultures.[75]

5.5.4   Dendrimer crosslinked collagen tissue-engineered corneal equivalent (Sheardown laboratory, Canada)

In order to increase the number of amine groups available for crosslinking, polypropyleneimine octaamine dendrimers were combined with collagen and crosslinked through EDC/NHS chemistry.[76] These materials demonstrated high mechanical strength, good optical clarity, biological stability and high crosslinking density.[76,77] Epithelial cell adhesion and growth was achieved *in vitro*,[77] and enhanced, as was neurite extension and nerve cell density, through the incorporation of an adhesion peptide, YIGSR.[78] Furthermore, incorporation of IKVAVYIGSR or YIGSRIKVAV peptides resulted in increased epithelial stratification, which was dependent on the peptide surface concentration.[79]

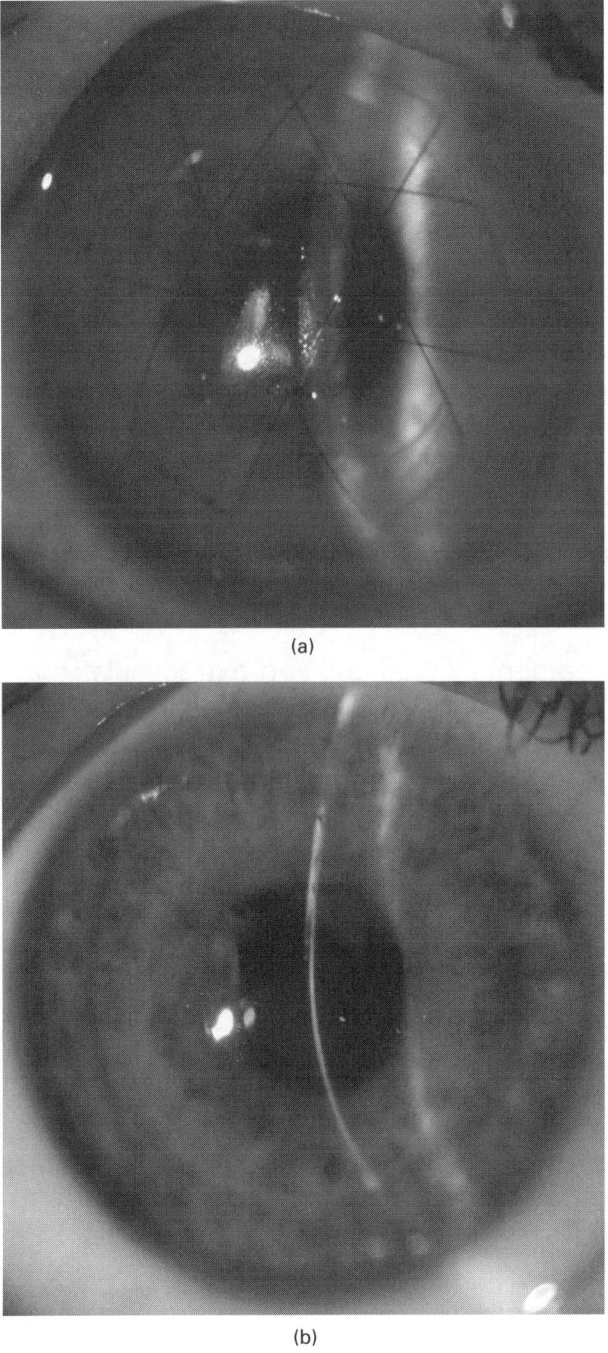

(a)

(b)

5.1 (a) Slit-lamp photograph of human cornea at 1 day post-transplantation and (b) 12 months postoperatively.

Heparin was also incorporated into dendrimer crosslinked collagen gels for the soluble delivery of basic fibroblast growth factor (FGF-2) and other heparin-binding growth factors.[80] Heparin did not compromise gel integrity, but opacity and FGF-2 retention were dependent on heparin concentration.[80]

5.5.5   Collagen–chitosan–glycosaminoglycan-based tissue-engineered corneal equivalent (Huang laboratory, China)

Collagen, chitosan and glycosaminoglycans were combined to form a degradable hydrogel for corneal replacement.[81] Chitosan was incorporated with collagen to decrease collagenase digestion and increase the mechanical strength of the resulting hydrogel, while glycosaminoglycans were also added for increased cell adhesion, flexibility and porosity.[81] Following implantation into 18 rabbits, re-epithelialization occurred after 5 days, clarity was maintained with only minor vessel hyperplasia after 10 days, and full degradation was achieved after 6 months with new corneal tissue and keratocytes replacement.[81]

5.5.6   Three-dimensional cell and extracellular matrix-based tissue-engineered corneal equivalent (LOEX group, Canada)

The three-dimensional collagen thermogel was developed by the Laboratoire d'Organogenese Experimentale (LOEX) group, whereby corneal epithelial cells are seeded atop of a previously cultured multi-layered fibroblast collagenous extracellular matrix to create a reconstructed corneal.[59,61,82]

5.6   Conclusions

The past decade has seen significant advances in the development of corneal substitutes. Extremely promising results have been obtained with synthetic artificial corneas, and a number of different prototypes are available. As a result, replacement of corneal tissue with artificial substitutes, while not commonplace, is certainly possible. The development of new tissue-engineered prototypes will only serve to enhance the potential of these systems for restoring the sight of visually compromised patients.

5.7   References

1 Chirila TA, Hicks CR, Dalton PD, Vijayasekaran S, Lou X, Hong Y, Clayton AB, Ziegelaar BW, Fitton JH, Platten S, Crawford GJ, Constable IJ (1998). Artificial cornea. *Prog Polym Sci.* **23**:447–473.

2 Griffith M, Hakim M, Shimmura S, Watsky MA, Li FF, Carlsson D, Doillon CJ, Nakamura M, Suuronen E, Shinozaki N, Nakata K, Sheardown H (2002). Artificial human corneas: Scaffolds for transplantation and host regeneration. *Cornea.* **21**:S54–S61.

3 Whitcher JP, Srinivasan M, Upadhyay MP (2001). Corneal blindness: A global perspective. *Bull World Health Organ.* **79**:214–221.

4 Carlsson DJ, Li F, Shimmura S, Griffith M (2003). Bioengineering corneas: How close are we? *Curr Opin Ophthalmol.* **14**:192–197.

5 Sit M, Weisbrod DJ, Naor J, Slomovic AR (2001). Corneal graft outcome study. *Cornea.* **20**:129–133.

6 Griffith M, Li F, Lohman C, Sheardown HD, Shimmura S, Carlsson DJ (2003). Tissue engineering of the cornea. In: Ma P, Ellsieff J, eds. *Scaffolds in Tissue Engineering.* USA: CRC Press, pp. 413–423.

7 Duan D, Klenkler BJ, Sheardown H (2006). Progress in the development of a corneal replacement: Keratoprosthesis and tissue-engineered corneas. *Expert Rev Med Devices.* **3**:59–72.

8 Khan B, Dudenhoefer EJ, Dohlman CH (2001). Keratoprosthesis: An update. *Curr Opin Ophthalmol.* **12**:282–287.

9 Hicks C, Crawford G, Chirila T, Wiffen S, Vijayasekaran S, Lou X, Fitton J, Maley M, Clayton A, Dalton P, Platten S, Ziegelaar B, Hong Y, Russo A, Constable I (2000). Development and clinical assessment of an artificial cornea. *Prog Retin Eye Res.* **19**:149–170.

10 Chirila TV (2001). An overview of the development of artificial corneas with porous skirts and the use of PHEMA for such an application. *Biomaterials.* **22**:3311–3317.

11 Lloyd AW, Faragher RGA, Denyer SP (2001). Ocular biomaterials and implants. *Biomaterials.* **22**:769–785.

12 Ilhan-Sarac O, Akpek EK (2005). Current concepts and techniques in keratoprosthesis. *Curr Opin Ophthalmol.* **16**:246–256.

13 Dudenhoefer EJ, Nouri M, Gipson IK, Baratz KH, Tisdale AS, Dryja TP, Abad JC, Dohlman CH (2003). Histopathology of explanted collar button keratoprostheses: A clinicopathologic correlation. *Cornea.* **22**:424–428.

14 Yaghouti F, Nouri M, Abad JC, Power WJ, Doane MG, Dohlman CH (2001). Keratoprosthesis: Preoperative prognostic categories. *Cornea.* **20**:19–23.

15 Aquavella JV, Qian Y, McCormick GJ, Palakuru JR (2005). Keratoprosthesis: The Dohlman-Doane device. *Am J Ophthalmol.* **140**:1032–1038.

16 Ray S, Khan BF, Dohlman CH, D'Amico DJ (2002). Management of vitreoretinal complications in eyes with permanent keratoprosthesis. *Arch Ophthalmol.* **120**:559–565.

17 Aquavella JV, Qian Y, McCormick GJ, Palakuru JR (2006). Keratoprosthesis: Current techniques. *Cornea.* **25**:656–662.

18 Falcinelli G, Falsini B, Taloni M, Colliardo P, Falcinelli G (2005). Modified osteo-odonto-keratoprosthesis for treatment of corneal blindness: Long-term anatomical and functional outcomes in 181 cases. *Arch Ophthalmol.* **123**:1319–1329.

19 Liu C, Paul B, Tandon R, Lee E, Fong K, Mavrikakis I, Herold J, Thorp S, Brittain P, Francis I, Ferrett C, Hull C, Lloyd A, Green D, Franklin V, Tighe B, Fukuda M, Hamada S (2005). The osteo-odonto-keratoprosthesis (OOKP). *Semin Ophthalmol.* **20**:113–128.

20 Viitala R, Franklin V, Green D, Liu C, Lloyd A, Tighe B (2009). Towards a synthetic osteo-odonto-keratoprosthesis. *Acta Biomater.* **5**: 438–452.

21 Kim MK, Lee JL, Wee WR, Lee JH (2002). Seoul-type keratoprosthesis: Preliminary results of the first 7 human cases. *Arch Ophthalmol.* **120**:761–766.

22 Kim MK, Lee JL, Wee WR, Lee JH (2002). Comparative experiments for in vivo fibroplasia and biological stability of four porous polymers intended for use in the Seoul-type keratoprosthesis. *Br J Ophthalmol.* **86**:809–814.

23 Kim MK, Lee SM, Lee JL, Chung TY, Kim YH, Wee WR, Lee JH (2007). Long-term outcome in ocular intractable surface disease with Seoul-type keratoprosthesis. *Cornea.* **26**:546–551.

24 Lee SM, Kim MK, Oh JY, Heo JW, Shin MS, Lee MS, Wee WR, Lee JH (2008). Endoscopic vitrectomy improves outcomes of seoul-type keratoprosthesis exchange in rabbit model. *Invest. Ophthalmol. Vis. Sci.* **49**:4407–4411.

25 Hicks CR, Crawford GJ, Dart JK, Grabner Holland EJ, Stulting RD, Tan DT, Bulsara M (2006). AlphaCor: Clinical outcomes. *Cornea.* **25**:1034–1042.

26 Hicks CR, Crawford GJ, Tan DT, Snibson GR, Sutton GL, Downie N, Gondhowiardjo TD, Lam DSC, Werner L, Apple D, Constable IJ (2003). AlphaCor cases: Comparative outcomes. *Cornea.* **22**:583–590.

27 Chow CC, Kulkarni AD, Albert DM, Darlington JK, Hardten DR (2007). Clinicopathologic correlation of explanted AlphaCor artificial cornea after exposure of implant. *Cornea.* **26**:1004–1007.

28 Coassin M, Zhang C, Green WR, Aquavella JV, Akpek EK (2007). Histopathologic and immunologic aspects of alphacor artificial corneal failure. *Am J Ophthalmol.* **144**:699–704.

29 Chalam KV, Chokshi A, Agarwal S, Edward DP (2007). Complications of AlphaCor keratoprosthesis: A clinicopathologic report. *Cornea.* **26**:1258–1260.

30 Ngakeng V, Hauck MJ, Price MO, Price FWJ (2008). AlphaCor keratoprosthesis: A novel approach to minimize the risks of long-term postoperative complications. *Cornea.* **27**:905–910.

31 Alio JL, Mulet ME, Haroun H, Merayo J, Ruiz Moreno JM (2004). Five year follow up of biocolonisable microporous fluorocarbon haptic (BIOKOP) keratoprosthesis implantation in patients with high risk of corneal graft failure. *Br J Ophthalmol.* **88**:1585–1589.

32 Legeais JM, Renard G, Parel JM, Serdarevic O, Mei-Mui M, Pouliquen Y (1994). Expanded fluorocarbon for keratoprosthesis cellular ingrowth and transparency. *Exp Eye Res.* **58**:41–51.

33 Legeais JM, Renard G, Parel JM, Savoldelli M, Pouliquen Y (1995). Keratoprosthesis with biocolonizable microporous fluorocarbon haptic. *Arch Opthamol.* **113**:757–763.

34 Legeais JM, Renard G (1998). A second generation of artificial cornea (biokpro II). *Biomaterials.* **19**:1517–1522.

35 Hollick EJ, Watson SL, Dart JK, Luthert PJ, Allan BD (2006). Legeais BioKpro III keratoprosthesis implantation: Long term results in seven patients. *Br J Ophthalmol.* **90**:1146–1151.

36 Stoiber J, Fernandez V, Kaminski S, Lamar PD, Dubovy S, Alfonso E, Parel JM (2004). Biological response to a supraDescemetic synthetic cornea in rabbits. *Arch Ophthalmol.* **122**:1850–1855.

37 Stoiber J, Fernandez V, Lamar PD, Kaminski S, Acosta AC, Dubovy S, Alfonso E, Parel JM (2005). Biocompatibility of a nonpenetrating synthetic cornea in vascularized rabbit cornea. *Cornea.* **24**:467–473.

38 Acosta AC, Espana EM, Stoiber J, Lamar PD, Marangon F, Alfonso E, Parel JM

(2006). Corneal stroma regeneration in felines after supradescemetic keratoprosthesis implantation. *Cornea*. **25**:1830–1838.

39 Langefeld S, Kompa S, Redbrake C, Brenman K, Kirchhof B, Schrage NF (2000). Aachen keratoprosthesis as temporary implant for combined vitreoretinal surgery and keratoplasty: Report on 10 clinical applications. *Graefe's Arch Clin Exp Ophthalmol*. **238**:722–726.

40 Kompa S, Langefeld S, Kirchhof B, Brenman K, Schrage N (2000). Aachen-keratoprosthesis as temporary implant. Case report on first clinical application. *Int J Artif Organs*. **23**:345–348.

41 Kompa S, Redbrake C, Langefeld S, Brenman K, Schrage N (2001). The type II aachen-keratoprosthesis in humans: Case report of the first prolonged application. *Int J Artif Organs*. **24**:110–114.

42 Krug A, Kompa S, Schrage NF (2002). The aachen-keratoprosthesis – a flexible KPro that permits intraocular pressure measurement. *Int J Artif Organs*. **25**:238–342.

43 Liu L, Sheardown H (2005). Glucose permeable poly(dimethyl siloxane) poly(*N*-isopropyl acrylamide) interpenetrating networks as ophthalmic biomaterials. *Biomaterials*. **26**:233–244.

44 Wu XY, Tsuk A, Leibowitz HM, Trinkaus-Randall V (1998). *In vivo* comparison of three different porous materials intended for use in a keratoprosthesis. *Br J Ophthalmol*. **82**:569–576.

45 Myung D, Farooqui N, Waters D, Schaber S, Koh W, Carrasco M, Noolandi J, Frank CW, Ta CN (2008). Glucose-permeable interpenetrating polymer network hydrogels for corneal implant applications: A pilot study. *Curr Eye Res*. **33**:29–43.

46 Myung D, Farooqui N, Zheng LL, Koh W, Gupta S, Bakri A, Noolandi J, Cochran JR, Frank CW, Ta CN (2009). Bioactive interpenetrating polymer network hydrogels that support corneal epithelial wound healing. *J Biomed Mater Res A*. **90**:70–81.

47 Myung D, Duhamel PE, Cochran JR, Noolandi J, Ta CN, Frank CW. (2008). Development of hydrogel-based keratoprostheses: A materials perspective. *Biotechnol Prog*. **24**:735–741.

48 Miyashita H, Shimmura S, Kobayashi H, Taguchi T, Asano-Kato N, Uchino Y, Kato M, Shimazaki J, Tanaka J, Tsubota K (2006). Collagen-immobilized poly(vinyl alcohol) as an artificial cornea scaffold that supports a stratified corneal epithelium. *J Biomed Mater Res B Appl Biomater*. **76**:56–63.

49 Uchino Y, Shimmura S, Miyashita H, Taguchi T, Kobayashi H, Shirnazaki J, Tanaka J, Tsubota K (2007). Amniotic membrane immobilized poly(vinyl alcohol) hybrid polymer as an artificial cornea scaffold that supports a stratified and differentiated corneal epithelium. *J Biomed Mater Res B Appl Biomater*. **81**:201–206.

50 Evans MD, Xie RZ, Fabbri M, Madigan MC, Chaouk H, Beumer GJ, Meijs GF, Griesser HJ, Steele JG, Sweeney DF (2000). Epithelialization of a synthetic polymer in the feline cornea: A preliminary study. *Invest Ophthalmol Vis Sci*. **41**:1674–1680.

51 Sweeney DF, Xie RZ, Evans MD, Vannas A, Tout SD, Griesser HJ, Johnson G, Steele JG (2003). A comparison of biological coatings for the promotion of corneal epithelialization of synthetic surface in vivo. *Invest Ophthalmol Vis Sci*. **44**:3301–3309.

52 Jacob JT, Rochefort JR, Bi J, Gebhardt BM (2005). Corneal epithelial cell growth over tethered-protein/peptide surface-modified hydrogels. *J Biomed Mater Res B Appl Biomater*. **72**:198–205.

53 Wallace C, Jacob JT, Stoltz A, Bi J, Bundy K (2005). Corneal epithelial adhesion

strength to tethered-protein/peptide modified hydrogel surfaces. *J Biomed Mater Res A Appl Biomater.* **72**:19–24.

54   Merrett K, Griffith CM, Deslandes Y, Pleizier G, Sheardown H (2001). Adhesion of corneal epithelial cells to cell adhesion peptide modified pHEMA surfaces. *J Biomater Sci Polym Ed.* **12**:647–671.

55   Klenkler BJ, Griffith M, Becerril C, West-Mays JA, Sheardown H (2005). EGF-grafted PDMS surfaces in artificial cornea applications. *Biomaterials.* **26**:7286–7296.

56   Klenkler BJ, Sheardown H. (2006) Characterization of EGF coupling to animated silicone rubber surfaces. *Biotechnol Bioeng.* 2006;**95**:1158–1166.

57   Klenkler BJ, Chen H, Chen Y, Brook MA, Sheardown H (2008). A high-density PEG interfacial layer alters the response to an EGF tethered polydimethylsiloxane surface. *J Biomater Sci Polym Ed.* **19**:1411–1424.

58   Merrett K, Griffith CM, Deslandes Y, Pleizier G, Dube MA, Sheardown H (2003). Interactions of corneal cells with transforming growth factor beta 2-modified poly-dimethyl siloxane surfaces. *J Biomed Mater Res A.* **67A**:981–993.

59   Auger FA, Rémy-Zolghadri M, Grenier G, Germain L (2002). A truly new approach fwor tissue engineering: The LOEX self-assembly technique. *Ernst Schering Res Found Workshop.* **35**:73.

60   Griffith M, Osborne R, Munger R, Xiong XJ, Doillon CJ, Laycock NLC, Hakim M, Song Y, Watsky MA (1999). Functional human corneal equivalents constructed from cell lines. *Science.* **286**:2169–2172.

61   Germain L, Auger FA, Grandbois E, Guignard R, Giasson M, Boisjoly H, Guerin SL (1999). Reconstructed human cornea produced in vitro by tissue engineering. *Pathobiology.* **67**:140–147.

62   Minami Y, Sugihara H, Oono S (1993). Reconstruction of cornea in three-dimensional collagen gel matrix culture. *Invest Ophthalmol Vis Sci.* **34**:2316–2324.

63   Orwin EJ, Hubel A (2000). In vitro culture characteristics of corneal epithelial, endothelial, and keratocyte cells in a native collagen matrix. *Tissue Eng.* **6**:307–319.

64   Yang J, Yamato M, Nishida K, Hayashida Y, Shimizu T, Kikuchi A, Tano Y, Okano T (2006). Corneal epithelial stem cell delivery using cell sheet engineering: Not lost in transplantation. *J Drug Target.* **14**:471–482.

65   Nishida K (2003). Tissue engineering of the cornea. *Cornea.* **22**:S28–S34.

66   Nozaki T, Yamato M, Inuma T, Nishida K, Okano T (2008). Transportation of transplantable cell sheets fabricated with temperature-responsive culture surfaces for regenerative medicine. *J Tissue Eng Regen Med.* **2**:190–195.

67   Orwin EJ, Borene ML, Hubel A (2003). Biomechanical and optical characteristics of a corneal stromal equivalent. *J Biomech Eng.* **125**:439–444.

68   Borene ML, Barocas VH, Hubel A (2004). Mechanical and cellular changes during compaction of a collagen-sponge-based corneal stroma equivalent. *Ann Biomed Eng.* **32**:274–283.

69   Crabb RA, Hubel A (2008). Influence of matrix processing on the optical and biomechanical properties of a corneal stroma equivalent. *Tissue Eng Part A.* **14**:173–182.

70   Liu Y, Gan L, Carlsson DJ, Fagerholm P, Lagali N, Watsky MA, Munger R, Hodge WD, Priest D, Griffith M (2006). A simple, cross-linked collagen tissue substitute for corneal implantation. *Invest Ophthalmol Vis Sci.* **47**:1869–1875.

71   Merrett K, Fagerholm P, McLaughlin CR, Dravida S, Lagali N, Shinozaki N, Watsky MA, Munger R, Kato Y, Li F, Marmo CJ, Griffith M (2008). Tissue engineered

recombinant human collagen-based corneal substitutes for implantation: performance of type I versus type III collagen *Invest Ophthalmol Vis Sci.* **49**:3887–3894.

72 Fagerholm P, Lagali N, Carlson DJ, Merrett K, Griffith M (2009). Corneal regeneration following implantation of a biomimetic tissue-engineered substitute *Clin Transl Sci*, **2**:162–164.

73 Li F, Carlsson D, Lohmann C, Suuronen E, Vascotto S, Kobuch K, Sheardown H, Munger R, Nakamura M, Griffith M (2003). Cellular and nerve regeneration within a biosynthetic extracellular matrix for corneal transplantation. *Proc Natl Acad Sci.* **100**:15346–15351.

74 Liu W, Deng C, McLaughlin C R, Fagerholm P, Watsky M A, Heyne B, Scaiano JC, Lagali NS, Munger R, Li F, Griffith, M (2009). Collagen-phosphorylcholine interpenetrating network hydrogels as corneal substitutes *Biomaterials.* **30**:1551–1559.

75 Dravida S, Gaddipati S, Griffith M, Merrett K, Lakshmi S, Sangwan VS, Veemuganti GK (2008). A biomimetic scaffold for culturing limbal stem cells: Promising alternative for clinical transplantation. *J Tissue Eng Regen Med.* **2**:263–271.

76 Duan X, Sheardown H (2005). Crosslinking of collagen with dendrimers. (2005) *J Biomed Mater Res.* **75A**:510–518.

77 Duan X, Sheardown H (2006). Dendrimer crosslinked collagen as a corneal tissue engineering scaffold: Mechanical properties and corneal epithelial cell interactions. *Biomaterials.* **27**:4608–4617.

78 Duan X, McLaughlin C, Griffith M, Sheardown H (2007). Biofunctionalization of collagen for improved biological response: Scaffolds for corneal tissue engineering. *Biomaterials.* **28**:78–88.

79 Duan X, Sheardown H (2007). Incorporation of cell-adhesion peptides into collagen scaffolds promotes corneal epithelial stratification. *J Biomater Sci Polym Ed.* **18**:701–711.

80 Princz MA, Sheardown H (2008). Heparin modified dendrimer crosslinked collagen matrices for the delivery of basic fibroblast growth factor (FGF-2). *J Biomater Sci Polymer Ed.* **19**:1201–1218.

81 Huang YX, Li QH (2007). An active artificial cornea with the function of inducing new corneal tissue generation in vivo – a new approach to corneal tissue engineering. *Biomed Mater.* **2**:S121–S125.

82 Germain L, Carrier P, Auger FA, Salesse C, Guerin SL (2000). Can we produce a human corneal equivalent by tissue engineering? *Prog Retin Eye Res.* **19**:497–527.

6
Tissue engineering of human cornea

S. PROULX, M. GUILLEMETTE, P. CARRIER,
F. A. AUGER, and L. GERMAIN,
Laval University, Canada;
C. J. GIASSON, Montréal University, Canada;
M. GAUDREAULT and S. L. GUÉRIN, CRCHUQ
Laval University, Canada

Abstract: The cornea is a well-organized tissue composed of three cell types (epithelial, stromal and endothelial cells), each having an important role for its functionality. This chapter will address different tissue engineering approaches to the reconstruction of either partial or full-thickness living corneal substitutes that can be used either as *in vitro* models for wound-healing studies, or *in vivo*, eventually replacing the donor cornea for transplantation in humans. Isolation of the proper cells, followed by appropriate culture conditions, and assembly into a three-dimensional tissue construct, are the first steps required for producing a functional corneal substitute.

Key words: corneal cell culture, limbal epithelial cells, endothelium, reconstructed tissue, integrin.

6.1   Introduction

6.1.1   The cornea

The transparent cornea is the main lens and the curved window of the human eye (Fatt and Weissman, 1992). The cornea is not vascularized except at its extreme periphery, the limbus, which is the transitional zone between the transparent cornea and the opaque sclera. The avascular nature of the cornea contributes to both the immune privilege of the anterior segment and to corneal transparency, but requires the circulation of the clear aqueous humor in the anterior chamber of the eye to supply it with essential elements and to evacuate metabolic wastes. The cornea is composed of three main layers, each with its resident cells. From outside to inside the eye: the corneal epithelium, which represents about 10% of the corneal thickness; the corneal stroma; and the corneal endothelium (Maurice, 1984) (Fig. 6.1).

The stratified, non-keratinized, squamous corneal epithelium acts as a barrier to protect corneal transparency. Deepest into the epithelium, basal cylindrical cells resting on the basal lamina (Maurice, 1984) are responsible in part for the renewal of epithelial cells: during mitosis (Fatt and Weissman,

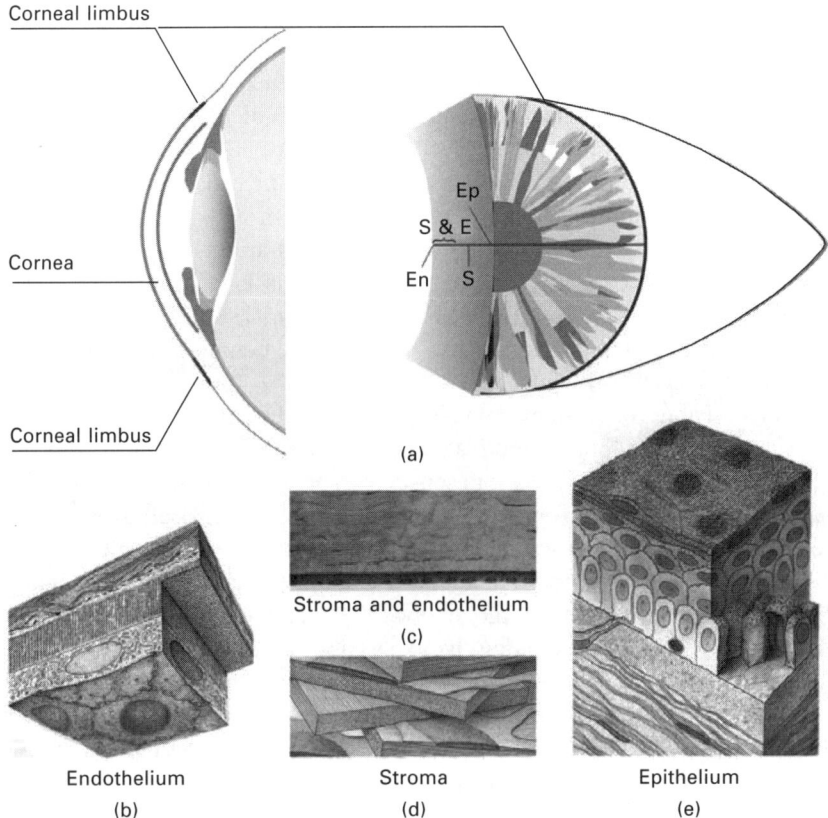

Corneal limbus

Cornea

Corneal limbus

(a)

Endothelium
(b)

Stroma and endothelium
(c)

Stroma
(d)

Epithelium
(e)

6.1 Anatomy and histology of the human cornea. (a) Side and frontal view of the cornea and the eye to show the epithelium (Ep), the stroma (S) and the endothelium (En). S & E is the back half of the corneal stroma with the endothelial layer, as represented in detail by the drawing and picture in panels (b) and (c). Panel (d) is a diagram of the corneal stroma representing a few corneal lamellae, each containing parallel collagen fibrils as well as corneal fibroblasts or keratocytes, represented by flat cells between these lamellae. (e) Drawing of the central corneal epithelium that shows the superficial, wing and basal cells of the anterior epithelium resting on Bowman's membrane and anterior stroma. (Panels (b), (c), (d) and (e) are reproduced courtesy of Elsevier and were originally published in Hogan *et al.*, 1971.)

1992), the daughter cells migrate towards the corneal surface and progressively flatten to become polygonal cells in the two or three intermediate epithelial cell layers and then differentiate into very flat cells in the most superficial couple of layers. With their continuous tight junctions, these superficial cells form a barrier between the tears and the cornea. They eventually desquamate into the tear film (Tripathi and Tripathi, 1984). It was initially believed that cell division of the basal cells accounted for the replacement of the whole corneal epithelium during the entire life of an individual. However, it was realized 25 years ago that this process alone was unable to account for the epithelial rate of desquamation, and that such a calculation required the contribution of the limbic stem cells (Thoft and Friend, 1983).

At the limbus, the corneal epithelium gradually thickens and becomes the conjunctival epithelium. The corneal epithelial stem cells are located deep into the limbic zone. Unlike basal cells, stem cells are undifferentiated and have an unlimited capacity for renewal (Cotsarelis *et al.*, 1989; Dua and Azuara-Blanco, 2000; Kruse, 1994; Schermer *et al.*, 1986). They also form a barrier to invasion of the cornea by cells from the conjunctival epithelium. Each cell is produced by successive divisions of the limbal epithelial cells. The first division from a stem cell is irreversible and asymmetric. It gives rise to a stem cell and a mid-differentiated cell (Schermer *et al.*, 1986), with the following characteristics: it is more sensitive to apoptosis than its mother cell, it has a limited potential for division, and migrates in the basal layer toward the center of the corneal epithelium in a centripetal movement (Thoft and Friend, 1983). After several rounds of cell division, cells reduce their contact with the basement membrane, move towards the epithelial surface, and enter terminal differentiation, initiating the expression of keratins 3 and 12 before desquamation and loss into the tear film (Dua *et al.*, 2003). In the central cornea, the daughter cells from the basal cell mitosis desquamate into the tear film after a period of 7 (Hanna and O'Brien, 1960) to 14 days (Haddad, 2000). The emergence of a new cell occurs before the old cell is removed (Klyce and Beuerman, 1998) in order to preserve the regularity of the corneal surface and the optical stability. The mitotic activity, which shows a rate of mitosis of 10–15% per day in the basal cell layer, allows the epithelium to ensure the tightness of the tissue (Edelhauser and Ubels, 2003). Experimentally, the mitotic activity of the limbic epithelium is higher than that of the epithelium at the periphery of the cornea, which is itself larger than the center.

The corneal epithelium lies on its basement membrane, which rests over the Bowman's membrane, a less organized form of corneal stroma. The corneal stroma represents 90% of the corneal thickness (Maurice, 1984). It is a pile of 300 superposed lamellae in the central cornea and 500 in the periphery (Hamada *et al.*, 1972). The lamellae extend from one end of the limbus to the other. Collagen molecules that form collagen fibrils are aligned parallel to each other within one lamella as well as to the corneal surface (Komai and Ushiki, 1991). The fibrils within adjacent lamellae are oriented at various angles (Klyce and Beuerman, 1998; Radner *et al.*, 1998). The angle between collagen fibers from two contiguous lamellae varies, having a mean of 60°. This arrangement not only provides extreme resistance to a tissue as thin as the corneal stroma, but also accounts for corneal transparency. Transparency arises from destructive interference that neutralizes reflections at the surface of the tissue; the relatively constant fibril diameter and density of the stroma act as a grating (Maurice, 1957). Laminin (LM), fibronectin (FN) and glycoaminoglycans (GAGs) are also found in the corneal stroma. The GAGs, which are located in the interfibrillar space, have a very strong tendency to attract water: under normal circumstances, the epithelium and the endothelium can maintain stromal hydration at 77% of water per corneal weight (Maurice, 1984). However, when these cell layers are compromised, the cornea swells. A significant edema disturbs the regular stromal arrangement and leads to loss of transparency and corneal blindness.

The keratocytes, dormant fibroblasts, are the most abundant stromal cells. From their cell bodies, which lie between lamellae of collagen fibrils (Klyce and Beuerman, 1998), emerge long cytoplasmic filaments that form a three-dimensional network of interconnected cells possibly involved in the process of healing and nutrition of the stroma (Watsky, 1995). The keratocytes closely regulate the synthesis and degradation of the extracellular matrix (ECM) with the synthesis of enzymes (please consult Maurice (1984)). During stromal trauma, the keratocytes lose their connections in order to repair the injury and become activated fibroblasts involved in the synthesis of procollagen and GAGs (Ham, 1974). The corneal stroma also contains other cells, especially during inflammation: dendritic cells, macrophages, lymphocytes as well as polymorphonuclear leucocytes.

The non-vascular corneal endothelium is a monolayer of cells. Their apical side with its discontinuous tight junctions (macula occludens) (Barry et al., 1995; Petroll et al., 1999) faces the aqueous humor contained within the anterior chamber (Hogan et al., 1971). This leaky barrier allows for a paracellular passive influx of water that contributes to supply all corneal layers with essential nutrients (Fatt and Weissman, 1992). The cornea can maintain its hydration and transparency only if this passive water influx is opposed by an active water outflux of the same magnitude. This concept is referred to as the 'pump and leak hypothesis' (Maurice, 1984). The ionic pumps from the corneal endothelium regulate corneal hydration through Na^+-, HCO_3^-- and Cl^-- dependent mechanisms. When the endothelium becomes unable to sustain this important function, because of insufficient cell density or disease, the cornea loses its transparency. Because the endothelium is unable to undergo mitosis in vivo, the endothelial cell density decreases steadily with age from 0.3 to 0.6% annually (Bourne et al., 1997; Murphy et al., 1984). This cell loss is usually compensated by the spreading and thinning of the remaining cells.

6.1.2 Clinical problems and progress in regenerative medicine

The need for corneal tissues is rising constantly in most developed countries. In 1996, 34 668 corneal transplantations were performed in the United States

(Barron, 1998), with a rise to 39 391 in 2007 (http://www.restoresight.org/ newsroom/newsroom.htm). On the other hand, the pool of donors is bound to decrease as a result of the popularity of refractive surgery and eventual improvements in selection criteria and in donor matching.

According to two studies of the keratoplasties conducted in Toronto from 1964 to 1997 (Maeno *et al.*, 2000), and in Philadelphia between 2001 and 2005 (Ghosheh *et al.*, 2008), the two groups of diseases for which keratoplasty was most frequently indicated were: (a) primary or secondary endotheliopathy, and (b) keratoconus. Whereas endothelial dysfunction causes edema and corneal blindness, keratoconus is characterized by a progressive dystrophic ectasia, which ultimately causes corneal thinning, scarring and deformation of corneal surfaces with complex optical problems. Both of these corneal disorders as well as their management are reviewed in textbooks (Kaufman *et al.*, 1998; Krachmer *et al.*, 2005).

Most corneal allogeneic transplantation involves a full thickness graft of a donor cornea from a deceased patient, a surgery called penetrating keratoplasty (PK) (Barron, 1998). Lamellar keratoplasty, a now rarely used type of procedure, involves a partial replacement of the cornea that is limited to the anterior cornea (epithelium with some stroma) (Hamilton and Wood, 1998). Recent improvements in surgical tools and techniques allow for the replacement of the endothelium with a thin supporting layer of stroma. This delicate procedure, called either Descemet stripping automated endothelial keratoplasty (DSAEK) or deep lamellar endothelial keratoplasty (DLEK), has much fewer side effects compared with PK for treating endotheliopathy (Price and Price, 2007; Terry, 2007) and this explains why it has become very popular among corneal surgeons.

The adaptation of techniques for cell culture of cells grown over a backing support (see also Section 6.3.3) with the advent of posterior lamellar surgery could open up efficient ways to treat patients with less rejection and better optical outcome compared with PK, while possibly allowing more than one recipient to be treated with a single donor cornea (Ishino *et al.*, 2004; Wencan *et al.*, 2007).

Tissue engineering methods have already been very successful in treating patients with limbal stem cell deficiency. The treatment of this condition is usually not successful with PK, as prognosis is not good for patients treated with PK alone (without a graft of limbal cells) (Whitson *et al.*, 1999). This is because the diameter of the corneal graft is insufficiently large to also include the stem cells (located at the limbus) from the donor's cornea, and these are necessary to treat corneal conjunctivalization. During this process, the absence of stem cells allows conjunctival epithelial cells to migrate over the limbus and invade the cornea. Neovascularization extends from the limbus and covers the whole cornea. Goblet cells, and their specific mucin product MUC5AC, are then present over a keratin 4 (K4)-expressing corneal epithelium. In normal eyes *in situ*, goblet cells and MUC5AC, as well as K4, are only associated with the conjunctiva (Meller *et al.*, 2002; Puangsricharern and Tseng, 1995, Tsai *et al.*, 1990). Limbal stem cell deficiency is either hereditary or acquired after disease or following a thermal or a chemical burn. Such a change in phenotype leads to loss of corneal transparency and visual disability. In the clinic, tissue engineering of the epithelium coupled with the classical treatment of limbal graft has been used to treat successfully patients with limbal stem cell deficiency (Pellegrini *et al.*, 2008; Shortt *et al.*, 2007). These treatments are covered in Section 6.5.

6.2   Cell source

Reconstructing a functional tissue *in vitro* first requires high-quality cells, like stem cells that have the property of self-renewal. Corneal stem cells, and progenitor cells that are already committed to a cell lineage, may be more appropriate for corneal tissue reconstruction, because such cells differentiate to produce their tissue of origin and do not have a tendency to produce multiple cell lineage such as multipotent stem cells. Thus, for many years, investigators have searched for the presence of corneal epithelial, stromal and endothelial stem/progenitor cells. Once located, cells have to be isolated and grown under appropriate conditions (substratum, culture medium) so that the tissue reconstructed with the cultured cells maintains functional and regenerative capacities.

6.2.1   Corneal epithelial cells

Best anatomic site

As discussed in Section 6.1.1, epithelial stem cells are located at the limbus. It is interesting to note that cells isolated from the limbus grow much better in culture than cells from the central cornea, suggesting that stem cells are preserved in culture. Cells from the central cornea have a short lifetime in culture as they can barely be subcultured. In contrast, limbal cells can be subcultured for several passages (up to seven passages depending on the donor). Moreover, cells isolated from the central cornea present morphological characteristics consistent with their low proliferative potential. They form small colonies containing large cells with a low nucleus to cytoplasm ratio, indicating that they are differentiated. In contrast, limbal cells produce large colonies constituted of small cells that possess a high nucleus to cytoplasm ratio. These characteristics are typical of less differentiated cells.

Within the limbus, a higher colony forming efficiency is attributed to cells that have been isolated from the superior and temporal quadrants compared with cells from nasal or inferior limbus (Deschambeault *et al.*,

2002; Pellegrini *et al.*, 1999a) or from limbal regions containing crypts and focal stromal projections, mostly present in the superior and inferior corneal limbal quadrants (Shortt *et al.*, 2007) suggesting that biopsies should preferably be taken from the superior quadrant. The preferential location of stem cells in the superior quadrants is consistent with the better protection against environmental and mechanical injuries provided by the eyelids in this region.

Culture of corneal epithelial cells

The use of the enzyme dispase for separating the epithelium from deeper tissues yields pure cultures without any contamination by stromal fibroblasts (Gipson and Grill, 1982). With this technique, epithelial cells may be detached from the basement membrane in order to detach a viable sheet of epithelium (Espana *et al.*, 2003) from which cells are isolated and cultures established (Germain *et al.*, 2000). The addition of a feeder layer is advantageous since large colonies can be grown from single cells under these conditions (Germain *et al.*, 2000; Green and Barrandon, 1988; Pellegrini *et al.*, 1999a).

Improved cultures with a feeder layer through stabilization of transcription factors

Human corneal epithelial cells reach senescence quickly, even in the primary culture (Lindberg *et al.*, 1993), and culturing them along with a lethally irradiated fibroblast feeder layer (such as i3T3) proved to be a major step forward as such mesenchymal cells not only provide an environment that limits invasion of the culture surface by contaminating living fibroblasts but also considerably improve both the cell morphological and growth properties (Pellegrini *et al.*, 1999a; Rheinwald and Green, 1975). Experiments that we recently conducted with both human skin keratinocytes and human corneal epithelial cells revealed that besides considerably improving the ability to sustain cell passages, the presence of a feeder layer also preserves the morphological and growth properties that typically characterize undifferentiated cells. Although we demonstrated that both secreted factors and cell–cell interactions are important for maintaining these feeder layer-mediated cell properties (Masson-Gadais *et al.*, 2006), the exact mechanism by which i3T3 improves cell behavior remains elusive. Recently, we reasoned that one possible way in which i3T3 may delay tissue-cultured cells reaching senescence is by altering either the expression or DNA binding of nuclear transcription factors which regulate the expression of a large array of genes in the human genome. Cell migration and proliferation, as observed with human corneal epithelial cells co-cultured along with i3T3, is dependent on cell cycle-related gene expression, the latter being modulated by the action of transcription factors that act either positively or negatively on the transcription of these genes. GC-boxes and related motifs are regulatory elements very frequently observed in the promoters and 5'-flanking sequences of many, if not all mRNA-encoding genes. The positive transcription factor Sp1 was one of the very first transcription factors to be identified and cloned by virtue of its ability to bind GC-rich motifs. Similarly, members from the nuclear factor I (NFI) family of transcription factors were also found to regulate a large number of human genes (although not as many as for Sp1) by interacting with a GC-rich motif (5'-TGGA/C(N)$_5$GCCAA-3') (Roulet et al., 2000; Roulet et al., 2002) distinct from that recognized by Sp1 (5'-GGGGCGGGG-3') (Dynan et al., 1985) and present in the promoter of the regulated target genes. Both Sp1 and NFI have been shown to play a critical role during cell cycle progression by acting on key regulators such as the cyclin-dependent kinase inhibitor 1A (CDKN1A), also known as p21 (WAF1/CIP1) that also participates in regulating apoptosis, senescence and differentiation besides a function in cell cycle modulation (Opitz and Rustgi, 2000; Ouellet et al., 2006; Watanabe et al., 1998). By exploiting the use of primary cultured skin keratinocytes grown with or without a feeder layer, we indeed provided evidence that i3T3 dramatically improves both the expression and DNA binding of the transcription factors Sp1 and Sp3 ((Masson-Gadais et al., 2006), see also Fig. 6.2). The process by which i3T3 acts on the properties of these transcription factors is believed to reside, at least for Sp1, in stabilizing them through post-translational modifications such as glycosylation which may prevent them from being degraded by the proteasome, as has been proposed for Sp1 (Bouwman and Philipsen, 2002; Han and Kudlow, 1997; Majumdar et al., 2003). Preserving expression of these transcription factors through an as yet unclear feeder layer-mediated influence will most certainly affect genes whose respective products are either related to the cell cycle or encode cell structural proteins, such as keratins and membrane-bound receptors, that are required for cell adhesion, migration and differentiation (Gaudreault et al., 2003; Masson-Gadais et al., 2006). In turn, improving these transcription factor properties is expected to also improve the quality of the epithelial layer overlaying the corneal stroma in the reconstructed corneas.

6.2.2   Corneal stromal keratocytes

Best anatomic site

In 2005, keratocyte progenitors were identified in adult bovine corneal stromas (Funderburgh et al., 2005). In this particular study, the authors reported that 3% of freshly isolated bovine stromal cells exhibited clonal growth. Using sphere-forming assays, stromal precursors from mouse (Yoshida et al., 2005), rabbit (Mimura et al., 2008) and human (Yamagami et al.,

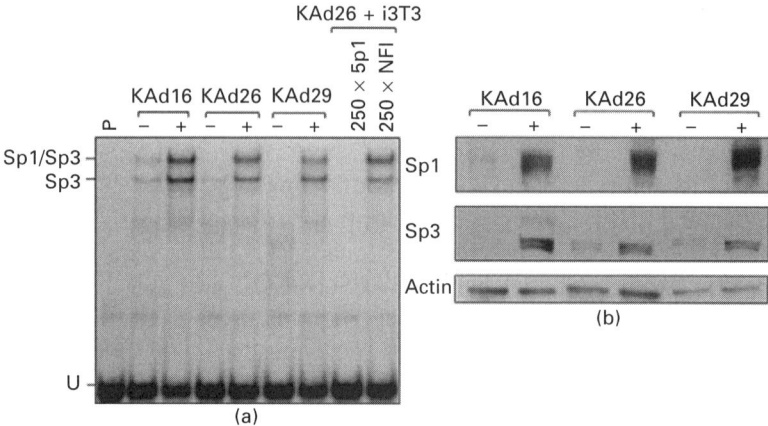

6.2 Expression and DNA binding of the transcription factors Sp1
and Sp3 isolated from skin keratinocytes co-cultured with i3T3. (a)
Electrophoretic mobility shift assay (EMSA) analyses of Sp1 binding
in human skin keratinocytes co-cultured with i3T3. Crude nuclear
proteins (5 μg) from skin keratinocytes cultured from skin biopsies of
16- (KAd16), 26-(KAd26) and 29-(KAd29) year-old human donors and
grown either alone (–) or in the presence of (+) i3T3 were incubated
with a 5′ end-labeled, double-stranded oligonucleotide bearing the
high affinity binding site for the transcription factor Sp1, either
alone or in the presence of a 250-fold molar excess of unlabeled
competitor oligonucleotides bearing target sites for either Sp1 or
NFI. The formation of DNA–protein complexes was then examined by
EMSA through a 6% native polyacrylamide gel. The position of the
DNA–protein complexes corresponding to the transcription factors
Sp1 and Sp3 is indicated along with that of the free probe (U). P,
labeled probe with no proteins. (b) Western blot analyses of Sp1
and Sp3 in human skin keratinocytes co-cultured with (+) or without
(–) i3T3. Approximately 30 μg of proteins from each of the nuclear
extracts used in panel (a) were examined in Western blot using
polyclonal antibodies directed against the transcription factors Sp1
and Sp3. As a normalization control, the membrane was also blotted
using a monoclonal antibody against human actin.

2007) corneas were isolated. Further studies showed that the cells from the
peripheral stroma possessed more precursors with a stronger proliferative
capacity than cells from the central stroma (Builles *et al.*, 2008; Mimura *et
al.*, 2008; Yamagami *et al.*, 2007).

Culture of stromal cells

Human corneal keratocyte cultures can be established from the corneal stroma
that is left after the removal of the epithelium and endothelium. Stromal
explants are seeded in DMEM (Dulbecco's modified Eagle's medium)
supplemented with 10% fetal calf serum and antibiotics (Germain *et al.*, 2000).

Stromal cells are subcultured in the same medium and can undergo more than nine passages. In this culture medium, stromal cells adopt a fibroblastic morphology after subculturing. Alternatively, human corneal keratocytes can be obtained after digestion of bare corneal stroma with collagenase (Carrier *et al.*, 2008; Germain *et al.*, 1999).

Keratocytes cultured in a protein-free culture medium adopt a dendritic morphology and maintain a differentiated phenotype. Keratan sulfate or keratokan protein expression is widely used as a marker for keratocyte differentiation (Beales *et al.*, 1999; Long *et al.*, 2000). Adding the growth factor fibroblast growth factor (FGF)-2 to the culture medium has been shown to upregulate keratan sulfate (Long *et al.*, 2000). Insulin supplementation stimulates proliferation while maintaining keratocan expression (Musselmann *et al.*, 2005). A recent study also showed that culturing keratocytes as substrate-independent spheroids preserved their differentiated phenotype and that addition of ascorbate-2 phosphate upregulated keratan sulfate protein levels (Funderburgh *et al.*, 2008).

Culturing these cells in the presence of serum alters the keratocyte phenotype to an activated cell, stromal fibroblasts, mimicking wound healing. Corneal fibroblasts, cultured in the presence of ascorbic acid, secrete and organize ECM which, when maintained in long-term cultures, can form sheets that can be assembled into three-dimenstional stromal substitutes (see also subsection 'self-assembly approach' in Section 6.3.2) (Carrier *et al.*, 2008; Carrier *et al.*, 2009; Ren *et al.*, 2008).

6.2.3   Corneal endothelial cells

Best anatomic site

In contrast to the epithelial side, where it is now largely accepted that epithelial corneal stem cells reside at the limbus, no clear evidence has demonstrated the presence and location of corneal endothelial stem/progenitor cells. Although they do not proliferate *in vivo*, it has been shown that corneal endothelial cells from both the central and peripheral areas retain potential proliferative capacity (Konomi *et al.*, 2005). However, Joyce's group (Mimura and Joyce, 2006) showed that human corneal endothelial cells from the peripheral area retain higher replication competence, regardless of donor age. Even though human corneal endothelial cells from the central area of corneas from older donors retained their replicative ability, the relative percentage of cells that were competent to replicate in vitro was significantly lower than in the periphery or in the central area of corneas from younger donors. This study was in accordance with a previous report demonstrating that corneal endothelial cells from the periphery undergo a higher number of population doublings than those from the center before reaching senescence (Bednarz *et al.*, 1996)

Sphere-forming assays have been used to isolate human corneal endothelial progenitor cells (Yamagami *et al.*, 2007; Yokoo *et al.*, 2005). A higher number of spheres were formed using cells from the periphery (Yamagami *et al.*, 2007). Using a panel of stem cell markers, a recent study (McGowan *et al.*, 2007) identified stem cells in the trabecular meshwork and in the transitional zone between the trabecular meshwork and the corneal endothelial periphery (including Schwalbe's line). Thus, all these observations indicate that, like corneal epithelial and stromal cells, the best anatomic site from which to isolate corneal endothelial cells for tissue reconstruction would be at the periphery.

Culture of endothelial cells from different species

Culture techniques and growth medium formulations for untransformed corneal endothelial cells have been previously developed for human (Bednarz *et al.*, 2001; Engelmann *et al.*, 1988; Engelmann and Friedl, 1989; Engelmann and Friedl, 1995; Joyce and Zhu, 2004; Zhu and Joyce, 2004) or animal (Giguere *et al.*, 1982; Gospodarowicz *et al.*, 1977; Lee *et al.*, 1991; Proulx *et al.*, 2007; Schultz *et al.*, 1992; Woost *et al.*, 1992a; Woost *et al.*, 1992b) cells. Using human cells, the effects of numerous growth-promoting agents were tested, such as: epidermal growth factor (EGF), fibroblast growth factor (FGF), nerve growth factor (NGF), bovine pituitary extract (BPE) and endothelial cell growth factor (Samples *et al.*, 1991); or ascorbic acid, insulin, selenium, transferrin, lipids and FGF (Engelmann and Friedl, 1995). Joyce's group (Joyce and Zhu, 2004; Zhu and Joyce, 2004) observed mitotic or morphologic changes in response to serum, EGF, NGF and BPE. Since animal models are required for pre-clinical studies, we have previously optimized the culture medium of porcine (Proulx *et al.*, 2007) and feline (Audet *et al.*, 2008) corneal endothelial cells. Human endothelial cell growth in our selected culture medium consistently generates cultures of small, polygonal-shaped cells (Fig. 6.3).

6.3   Corneal tissue reconstruction

6.3.1   Reconstruction of the anterior cornea

Amniotic membranes

Limbic cells can be grown over a support of amniotic membrane in the presence or absence of feeder cells (Dua *et al.*, 2004). Limbal cells cultured on plastic in the presence of a feeder layer retain great potential for proliferation and regeneration suggesting the conservation of stem cells (Lindberg *et al.*, 1993). When limbic human cells are cultured on amniotic membranes, they retain their native characteristics (Du *et al.*, 2003; Hernandez Galindo *et al.*, 2003), and present, compared with the corresponding cells grown on

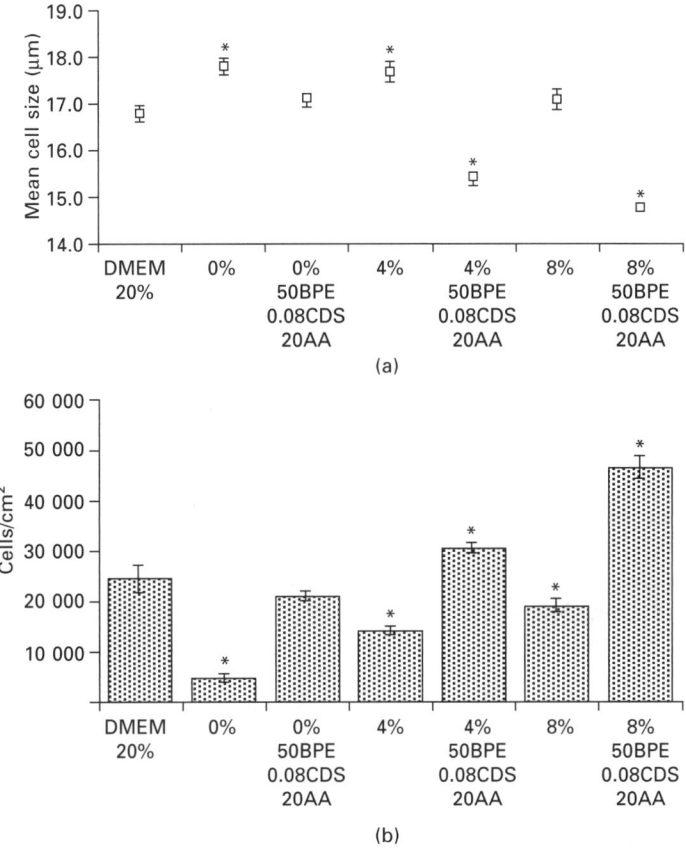

6.3 Effect of different culture media formulations on cell number, size and morphology of porcine corneal endothelial cells (PCECs). Representative results of the additive effect of 50 µg/ml bovine pituitary extract (50-BPE), 0.08% chondroitin sulfate (0.08CDS) and 20 µg/ml ascorbic acid (20AA) on (a) mean cell size and (b) cell number at day 4 on PCECs grown in Opti-MEM I supplemented with 0, 4 or 8% fetal bovine serum (FBS), and compared with the classic Dulbecco's modified Eagle's medium (DMEM) 20% FBS (diagonal dashed bar; mean ± standard deviation). The asterisks indicate a significance of $p < 0.001$ compared with DMEM 20% FBS (cell number and cell size). Lower panels show the morphology of PCECs grown in (c) DMEM 20% FBS or (d) the selected medium, consisting of Opti-MEM I supplemented with 8% FBS, 50 µg/ml BPE, 0.08% chondroitin sulfate and 20 µg/ml ascorbic acid. Cells were left in culture 1 week passed confluence to assess cell morphology of postconfluent cultures. The scale bar is equal to 100 µm. Note that in panel (c), endothelial cells are elongated and of different size, whereas in panel (d) they are small and cuboidal and have a morphology more characteristic of native cells. (Taken from Proulx *et al.* (2007) with permission.)

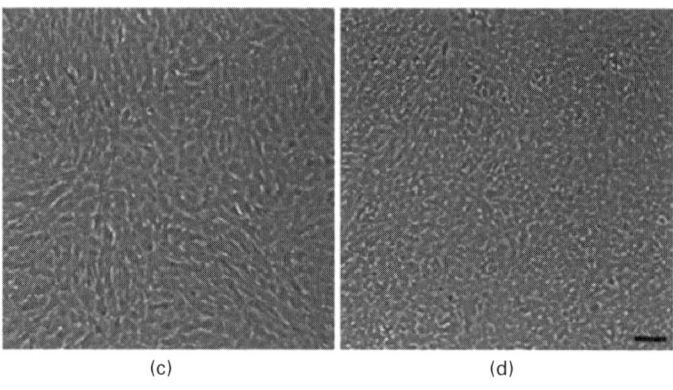

(c)   (d)

6.3 (Continued)

plastic, smaller proportions of K3+ and Cx43+ cells and larger proportions of cells positive for the transcription factor p63 or its isotype ΔNp63 (Du *et al.*, 2003; Hernandez Galindo *et al.*, 2003; Hernandez Galindo *et al.*, 2003). This transcription factor, expressed in basal cells of stratified epithelia, is crucial for the development and differentiation of epithelia. An homologue of the tumor-suppressor p53, p63, is localized in limbal basal epithelial cells of the cornea. The p63 isotype ΔNp63 has been proposed as a marker of corneal stem cells (Pellegrini *et al.*, 2001). For clinical applications regarding transplantation of epithelial cells seeded on amniotic membranes, see Section 6.5.1.

Fibrin gels

Fibrin gels, prepared from proteins that cause blood coagulation, have long been used clinically to prevent bleeding and promote wound healing. Their mechanical compliance as well as their biological features make fibrin gels a good carrier for cell transplantation, and their use has been reported for skin (Pellegrini *et al.*, 1999b) and cornea (Rama *et al.*, 2001). Limbal epithelial cells can easily be grown on fibrin gels (Rama *et al.*, 2001; Talbot *et al.*, 2006). The phenotype of rabbit limbal epithelial cells attached on fibrin gels and the negative immunostaining for both K3 and K4 suggest a low differentiation status, as the only cells with this phenotype *in situ* are the basal cells from the limbus where stem cells are located (Fig. 6.4).

In vivo experimental applications: transplantation of a reconstructed corneal epithelium

In order to assess whether cultured limbal epithelial cells are able to reform a corneal epithelium, the cultured cells seeded on a fibrin gel were

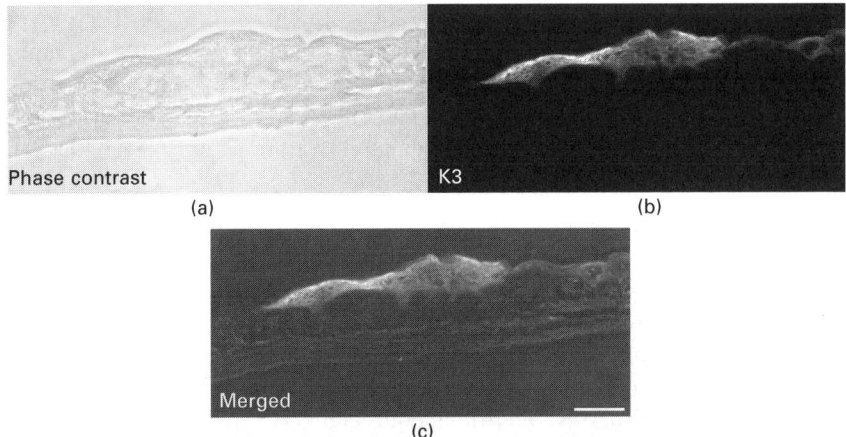

6.4 Keratin 3 staining of rabbit limbal epithelial cells cultured on a fibrin gel *in vitro*. (a) Phase contrast of confluent rabbit limbal epithelial cells (RLECs) cultured on fibrin gel. (b) Keratin 3 (K3) immunostaining of the same confluent RLECs cultured on fibrin gel. (c) A merger of the phase contrast (a) and K3 immunostaining (b). At this step, the RLECs cultured on fibrin gels were ready for grafting. Scale bar, 50 μm. (Taken from Talbot *et al.* (2006) with permission.)

autologously grafted on to a denuded conjunctivalized cornea of a limbal stem cell deficiency rabbit model (Talbot *et al.*, 2006). Results show that 1 month post-transplantation, neither goblet cells nor MUC5AC staining were observed in the central cornea of experimental animals, as opposed to untreated control rabbits that had goblet cells and stained positive for MUC5AC over the whole cornea in all epithelial layers. Therefore, the grafted epithelium most certainly adheres to the bare cornea, and the grafted epithelial cells proliferate and regenerate the corneal epithelium. For clinical applications regarding transplantation of human limbal epithelial cells, see subsection on 'Fibrin gels' in Section 6.5.1.

6.3.2   Reconstruction of the corneal stroma

Collagen gels

The unique properties of the cornea require that an engineered corneal stroma must be transparent and strong, and have an appropriate curvature. Since the corneal stroma is mostly made out of type 1 collagen (Klyce and Beuerman, 1998) many investigators have produced a corneal stroma by mixing cultured keratocytes into a collagen gel. The many drawbacks of this technique include, for instance: the important contraction that the collagen gel undergoes (Germain and Auger, 1995; Germain *et al.*, 2000; Germain *et al.*, 2004; Reichl and Muller-Goymann, 2003; Reichl *et al.*, 2004; Tegtmeyer *et al.*, 2001); the poor stability and strength of the matrix as well as its rapid degradation (Kondo *et al.*, 2008). The type of collagen used to produce the matrix also influences the end result, bovine collagen gels being softer and more fragile than rat tail tendon collagen gels (Doillon *et al.*, 2003), although all of them remain weak.

Hydrogels

In order to stabilize the collagen matrix, different cross-linking agents can be added to the collagen solution. The composition, cross-linking and configuration of collagen matrices were all shown to influence the optical and biochemical properties of stromal equivalents (Crabb and Hubel, 2008). Stromal substitutes, made from cross-linked porcine collagen or from recombinant collagen, have been shown to sustain epithelial and nerve regeneration both *in vitro* and *in vivo* (Dravida *et al.*, 2008; Lagali *et al.*, 2008; Liu *et al.*, 2008b; Liu *et al.*, 2009; McLaughlin *et al.*, 2008; Merrett *et al.*, 2008; Rafat *et al.*, 2008). Biosynthetic corneal substitutes fabricated using recombinant human collagen have the advantage of lowering the risk of pathogen transfer or xenogeneic immuno-responses posed by animal collagens. They have recently been reported to be biocompatible and to promote epithelial, stromal and nerve regeneration in phase 1 human clinical trials (Griffith *et al.*, 2009).

Keratocytes or stromal fibroblasts can be photoencapsulated into hydrogels (Garagorri *et al.*, 2008). Depending on the intended goal, the surface of the hydrogel can be modified to promote (Zainuddin *et al.*, 2008) or reduce cell attachment (Rafat *et al.*, 2009), or even to gradually release growth factors (Princz and Sheardown, 2008) or drugs (Liu *et al.*, 2008a), which could help in the healing or the long-term implant success of the grafted stromal equivalent.

Self-assembly approach

The self-assembly approach constitutes a truly new concept for tissue engineering. We originally designed it to reconstruct tissues as similar as possible to their physiological *in vivo* counterparts. In this approach, cells produce their own ECM and organize it into a structured three-dimensional network, without adding exogenous collagen or synthetic material (Auger *et al.*, 2002). Combined with the use of adequate cell types, the self-assembly approach results in the production of complex tissues with the expected histological, mechanical and functional properties as has been previously demonstrated by our group for blood vessels and skin (L'Heureux *et al.*, 1998; Michel *et al.*, 1999). The vascularization system can also be reconstructed as demonstrated by the formation of a capillary-like network in our skin construct. This new technology has recently given rise to very promising results for the reconstruction of human corneas (stroma and epithelium) in that corneal substitutes made out of corneal fibroblasts and corneal epithelial cells yielded a translucent tissue comparable to a native cornea, and dermal substitutes made out of dermal fibroblasts and dermal epithelial cells yielded an opaque tissue (Carrier *et al.*, 2008; Carrier *et al.*, 2009). In these tissue-engineered corneas, the stromal cells produced a dense matrix and the epithelial–mesenchymal interactions led to the formation of a complete basement membrane with all the expected ultrastructural components (lamina lucida, lamina densa, hemidesmosomes). Moreover, a new technology allowed the formation of oriented consecutive collagen lamellae (see Section 6.6).

6.3.3   Reconstruction of the posterior cornea

For many years, researchers have evaluated the feasibility of reconstructing a corneal endothelium from cultured corneal endothelial cells seeded on a carrier for eventual transplantation in humans. Different carriers have been proposed, such as hydrogels (Doillon *et al.*, 2003; Griffith *et al.*, 1999; Mimura *et al.*, 2004b Mohay *et al.*, 1994; Mohay *et al.*, 1997), vitrigel (Koizumi *et al.*, 2007), thin carriers such as Descemet's membranes (Lange *et al.*, 1993), amniotic membranes, (Ishino *et al.*, 2004; Wencan *et al.*, 2007) or gelatin membranes (Jumblatt *et al.*, 1980; Lai *et al.*, 2007; McCulley *et al.*, 1980; Schwartz and McCulley, 1981), as well as living or devitalized native corneas (see following two subsections).

Seeding cultured endothelial cells on living native stromas

The native corneal stroma is an ideal carrier primarily because it is transparent, has the right curvature, is naturally biocompatible and is mechanically stable. For these reasons, many investigators have used fresh native corneas as carriers for *in vitro* studies (Aboalchamat *et al.*, 1999; Amano, 2003; Amano *et al.*, 2005; Bohnke *et al.*, 1999; Chen *et al.*, 2001; Engelmann *et al.*, 1999; Gospodarowicz and Greenburg, 1979) or for transplantation in rats (Mimura *et al.*, 2004a; Tchah, 1992), mice (Joo *et al.*, 2000), rabbits (Jumblatt *et al.*, 1978), cats (Bahn *et al.*, 1982; Gospodarowicz *et al.*, 1979b) and monkeys (Insler and Lopez, 1986; Insler and Lopez, 1991a; Insler and Lopez, 1991b). Descemet's membrane was denuded of its endothelium using a cotton-swab. Cultured allogeneic or xenogeneic corneal endothelial cells were then seeded on top and cultured for times varying from 30 minutes (Joo *et al.*, 2000) to 7 days (Tchah, 1992). However, the high risk of contamination of the endothelium by the proliferating native epithelium of the living carrier impedes the use of prolonged periods of culture with fresh corneas.

Seeding cultured endothelial cells on devitalized native stromas

An alternative to fresh native corneas is the use of devitalized frozen corneas as carriers (Amano *et al.*, 2008; Bohnke *et al.*, 1999; Engelmann *et al.*, 1999; Proulx *et al.*, 2009a). Various methods have been reported for the initial removal of the native corneal endothelium. Most groups denude the Descemet's membrane mechanically using a cotton-swab (Alvarado *et al.*, 1981; Amano, 2003; Bahn *et al.*, 1982; Bohnke *et al.*, 1999; Engelmann *et al.*, 1999; Gospodarowicz and Greenburg, 1979; Gospodarowicz *et al.*, 1979a; Gospodarowicz *et al.*, 1979b; Insler and Lopez, 1986; Insler and Lopez, 1991a; Insler and Lopez, 1991b; Joo *et al.*, 2000; Jumblatt *et al.*, 1978; Mimura *et al.*, 2004a; Tchah, 1992). Other studies have reported denuding Descemet's membrane chemically using ammonium hydroxide (Bohnke *et al.*, 1999; Chen *et al.*, 2001; Engelmann *et al.*, 1999) or physically using one freeze–thaw cycle (Bohnke *et al.*, 1999; Engelmann *et al.*, 1999). In their comparative study of these three techniques, Engelman *et al.* found that the best method was denuding Descemet's membrane using one freeze (–80 °C)–thaw cycle (Engelmann *et al.*, 1999), as endothelial cells did not adhere well on to corneas treated chemically with ammonium hydroxide, and mechanical debridement with a cotton-swab left abundant residual components on the Descemet's membrane. We used the freeze–thaw technique to denude the Descemet's membrane and also found good preservation of that membrane after three cycles (Proulx *et al.*, 2009a).

We previously reported the production of a tissue-engineered corneal endothelium reconstructed from cultured feline corneal endothelial cells seeded on a devitalized stromal carrier (Proulx *et al.*, 2009a). Native cells of the carrier were eliminated through three freeze–thaw cycles. Devitalization eliminates any potential risk of contamination of the seeded endothelial cells by epithelial cells or keratocytes, while maintaining normal corneal shape and transparency. The destruction of all native cells by the three freeze–thaw cycles is also expected to reduce the immunogenicity of the carrier (Hori and Niederkorn, 2007; Quantock *et al.*, 2005). Most of all, corneas traditionally discarded because of the poor quality of their epithelium or endothelium could eventually be used and even kept frozen until needed, thus increasing tissue availability and decreasing wastage.

In vivo experimental applications: transplantation of a reconstructed corneal endothelium

Our laboratory has demonstrated that these cultured endothelial cells seeded on a devitalized stromal carrier can recover an active pump function and restore and maintain normal corneal thickness as well as crystal clear transparency over a 7-day observation period after transplantation (Proulx *et al.*, 2009b).

Assessment of the long-term functional outcome in the feline model will be the next necessary step in the development of this bioengineered living tissue, thereby representing a very promising approach for the treatment of endothelial dysfunctions.

6.3.4   Reconstruction of a complete cornea with all three corneal cell types

Reconstructing a complete cornea that mimics the structure and function of the normal tissue is a major bioengineering challenge. An approach that has been previously used by many investigators is a step-by-step procedure consisting of first culturing corneal endothelial cells on a culture insert, then pouring over either a collagen or a fibrin–agarose gel (cross-linked or not) embedded with stromal fibroblasts and, finally, culturing corneal epithelial cells on top of the polymerized gel (Alaminos *et al.*, 2006; Doillon *et al.*, 2003; Griffith *et al.*, 1999; Reichl and Muller-Goymann, 2003; Reichl *et al.*, 2004; Tegtmeyer *et al.*, 2001; Zieske *et al.*, 1994). Using an ouabain test assay, Griffith *et al.* (1999) have shown that their immortalized endothelial cells seeded on a collagen-chondroitin sulfate hydrogel were actively pumping fluid out of their stromal substitute.

More recently, a collagen–chondroitin sulfate foam was used to reconstruct a complete cornea. The scaffold was first seeded with stromal keratocytes and then successively with epithelial and endothelial cells (Vrana *et al.*, 2008). Other than demonstrating the feasibility of reconstructing a complete corneal equivalent containing all three cell types, two studies have shown that adding endothelial cells to the epithelial/stroma construct had an effect on epithelial cell differentiation and basement membrane quality. Indeed, in a rabbit model, constructs with endothelial cells showed a more defined LM and collagen VII staining and an improved epithelial differentiation (Zieske *et al.*, 1994). Using a human model, this influence was shown to be mediated through soluble factors secreted from the underlying corneal endothelium (Orwin and Hubel, 2000).

6.4   *In vitro* experimental applications

6.4.1   Re-epithelialization in a three-dimensional wound-healing model

Because of its anatomical localization, the cornea is more likely to be injured due to exposure to abrasive forces and occasional mechanical trauma, leading to wounding and scarring. Scarring of the corneal surface can result in the loss of transparency and even blindness. Many of these wound-healing problems are associated with the inability to reorganize a complete and mature smooth epithelium. Therefore, several models of wound healing have been developed in order to better understand the corneal mechanisms of re-epithelialization (Boisjoly *et al.*, 1993; Grant *et al.*, 1992; Maldonado and Furcht, 1995; Nelson *et al.*, 1990; Simmons *et al.*, 1987). However, the *in vitro* models of wound healing using cell monolayers lack the epithelial–mesenchymal interactions and are limited by the absence of multiple epithelial cell layers. Corneal wound healing has also been studied using human *ex vivo* organ culture models (Chuck *et al.*, 2001; Collin *et al.*, 1995; Foreman *et al.*, 1996; Lin and Boehnke, 1997; Hardarson *et al.*, 2004; Tanelian and Bisla, 1992; Zagon *et al.*, 2000). However, the availability of normal human donor corneas is limited and results can be influenced by factors such as variable delays between death and reception (Zhao *et al.*, 2003), reduction in epithelial cell layers, incomplete epithelium and stromal edema (Richard *et al.*, 1991; Tanelian and Bisla, 1992; Van Horn *et al.*, 1975).

The *in vivo* animal models of corneal wound healing using rabbits, rodents and horses (Brazzell *et al.*, 1991 Burling *et al.*, 2000; Kim *et al.*, 2001; Zieske *et al.*, 2001) are difficult to extrapolate to humans because, in contrast to humans, animal corneas have been shown to possess many stem cells in their central cornea, certainly affecting their response to wound healing (Majo *et al.*, 2008). Thus, there is a need for a new human three-dimensional corneal wound-healing model comprising both a well-differentiated epithelium and living fibroblasts. Using the previously described self-assembly approach (see subsection 'Self-assembly approach' in Section 6.3.2), we developed a fully human three-dimensional and completely biological anterior cornea, comprising both living fibroblasts and epithelial cells, thus allowing epithelial–mesenchymal interactions (Carrier *et al.*, 2008). In this *in vitro* model, human corneal epithelial cells migrate over a natural ECM (Fig. 6.5). This model also allows the study of a single parameter at a time as a result of controlled and reproducible *in vitro* conditions. Results showed that, during re-epithelialization, epithelial cell migration followed a consistent wave-like pattern (Fig. 6.6) (Carrier *et al.*, 2008) similar to that reported for human corneal wound healing *in vivo* (Dua and Forrester, 1987). It also allowed quantification of the re-epithelialization rate, which was significantly accelerated in the presence of fibrin or EGF. Therefore, this model offers a tool to compare and evaluate, under standard conditions, the effects of various exogenous factors on the rate and quality of re-epithelialization of the cornea.

This completely biological three-dimensional model sounds very promising for further studies on the mechanisms involved in the corneal re-epithelialization process, such as investigation of the expression, distribution and characterization of the role of growth factors, their receptors and extracellular matrix proteins.

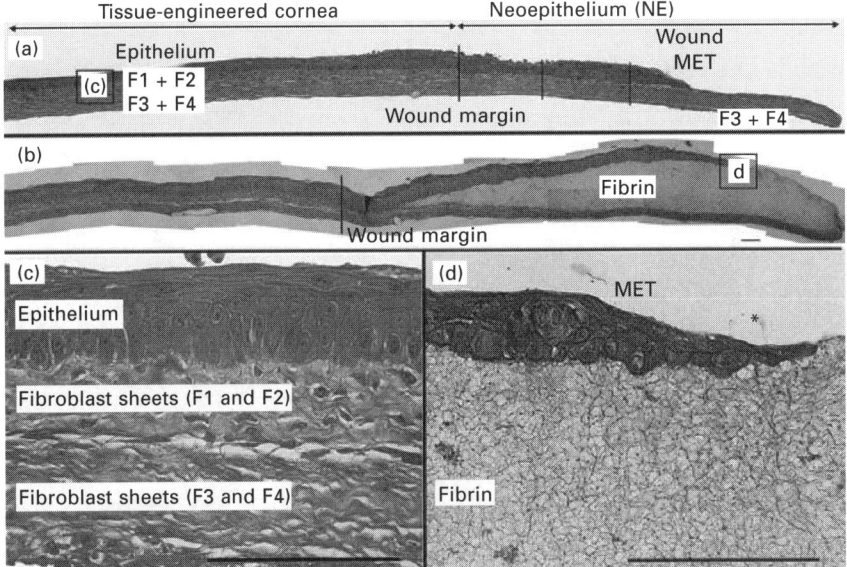

6.5 Histology of the *in vitro* human tissue-engineered corneal wound healing (hTECWH) model 3 days after wounding and treated ((b), (d)) or not treated ((a), (c)) with fibrin. MET, migrating epithelial tongue. Sections were stained with Masson trichrome. (a) Composite image showing a complete view of the hTECWH. (b) When a fibrin clot was added to the wounds, re-epithelialization was accelerated. (c) Higher magnification shows the histological organization of the unwounded side of the hTECWH. (d) Suprabasal epithelial cells at the tip of the migrating epithelial tongue (MET) (asterisk) elongated over the basal cells to make contact with the fibrin matrix. Scale bar, 100 μm. (Taken from Carrier *et al.* (2008) with permission.)

6.4.2   Extracellular matrix and cell adhesion in wound healing

Remodeling of the extracellular matrix during corneal wound healing

The ECM is a complex cross-linked structure made up of various proteins – such as FN, LM, collagens and vitronectin – as well as other polysaccharides (reviewed in Aumailley and Gayraud (1998) and Bosman and Stamenkovic (2003)). Attachment to the matrix not only enables cells to respond to soluble growth factors and cytokines, but also determines the nature of the response. This close, intimate contact with the matrix exerts an extraordinary control on the behavior of cells, determining whether they move or stay put, proliferate or remain quiescent, and even live or die. Many biological processes that typically characterize any given tissues – such as embryogenesis, cell differentiation as well as wound healing – will dictate which of these states the

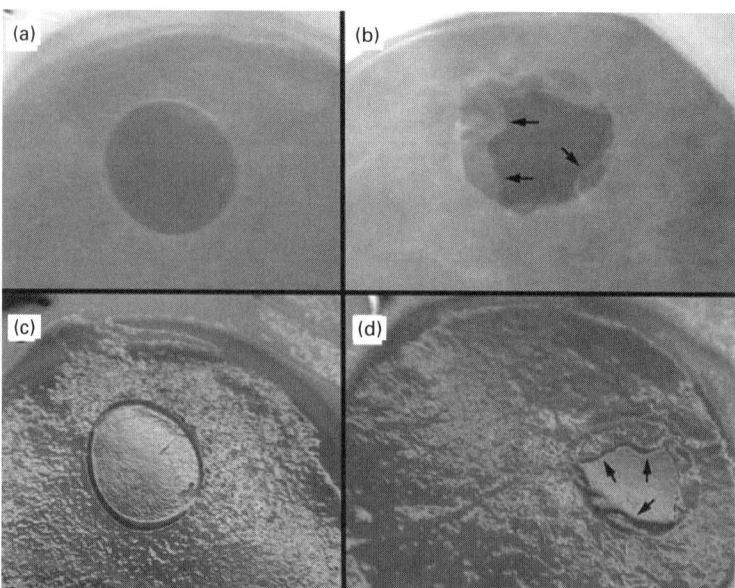

6.6 Macroscopic aspect of the wound in the hTECWH model. hTECWH immediately (a), (c) and 2 days (b), (d) after wounding with a 6-mm punch biopsy. Two days after wounding, the re-epithelialization progressing from the wound margin toward the center can be observed macroscopically (arrows). Note that in panels (c) and (d), the angle of the camera and the omission of the flash allowed us to visualize properly the extent of re-epithelialization from the surrounding epithelium. (Taken from Carrier *et al.* 2008 with permission.)

cell should get into. For instance, wound healing of any of the eye structures not only requires the formation of scar tissues but also the restoration and maintenance of the tissue's integrity, such as transparency for the cornea. In order to heal properly, the damaged corneal epithelium or any given epithelial tissue such as that of the skin, cells must first release themselves from the basement membrane through hemidesmosomes dissociation, and then reorganize their cell–substrate contacts to allow migration (Crosson, 1989). As hemidesmosomes are disassembled, important basement membrane remodeling is occurring that is chiefly characterized by the massive secretion of FN which is then used by the epithelial cells bordering the injured area as a provisional matrix over which they can migrate (Berman *et al.*, 1983; Gipson *et al.*, 1993). Expression of this provisional FN matrix peaks at between 3 and 12 hours following damage to the corneal epithelium and starts disappearing 1 week later (Kang *et al.*, 1999; Murakami *et al.*, 1992). As FN staining progressively diminishes, secretion of LM increases to reach maximal expression 1 week after corneal damage (Murakami *et al.*, 1992).

These clinical findings suggest that FN might promote cell migration and proliferation in response to tissue injury whereas LM would signal exactly the opposite by restricting both these properties and forcing the cells to either progress into growth arrest or differentiate (Gaudreault *et al.*, 2007; Gingras *et al.*, 2009). The primary function of both FN and LM is in cell–matrix attachment, but many additional biological activities – including promotion of cell migration, wound repair and ECM-mediated cell-signaling events – have been demonstrated (Kurpakus *et al.*, 1999; Malinda and Kleinman, 1996). As with FN, tenascin (TN), a large hexameric protein from the ECM whose expression has been correlated with development and wound healing, was shown to accumulate beneath the migrating epithelial cells 3 days after damage to the corneal epithelium in a mouse wound debridement model (Stepp and Zhu, 1997). TN accumulation in the corneal basement membrane reached a peak 6 days after injury and then progressively decreased to undetectable levels as it is normally absent from the normal, unwounded cornea. Unlike FN, LM and TN, collagen type IV, also a major basement membrane component (Nakayasu *et al.*, 1986; Philipp *et al.*, 2003; Zimmermann *et al.*, 1986), disappears during the early steps of the wounding process until the denuded area is completely covered, and then sequentially reappears beneath the newly produced epithelium (Ljubimov *et al.*, 1998). Major remodeling of the ECM, affecting nearly all of its constituents, therefore occurs suddenly over a very restricted period of time during corneal wound healing.

The role of integrins in corneal wound healing

Integrins are widely expressed, glycosylated, heterodimeric transmembrane adhesion receptors made up of non-covalently bound α and β subunits that link the ECM to the cell's cytoskeleton. They can promote either cell–ECM or cell–cell interactions (Hynes, 1992; Ruoslahti, 1996). To date, 18 α- and 8 β-subunits that can heterodimerize into the 24 known integrins have been reported (Clark and Brugge, 1995; Hynes, 1987; Hynes, 1992; Plow *et al.*, 2000). The rapid changes in the composition of the ECM that occur during the wound-healing process also translate into similar changes in the expression of many integrin subunits at the cell surface of corneal epithelial cells, which have been reported to express the integrin subunits $\alpha 2$, $\alpha 3$, $\alpha 4$, $\alpha 5$, $\alpha 6$, αv, $\alpha 9$, $\beta 1$, $\beta 4$ and $\beta 5$ (Huttenlocher *et al.*, 1995; Latvala *et al.*, 1995; Lauweryns *et al.*, 1991; Lauweryns *et al.*, 1993; Maldonado and Furcht, 1995; Paallysaho *et al.*, 1992; Stepp *et al.*, 1993; Stepp *et al.*, 1995; Tervo *et al.*, 1991; Tuori *et al.*, 1996; Vorkauf *et al.*, 1995) (also reviewed in Stepp, 2006 and Vigneault *et al.*, 2007). Indeed, the massive increase in FN secretion that typically characterizes this process was postulated to be coordinated with the expression of the $\alpha 4$ subunit (Lauweryns *et al.*, 1991). Cell surface expression of $\alpha 4$ has also been suggested to increase during cell migration (Clark, 1990; Stepp *et al.*, 1993). Although expression of α4 has recently been found to be modulated by cell density in primary cultures of rabbit corneal epithelial cells (Zaniolo *et al.*, 2004), yet no *in vivo* data support a role for this integrin in re-epithelialization of the damaged corneal epithelium. On the other hand, the integrin α5β1 was shown to be present during corneal wound healing after radial keratectomy (Garana *et al.*, 1992). As expression of α5β1 was shown to increase in corneal fibroblasts grown on three-dimensional collagen gels when FN was also present, Liu and coworkers postulated that FN then actively participates in the corneal fibroblast-mediated contraction of the collagen gel (Liu *et al.*, 2006). The use of a debridement wound-healing model in mouse cornea showed that expression of both α6 and α9, as well as that of β4, is closely associated with wound repair, resulting in a significant increase in the level of expression of these integrins at both the mRNA and protein levels (Stepp and Zhu, 1997). Appearance and disappearance of the integrin subunits are thus well coordinated with the changes in the secretion of the ECM components during wound healing of the cornea. The complete closure of the wound typically coincides with the diminution of FN secretion and the beginning of LM accumulation beneath the leading edge. The signal transduction pathway that is then activated upon binding of the α6β1 and α6β4 integrins to their ligand LM is expected to trigger growth regulatory signals, most probably negative ones, totally distinct from those resulting from the binding of FN to the α5β1 integrin (Gaudreault *et al.*, 2007; Gingras *et al.*, 2003; Vigneault *et al.*, 2007).

Three-dimensional tissue-engineered human cornea as a model for studying integrin genes expression during corneal wound healing

As it is often exposed to injuries, the cornea has become a particularly attractive tissue for studying wound healing. Indeed, corneal wounds account for a large proportion of all visual disabilities (approximately 37%) and medical consultations (estimated to be about 23%) for ocular problems in North America (Reim *et al.*, 1997). Because of their close association with the ECM components, integrins act as sensors that can alter the transcriptome of a given adherent cell in response to any changes that may occur in its outside environment. This is ensured by the activation of one, or a few, of the signal transduction pathways that integrins use to transmit these environmental changes down to the nucleus of the cell (Juliano, 2002; Lee and Juliano, 2004). However, most of these studies, if not all of them, have been conducted in either transformed or primary cultured cells that are grown as monolayers on a plastic tissue culture support. For instance, primary culturing of corneal epithelial cells (from either human or rabbit) at varying cell densities as monolayers on tissue culture plates proved to be a very informative, and a particularly practical *in vitro* model for studying integrin gene expression in conditions (such as subconfluence) that closely resemble those of corneal epithelial cells during healing (Audet *et al.*, 1994; Gaudreault *et al.*, 2007; Gingras *et al.*, 2003; Larouche *et al.*, 2000; Vigneault *et al.*, 2007; Zaniolo *et al.*, 2004; Zaniolo *et al.*, 2006). However, despite their relative ease of use, monolayers of primary cultured cells also have their limitations as they lack a properly organized basement membrane and are therefore unable to adopt the appropriate behavior that is typical of their corresponding intact tissues.

Considering the limitations linked to the use of cell monolayers, the tissue-engineered corneal substitute described in subsection 'Self-assembly approach.' in Section 6.3.2 is therefore viewed as an outstanding tool for gene expression studies and can be used to study the expression of integrins and other participating genes during wound healing. Furthermore, tissue-engineered human corneas also render possible the study of the influence exerted by human stromal keratocytes on integrin gene expression as interaction between these two types of cells is now recognized as an important factor in corneal wound healing (Daniels and Khaw, 2000; Mishima *et al.*, 1998; Nakamura *et al.*, 2002) (also reviewed in Lim *et al.* (2003)). Indeed, signaling from the stromal keratocytes was suggested to play a significant role in the growth and proliferative response of the corneal epithelium (Wilson, 1998; Wilson *et al.*, 1999). Recently, the use of the self-assembly approach of tissue engineering using both epithelial cells and fibroblasts originating from either the cornea or the skin shed new light on the role of fibroblast in the homeostasis of the epithelium (Carrier *et al.*, 2009). Quite remarkably, these experiments revealed that the tissue origin of the fibroblasts that are used to generate the stroma on which the epithelial cells are deposited does indeed dictate the stratification and differentiation properties of these epithelial cells. Besides examining the expression of endogenous integrins in the epithelial cells, the use of tissue-engineered human corneal substitutes is also particularly attractive in that it can be exploited as a tool to virtually dissect the regulatory sequences (both the promoter and 5'-flanking region) of any given integrin gene (for instance, those of the $\alpha 5$ and $\alpha 6$ genes) and define precisely how they behave functionally when introduced into corneal epithelial cells that are re-allowed to grow and expand on the keratocytes-containing collagen matrix. By exploiting lentiviral technology to ensure a high level of stable transduction and expression of integrin gene promoters (for reviews see Kafri, 2004, and Stevenson, 2002) in corneal epithelial cells prior to their seeding on the reconstructed corneal stroma, one can easily bypass the limitations of commonly used transfection procedures such as low efficiency of transfection and transient expression of the recombinant construct. The use of tissue-engineered human corneas constructed using recombinant lentivirus-infected corneal epithelial cells will render possible the direct survey of integrin gene promoter activity into the completely stratified lentivirus-infected epithelium in response to wounds produced with a biopsy punch (Carrier *et al.*, 2008), a type of analysis that otherwise could not be conducted in intact human corneas.

In summary, tissue-engineered human corneal substitutes as a tool for studying gene expression will most certainly contribute to bring integrins to the forefront of components required to ensure proper healing of the injured cornea. As the understanding of the potential roles and implications of each integrin gene increases, the possibility of modifying the transcription of each of these subunits becomes quite interesting. Promising new technologies that directly affect the outcomes of a gene product are being developed and these represent potential therapeutic means to address wound healing directly. Interesting advances in the use of small interfering RNAs (siRNAs) are being proposed as a promising way to knockout the transcript of any chosen gene, but they could also be used against any transcription factors that regulate a particular gene (such as those encoding integrin subunits) to alleviate a repressionnal state that could be induced by a repressor on the core promoter of an integrin gene, for instance. Lentivirus-mediated RNA interference therapy is also considered to be a promising method for efficiently delivering stable expression and control of gene expression (reviewed in Morris and Rossi (2006)). Stably altering specific integrin expression in corneal epithelial cells may prove useful for improving the growth properties and stability of the tissue-engineered corneas, thereby reducing the risks of scar formation upon grafting on patients afflicted with corneal diseases.

6.5   Clinical applications

In ophthalmology, the most successful clinical application of tissue-engineering techniques has been in the treatment of patients with limbal stem cell deficiency (Pellegrini *et al.*, 2008; Shortt *et al.*, 2007). In this procedure, limbal cells that have been sampled and expanded in culture are autologously or heterologously grafted to patients on a support material (a polymer, an amniotic membrane or a gel). When a fibro-vascular outgrowth is present, it is necessary to remove it before transplanting corneal stem cells on a support of amniotic membrane or fibrin gel. An autologous limbal graft is considered in cases of unilateral lesions (Coster, 1998). In this case, a limbal biopsy as small as 1 mm^2 proved sufficient to cover the entire corneal surface (Pellegrini *et al.*, 2008). However, limbal sampling bears the potential risk of causing limbal stem cell deficiency in the healthy contralateral eye (Chen and Tseng, 1991), unless cells are expanded in culture prior to transplantation. Limbal allograft with systemic immunosuppression is another option; however, the risk of significant side effects from long-term immunosuppression is a major drawback of this technique.

6.5.1   Cultured epithelium grafting

Amniotic membrane

The amniotic membrane has been used as a biological dressing or as a substrate for epithelial growth in the management of various ocular surface conditions (Bouchard and John, 2004). The amnion abounds in cytokines that have antalgic, anti-bacterial, anti-inflammatory and anti-immunogenic properties; in addition the amnion allows, as fetal skin does, wound healing with reduced scar formation (for review, see Dua *et al.*, 2004). Specifically, the amnion is used to: (a) limit formation of adhesive bands between eyelids and eyeball (symblepharon) or the progression of a fibrovascular outgrowth towards the cornea (pterygium) or (b) facilitate the healing of corneal ulcers, bullous keratopathy, and corneal stem cell deficiency. For this last condition, the amniotic membrane is used with a limbal transplantation (Gomes *et al.*, 2003).

The limbal corneal and conjunctival cells may also be cultured separately on amniotic membrane before being transplanted to patients with eye burns. As burns destroy conjunctival and corneal stem cells, the addition of these two cell types stabilizes the ocular surface and prepares it for possible penetrating keratoplasty after the initial reconstruction (Sangwan *et al.*, 2003).

The amnion is also used to treat disorders of the eyelid and bulbar conjunctiva, and corneal diseases, and as a replacement tissue used in the management of corneal or scleral ulcers (Bouchard and John, 2004). It is indicated for treating persistent epithelial defects due to a neurotrophic keratopathy, bullous or exposure keratopathy, or during atopic keratoconjunctivitis and severe ocular pemphigoid (Bouchard and John, 2004). The use of amnion in patients suffering from Stevens–Johnson syndrome has produced mixed results (Gomes *et al.*, 2003; Shimazaki *et al.*, 2002). Finally, after a trauma, the amniotic membrane has been used as an alternative dressing to a bandage contact lens in order to reduce the friction between the eyelid and the injured surface epithelium and pain during blinking (Baum, 2002).

Fibrin gels

Pellegrini and coworkers reported the use of fibrin gels as a substrate for supporting cultured epithelial cells for the treatment of patients with severe skin burns (Pellegrini *et al.*, 1999b), and later for patients suffering from limbal stem cell deficiency (Rama *et al.*, 2001). The fibrin gel acts as a substrate that helps to support the cultured epithelial cells before and during grafting. In addition, its adhesive properties help to glue the sheet of epithelial cells to the underlying stroma. In contrast to the amniotic membrane, which lasts 10 days after grafting, the fibrin gel is degraded very rapidly within 24 hours without any deleterious effect on the survival of the cultured epithelial cells (Nakamura *et al.*, 2003). Fibrin is the only substrate for which the maintenance of stem cells and long-term proliferation of limbal cells have been demonstrated (Pellegrini *et al.*, 2008; Rama *et al.*, 2001).

6.6   Future trends

6.6.1   Stromal cell/collagen orientation

In the corneal stroma, the specific arrangement of collagen fibers is important for transparency and strength. Various methods of cell and ECM component alignment have been described and have recently been applied to corneal fibroblasts in culture. Corneal fibroblasts, as with many other cell types, will follow a specific orientation if cultured on microgrooved substrates (Crabb and Hubel, 2008; Guillemette *et al.*, 2009; Teixeira *et al.*, 2004; Vrana *et al.*, 2007) or on magnetically aligned collagen scaffold (Torbet *et al.*, 2007), a process called 'contact guidance'. Some local cell alignment over small areas has also been reported using cells grown over disorganized collagen substrates (Ren *et al.*, 2008) or without scaffolds (Du *et al.*, 2007; Guo *et al.*, 2007). The resulting aligned fibroblasts then secrete GAGs and aligned collagen fibrils over small surface areas. Furthermore, fibril size and interfibrillar spacing can be modified by adding epithelial cells (Builles *et al.*, 2007a; Builles *et al.*, 2007b).

A thermoplastic elastomer engraved with a depth of 1 µm and a grating period ranging from 1 to 4 µm was used to cultivate corneal fibroblasts (Guillemette *et al.*, 2009). Results show that cells grew aligned to the grooves and that cell–cell interactions were possible over the entire sample, leading to ECM secretion and organization following cell orientation. The second overlying cell layer was also oriented with a mean angle shift of 53 ± 8° relative to the first corneal fibroblast layer (Fig. 6.7(a) and (b)). This cell organization reflects the physiological organization within a human corneal stroma. Both cells and the cell-secreted ECM (mainly type I collagen) layer were highly organized. Transmission electron microscopy was used to visualize the regularly spaced rows of lines alternating with dots in the microstructured samples, indicating that the stromal sheets comprised lamellae of aligned collagen fibers shifting from plane to plane (Fig. 6.7(c) and (d)). Furthermore, results showed that oriented self-assembled stromal sheets exhibited a better transparency compared with the same nonstructured tissue. In contrast, tissues produced from skin fibroblasts did not show organization of the second overlaying cell layer.

Thus, stromal cells and corneal fibroblasts retain the potential to organize into a multilayered and aligned stromal tissue *in vitro*. Taking advantage of this ability using various cell culture techniques may ultimately lead to higher quality tissue-engineered corneal stromas.

Control corneal substitute   Oriented corneal substitute

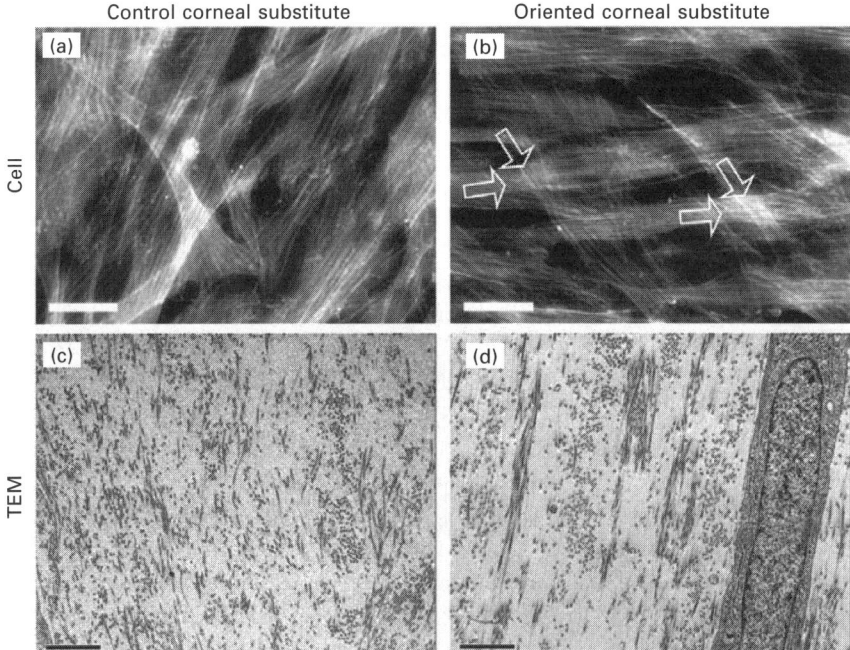

6.7 Cell and ECM alignment imaging. Actin filaments immunofluorescence staining of corneal fibroblasts grown on control (a) and oriented (b) substrates. Cells that have been cultured on control substrates have a random orientation compared with cells grown over microgrooved substrates where the cell shift in between layers can be observed. Transmission electronic microscopy (TEM) images of the corneal stroma. TEM images of control (c) and oriented (d) corneal stroma that have been cultured on microgrooved substrates, dots represents collagen fibres perpendicular to the plane and striated lines represents angled collagen fibres, they do not run longitudinally on the plane since they have about a 53° shift between each layer. Scale bars. (a) and (b), 50 μm; (c) and (d), 1 μm.

6.6.2   Future clinical applications

The fibrin support that has been used mainly for treating limbal stem cell deficiency could eventually be used to grow the endothelium *in vitro* and could be coupled with posterior lamellar keratoplasty such as DLEK or DSEAK in order to treat endotheliopathies.

6.7   Sources of futher information and advice

For more information on the various models of reconstructed corneas and their potential after grafting *in vivo*, readers are invited to consult the following reviews: Shortt *et al.* (2007), McLaughlin *et al.* (2009), Shah *et al.* (2008) and Ruberti and Zieske, (2008) and Griffith *et al.* (2009). For an in-depth review of the integrins, see Vigeault *et al.* (2007). More information on tissue engineering and regenerative medicine can be found at www.loex.qc.ca.

6.8   Acknowledgements

The authors would like to thank Elsevier, *Molecular Vision* and *Investigative Ophthalmology and Visual Science* for their permission to use previously published figures. This work was supported by the Canadian Institutes of Health Research (CIHR), Ottawa, Canada (L.G., S.L.G., F.A.A.), the Fonds de recherche en santé du Québec (FRSQ) Research in Vision Health Network, Montreal, Canada (L.G., S.L.G., C.G.J., F.A.A.), and the Centre de recherche FRSQ du CHA de Québec (L.G., F.A.A.). S.P. holds a postdoctoral fellowship from the Natural Sciences and Engineering Research Council of Canada (NSERC), Ottawa, Canada. L.G. is the recipient of a Canadian Research Chair from the CIHR in Stem Cells and Tissue Engineering. The authors would like to thank Alexandre Deschambeault, Caroline Audet, Alain Lapante, and the members of the LOEX who have participated in these studies.

6.9   References

Aboalchamat, B., Engelmann, K., Bohnke, M., Eggli, P. & Bednarz, J. (1999) Morphological and functional analysis of immortalized human corneal endothelial cells after transplantation. *Exp Eye Res*, **69**, 547–53.

Alaminos, M., Del Carmen Sanchez-Quevedo, M., Munoz-Avila, J. I., Serrano, D., Medialdea, S., Carreras, I. & Campos, A. (2006) Construction of a complete rabbit cornea substitute using a fibrin–agarose scaffold. *Invest Ophthalmol Vis Sci*, **47**, 3311–7.

Alvarado, J. A., Gospodarowicz, D. & Greenburg, G. (1981) Corneal endothelial replacement. I. In vitro formation of an endothelial monolayer. *Invest Ophthalmol Vis Sci*, **21**, 300–16.

Amano, S. (2003) Transplantation of cultured human corneal endothelial cells. *Cornea*, **22**, S66–74.

Amano, S., Mimura, T., Yamagami, S., Osakabe, Y. & Miyata, K. (2005) Properties of corneas reconstructed with cultured human corneal endothelial cells and human corneal stroma. *Jpn J Ophthalmol*, **49**, 448–52.

Amano, S., Shimomura, N., Yokoo, S., Araki-Sasaki, K. & Yamagami, S. (2008) Decellularizing corneal stroma using N_2 gas. *Mol Vis*, **14**, 878–82.

Audet, C., Proulx, S., Uwamaliya, J., Deschambeault, A., Carrier, P., Brunette, I. & Germain, L. (2008) Optimization of the culture conditions for feline corneal endothelial cell cultures. *Invest Ophthalmol Vis Sci*, **49**, E-Abstract 3944.

Audet, J. F., Masson, J. Y., Rosen, G. D., Salesse, C. & Guerin, S. L. (1994) Multiple regulatory elements control the basal promoter activity of the human alpha 4 integrin gene. *DNA Cell Biol*, **13**, 1071–85.

Auger, F. A., Remy-Zolghadri, M., Grenier, G. & Germain, L. (2002) A truly new approach for tissue engineering: the LOEX self-assembly technique. *Ernst Schering Res Found Workshop*, 73–88.

Aumailley, M. & Gayraud, B. (1998) Structure and biological activity of the extracellular matrix. *J Mol Med*, **76**, 253–65.

Bahn, C. F., Maccallum, D. K., Lillie, J. H., Meyer, R. F. & Martonyi, C. L. (1982) Complications associated with bovine corneal endothelial cell-lined homografts in the cat. *Invest Ophthalmol Vis Sci*, **22**, 73–90.

Barron, B. (1998) Penetrating keratoplasty. In Kaufman, H., Barron, B. & Mcdonald, M. (Eds) *The Cornea*. 2nd edn. Boston, Butterworth-Heinemann, pp. 809–13.

Barry, P. A., Petroll, W. M., Andrews, P. M., Cavanagh, H. D. & Jester, J. V. (1995) The spatial organization of corneal endothelial cytoskeletal proteins and their relationship to the apical junctional complex. *Invest Ophthalmol Vis Sci*, **36**, 1115–24.

Baum, J. (2002) Thygeson lecture. Amniotic membrane transplantation: why is it effective? *Cornea*, **21**, 339–41.

Beales, M. P., Funderburgh, J. L., Jester, J. V. & Hassell, J. R. (1999) Proteoglycan synthesis by bovine keratocytes and corneal fibroblasts: maintenance of the keratocyte phenotype in culture. *Invest Ophthalmol Vis Sci.*, **40**, 1658–63.

Bednarz, J., Doubilei, V., Wollnik, P. C. & Engelmann, K. (2001) Effect of three different media on serum free culture of donor corneas and isolated human corneal endothelial cells. *Br J Ophthalmol*, **85**, 1416–20.

Bednarz, J., Richard, G., Bohnke, M. & Engelmann, K. (1996) Differences in proliferation and migration of corneal endothelial cells [correction of epithelial cells] after cell transplantation in vitro. *Ger J Ophthalmol*, **5**, 346–51.

Berman, M., Manseau, E., Law, M. & Aiken, D. (1983) Ulceration is correlated with degradation of fibrin and fibronectin at the corneal surface. *Invest Ophthalmol Vis Sci*, **24**, 1358–66.

Bohnke, M., Eggli, P. & Engelmann, K. (1999) Transplantation of cultured adult human or porcine corneal endothelial cells onto human recipients in vitro. Part II: Evaluation in the scanning electron microscope. *Cornea*, **18**, 207–13.

Boisjoly, H. M., Laplante, C., Bernatchez, S. F., Salesse, C., Giasson, M. & Joly, M. C. (1993) Effects of EGF, IL-1 and their combination on in vitro corneal epithelial wound closure and cell chemotaxis. *Exp Eye Res*, **57**, 293–300.

Bosman, F. T. & Stamenkovic, I. (2003) Functional structure and composition of the extracellular matrix. *J Pathol*, **200**, 423–8.

Bouchard, C. S. & John, T. (2004) Amniotic membrane transplantation in the management of severe ocular surface disease: indications and outcomes. *Ocul Surf*, **2**, 201–11.

Bourne, W. M., Nelson, L. R. & Hodge, D. O. (1997) Central corneal endothelial cell changes over a ten-year period. *Invest Ophthalmol Vis Sci*, **38**, 779–82.

Bouwman, P. & Philipsen, S. (2002) Regulation of the activity of Sp1-related transcription factors. *Mol Cell Endocrinol*, **195**, 27–38.

Brazzell, R. K., Stern, M. E., Aquavella, J. V., Beuerman, R. W. & Baird, L. (1991) Human recombinant epidermal growth factor in experimental corneal wound healing. *Invest Ophthalmol Vis Sci*, **32**, 336–40.

Builles, N., Bechetoille, N., Justin, V., Andre, V., Barbaro, V., Di Iorio, E., Auxenfans, C., Hulmes, D. J. & Damour, O. (2007a) Development of a hemicornea from human primary cell cultures for pharmacotoxicology testing. *Cell Biol Toxicol*, **23**, 279–92.

Builles, N., Bechetoille, N., Justin, V., Andre, V., Burillon, C. & Damour, O. (2008) Variations in the characteristics of keratocytes in culture in relation to their location in human cornea. *Biomed Mater Eng*, **18**, S87–98.

Builles, N., Justin, V., Andre, V., Burillon, C. & Damour, O. (2007b) Reconstructed corneas: effect of three-dimensional culture, epithelium, and tetracycline hydrochloride on newly synthesized extracellular matrix. *Cornea*, **26**, 1239–48.

Burling, K., Seguin, M. A., Marsh, P., Brinkman, K., Madigan, J., Thurmond, M., Moon-Massat, P., Mannis, M. & Murphy, C. J. (2000) Effect of topical administration of epidermal growth factor on healing of corneal epithelial defects in horses. *Am J Vet Res*, **61**, 1150–5.

Carrier, P., Deschambeault, A., Audet, C., Talbot, M., Gauvin, R., Giasson, C. J., Auger, F. A., Guérin, S. L. & Germain, L. (2009) Impact of cell source on human cornea reconstructed by tissue engineering. *Invest Ophthalmol Vis Sci*, **50**, 2645–52.

Carrier, P., Deschambeault, A., Talbot, M., Giasson, C. J., Auger, F. A., Guerin, S. L. & Germain, L. (2008) Characterization of wound reepithelialization using a new human tissue-engineered corneal wound healing model. *Invest Ophthalmol Vis Sci*, **49**, 1376–85.

Chen, J. J. & Tseng, S. C. (1991) Abnormal corneal epithelial wound healing in partial-thickness removal of limbal epithelium. *Invest Ophthalmol Vis Sci.*, **32**, 2219–2233.

Chen, K. H., Azar, D. & Joyce, N. C. (2001) Transplantation of adult human corneal endothelium ex vivo: a morphologic study. *Cornea*, **20**, 731–7.

Chuck, R. S., Behrens, A., Wellik, S., Liaw, L. L., Dolorico, A. M., Sweet, P., Chao, L. C., Osann, K. E., Mcdonnell, P. J. & Berns, M. W. (2001) Re-epithelialization in cornea organ culture after chemical burns and excimer laser treatment. *Arch Ophthalmol*, **119**, 1637–42.

Clark, E. A. & Brugge, J. S. (1995) Integrins and signal transduction pathways: the road taken. *Science*, **268**, 233–9.

Clark, R. A. (1990) Fibronectin matrix deposition and fibronectin receptor expression in healing and normal skin. *J Invest Dermatol*, **94**, 128S–134S.

Collin, H. B., Anderson, J. A., Richard, N. R. & Binder, P. S. (1995) In vitro model for corneal wound healing; organ-cultured human corneas. *Curr Eye Res*, **14**, 331–9.

Coster, D. J. (1998) Surgical procedures to restore the corneal epithelium. In Kaufman, H. E., Barron, B. A. & Mcdonald, M. B. (Eds) *The Cornea*. 2nd edn. Boston, Butterworth-Heinemann, pp. 715–26.

Cotsarelis, G., Cheng, S. Z., Dong, G., Sun, T. T. & Lavker, R. M. (1989) Existence of slow-cycling limbal epithelial basal cells that can be preferentially stimulated to proliferate: implications on epithelial stem cells. *Cell*, **57**, 201–9.

Crabb, R. A. & Hubel, A. (2008) Influence of matrix processing on the optical and biomechanical properties of a corneal stroma equivalent. *Tissue Eng Part A*, **14**, 173–82.

Crosson, C. E. (1989) Cellular changes following epithelial abrasion. In Beuerman R. W., H. E. (Rosson, C. E. & Kaufmann, H. E. (Eds) *Healing Processes in the Cornea*. The Woodlands, Texas, Portofolio Publishing, pp. 3–14.

Daniels, J. T. & Khaw, P. T. (2000) Temporal stimulation of corneal fibroblast wound healing activity by differentiating epithelium in vitro. *Invest Ophthalmol Vis Sci*, **41**, 3754–62.

Deschambeault, A., Carrier, P., Talbot, M., Guérin, S. L., Auger, F. A. & Germain, L. (2002) Regional variation in the localization of limbal stem cells. *Invest Ophthalmol Vis Sci*, **43**, E-Abstract 1621.

Doillon, C. J., Watsky, M. A., Hakim, M., Wang, J., Munger, R., Laycock, N., Osborne, R. & Griffith, M. (2003) A collagen-based scaffold for a tissue engineered human cornea: physical and physiological properties. *Int J Artif Organs*, **26**, 764–73.

Dravida, S., Gaddipati, S., Griffith, M., Merrett, K., Lakshmi Madhira, S., Sangwan, V. S. & Vemuganti, G. K. (2008) A biomimetic scaffold for culturing limbal stem cells: a promising alternative for clinical transplantation. *J Tissue Eng Regen Med*, **2**, 263–71.

Du, Y., Chen, J., Funderburgh, J. L., Zhu, X. & Li, L. (2003) Functional reconstruction of rabbit corneal epithelium by human limbal cells cultured on amniotic membrane. *Mol Vis*, **9**, 635–43.

Du, Y., Sundarraj, N., Funderburgh, M. L., Harvey, S. A., Birk, D. E. & Funderburgh, J. L. (2007) Secretion and organization of a cornea-like tissue in vitro by stem cells from human corneal stroma. *Invest Ophthalmol Vis Sci*, **48**, 5038–45.

Dua, H. S. & Azuara-Blanco, A. (2000) Limbal stem cells of the corneal epithelium. *Surv Ophthalmol*, **44**, 415–425.

Dua, H. S. & Forrester, J. V. (1987) Clinical patterns of corneal epithelial wound healing. *Am J Ophthalmol*, **104**, 481–9.

Dua, H. S., Gomes, J. A., King, A. J. & Maharajan, V. S. (2004) The amniotic membrane in ophthalmology. *Surv Ophthalmol*, **49**, 51–77.

Dua, H. S., Joseph, A., Shanmuganathan, V. A. & Jones, R. E. (2003) Stem cell differentiation and the effects of deficiency. *Eye*, **17**, 877–85.

Dynan, W. S., Saffer, J. D., Lee, W. S. & Tjian, R. (1985) Transcription factor Sp1 recognizes promoter sequences from the monkey genome that are simian virus 40 promoter. *Proc Natl Acad Sci U S A*, **82**, 4915–9.

Edelhauser, H. F. & Ubels, J. L. (2003) The cornea and the sclera. In Kaufman, P. L. & Alm, A. (Eds) *Adler's Physiology of the Eye*. St Louis, Mosby, pp. 47–114.

Engelmann, K., Bohnke, M. & Friedl, P. (1988) Isolation and long-term cultivation of human corneal endothelial cells. *Invest Ophthalmol Vis Sci*, **29**, 1656–62.

Engelmann, K., Drexler, D. & Bohnke, M. (1999) Transplantation of adult human or porcine corneal endothelial cells onto human recipients in vitro. Part I: Cell culturing and transplantation procedure. *Cornea*, **18**, 199–206.

Engelmann, K. & Friedl, P. (1989) Optimization of culture conditions for human corneal endothelial cells. *In Vitro Cell Dev Biol*, **25**, 1065–72.

Engelmann, K. & Friedl, P. (1995) Growth of human corneal endothelial cells in a serum-reduced medium. *Cornea*, **14**, 62–70.

Espana, E. M., Romano, A. C., Kawakita, T., Di Pascuale, M., Smiddy, R. & Tseng, S. C. (2003) Novel enzymatic isolation of an entire viable human limbal epithelial sheet. *Invest Ophthalmol Vis Sci*, **44**, 4275–81.

Fatt, I. & Weissman, B. A. (1992) *Physiology of the Eye: An Introduction to the Vegetative Functions*. Boston, Butterworth-Heinemann.

Foreman, D. M., Pancholi, S., Jarvis-Evans, J., Mcleod, D. & Boulton, M. E. (1996) A simple organ culture model for assessing the effects of growth factors on corneal re-epithelialization. *Exp Eye Res*, **62**, 555–64.

Funderburgh, M. L., Du, Y., Mann, M. M., Sundarraj, N. & Funderburgh, J. L. (2005) PAX6 expression identifies progenitor cells for corneal keratocytes. *FASEB J*, **19**, 1371–3.

Funderburgh, M. L., Mann, M. M. & Funderburgh, J. L. (2008) Keratocyte phenotype is enhanced in the absence of attachment to the substratum. *Mol Vis*, **14**, 308–17.

Garagorri, N., Fermanian, S., Thibault, R., Ambrose, W. M., Schein, O. D., Chakravarti, S. & Elisseeff, J. (2008) Keratocyte behavior in three-dimensional photopolymerizable poly(ethylene glycol) hydrogels. *Acta Biomater*, **4**, 1139–47.

Garana, R. M., Petroll, W. M., Chen, W. T., Herman, I. M., Barry, P., Andrews, P.,

Cavanagh, H. D. & Jester, J. V. (1992) Radial keratotomy. II. Role of the myofibroblast in corneal wound contraction. *Invest Ophthalmol Vis Sci*, **33**, 3271–82.

Gaudreault, M., Carrier, P., Larouche, K., Leclerc, S., Giasson, M., Germain, L. & Guerin, S. L. (2003) Influence of sp1/sp3 expression on corneal epithelial cells proliferation and differentiation properties in reconstructed tissues. *Invest Ophthalmol Vis Sci*, **44**, 1447–57.

Gaudreault, M., Vigneault, F., Leclerc, S. & Guerin, S. L. (2007) Laminin reduces expression of the human alpha6 integrin subunit gene by altering the level of the transcription factors Sp1 and Sp3. *Invest Ophthalmol Vis Sci*, **48**, 3490–505.

Germain, L. & Auger, F. A. (1995) Tissue engineered biomaterials: biological and mechanical characteristics. In Wise, D. L., Trantolo, D. J., Altobelli, D. E., Yaszemski, M. J., Gresser, J. D. & Schwartz, E. R. (Eds) *Encyclopedic Handbook of Biomaterials and Bioengineering, Part B; Applications*. New York, USA, Marcel Dekker, Inc., pp. 699–734.

Germain, L., Auger, F. A., Grandbois, E., Guignard, R., Giasson, M., Boisjoly, H. & Guerin, S. L. (1999) Reconstructed human cornea produced in vitro by tissue engineering. *Pathobiology*, **67**, 140–7.

Germain, L., Carrier, P., Auger, F. A., Salesse, C. & Guerin, S. L. (2000) Can we produce a human corneal equivalent by tissue engineering? *Prog Retin Eye Res*, **19**, 497–527.

Germain, L., Giasson, C. J., Carrier, P., Guérin, S. L., Salesse, C. & Auger, F. A. (2004) Tissue engineering of cornea. In Wnek, G. E. & Bowlin, G. L. (Eds) *Encyclopedia of Biomaterials and Biomedical Engineering*. New York, USA, Marcel Dekker, Inc., pp. 2707–18.

Ghosheh, F. R., Cremona, F., Ayres, B. D., Hammersmith, K. M., Cohen, E. J., Raber, I. M., Laibson, P. R. & Rapuano, C. J. (2008) Indications for penetrating keratoplasty and associated procedures, 2001–2005. *Eye Contact Lens*, **34**, 211–4.

Giguere, L., Cheng, J. & Gospodarowicz, D. (1982) Factors involved in the control of proliferation of bovine corneal endothelial cells maintained in serum-free medium. *J Cell Physiol*, **110**, 72–80.

Gingras, M. E., Larouche, K., Larouche, N., Leclerc, S., Salesse, C. & Guerin, S. L. (2003) Regulation of the integrin subunit alpha5 gene promoter by the transcription factors Sp1/Sp3 is influenced by the cell density in rabbit corneal epithelial cells. *Invest Ophthalmol Vis Sci*, **44**, 3742–55.

Gingras, M. E., Masson-Gadais, B., Zaniolo, K., Leclerc, S., Drouin, R., Germain, L. & Guerin, S. L. (2009) Differential binding of the transcription factors Sp1, AP-1 and NFI to the promoter of the human alpha5 integrin gene dictates its transcriptional activity. *Invest Ophthalmol Vis Sci*, **50**, 57–67.

Gipson, I. K. & Grill, S. M. (1982) A technique for obtaining sheets of intact rabbit corneal epithelium. *Invest Ophthalmol Vis Sci*, **23**, 269–273.

Gipson, I. K., Watanabe, H. & Zieske, J. D. (1993) Corneal wound healing and fibronectin. *Int Ophthalmol Clin*, **33**, 149–63.

Gomes, J. A., Santos, M. S., Ventura, A. S., Donato, W. B., Cunha, M. C. & Hofling-Lima, A. L. (2003) Amniotic membrane with living related corneal limbal/conjunctival allograft for ocular surface reconstruction in Stevens–Johnson syndrome. *Arch Ophthalmol*, **121**, 1369–74.

Gospodarowicz, D. & Greenburg, G. (1979) The coating of bovine and rabbit corneas denuded of their endothelium with bovine corneal endothelial cells. *Exp Eye Res*, **28**, 249–65.

Gospodarowicz, D., Greenburg, G. & Alvarado, J. (1979a) Transplantation of cultured bovine corneal endothelial cells to rabbit cornea: clinical implications for human studies. *Proc Natl Acad Sci U S A*, **76**, 464–8.

Gospodarowicz, D., Greenburg, G. & Alvarado, J. (1979b) Transplantation of cultured bovine corneal endothelial cells to species with nonregenerative endothelium. The cat as an experimental model. *Arch Ophthalmol*, **97**, 2163–9.

Gospodarowicz, D., Mescher, A. L. & Birdwell, C. R. (1977) Stimulation of corneal endothelial cell proliferations *in vitro* by fibroblast and epidermal growth factors. *Exp Eye Res*, **25**, 75–89.

Grant, M. B., Khaw, P. T., Schultz, G. S., Adams, J. L. & Shimizu, R. W. (1992) Effects of epidermal growth factor, fibroblast growth factor, and transforming growth factor-beta on corneal cell chemotaxis. *Invest Ophthalmol Vis Sci*, **33**, 3292–301.

Green, H. & Barrandon, Y. (1988) Cultured epidermal cells and their use in the generation of epidermis. *News Physiol Sci*, **3**, 53–6.

Griffith, M., Jackson, W. B., Lagali, N., Merrett, K., Li, F. & Fagerholm, P. (2009) Artificial corneas: a regenerative medicine approach. *Eye*, 1–5.

Griffith, M., Osborne, R., Munger, R., Xiong, X., Doillon, C. J., Laycock, N. L., Hakim, M., Song, Y. & Watsky, M. A. (1999) Functional human corneal equivalents constructed from cell lines. *Science*, **286**, 2169–72.

Guillemette, M. D., Cui, B., Roy, E., Gauvin, R., Giasson, C. J., Esch, M. B., Carrier, P., Deschambeault, A., Dumoulin, M., Toner, M., Germain, L., Veres, T. & Auger, F. A. (2009) Surface topography induces 3D self-orientation of cells and extracellular matrix resulting in improved tissue function. *Integr Biol*, **1**, 196–204.

Guo, X., Hutcheon, A. E., Melotti, S. A., Zieske, J. D., Trinkaus-Randall, V. & Ruberti, J. W. (2007) Morphologic characterization of organized extracellular matrix deposition by ascorbic acid-stimulated human corneal fibroblasts. *Invest Ophthalmol Vis Sci*, **48**, 4050–60.

Haddad, A. (2000) Renewal of the rabbit corneal epithelium as investigated by autoradiography after intravitreal injection of ^{3}H-thymidine. *Cornea*, **19**, 378–83.

Ham, A. W. (1974) *Histology*. Philadelphia, Lippincott.

Hamada, R., Giraud, J. P., Graf, B. & Pouliquen, Y. (1972) [Analytical and statistical study of the lamellae, keratocytes and collagen fibrils of the central region of the normal human cornea. (Light and electron microscopy)]. *Arch Ophtalmol Rev Gen Ophtalmol*, **32**, 563–70.

Hamilton, W. & Wood, T. (1998) Inlay lamellar keratoplasty. In Kaufman, H. E., Barron, B. A. & Mcdonald, M. B. (Eds) *The Cornea*. 2nd edn. Boston, Butterworth-Heinemann, 761–68.

Han, I. & Kudlow, J. E. (1997) Reduced O glycosylation of Sp1 is associated with increased proteasome susceptibility. *Mol Cell Biol*, **17**, 2550–8.

Hanna, C. & O'brien, J. E. (1960) Cell production and migration in the epithelial layer of the cornea. *Arch Ophthalmol*, **64**, 536–9.

Hardarson, T., Hanson, C., Claesson, M. & Stenevi, U. (2004) Time-lapse recordings of human corneal epithelial healing. *Acta Ophthalmol Scand*, **82**, 184–8.

Hernandez Galindo, E. E., Theiss, C., Steuhl, K. P. & Meller, D. (2003) Expression of Delta Np63 in response to phorbol ester in human limbal epithelial cells expanded on intact human amniotic membrane. *Invest Ophthalmol Vis Sci*, **44**, 2959–65.

Hogan, M. J., Alvarado, J. A. & Weddel, J. E. (1971) The cornea. In Hogan, M. J., Alvarado, J. A. & Weddel, J. E. (Eds) *Histology of the Human Eye: An Atlas and Textbook*. Philadelphia, W.B. Saunders, pp. 55–111.

Hori, J. & Niederkorn, J. Y. (2007) Immunogenicity and immune privilege of corneal allografts. *Chem Immunol Allergy*, **92**, 290–9.

Huttenlocher, A., Sandborg, R. R. & Horwitz, A. F. (1995) Adhesion in cell migration. *Curr Opin Cell Biol*, **7**, 697–706.

Hynes, R. O. (1987) Integrins: a family of cell surface receptors. *Cell*, **48**, 549–54.

Hynes, R. O. (1992) Integrins: versatility, modulation, and signaling in cell adhesion. *Cell*, **69**, 11–25.

Insler, M. S. & Lopez, J. G. (1986) Transplantation of cultured human neonatal corneal endothelium. *Curr Eye Res*, **5**, 967–72.

Insler, M. S. & Lopez, J. G. (1991a) Extended incubation times improve corneal endothelial cell transplantation success. *Invest Ophthalmol Vis Sci*, **32**, 1828–36.

Insler, M. S. & Lopez, J. G. (1991b) Heterologous transplantation versus enhancement of human corneal endothelium. *Cornea*, **10**, 136–48.

Ishino, Y., Sano, Y., Nakamura, T., Connon, C. J., Rigby, H., Fullwood, N. J. & Kinoshita, S. (2004) Amniotic membrane as a carrier for cultivated human corneal endothelial cell transplantation. *Invest Ophthalmol Vis Sci*, **45**, 800–6.

Joo, C. K., Green, W. R., Pepose, J. S. & Fleming, T. P. (2000) Repopulation of denuded murine Descemet's membrane with life-extended murine corneal endothelial cells as a model for corneal cell transplantation. *Graefes Arch Clin Exp Ophthalmol*, **238**, 174–80.

Joyce, N. C. & Zhu, C. C. (2004) Human corneal endothelial cell proliferation: potential for use in regenerative medicine. *Cornea*, **23**, S8–S19.

Juliano, R. L. (2002) Signal transduction by cell adhesion receptors and the cytoskeleton: functions of integrins, cadherins, selectins, and immunoglobulin-superfamily members. *Annu Rev Pharmacol Toxicol*, **42**, 283–323.

Jumblatt, M. M., Maurice, D. M. & Mcculley, J. P. (1978) Transplantation of tissue-cultured corneal endothelium. *Invest Ophthalmol Vis Sci*, **17**, 1135–41.

Jumblatt, M. M., Maurice, D. M. & Schwartz, B. D. (1980) A gelatin membrane substrate for the transplantation of tissue cultured cells. *Transplantation*, **29**, 498–9.

Kafri, T. (2004) Gene delivery by lentivirus vectors: an overview. *Methods Mol Biol*, **246**, 367–90.

Kang, S. J., Kim, E. K. & Kim, H. B. (1999) Expression and distribution of extracellular matrices during corneal wound healing after keratomileusis in rabbits. *Ophthalmologica*, **213**, 20–4.

Kaufman, H. E., Barron, B. A. & Mcdonald, M. B. (Eds) (1998) *The Cornea*. 2nd edn. Boston, Butterworth-Heinemann.

Kim, M. J., Jun, R. M., Kim, W. K., Hann, H. J., Chong, Y. H., Park, H. Y. & Chung, J. H. (2001) Optimal concentration of human epidermal growth factor (hEGF) for epithelial healing in experimental corneal alkali wounds. *Curr Eye Res*, **22**, 272–9.

Klyce, S. D. & Beuerman, R. W. (1998) Structure and function of the cornea. In Kaufman, H. E., Barron, B. A. & Mcdonald, M. B. (Eds) *The Cornea*. 2nd edn. Boston, Butterworth–Heinemann, pp. 3–50.

Koizumi, N., Sakamoto, Y., Okumura, N., Okahara, N., Tsuchiya, H., Torii, R., Cooper, L. J., Ban, Y., Tanioka, H. & Kinoshita, S. (2007) Cultivated corneal endothelial cell sheet transplantation in a primate model. *Invest Ophthalmol Vis Sci*, **48**, 4519–26.

Komai, Y. & Ushiki, T. (1991) The three-dimensional organization of collagen fibrils in the human cornea and sclera. *Invest Ophthalmol Vis Sci*, **32**, 2244–58.

Kondo, Y., Fukuda, K., Adachi, T. & Nishida, T. (2008) Inhibition by a selective IkappaB kinase-2 inhibitor of interleukin-1-induced collagen degradation by corneal fibroblasts in three-dimensional culture. *Invest Ophthalmol Vis Sci*, **49**, 4850–7.

Konomi, K., Zhu, C., Harris, D. & Joyce, N. C. (2005) Comparison of the proliferative capacity of human corneal endothelial cells from the central and peripheral areas. *Invest Ophthalmol Vis Sci*, **46**, 4086–91.

Krachmer, J. H., Mannis, M. J. & Holland, E. J. (2005) *Cornea*. Philadelphia, Toronto, Elsevier Mosby.

Kruse, F. E. (1994) Stem cells and corneal epithelial regeneration. *Eye*, 8(Pt 2), 170–83.

Kurpakus, M. A., Daneshvar, C., Davenport, J. & Kim, A. (1999) Human corneal epithelial cell adhesion to laminins. *Curr Eye Res*, **19**, 106–14.

Lagali, N., Griffith, M., Fagerholm, P., Merrett, K., Huynh, M. & Munger, R. (2008) Innervation of tissue-engineered recombinant human collagen-based corneal substitutes: a comparative in vivo confocal microscopy study. *Invest Ophthalmol Vis Sci*, **49**, 3895–902.

Lai, J. Y., Chen, K. H. & Hsiue, G. H. (2007) Tissue-engineered human corneal endothelial cell sheet transplantation in a rabbit model using functional biomaterials. *Transplantation*, **84**, 1222–32.

Lange, T. M., Wood, T. O. & Mclaughlin, B. J. (1993) Corneal endothelial cell transplantation using Descemet's membrane as a carrier. *J Cataract Refract Surg*, **19**, 232–5.

Larouche, K., Leclerc, S., Salesse, C. & Guerin, S. L. (2000) Expression of the alpha 5 integrin subunit gene promoter is positively regulated by the extracellular matrix component fibronectin through the transcription factor Sp1 in corneal epithelial cells in vitro. *J Biol Chem*, **275**, 39182–92.

Latvala, T., Tervo, K., Mustonen, R. & Tervo, T. (1995) Expression of cellular fibronectin and tenascin in the rabbit cornea after excimer laser photorefractive keratectomy: a 12 month study. *Br J Ophthalmol*, **79**, 65–9.

Lauweryns, B., Van Den Oord, J. J. & Missotten, L. (1993) The transitional zone between limbus and peripheral cornea. An immunohistochemical study. *Invest Ophthalmol Vis Sci*, **34**, 1991–9.

Lauweryns, B., Van Den Oord, J. J., Volpes, R., Foets, B. & Missotten, L. (1991) Distribution of very late activation integrins in the human cornea. An immunohistochemical study using monoclonal antibodies. *Invest Ophthalmol Vis Sci*, **32**, 2079–85.

Lee, H. J., Lin, C. P. & Chen, C. W. (1991) The effects of epidermal growth factor and chondroitin sulfate on the animal corneal endothelial cell culture. *Gaoxiong Yi Xue Ke Xue Za Zhi*, **7**, 614–21.

Lee, J. W. & Juliano, R. (2004) Mitogenic signal transduction by integrin- and growth factor receptor-mediated pathways. *Mol Cells*, **17**, 188–202.

L'heureux, N., Paquet, S., Labbe, R., Germain, L. & Auger, F. A. (1998) A completely biological tissue-engineered human blood vessel. *FASEB J*, **12**, 47–56.

Lim, M., Goldstein, M. H., Tuli, S. & Schultz, G. S. (2003) Growth factor, cytokine and protease interactions during corneal wound healing. *Ocul Surf*, **1**, 53–65.

Lin, C. P. & Boehnke, M. (1997) A new model for in vitro corneal epithelial wound healing study. *Kaohsiung J Med Sci*, **13**, 475–9.

Lindberg, K., Brown, M. E., Chaves, H. V., Kenyon, K. R. & Rheinwald, J. G. (1993) *In vitro* propagation of human ocular surface epithelial cells for transplantation. *Invest Ophthalmol Vis Sci*, **34**, 2672–9.

Liu, W., Deng, C., Mclaughlin, C. R., Fagerholm, P., Lagali, N. S., Heyne, B., Scaiano, J. C., Watsky, M. A., Kato, Y., Munger, R., Shinozaki, N., Li, F. & Griffith, M. (2009) Collagen-phosphorylcholine interpenetrating network hydrogels as corneal substitutes. *Biomaterials*, **30**, 1551–9.

Liu, W., Griffith, M. & Li, F. (2008a) Alginate microsphere–collagen composite hydrogel for ocular drug delivery and implantation. *J Mater Sci Mater Med*, **19**, 3365–71.

Liu, W., Merrett, K., Griffith, M., Fagerholm, P., Dravida, S., Heyne, B., Scaiano, J. C., Watsky, M. A., Shinozaki, N., Lagali, N., Munger, R. & Li, F. (2008b) Recombinant human collagen for tissue engineered corneal substitutes. *Biomaterials*, **29**, 1147–58.

Liu, Y., Yanai, R., Lu, Y., Kimura, K. & Nishida, T. (2006) Promotion by fibronectin of collagen gel contraction mediated by human corneal fibroblasts. *Exp Eye Res*, **83**, 1196–204.

Ljubimov, A. V., Alba, S. A., Burgeson, R. E., Ninomiya, Y., Sado, Y., Sun, T. T., Nesburn, A. B., Kenney, M. C. & Maguen, E. (1998) Extracellular matrix changes in human corneas after radial keratotomy. *Exp Eye Res*, **67**, 265–72.

Long, C. J., Roth, M. R., Tasheva, E. S., Funderburgh, M., Smit, R., Conrad, G. W. & Funderburgh, J. L. (2000) Fibroblast growth factor-2 promotes keratan sulfate proteoglycan expression by keratocytes in vitro. *J Biol Chem*, **275**, 13918–23.

Maeno, A., Naor, J., Lee, H. M., Hunter, W. S. & Rootman, D. S. (2000) Three decades of corneal transplantation: indications and patient characteristics. *Cornea*, **19**, 7–11.

Majo, F., Rochat, A., Nicolas, M., Jaoude, G. A. & Barrandon, Y. (2008) Oligopotent stem cells are distributed throughout the mammalian ocular surface. *Nature*, **456**, 250–4.

Majumdar, G., Harmon, A., Candelaria, R., Martinez-Hernandez, A., Raghow, R. & Solomon, S. S. (2003) O-glycosylation of Sp1 and transcriptional regulation of the calmodulin gene by insulin and glucagon. *Am J Physiol Endocrinol Metab*, **285**, E584–91.

Maldonado, B. A. & Furcht, L. T. (1995) Involvement of integrins with adhesion-promoting, heparin-binding peptides of type IV collagen in cultured human corneal epithelial cells. *Invest Ophthalmol Vis Sci*, **36**, 364–72.

Malinda, K. M. & Kleinman, H. K. (1996) The laminins. *Int J Biochem Cell Biol*, **28**, 957–9.

Masson-Gadais, B., Fugere, C., Paquet, C., Leclerc, S., Lefort, N. R., Germain, L. & Guerin, S. L. (2006) The feeder layer-mediated extended lifetime of cultured human skin keratinocytes is associated with altered levels of the transcription factors Sp1 and Sp3. *J Cell Physiol*, **206**, 831–42.

Maurice, D. M. (1957) The structure and transparency of the cornea. *J Physiol Lond*, **136**, 263–86.

Maurice, D. M. (1984) The cornea and sclera. In Davison, H. (Ed.) *The Eye. Vegetative Physiology and Biochemistry*. 3rd edn. Orlando, Florida, Academic Press.

Mcculley, J. P., Maurice, D. M. & Schwartz, B. D. (1980) Corneal endothelial transplantation. *Ophthalmology*, **87**, 194–201.

Mcgowan, S. L., Edelhauser, H. F., Pfister, R. R. & Whikehart, D. R. (2007) Stem cell markers in the human posterior limbus and corneal endothelium of unwounded and wounded corneas. *Mol Vis*, **13**, 1984–2000.

Mclaughlin, C. R., Fagerholm, P., Muzakare, L., Lagali, N., Forrester, J. V., Kuffova, L., Rafat, M. A., Liu, Y., Shinozaki, N., Vascotto, S. G., Munger, R. & Griffith, M. (2008) Regeneration of corneal cells and nerves in an implanted collagen corneal substitute. *Cornea*, **27**, 580–9.

Mclaughlin, C. R., Tsai, R. J., Latorre, M. A. & Griffith, M. (2009) Bioengineered corneas for transplantation and in vitro toxicology. *Front Biosci*, **14**, 3326–37.

Meller, D., Dabul, V. & Tseng, S. C. (2002) Expansion of conjunctival epithelial progenitor cells on amniotic membrane. *Exp Eye Res*, **74**, 537–45.

Merrett, K., Fagerholm, P., Mclaughlin, C. R., Dravida, S., Lagali, N., Shinozaki, N., Watsky, M. A., Munger, R., Kato, Y., Li, F., Marmo, C. J. & Griffith, M. (2008) Tissue-engineered recombinant human collagen-based corneal substitutes for implantation: performance of type I versus type III collagen. *Invest Ophthalmol Vis Sci*, **49**, 3887–94.

Michel, M., L'heureux, N., Pouliot, R., Xu, W., Auger, F. A. & Germain, L. (1999) Characterization of a new tissue-engineered human skin equivalent with hair. *In Vitro Cell Dev Biol Anim*, **35**, 318–26.

Mimura, T., Amano, S., Usui, T., Araie, M., Ono, K., Akihiro, H., Yokoo, S. & Yamagami, S. (2004a) Transplantation of corneas reconstructed with cultured adult human corneal endothelial cells in nude rats. *Exp Eye Res*, **79**, 231–7.

Mimura, T., Amano, S., Yokoo, S., Uchida, S., Usui, T. & Yamagami, S. (2008) Isolation and distribution of rabbit keratocyte precursors. *Mol Vis*, **14**, 197–203.

Mimura, T. & Joyce, N. C. (2006) Replication competence and senescence in central and peripheral human corneal endothelium. *Invest Ophthalmol Vis Sci*, **47**, 1387–96.

Mimura, T., Yamagami, S., Yokoo, S., Usui, T., Tanaka, K., Hattori, S., Irie, S., Miyata, K., Araie, M. & Amano, S. (2004b) Cultured human corneal endothelial cell transplantation with a collagen sheet in a rabbit model. *Invest Ophthalmol Vis Sci*, **45**, 2992–7.

Mishima, H., Hibino, T., Hara, H., Murakami, J. & Otori, T. (1998) SPARC from corneal epithelial cells modulates collagen contraction by keratocytes. *Invest Ophthalmol Vis Sci*, **39**, 2547–53.

Mohay, J., Lange, T. M., Soltau, J. B., Wood, T. O. & Mclaughlin, B. J. (1994) Transplantation of corneal endothelial cells using a cell carrier device. *Cornea*, **13**, 173–82.

Mohay, J., Wood, T. O. & Mclaughlin, B. J. (1997) Long-term evaluation of corneal endothelial cell transplantation. *Trans Am Ophthalmol Soc*, **95**, 131–48; discussion 149–51.

Morris, K. V. & Rossi, J. J. (2006) Lentivirus-mediated RNA interference therapy for human immunodeficiency virus type 1 infection. *Hum Gene Ther*, **17**, 479–86.

Murakami, J., Nishida, T. & Otori, T. (1992) Coordinated appearance of beta 1 integrins and fibronectin during corneal wound healing. *J Lab Clin Med*, **120**, 86–93.

Murphy, C., Alvarado, J., Juster, R. & Maglio, M. (1984) Prenatal and postnatal cellularity of the human corneal endothelium. A quantitative histologic study. *Invest Ophthalmol Vis Sci*, **25**, 312–22.

Musselmann, K., Alexandrou, B., Kane, B. & Hassell, J. R. (2005) Maintenance of the keratocyte phenotype during cell proliferation stimulated by insulin. *J Biol Chem*, **280**, 32634–9.

Nakamura, K., Kurosaka, D., Yoshino, M., Oshima, T. & Kurosaka, H. (2002) Injured corneal epithelial cells promote myodifferentiation of corneal fibroblasts. *Invest Ophthalmol Vis Sci*, **43**, 2603–8.

Nakamura, T., Endo, K., Cooper, L. J., Fullwood, N. J., Tanifuji, N., Tsuzuki, M., Koizumi, N., Inatomi, T., Sano, Y. & Kinoshita, S. (2003) The successful culture and autologous transplantation of rabbit oral mucosal epithelial cells on amniotic membrane. *Invest Ophthalmol Vis Sci*, **44**, 106–16.

Nakayasu, K., Tanaka, M., Konomi, H. & Hayashi, T. (1986) Distribution of types I, II, III, IV and V collagen in normal and keratoconus corneas. *Ophthalmic Res*, **18**, 1–10.

Nelson, J. D., Silverman, V., Lima, P. H. & Beckman, G. (1990) Corneal epithelial wound healing: a tissue culture assay on the effect of antibiotics. *Curr Eye Res*, **9**, 277–85.

Opitz, O. G. & Rustgi, A. K. (2000) Interaction between Sp1 and cell cycle regulatory proteins is important in transactivation of a differentiation-related gene. *Cancer Res*, **60**, 2825–30.

Orwin, E. J. & Hubel, A. (2000) In vitro culture characteristics of corneal epithelial, endothelial, and keratocyte cells in a native collagen matrix. *Tissue Eng*, **6**, 307–19.

Ouellet, S., Vigneault, F., Lessard, M., Leclerc, S., Drouin, R. & Guerin, S. L. (2006) Transcriptional regulation of the cyclin-dependent kinase inhibitor 1A (p21) gene by NFI in proliferating human cells. *Nucleic Acids Res*, **34**, 6472–87.

Paallysaho, T., Tervo, K., Tervo, T., Van Setten, G. B. & Virtanen, I. (1992) Distribution of integrins alpha 6 and beta 4 in the rabbit corneal epithelium after anterior keratectomy. *Cornea*, **11**, 523–8.

Pellegrini, G., Dellambra, E., Golisano, O., Martinelli, E., Fantozzi, I., Bondanza, S., Ponzin, D., Mckeon, F. & De Luca, M. (2001) p63 identifies keratinocyte stem cells. *Proc Natl Acad Sci USA*, **98**, 3156–61.

Pellegrini, G., Golisano, O., Paterna, P., Lambiase, A., Bonini, S., Rama, P. & De Luca, M. (1999a) Location and clonal analysis of stem cells and their differentiated progeny in the human ocular surface. *J Cell Biol*, **145**, 769–82.

Pellegrini, G., Rama, P., Mavilio, F. & Luca, M. D. (2008) Epithelial stem cells in corneal regeneration and epidermal gene therapy. *J Pathol*, **217**, 217–28.

Pellegrini, G., Ranno, R., Stracuzzi, G., Bondanza, S., Guerra, L., Zambruno, G., Micali, G. & De Luca, L. M. (1999b) The control of epidermal stem cells (holoclones) in the treatment of massive full-thickness burns with autologous keratinocytes cultured on fibrin. *Transplantation*, **68**, 868–79.

Petroll, W. M., Hsu, J. K., Bean, J., Cavanagh, H. D. & Jester, J. V. (1999) The spatial organization of apical junctional complex-associated proteins in feline and human corneal endothelium. *Curr Eye Res*, **18**, 10–19.

Philipp, W. E., Speicher, L. & Gottinger, W. (2003) Histological and immunohistochemical findings after laser in situ keratomileusis in human corneas. *J Cataract Refract Surg*, **29**, 808–20.

Plow, E. F., Haas, T. A., Zhang, L., Loftus, J. & Smith, J. W. (2000) Ligand binding to integrins. *J Biol Chem*, **275**, 21785–8.

Price, M. O. & Price, F. W. (2007) Descemet's stripping endothelial keratoplasty. *Curr Opin Ophthalmol*, **18**, 290–4.

Princz, M. A. & Sheardown, H. (2008) Heparin-modified dendrimer cross-linked collagen matrices for the delivery of basic fibroblast growth factor (FGF-2). *J Biomater Sci Polym Ed*, **19**, 1201–18.

Proulx, S., Audet, C., D'arc Uwamaliya, J., Deschambeault, A., Carrier, P., Giasson, C. J., Brunette, I. & Germain, L. (2009a) Tissue engineering of feline corneal endothelium using devitalized human corneas as carrier. *Tissue Eng Part A*, Jan 6 [Epub ahead of print].

Proulx, S., Bensaoula, T., Nada, O., Audet, C., Uwamaliya, J., Devaux, A., Allaire, G., Germain, L. & Brunette, I. (2009b) Transplantation of a tissue-engineered corneal endothelium reconstructed on a devitalized carrier in the feline model. *Invest Ophthalmol Vis Sci*, **50**, 2686–94.

Proulx, S., Bourget, J. M., Gagnon, N., Martel, S., Deschambeault, A., Carrier, P., Giasson, C. J., Auger, F. A., Brunette, I. & Germain, L. (2007) Optimization of culture conditions for porcine corneal endothelial cells. *Mol Vis*, **13**, 524–33.

Puangsricharern, V. & Tseng, S. C. (1995) Cytologic evidence of corneal diseases with limbal stem cell deficiency. *Ophthalmology*, **102**, 1476–85.

Quantock, A. J., Sano, Y., Young, R. D. & Kinoshita, S. (2005) Stromal architecture and immune tolerance in additive corneal xenografts in rodents. *Acta Ophthalmol Scand*, **83**, 462–6.

Radner, W., Zehetmayer, M., Aufreiter, R. & Mallinger, R. (1998) Interlacing and cross-angle distribution of collagen lamellae in the human cornea. *Cornea*, **17**, 537–43.

Rafat, M., Li, F., Fagerholm, P., Lagali, N. S., Watsky, M. A., Munger, R., Matsuura, T. & Griffith, M. (2008) PEG-stabilized carbodiimide crosslinked collagen–chitosan hydrogels for corneal tissue engineering. *Biomaterials*, **29**, 3960–72.

Rafat, M., Matsuura, T., Li, F. & Griffith, M. (2009) Surface modification of collagen-based artificial cornea for reduced endothelialization. *J Biomed Mater Res A*, **88**, 755–68.

Rama, P., Bonini, S., Lambiase, A., Golisano, O., Paterna, P., De Luca, M. & Pellegrini, G. (2001) Autologous fibrin-cultured limbal stem cells permanently restore the corneal surface of patients with total limbal stem cell deficiency. *Transplantation*, **72**, 1478–1485.

Reichl, S., Bednarz, J. & Muller-Goymann, C. C. (2004) Human corneal equivalent as cell culture model for in vitro drug permeation studies. *Br J Ophthalmol*, **88**, 560–5.

Reichl, S. & Muller-Goymann, C. C. (2003) The use of a porcine organotypic cornea construct for permeation studies from formulations containing befunolol hydrochloride. *Int J Pharm*, **250**, 191–201.

Reim, M, Kottek, A, Schrage, N, (1997) The cornea surface and wound healing. *Prog Ret Eye Res.* **16**, 183–225.

Ren, R., Hutcheon, A. E., Guo, X. Q., Saeidi, N., Melotti, S. A., Ruberti, J. W., Zieske, J. D. & Trinkaus-Randall, V. (2008) Human primary corneal fibroblasts synthesize and deposit proteoglycans in long-term 3-D cultures. *Dev Dyn*, **237**, 2705–15.

Rheinwald, J. G. & Green, H. (1975) Serial cultivation of strains of human epidermal keratinocytes: the formation of keratinizing colonies from single cells. *Cell*, **6**, 331–43.

Richard, N. R., Anderson, J. A., Weiss, J. L. & Binder, P. S. (1991) Air/liquid corneal organ culture: a light microscopic study. *Curr Eye Res*, **10**, 739–49.

Roulet, E., Bucher, P., Schneider, R., Wingender, E., Dusserre, Y., Werner, T. & Mermod, N. (2000) Experimental analysis and computer prediction of CTF/NFI transcription factor DNA binding sites. *J Mol Biol*, **297**, 833–48.

Roulet, E., Busso, S., Camargo, A. A., Simpson, A. J., Mermod, N. & Bucher, P. (2002) High-throughput SELEX SAGE method for quantitative modeling of transcription-factor binding sites. *Nat Biotechnol*, **20**, 831–5.

Ruberti, J. W. & Zieske, J. D. (2008) Prelude to corneal tissue engineering – gaining control of collagen organization. *Prog Retin Eye Res*, **27**, 549–77.

Ruoslahti, E. (1996) RGD and other recognition sequences for integrins. *Annu Rev Cell Dev Biol*, **12**, 697–715.

Samples, J. R., Binder, P. S. & Nayak, S. K. (1991) Propagation of human corneal endothelium in vitro effect of growth factors. *Exp Eye Res*, **52**, 121–8.

Sangwan, V. S., Vemuganti, G. K., Singh, S. & Balasubramanian, D. (2003) Successful reconstruction of damaged ocular outer surface in humans using limbal and conjuctival stem cell culture methods. *Biosci Rep*, **23**, 169–74.

Schermer, A., Galvin, S. & Sun, T.-T. (1986) Differentiation-related expression of a major 64K corneal keratin *in vivo* and in culture suggests limbal location of corneal epithelial stem cells. *J Cell Biol*, **103**, 49–62.

Schultz, G., Cipolla, L., Whitehouse, A., Eiferman, R., Woost, P. & Jumblatt, M. (1992) Growth factors and corneal endothelial cells: III. Stimulation of adult human corneal endothelial cell mitosis *in vitro* by defined mitogenic agents. *Cornea*, **11**, 20–7.

Schwartz, B. D. & Mcculley, J. P. (1981) Morphology of transplanted corneal endothelium derived from tissue culture. *Invest Ophthalmol Vis Sci*, **20**, 467–80.

Shah, A., Brugnano, J., Sun, S., Vase, A. & Orwin, E. (2008) The development of a tissue-engineered cornea: biomaterials and culture methods. *Pediatr Res*, **63**, 535–44.

Shimazaki, J., Aiba, M., Goto, E., Kato, N., Shimmura, S. & Tsubota, K. (2002) Transplantation of human limbal epithelium cultivated on amniotic membrane for the treatment of severe ocular surface disorders. *Ophthalmology*, **109**, 1285–90.

Shortt, A. J., Secker, G. A., Notara, M. D., Limb, G. A., Khaw, P. T., Tuft, S. J. & Daniels, J. T. (2007) Transplantation of ex vivo cultured limbal epithelial stem cells: a review of techniques and clinical results. *Surv Ophthalmol*, **52**, 483–502.

Simmons, S. J., Jumblatt, M. M. & Neufeld, A. H. (1987) Corneal epithelial wound closure in tissue culture: an in vitro model of ocular irritancy. *Toxicol Appl Pharmacol*, **88**, 13–23.

Stepp, M. A. (2006) Corneal integrins and their functions. *Exp Eye Res*, **83**, 3–15.

Stepp, M. A., Spurr-Michaud, S. & Gipson, I. K. (1993) Integrins in the wounded and unwounded stratified squamous epithelium of the cornea. *Invest Ophthalmol Vis Sci*, **34**, 1829–44.

Stepp, M. A. & Zhu, L. (1997) Upregulation of alpha 9 integrin and tenascin during epithelial regeneration after debridement in the cornea. *J Histochem Cytochem*, **45**, 189–201.

Stepp, M. A., Zhu, L., Sheppard, D. & Cranfill, R. L. (1995) Localized distribution of alpha 9 integrin in the cornea and changes in expression during corneal epithelial cell differentiation. *J Histochem Cytochem*, **43**, 353–62.

Stevenson, M. (2002) Molecular biology of lentivirus-mediated gene transfer. *Curr Top Microbiol Immunol*, **261**, 1–30.

Talbot, M., Carrier, P., Giasson, C. J., Deschambeault, A., Guerin, S. L., Auger, F. A., Bazin, R. & Germain, L. (2006) Autologous transplantation of rabbit limbal epithelia cultured on fibrin gels for ocular surface reconstruction. *Mol Vis*, **12**, 65–75.

TANELIAN, D. L. & BISLA, K. (1992) A new in vitro corneal preparation to study epithelial wound healing. *Invest Ophthalmol Vis Sci*, **33**, 3024–8.

Tchah, H. (1992) Heterologous corneal endothelial cell transplantation – human corneal endothelial cell transplantation in Lewis rats. *J Korean Med Sci*, **7**, 337–42.

Tegtmeyer, S., Papantoniou, I. & Muller-Goymann, C. C. (2001) Reconstruction of an in vitro cornea and its use for drug permeation studies from different formulations containing pilocarpine hydrochloride. *Eur J Pharm Biopharm*, **51**, 119–25.

Teixeira, A. I., Nealey, P. F. & Murphy, C. J. (2004) Responses of human keratocytes to micro- and nanostructured substrates. *J Biomed Mater Res A*, **71**, 369–76.

Terry, M. A. (2007) Endothelial keratoplasty: clinical outcomes in the two years following deep lamellar endothelial keratoplasty (an American Ophthalmological Society thesis). *Trans Am Ophthalmol Soc*, **105**, 530–63.

Tervo, K., Tervo, T., Van Setten, G. B. & Virtanen, I. (1991) Integrins in human corneal epithelium. *Cornea*, **10**, 461–5.

Thoft, R. A. & Friend, J. (1983) The X, Y, Z hypothesis of corneal epithelial maintenance. *Invest Ophthalmol Vis Sci*, **24**, 1442–3.

Torbet, J., Malbouyres, M., Builles, N., Justin, V., Roulet, M., Damour, O., Oldberg, A., Ruggiero, F. & Hulmes, D. J. (2007) Orthogonal scaffold of magnetically aligned collagen lamellae for corneal stroma reconstruction. *Biomaterials*, **28**, 4268–76.

Tripathi, R. C. & Tripathi, B. J. (1984) Anatomy of the eye, orbit and adnexa. In Davson, H. (Ed.) *The Eye. Vegetative Physiology and Biochemistry*. 3rd edn. London, Academic Press, pp. 1–268.

Tsai, R. J., Sun, T.-T. & Tseng, S. C. (1990) Comparison of limbal and conjunctival autograft transplantation in corneal surface reconstruction in rabbits. *Ophthalmology*, **97**, 446–55.

Tuori, A., Uusitalo, H., Burgeson, R. E., Terttunen, J. & Virtanen, I. (1996) The immunohistochemical composition of the human corneal basement membrane. *Cornea*, **15**, 286–94.

Van Horn, D. L., Doughman, D. J., Harris, J. E., Miller, G. E., Lindstrom, R. & Good, R. A. (1975) Ultrastructure of human organ-cultured cornea. II. Stroma and epithelium. *Arch Ophthalmol*, **93**, 275–7.

Vigneault, F., Zaniolo, K., Gaudreault, M., Gingras, M. E. & Guerin, S. L. (2007) Control of integrin genes expression in the eye. *Prog Retin Eye Res*, **26**, 99–161.

Vorkauf, W., Vorkauf, M., Nolle, B. & Duncker, G. (1995) Adhesion molecules in normal and pathological corneas. An immunohistochemical study using monoclonal antibodies. *Graefes Arch Clin Exp Ophthalmol*, **233**, 209–19.

Vrana, N. E., Builles, N., Justin, V., Bednarz, J., Pellegrini, G., Ferrari, B., Damour, O., Hulmes, D. J. & Hasirci, V. (2008) Development of a reconstructed cornea from collagen–chondroitin sulfate foams and human cell cultures. *Invest Ophthalmol Vis Sci*, **49**, 5325–31.

Vrana, N. E., Elsheikh, A., Builles, N., Damour, O. & Hasirci, V. (2007) Effect of human corneal keratocytes and retinal pigment epithelial cells on the mechanical properties of micropatterned collagen films. *Biomaterials*, **28**, 4303–10.

Watanabe, G., Albanese, C., Lee, R. J., Reutens, A., Vairo, G., Henglein, B. & Pestell, R. G. (1998) Inhibition of cyclin D1 kinase activity is associated with E2F-mediated inhibition of cyclin D1 promoter activity through E2F and Sp1. *Mol Cell Biol*, **18**, 3212–22.

Watsky, M. A. (1995) Keratocyte gap junctional communication in normal and wounded rabbit corneas and human corneas. *Invest Ophthalmol Vis Sci*, **36**, 2568–76.

Wencan, W., Mao, Y., Wentao, Y., Fan, L., Jia, Q., Qinmei, W. & Xiangtian, Z. (2007) Using basement membrane of human amniotic membrane as a cell carrier for cultivated cat corneal endothelial cell transplantation. *Curr Eye Res*, **32**, 199–215.

Whitson, W. E., Weisenthal, R. W. & Krachmer, J. H. (1999) Penetrating keratoplasty and keratoprosthesis. In Tasman W. & Jaeger, E. A. (Eds) *Duane's Clinical Ophthalmology on CD-ROM*. Philadelphia, Lippincott Williams & Wilkins.

Wilson, S. E. (1998) Everett Kinsey Lecture. Keratocyte apoptosis in refractive surgery. *CLAO J*, **24**, 181–5.

Wilson, S. E., Liu, J. J. & Mohan, R. R. (1999) Stromal–epithelial interactions in the cornea. *Prog Retin Eye Res*, **18**, 293–309.

Woost, P. G., Jumblatt, M. M., Eiferman, R. A. & Schultz, G. S. (1992a) Growth factors and corneal endothelial cells: I. Stimulation of bovine corneal endothelial cell DNA synthesis by defined growth factors. *Cornea*, **11**, 1–10.

Woost, P. G., Jumblatt, M. M., Eiferman, R. A. & Schultz, G. S. (1992b) Growth factors and corneal endothelial cells: II. Characterization of epidermal growth factor receptor from bovine corneal endothelial cells. *Cornea*, **11**, 11–19.

Yamagami, S., Yokoo, S., Mimura, T., Takato, T., Araie, M. & Amano, S. (2007) Distribution of precursors in human corneal stromal cells and endothelial cells. *Ophthalmology*, **114**, 433–9.

Yokoo, S., Yamagami, S., Yanagi, Y., Uchida, S., Mimura, T., Usui, T. & Amano, S. (2005) Human corneal endothelial cell precursors isolated by sphere-forming assay. *Invest Ophthalmol Vis Sci*, **46**, 1626–31.

Yoshida, S., Shimmura, S., Shimazaki, J., Shinozaki, N. & Tsubota, K. (2005) Serum-free spheroid culture of mouse corneal keratocytes. *Invest Ophthalmol Vis Sci*, **46**, 1653–8.

Zagon, I. S., Sassani, J. W. & Mclaughlin, P. J. (2000) Reepithelialization of the human cornea is regulated by endogenous opioids. *Invest Ophthalmol Vis Sci*, **41**, 73–81.

Zainuddin, Barnard, Z., Keen, I., Hill, D. J., Chirila, T. V. & Harkin, D. G. (2008) PHEMA hydrogels modified through the grafting of phosphate groups by ATRP support the attachment and growth of human corneal epithelial cells. *J Biomater Appl*, **23**, 147–68.

Zaniolo, K., Gingras, M. E., Audette, M. & Guerin, S. L. (2006) Expression of the gene encoding poly(ADP-ribose) polymerase-1 is modulated by fibronectin during corneal wound healing. *Invest Ophthalmol Vis Sci*, **47**, 4199–210.

Zaniolo, K., Leclerc, S., Cvekl, A., Vallieres, L., Bazin, R., Larouche, K. & Guerin, S. L. (2004) Expression of the alpha4 integrin subunit gene promoter is modulated by the transcription factor Pax-6 in corneal epithelial cells. *Invest Ophthalmol Vis Sci*, **45**, 1692–704.

Zhao, M., Song, B., Pu, J., Forrester, J. V. & Mccaig, C. D. (2003) Direct visualization of a stratified epithelium reveals that wounds heal by unified sliding of cell sheets. *FASEB J*, **17**, 397–406.

Zhu, C. & Joyce, N. C. (2004) Proliferative response of corneal endothelial cells from young and older donors. *Invest Ophthalmol Vis Sci*, **45**, 1743–51.

Zieske, J. D., Hutcheon, A. E., Guo, X., Chung, E. H. & Joyce, N. C. (2001) TGF-beta receptor types I and II are differentially expressed during corneal epithelial wound repair. *Invest Ophthalmol Vis Sci*, **42**, 1465–71.

Zieske, J. D., Mason, V. S., Wasson, M. E., Meunier, S. F., Nolte, C. J., Fukai, N., Olsen, B. R. & Parenteau, N. L. (1994) Basement membrane assembly and differentiation of cultured corneal cells: importance of culture environment and endothelial cell interaction. *Exp Cell Res*, **214**, 621–33.

Zimmermann, D. R., Trueb, B., Winterhalter, K. H., Witmer, R. & Fischer, R. W. (1986) Type VI collagen is a major component of the human cornea. *FEBS Lett*, **197**, 55–8.

7

Engineering the corneal epithelial cell response to materials

J. T. JACOB, Louisiana State University, Health Sciences
Center, USA

Abstract: The epithelial cell layer of the cornea plays an important role
not only as a refracting surface and a barrier to pathogens, but also in the
maintenance of tear film spreading and stability. Any device used to replace
or augment the cornea must support a healthy anterior epithelial cell layer
in order to maintain these precorneal functions. The objective is to translate
fundamental knowledge from the cell-biology laboratory to the engineering
of synthetic corneas that stimulate integrative biological responses when
transplanted to a needy eye. Cells rely on the extrinsic meso-, micro-, and
nano-scale chemistry and topography of their surroundings to provide the
necessary physiological cues for their development and survival. Signals,
in the form of peptide sequences, from the extracellular matrix milieu
trigger integrins and receptors on the cell membrane to initiate diverse
cell functions. The natural immobilization of signaling ligands within
the extracellular environment provides a basis to engineer synthetic cell-
surface interfaces that enhance cellular migration and proliferation. These
surfaces will provide the basis for future clinical interventions that employ
the substrates developed as biomimetic surfaces which generate normal
corneal epithelial cell wound healing when used for corneal replacement/
augmentation.

Key words: biomimetic surfaces, cell adhesion, corneal augmentation,
corneal epithelium, tissue engineering, keratoprosthesis.

7.1   Surface properties influencing cell adhesion

Cells rely on the extrinsic meso-, micro-, and nano-scale chemistry and
topography of their surroundings to provide the necessary physiological
cues for their development and survival. Throughout their lifespan, almost
all cells adhere to an underlying extracellular matrix (ECM). The ECM is a
complex structure composed of numerous cross-linked collagens, vitronectins,
proteins, and polysaccharides.[1, 2] Adherence to an ECM is generally required
for cells to respond to endogenous signals. Signals, in the form of peptide
sequences from the extracellular milieu, including soluble growth factors and
cytokines, trigger integrins and receptors on the cell membrane to initiate
diverse cell functions. Cell adhesion to a material, whether that material
is the naturally occurring ECM of the basement membrane or a synthetic
biomaterial, is mediated primarily by the interaction between surface-bound

proteins/biological factors and the corresponding receptors on the cell membrane. The type and degree of contact between the cell and underlying matrix is the primary factor that determines cell behavior such as growth, migration, and health.[3]

7.1.1   Surface energy

Many years of biomaterial research have focused on determining the material surface characteristics – such as charge, energy, and roughness – that influence specific protein deposition, in the hope of developing the ability to tailor the Vroman effect to the specific type of cellular adhesion desired.[4] Studies involving both fibroblasts and endothelial cells in culture have shown that positively charged surfaces enhance cellular proliferation and adhesion significantly better than negatively charged or non-ionic hydrogel surfaces.[5, 6] The interfacial surface energy of the material also plays an important role in the thermodynamic free energy of adhesion for solutes in the surrounding media in the absence of any specific biochemical interactions (i.e. ligand–receptor interactions).[7–9] High surface energy or wettability has been shown to interfere with both human fibroblast[10, 11] and endothelial cell[12, 13] attachment, and low surface energy or wettability has been shown to interfere with plasma protein adsorption.[9, 14,15] In general, non-wettable materials have been shown to inhibit the attachment and growth of anchorage-dependent cells.[16]

7.1.2   Topography

Studies have also shown that microscopically roughened surfaces of a given material demonstrate enhanced vascular cell adhesion and migration rates, compared with smooth surfaces of the same material.[17, 18] Indeed, an atomic force microscopy study has quantified the fine structure of the basement membrane underlying the corneal epithelium as a complex topographical structure composed of pores and networks of fibers with diameters around 70 nm.[19] Steele and colleagues[20, 21] have shown that corneal epithelial cell migration was enhanced across surfaces with 0.1 μm track-etched pores over non-porous surfaces and that the effects were additive with hydrophilicity; however, pores greater than 0.9 μm inhibited migration even on hydrophilic surfaces. Other investigations have focused on the nanoscale roughness patterning of the substrate surface: smooth muscle cells have been shown to align preferentially to nanopatterned gratings (350 nm line width, 700 nm pitch, and 350 nm depth) on both polymethyl methacrylate and polydimethyl siloxane surfaces.[22]

7.1.3   Adsorbed protein conformation

Although these investigations have helped to define some of the characteristics necessary for an optimal surface, they have also revealed that it is not only the type of protein at the surface that is important for good cellular response, but also the conformation of the protein and the ability of the cell to interact with it. Generally, proteins are intrinsically surface active and tend to concentrate at interfaces, in part because of their polymeric structure and in part because of their amphoteric nature.[23] The opportunity for multiple modes of binding with many different types of surfaces is provided by the polar, charged, and non-polar amino acid side chains of the proteins. It has been observed that the general tendency for non-polar residues to be internalized in the native protein often requires structural alterations of the protein upon adsorption, in order to maximize the number of contacts with the surface.[24] For example, protein adsorption on a hydrophobic surface could involve entropically driven, conformational changes to optimize the various bonding interactions between the hydrophobic and hydrophilic sites of the protein and the surface and water phases of the interface, respectively. Real-time Fourier transform infrared spectroscopy (FTIR) analysis of proteins binding to surfaces has demonstrated conformational changes in the proteins as they first adhere and then adsorb to the material surface.[25–27]

Studies have shown that ECM proteins such as fibronectin (FN) and vitronectin must be adsorbed from the plasma or serum on to biomaterial surfaces as a prerequisite for successful cell adhesion and spreading.[28–30] However, adsorption of FN on to hydrophobic materials is followed by a decrease in cell adhesion and adhesion strength, and diminished cell spreading,[31–33] a fact that has been attributed to the possible conformation changes in the protein induced upon adsorption.[31, 33] Extensive research evaluating the cellular response to different proteins pre-adsorbed on to surfaces varying in hydrophilicity has determined that the reason for the hydrophobic effect may be the mode of adsorption of attachment proteins (e.g. FN), resulting in an impaired interaction with the corresponding integrin receptor, as well as the lack of a possible rearrangement of FN into ECM-like structures.[16, 34–43] The results of these studies indicate that synthetic materials must adsorb FN or other proteins in a relatively native conformation to improve their interaction with cells.[44–47] If this is the case, the material surface may interact with adhering cells in a manner similar to that of the native ECM.[34] However, the overwhelming evidence indicating that protein biological functions are often mediated by specific amino acid sequences (exposed surface epitopes or peptides released by proteolysis) has focused the majority of biomaterial development on direct chemical attachment of proteins and/or peptides to the polymer surface.[48, 49]

7.2   Engineering cellular adhesion

Over the last two decades, material science research has focused on specifically engineering the polymer surface to have the ability to interact actively with receptors on target cell membranes through the use of ligand-specific chemical sequences and tethered biological molecules. Short peptide sequences (such as YIGSR and RGD) responsible for cell-surface adhesion binding activity in extracellular adhesion proteins such as FN and laminin (LM) have proven to be sufficient for *in vitro* cell adhesion and spreading when chemically incorporated on to the surfaces in adequate numbers.[48–55] Although these minimal binding sequences have only a fraction of the activity of the entire protein, their small size allows them to be incorporated at much higher concentrations than would be possible with entire protein structures. The short peptide sequences have the advantage of being relatively stable, and their synthetic nature renders them more amenable to chemical derivatization and covalent attachment.

7.2.1   Direct attachment

Direct attachment of these cell-surface receptor recognition sequences has been associated with an increase in cell culture adhesion of a variety of cell types, including human foreskin fibroblasts, bovine pulmonary endothelial cells, human umbilical vein endothelial cells, and porcine pulmonary aortic endothelial cells.[48–55] However, the increase in cell adhesion in these systems, while significant, was not as high as was anticipated and did not reach the levels seen in natural systems. Generally, the increase seemed to be of a non-specific nature and was not found for all cell types tested.[56] Use of these sequences on surfaces cultured with rabbit corneal epithelial cells has not demonstrated the same marked increase in cell adhesion as has been reported for other cellular systems.[38, 57]

The reason for the limited results may be threefold: (a) the attached short peptide sequence is held very close to the surface and may be sterically hindered from orienting itself into optimal attachment positions; (b) the short peptide sequence is not of sufficient length to extend out and away from proteins non-specifically adsorbing to the surface and, therefore, is obscured to some extent from the cell receptor (Fig. 7.1); and (c) the single short peptide sequence does not adequately mimic the complex adhesion-promoting abilities found in a protein with quaternary structure. Several studies support these hypotheses.

7.2.2   Spacers

Kugo *et al.*[58] and others[56] have shown that attaching the peptide sequence to a poly(ethylene glycol) (PEG) spacer arm (molecular weight (MW)

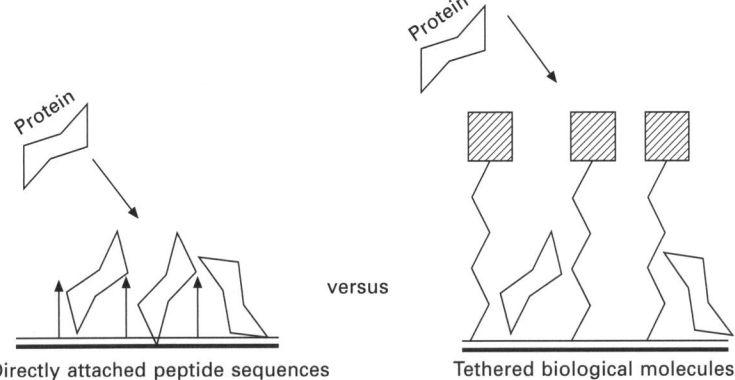

Directly attached peptide sequences   Tethered biological molecules

7.1 Directly attached RGD peptide sequences (triangles) can be obscured by non-specifically adsorbed proteins, whereas the tethered biological molecules (squares) are held away from the adsorbed proteins.

3400) results in a 50% increase in specific cell attachment, compared with the response to a surface with directly attached peptides. PEG is widely recognized for its lack of interactions with macromolecules found in body fluids.[59–61] Use of PEG as a spacer arm or tether has been shown to increase the activity of bound enzymes. D'Urso et al.[62] found that the K_m (concentration of substrate that gives 'half-maximal' activity) of enzymes bound to a surface by a PEG tether is increased 10–20 times over that of the native enzyme. Tethering of the active molecule decreases unproductive diffusion and increases the probability of successful interactions with target molecules or cells. Further investigations[59, 63] have reported the tethering of biologically active protein molecules to polymer scaffolds for tissue regeneration. By covalently linking epidermal growth factor (EGF) on to a star-poly(ethylene oxide) tether and then anchoring the tether on to the surface of a biodegradable scaffold, Griffith-Cima[64] showed a 40% increase in rat hepatocyte cell adhesion and migration; this investigator also reported that DNA synthesis within the cells was comparable with the levels found when the medium contained free EGF.

Although the use of the PEG spacer arm diminishes the steric constraints and the effects of non-specifically adsorbed proteins, it does not address the problem of the need for adhesion of a specifically targeted cell type and exclusion all other cell types. For example, five peptide sequences on the LM α1 chain carboxyl-terminal globular domain have been found to exhibit cell-type-specific attachment activities, including SIYITRF, IAFQRN, and LQVQLSIR.[65] PHSRN (from the ninth type II repeating unit), a synergistic peptide that enhances the activity of RGD, has been found in the central cell-adhesive domain of FN.[66] Additionally, Cameron et al.[67] have shown that rabbit corneal epithelial cells interact with FN via multiple adhesion-promoting sequences within the intact FN molecule. Another study using osteoblasts showed that, by linking PHSRN and RGD sequences to recapitulate the native spacing of FN prior to surface tethering cell adhesion, spreading and focal contact formation was increased compared with RGD alone.[68] It is apparent that for most cells the use of just one peptide sequence is insufficient to mimic these complex matrix binding proteins.

7.3   Engineering corneal epithelium attachment and growth

7.3.1   Synthetic replacement/augmentation of the cornea

Synthetic augmentation of the cornea to produce refractive change has been investigated by a number of researchers during the past 30 years,[69–72] while complete synthetic replacement of diseased and opacified corneas has been investigated for more than 200 years.[73, 74] Initial replacement studies included the use of glass, metal, and bone as substitute materials;[75–77] studies over the past 50 years have focused on the use of polymers.[78–82] As the field of polymer chemistry and its medical applications grew in the mid 1980s, there was a shift from the use of hard polymers such as poly(methyl methacrylate) (PMMA) to soft hydrogels such as collagen, polyurethanes, and poly(2-hydroxyethyl methacrylate) and co-polymers thereof.[83–90] Hydrogels are used not only because their compliance (softness) allows them to respond to the pressure fluctuations caused during blink without inducing high shear forces at the material–tissue interface and damaging surrounding tissue, but also because of their ability to maintain a hydrated environment similar to that of the natural tissues.

In the past decade there has been some clinical success in both corneal augmentation and replacement. For replacement devices, the use of a soft, porous polymer attachment skirt has improved anchoring of the central optic and decreased extrusion of the devices.[88, 91–96] The AlphaCor keratoprosthesis (KPro) (Addition Technology Inc., Des Plaines, IL, USA) has been successful in a number of uncomplicated corneal replacement cases; however, the list of exclusion criteria for its implantation is extensive and long-term viability is uncertain.[93] For augmentation devices, the use of hydrogels that allow nutrients to permeate the material to supply the tissue anterior to the implant has significantly increased the functional life of these devices.[97–99] Both synthetic replacement and augmentation devices share the requirement that corneal epithelial cells must be able to form a viable confluent layer across the anterior surface of the optical material.[96, 99] However, corneal epithelial cell attachment to, and growth over, these hydrogel surfaces is generally minimal.[94]

7.3.2   Corneal epithelium/extracelllular matrix structure and repair

The corneal epithelium is composed of three types of cells: basal cells (one layer), wing cells (one to three layers), and squamous cells (three to four layers) – all of which tightly adhere to one another. The basal cells also form strong adhesion complexes with the underlying ECM and, ultimately, with Bowman's layer.[100] Only the basal cells have mitotic capabilities. Like all stratified epithelia in the body, the corneal epithelium is self-renewing; complete cellular turnover occurs every 5–7 days.[101] Generally, after the basal cells undergo mitosis, the daughter cells begin to move upward toward terminal differentiation and eventual desquamation from the apical surface.

As part of its protective function, the corneal epithelium also has a strong wound-healing response. After corneal wounding, growth factor and cytokine levels increase in the tear fluid and stromal layers, and a provisional ECM is elaborated. Previous research has shown that epithelial recovery following an external injury is a complex process characterized by three overlapping phases.[1] In the first phase, a single layer of epithelial cells at the wound margin becomes motile by forming cellular processes at the wound edge, releasing the hemidesmosomal attachments to the basement membrane and forming a provisional attachment complex called 'focal contacts'. During this phase, the epithelial cells flatten and migrate as an intact sheet to cover the wound.

Adhesion of the migrating epithelial monolayer to the stroma is thought to be mediated by the glycoprotein FN.[102] FN is normally not present beneath corneal epithelial cells but appears after injury and persists until migration is complete. FN contains both cell-specific binding sequences and a binding region for heparin sulfate and type IV collagen (basement membrane components).[103] FN provides a temporary, subepithelial matrix on which the epithelial cells can migrate; this occurs in repetitive cycles, during which the cells cleave their attachments, advance, and then form new attachments. Recently, it has become known that a variety of other matrix components – such as LM-5, lumican, fibrin, and perlecan – are found in a temporary or 'provisional' matrix in response to wounding.[104] A number of LM isoforms have been identified in the wounded cornea, indicating that, not only is LM important in the corneal epithelial cell–substrate adhesion complex, but it may play a role in cell migration during corneal wound healing.

In the second phase of corneal epithelial wound healing, cells distal to the original wound begin to proliferate to repopulate the wound area, and cell stratification and differentiation occur. In the third phase, the epithelium attaches to the basement membrane more firmly, via newly synthesized hemidesmosomes and associated type VII collagen containing anchoring filaments.[105] The anchoring filaments pass through the basement membrane and are contiguous with anchoring fibrils that terminate as anchoring plaques in Bowman's layer.

Integrins expressed on the corneal epithelial cell surface change during wound healing.[106] Among the expressed integrins, α2β1, α3β1, and αvβ1 bind LM, collagen, and FN. Epithelial expression of β1 integrins has been shown to increase as FN in the wound increases and then decreases as wound healing becomes complete. α6β4 integrin is synthesized and redistributed in wound healing and binds LM-5, whereas LM-10 promotes reorganization of filamentous actin (F-actin) in corneal epithelial cells. The proteins LM (isoforms 1, 5, and 10), k-LM, talin, integrin, and kalinin also play roles in the attachment of the epithelium to the stroma. Although much is known about the factors that make up the adhesion complexes, the precise sequence by which these adhesion complex components are assembled has not yet been fully elucidated. Certain growth factors, such as EGF,[107] fibroblast growth factor (FGF)[108] and transforming growth factor (TGF)-β1,[109] enhance the rate of epithelial wound healing, and human EGF has been specifically shown to induce a dose-dependent increase in epithelial replication in the epithelial stem cells of the corneoscleral limbus.[110]

Extracellular gradients of growth factors, FN, or LM also may be important. The ECM contains a complex array of fixed charges, and the ionic charge of substrates has been shown to modulate corneal cell integrin expression, cell spreading, and cell motility. Thus, reorganization of cell surface receptors or extracellular molecules to induce a gradient of either receptor or ligand, respectively, is likely an initial event that activates cells asymmetrically, drives subsequent cytoskeletal reorganization, and directs cell migration.

7.3.3   Corneal epithelial cell repair and growth ligands

Elucidation of signaling events and the underlying biological factors that produce them is key to understanding the fundamental elements required to produce an ECM-like environment. Identification of these important moieties for corneal epithelial cells has been substantial to date. LM and FN are multifunctional ECM proteins that play a central role in cell adhesion and migration. Expression of integrin receptors for both of these proteins has been shown to occur within hours of the ligands being detected in the matrix.[37] LM is a major component of the intact basal lamina and has been shown to enhance epithelial cell adhesion and spreading on surfaces. Twelve isoforms of LM have been identified; however, only three isoforms – LM-1, LM-5, and LM-10 – have been consistently found within the basement membrane of the cornea.[111, 112] In unwounded corneas, expression of lumican is limited to stromal keratocytes. The expressed lumican molecules are glycanated with keratin sulfate. In healing corneal wounds, a non-glycanated form of lumican is produced and has been shown to significantly enhance epithelial cell migration and proliferation.[113]

FN, seen on the surface of healing epithelial wounds, is an insoluble glycoprotein dimer (unlike the soluble disulfide linked dimer) found in plasma. The primary transcript of FN is alternatively spliced and, therefore, different isoforms, such as EDA-, EDB-, CS1-, and a further isoform, Onc-Fn, are expressed by alternative glycosylation.[114] Exogenous FN has been shown to promote the healing of corneal epithelial wounds experimentally *in vivo* and *in vitro*, and the healing of persistent corneal epithelial defects in humans.[115] FN is widely expressed in the cornea and EDA-FN emerges during wound healing.[116] In addition, studies have concluded that the cell adhesion properties of FN can be generated using only peptide fragments of the molecule.[103] FN peptide sequences, RGD (the central cell binding domain) and PHSRN (from the ninth type II repeating unit), when co-localized, have been found to enhance the cell-adhesive activity of RGD.[68] Fibronection adhesion peptide (FAP), the carboxy-terminal heparin binding and cell adhesion-promoting domain, from within the FN molecule, has been shown to promote attachment and spreading of several cultured cell lines including corneal epithelial cells.[117, 118] YIGSR is a peptide sequence from the LM A chain that has also demonstrated the ability to promote cell attachment and spreading in corneal epithelial cells.[119]

7.3.4   Engineering surfaces for corneal epithelial growth and health

A number of different surface modification techniques have been investigated in the attempt to foster productive biological interactions between the modified elastomer/hydrogel surface and the corneal epithelial cell membrane. Franco *et al.*[120] evaluated the interactive effects of different surface functionalities with corneal epithelial cells using self-assembled monolayers of alkanethiols and alkylsiloxanes. In addition, several investigators have used plasma modification of various surfaces including silicone rubber[121–123] and polyvinyl alcohol[124] to improve the corneal epithelial cell response with limited success.

Adsorption and direct covalent attachment of ECM proteins such as FN and LM, as well as collagens types I and IV, to various surfaces have also been investigated. Hydrogels pre-adsorbed with types I and IV collagen showed a more rapid rate of cell growth than those coated with either FN or LM.[125, 126] Adsorption of FN to a collagen-modified surface resulted in further acceleration of corneal cell attachment.[127, 128] Collagen-modified corneal inlays also maintained a healthy, differentiated, and stratified epithelium with focal attachments for over 6 weeks in feline corneas.[129] More recent studies with polyvinyl alcohol substrates modified with collagen and amniotic membrane also resulted in stratified corneal epithelium over finite time periods.[130, 131]

However, collagen-modified surfaces have been shown to be susceptible to collagenase activity over time. The ability of these modified surfaces to exist over the lifetime of the implant is not clear.

Cell adhesion peptides – including RGD, YIGSR, and a novel collagen peptoid Gly-Pro-nLeu – directly attached to surfaces have also been studied, but these peptide/peptoid modifications have produced only modest increases in the rate of epithelialization *in vitro*.[38, 132–135] However, direct attachment of YIGSR throughout a collagen matrix increased not only epithelialization rates and produced some stratification of the epithelium but also neurite in-growth after 6 weeks of implantation in porcine corneas.[119] In general, although a few replacement materials with either coating and/or direct attachment of biological factors (both proteins and peptides) to their surfaces have had some short-term success in maintaining a somewhat normal epithelial layer, long-term analysis (up to 8 years) has shown that the density of the epithelial layer is not maintained.[135–139]

Investigations into the use of spacers or tethers to increase the long-term corneal epithelial cell health over hydrogel materials have been reported. These include studies to develop and test a wet chemistry method to covalently bond PEG-tethered ECM proteins and/or peptides on to the surface of a hydrogel.[140, 141] The resultant hydrogels were biologically active and possessed physical characteristics similar to the natural cornea. Analysis of the corneal epithelial cell response to six different tether-modified hydrogels showed that, while little to no cell growth occurred on plain (unmodified) hydrogels, and only a maximum confluence of 20% occurred on protein/ peptide-coated hydrogels, three types of tether-modified hydrogels (LM, an FN adhesion peptide sequence (FAP), and FN/LM (1:1)) all achieved 100% confluence at the end of the same culture period.[142] However, the rate of cell confluence was considerably different for the three different tether-modified hydrogels. LM-only-tethered surfaces initially had significantly less cell growth than the surfaces with FAP-only or FN/LM. However, during the last third of the culture period, the rate of epithelial cell confluence over the LM-only modified surfaces surpassed that of the FN/LM surface. This result indicates that FN or a ligand within the FN molecule is a key component for early epithelial cell adhesion and replication in cell culture. The relative strength of the cellular attachment to the tether-modified hydrogel surfaces was determined with jet impingement. Epithelial cells grown on LM- and FAP-tethered hydrogel surfaces attached with significantly higher adhesion strengths than any other type of tether-modified hydrogel.[143] There are several possible explanations for the significantly lower adhesion strength to the FN-modified surfaces: (1) the modified surfaces presented too little FN to provide the ligand surface concentration necessary for the formation of stable epithelial cell receptor–ligand bonds; (b) the percentage of FN-bound molecules bound to the surface with the appropriate receptor binding sites exposed to the epithelial cells was inadequate for strong cell adhesion; and (c) the tethering technique presented competitive ligand sites on the FN molecule that have a down-regulating effect on epithelial cell adhesion. Further studies are needed to clarify these issues. Addition of PEG-tethered EGF to allylamine-activated polydimethylsiloxane (PDMS) by other investigators also showed increased epithelial cell coverage rates as compared with unmodified controls in both serum-free and EGF-free medium studies.[144] Overall these studies support the hypothesis that tethering proteins and peptides increases their ability to interact with cell membrane receptors and, therefore, only very small amounts (<0.1 $\mu g/cm^2$) of proteins and/or peptides are necessary to elicit a cellular response.

In addition to which biological factors are added to the surface and by what method, the spatial density of the addition is important. The natural substrate has a variety of biological factors spatially distributed for cell signaling. Therefore, the optimal biomimetic surface for engineering the cell response would have a nanopatterned distribution of biological factors over its surface. There are three main methods for providing reactive groups on the surface for addition of the tethered moieties including (a) monomer pendant groups within the base polymer;[140] (b) addition of reactive groups (acetaldehyde or allylamine) or reactive polymers through plasma addition;[144] and addition of reactive groups through photopatterning.[145] The ability to specifically populate a surface with combinations of signaling moieties can require extensive blocking chemistry unless specific patterning techniques are used. Spatially controlled patterning of the surface, by masking during the plasma polymerization, for increased corneal epithelial outgrowth recently showed preferential binding of collagen I and cell growth on those areas.[146] However, the areas of photopatterning in this study were very large (13 mm) in relation to cell size. Continued research into developing nano-scale patterning methods for the spatial addition of specific cell-activating moieties will be important in furthering developments in this area.

Engineering of corneal epithelial cell attachment and growth should focus not only on the structure of the normal epithelial ECM but also on how the natural cornea heals a de-epithelialized stroma. Knowledge of the important cell signaling events and the biological factors that produce them provides the researcher with the fundamental elements needed to produce an ECM-like environment. Engineering a surface to mimic the natural corneal epithelial ECM and basement membrane sufficiently involves populating the surface with enough cellular signals (proteins/peptides) to initiate cell attachment, migration, differentiation, and stratification and then maintain the stratified epithelium over time. As more detailed information on the specific isoforms of proteins and functions of peptide sequences becomes available, more advanced surfaces can be developed. In addition to further refinement of the type of tethered moieties, optimization of their exact quantity and spatial distribution is needed to develop a truly biomimetic surface.

7.4   References

1 Zieske JD: Extracellular matrix and wound healing. *Curr Opinion Ophthalmol* **12**(4), 237–241, 2001.
2 Aumailley M, Gayraud B: Structure and biological activity of the extracellular matrix. *J Mol Med* **76**, 253–65, 1998.
3 Bosman FT, Stamenkovic I: Functional structure and composition of the extracellular matrix. *Pathology* **200**, 423–428, 2003.
4 Horbett TA: The role of adsorbed proteins in animal cell adhesion. *Colloids Surf B Biointerfaces* **2**, 225–240, 1994.
5 Hattori S, Andrade JD, Hibbs JB Jr, Gregonis DE, King RN: Fibroblast cell proliferation on charged hydroxyethyl methacrylate copolymers. *J Colloid Interface Sci* **104**, 72–78, 1985.
6 Wu XY, Cornell-Bell A, Davies TA, Simons ER, Trinkaus-Randall V: Expression of integrin and organization of F-actin in epithelial cells depends on the underlying surface. *Invest Ophthalmol Vis Sci* **35**, 878–890, 1994.
7 Lymann DJ, Muir WM, Lee IT: The effect of chemical structure and surface properties of polymers on the coagulation of blood. I. Surface free energy effects. *Trans Am Soc Artific Intern Organs* **11**, 301–306, 1965.
8 Andrade JD, Hattori S, King RN: Surface characterization of poly (hydroxyethyl methacrylate) and related polymers I. Contact angle method in water. *J Polym Sci: Polym Symp* **66**, 313–319, 1979.
9 Absolom DR, Zing W, van Oss CJ, Neumann AW: Protein and platelet interaction with polymer surfaces. *Biomater Med Devices Artif Organs* **12**, 235–266, 1984/85.
10 Ruardy TG, Schakenraad JM, van der Mei HC, Busscher HJ: Adhesion and spreading of human skin fibroblasts on physicochemically characterized gradient surfaces. *J Biomed Mater Res* **29**, 1415–1423, 1995.
11 Bohnert JL, Horbett TA, Ratner DB, Royce FH: Adsorption of proteins from artificial tear solutions to contact lens materials. *Invest Ophthalmol Vis Sci* **29**, 362–373, 1988.
12 Yasuda H, Yamanashi BS, Devito DP: The rate of adhesion of melanoma cells onto nonionic polymer surfaces. *J Biomed Mater Res* **12**, 701–706, 1978.
13 van Wachem PB, Hogt AH, Beugeling T, Freijen J, Bantjes A, Detmer JP, van Aken WG: Adhesion of cultured human endothelial cells onto methacrylate polymers with varying surface wettability and charge. *Biomaterials* **8**, 323–328, 1987.
14 Kothari S, Hatton PV, Danglas CWI: Protein adsorption to titanic surface. *J Mater Sci* **6**, 695–698, 1995.
15 Altankov G, Groth T: Reorganization of substratum on hydrophilic and hydrophobic materials is related to biocompatibility. *J Mater Sci* **5**, 732–737, 1994.
16 Groth T, Altankov G: Studies on cell-biomaterial interaction: role of tyrosine phosphorylation during fibroblast spreading on surfaces varying in wettability. *Biomaterials* **17**, 1227–1234, 1996.
17 Lampin M, Werocquier-Clérout R, Legris C, Degrange M, Sigot-Luizard MF: Correlation between substratum roughness and wettability, cell adhesion, and cell migration. *J Biomed Mater Res* **36**, 99–108, 1997.

18 Goodman SL, Sims PA, Albrecht RM: Three-dimensional extracellular matrix textured biomaterials. *Biomaterials* **17**, 2087–2095, 1996.

19 Abrams GA, Goodman SL, Nealey PF, Franco M, Murphy CJ. Nanoscale topography of the basement membrane underlying the corneal epithelium of the rhesus macaque. *Cell Tissue Res* **299**, 39–46.

20 Fitton JH, Dalton BA, Beumer G, Johnson G, Griesser HJ, Steele JG: Surface topography can interfere with epithelial tissue migration. *J Biomed Mater Res* **42**, 245–257, 1998.

21 Steele JG, Johnson G, McLean KM, Beumer GJ, Griesser HJ: Effect of porosity and surface hydrophilicity on migration of epithelial tissue over synthetic polymer. *J Biomed Mater Res* **50**, 475–482, 2000.

22 Yim EKF, Reano RM, Pang SW, Yee AF, Chen CS, Leong KW: Nanopattern-induced changes in morphology and motility of smooth muscle cells. *Biomaterials* **26**, 5405–5413, 2005.

23 MacRitchie R: The adsorption of proteins at the solid/liquid interface. *J Colloid Interface Sci* **38**, 484–488, 1972.

24 Hoffman AS: Blood–biomaterial interactions: an overview. In: *Biomaterials: Interfacial Phenomena and Applications*. Cooper SL, Peppas NA (eds). Advances in Chemistry Series 199, Oxford University Press, New York, 1982, p. 3.

25 Castillo EJ, Koenig JL, Anderson JM, Lo J: Protein adsorption on hydrogels. II. Reversible and irreversible interactions between lysozyme and soft contact lens surfaces. *Biomaterials* **6**, 338–344, 1985.

26 Castillo EJ, Koenig JL, Anderson JM, Lo J: Characterization of protein adsorption on soft contact lenses. I. Conformational changes of adsorbed human serum albumin. *Biomaterials* **5**, 319–325, 1984.

27 Pitt WG, Spiegelberg SH, Cooper SL: Adsorption of fibronectin to polyurethane surfaces: Fourier transformed infrared spectroscopic studies. In: *Proteins and Interfaces: Physicochemical and Biochemical Studies*. Brash JL, Horbett TA (*eds). ACS Symposium Series 343, Oxford University Press, New York, 1977, pp. 324–338.

28 Grinnell F, Feld MK: Adsorption characteristics of plasma fibronectin in relationship to biological activity. *J Biomed Mater Res* **15**, 363–381, 1981.

29 Steele JG, McFarland C, Dalton BA, Johnson G, Evans MD, Howlett CR, Underwood PA: Attachment of human bone cells to tissue culture polystyrene: the effect of surface chemistry upon initial cell attachment. *J Biomater Sci Polymer Edn* **5**, 245–257, 1993.

30 Howlett CR, Evans MDM, Walsh WR, Johnson G, Steele JG: Mechanism of initial attachment of cells derived from human bone to commonly used prosthetic materials during cell culture. *Biomaterials* **15**, 213–222, 1994.

31 Juliano DJ, Saavedra SS, Truskey GA: Effect of the conformation and orientation of adsorbed fibronectin on endothelial cell spreading and the strength of adhesion. *J Biomed Mater Res* **27**, 1103–1113, 1993.

32 Groth TH, Zlatanov I, Altankov G: Adhesion of human peripheral lymphocytes on biomaterials preadsorbed with fibronectin and vitronectin. *J Biomater Sci Polymer Edn* **6**, 729–739, 1994.

33 Truskey GA, Proulx TL: Relationship between 3T3 cell spreading and the strength of adhesion on glass and silane surfaces. *Biomaterials* **14**, 243–254, 1993.

34 Andrade JD, Hlady V: Protein adsorption and materials biocompatibility: A tutorial review and suggested hypothesis. *Prog Surface Sci* **79**, 1–64, 1986.

35 Norde W, Lyklema J: Why proteins prefer interfaces. *J Biomater Sci Polymer Edn* **2**, 183–202, 1991.

36 Kirkham SM, Dangel ME: The keratoprosthesis: improved biocompatibility through design and surface modification. *Ophthalmic Surg* **22**, 455–461, 1991.

37 Grushkin-Lerner LS, Kewalramani R, Trinkaus-Randall V: Expression of integrin receptors on plasma membranes of primary corneal epithelial cells is matrix specific. *Exp Eye Res* **64**, 323–334, 1997.

38 Trinkaus-Randall V, Vural M, Capecchi J, Franzblau C, Leibowitz HM: Modification of polymers for synthesis by corneal epithelial cells. *Invest Ophthalmol Vis Sci* **32**(suppl), 1072, 1991.

39 Steele JG, Johnson G, Griesser HJ, Underwood PA: Mechanism of initial attachment of corneal epithelial cells to polymeric surfaces. *Biomaterials* **18**, 1541–1551, 1997.

40 Paulsson M, Kober M, Freij-Larsson C, Stollenwerk M, Wesslen B and Ljungh Å: Adhesion of staphylococci to chemically modified and native polymers, and the influence of preadsorbed fibronectin, vitronectin and fibrinogen. *Biomaterials* **14**, 845–853, 1993.

41 Pettit DK, Horbett TA, Hoffman AS: Influence of the substrate binding characteristics of fibronectin on corneal epithelial cell outgrowth. *J Biomed Mater Res* **26**, 1259–1275, 1992.

42 Pettit DK, Hoffman AS, Horbett TA: Correlation between corneal epithelial cell outgrowth and monoclonal antibody binding to the cell binding domain of adsorbed fibronectin. *J Biomed Mater Res* **28**, 685–691, 1994.

43 Altankov G, Grinnell F, Groth TH: Studies on the biocompatibility of materials: fibroblast reorganization of substratum-bound fibronectin on surfaces varying in wettability. *J Biomed Mater Res* **33**, 494–499, 1999.

44 Grinnell F, Feld M: Fibronectin adsorption on hydrophilic and hydrophobic surfaces detected by antibody binding and analyzed during cell adhesion in serum containing medium. *J Biol Chem* **257**, 4888–4893, 1982.

45 van Wachem PB, Beugeling T, Feijen J, Bantjes A, Detmers JP, van Aken WG: Interaction of cultured human endothelial cells with polymeric surfaces of different wettabilities. *Biomaterials* **6**, 403–408, 1985.

46 van Koten TG, Schakenraad A, van der Mei HC, Busscher HJ: Influence of substratum wettability on the strength of adhesion of human fibroblasts. *Biomaterials* **12**, 897, 1992.

47 Chen W, Hasegawa C, Hasegawa T, Wenstock C, Yamada K: Development of cell surface linkage complexes in cultured fibroblasts. *J Cell Biol* **100**(4), 1103–1114, 1985.

48 Massia SP, Hubbell JA: Covalent surface immobilization of Arg-Gly-Asp- and Tyr-Ile-Gly-Ser-Arg-containing peptides to obtain well-defined cell-adhesive substrates. *Analyt Biochem* **187**, 292–301, 1990.

49 Murphy WL, Mercurius KO, Koide S, Mrksich M: Substrates for cell adhesion prepared via site-directed immobilization of a protein domain. *Langmuir* **20**, 1026–1030, 2004.

50 Massia SP, Hubbell JA: An RGD spacing of 440 nm is sufficient for integrin $\alpha_v\beta_3$-mediated fibroblast spreading and 140 nm for focal contact and stress fiber formation. *J Cell Biol* **12**, 1089–1100, 1991.

51 Tashiro K-I, Sephel GC, Greatorex D, Sasaki M, Shirashi N, Martin GR, Kleinman HK, Yamada Y: The RGD containing site of the mouse laminin A chain is active

for cell attachment, spreading, migration and neurite outgrowth. *J Cell Physiol* **146**, 451–459, 1991.

52 Massia SP, Rao SS, Hubbell JA: Covalently immobilized laminin peptide Tyr-Ile-Gly-Ser-Arg (YIGSR) supports cell spreading and co-localization of the 67-kilodalton laminin receptor with α-actinin and vinculin. *J Biol Chem* **268**, 8053–8059, 1993.

53 Lin H-B, Sun W, Mosher DF, Garcia-Echeverría C, Schaufelberger K, Lelkes PI, Cooper SL: Synthesis, surface, and cell-adhesion properties of polyurethanes containing covalently grafted RGD-peptides. *J Biomed Mater Res* **28**, 329–342, 1994.

54 Olbrich KC, Andersen TT, Blumenstock FA, Bizios R: Surfaces modified with covalently-immobilized adhesive peptides affect fibroblast population motility. *Biomaterials* **17**, 759–764, 1996.

55 Glass JR, Dickerson KT, Stecker K, Polarek JW: Characterization of a hyaluronic acid–Arg–Gly–Asp peptide cell attachment matrix. *Biomaterials* **17**, 1101–1108, 1996.

56 Hern DL, Hubbell JA: Incorporation of adhesion peptides into nonadhesive hydrogels useful for tissue resurfacing. *J Biomed Mater Res* **39**, 266–276, 1998.

57 Watanabe K, Berman M: Mechanisms of persistent epithelial defect formation: peptide from the cell-domain (GRGDS) inhibits corneal epithelial cell migration. *Invest Ophthalmol Vis Sci* **29**(suppl), 192, 1988.

58 Kugo K, Okuno M, Masusa K, Nishino J, Masufa H, Iwatsuki M: Fibroblast attachment to Arg–Gly–Asp peptide-immobilized poly(gamma-methyl L-glutamate). *J Biomater Sci Polymer Edn* **5**, 325–327, 1994.

59 Griffith-Cima L: Polymer substrates for controlled biological interactions. *J Cell Biochem* **56**, 155–161, 1994.

60 Jeon SI, Lee JH, Andrade JD, DeGennes PG: Protein–surface interactions in the presence of polyethylene oxide. I. Simplified theory. *J Colloid Interface Sci* **142**, 149–158, 1991.

61 Bergstrom K, Holmberg K, Safranj A, Hoffman AS, Edgell MJ, Kozlowski A, Hovanas BA, Harris JM: Reduction of fibrinogen adsorption on PEG-coated polystyrene surfaces. *J Biomed Mater Res* **26**, 779–790, 1992.

62 D'Urso EM, Jean-Francois J, Fortier G: Bioapplication of poly(ethylene glycol)-albumin hydrogels: Matrix for enzyme immobilization. In: *Hydrogels and Biodegradable Polymers for Bioapplications*. Ottenbrite RM, Huang SJ, Park K (eds). American Chemical Society, Washington, 1996, pp. 25–41.

63 Kuhl PR, Griffith-Cima LG: Tethered epidermal growth factor as a paradigm for growth factor-induced stimulation from the solid phase. *Nat Med* **2**, 1022–1027, 1996.

64 Griffith-Cima L: Tissue engineered scaffolds for liver regeneration. Presented at Molecular Engineering of Polymers Workshop: *Directing Biological Response*. American Chemical Society, Washington November, 1996.

65 Nomizu M, Kim WH, Yamamura K, Utani A, Song SY, Ottaka A, Roller PP: Identification of cell binding sites in the laminin alpha 1 chain carboxyl-terminal globular domain by systemic screening of synthetic peptides. *J Biol Chem* **270**, 20583–20590, 1995.

66 Aota S, Nomizu M, Yamada K: The short amino acid sequence Pro–His–Ser–Arg–Asn in human fibronectin enhances cell-adhesive function. *J Biol Chem* **269**, 24756–24761, 1994.

67 Cameron JD, Mooradian DL, Furcht LT: Rabbit corneal epithelial cell adhesion to proteolytic fragments and synthetic peptides of fibronectin. *Invest Ophthalmol Vis Sci* **32**(suppl), 1072, 1991.

68 Benoit DS, Anseth KS: The effect on osteoblast function of colocalized RGD and PHSRN epitopes on PEG surfaces. *Biomaterials* **26**, 5209–5220, 2005.

69 Gasset AR, Kaufman H: Epikeratoprosthesis. Replacement of superficial cornea by methyl methacrylate. *Am J Ophthalmol* **66**, 641–645, 1968.

70 Binder PS, Deg JK, Zavala EY, Grossman RG: Hydrogel keratophakia in non-human primates. *Curr Eye Res* **1**, 535, 1981/82.

71 Samples JR, Binder PS, Zavala EY, Baumgartner SD, Deg JK: Morphology of hydrogel implants used for refractive keratoplasty. *Invest Ophthalmol Vis Sci* **25**, 843–850, 1984.

72 Werblin TP, Fryczkowski AW, Peiffer RL: Myopic correction using alloplastic implants in non-human primates – a preliminary report. *Ann Ophthalmol* **16**(12), 1127–1130, 1984.

73 Quengsy Pellier de: *Precis ou cours d'operations sur la chirurgie de yeux.* Didot, Paris, 1789.

74 Nussbaum A: *Corn Artef.* Munich, 1853.

75 Cuperus PL, Jongebloed WL, van Andel P, Worst JGF: Glass–metal keratoprosthesis: light and electron microscopical evaluation of experimental surgery on rabbit eyes. *Doc Ophthalmol* **71**, 29–47, 1989.

76 Linnola RJ, Happonen RP, Andersson OH, Vedel E, Yli-Urpo AU, Krause U, Laatikainen L: Titanium and bioactive glass-ceramic coated titanium as materials for keratoprosthesis. *Exp Eye Res* **63**, 471–478, 1996.

77 Ricci R, Pecorella I, Ciardi A, Della Rocca C, Di Tondo U, Marchi V: Strampelli's osteo-odonto-keratoprosthesis. Clinical and histological long-term features of three prostheses. *Br J Ophthalmol* **76**, 232–234, 1992.

78 Sommer G: Neue Versuche sur Allopastic der Kornea. *Klin Monatsbl Augenheilkd* **122**, 545–554, 1953.

79 Stone W Jr, Herbert E: Experimental study of plastic material as replacement for the cornea. *Am J Ophthalmol* **36**, 168–173, 1953.

80 Cardona H: Keratoprosthesis. Acrylic optical cylinder with supporting intralamellar plate. *Am J Ophthalmol* **54**, 284–294, 1962.

81 Girard LJ, Hawkins RS, Nieves R, Borodofsky T, Grant C: Keratoprosthesis: A 12-year follow-up. *Trans Am Acad Ophthalmol Otolaryngol* **83**, 525–267, 1977.

82 Cardona H: The Cardona keratoprosthesis: 40 years experience. *Refract Corneal Surg* **7**, 468–471, 1991.

83 Jacob-LaBarre JT, Caldwell DR: Development of a practical artificial cornea for end stage corneal diseases. *Transactions of the Thirteenth Annual Meeting for the Society for Biomaterials*, New York City. Volume X, 1987, p. 57.

84 Jacob-LaBarre JT, Caldwell DR: Development of a soft artificial cornea for end stage corneal diseases. *Proceedings of the American Chemical Society Division of Polymeric Materials: Science and Engineering*, Los Angeles, California, Volume **59**, 1988, pp. 95–99.

85 Trinkaus-Randall V, Capecchi J, Newton A, Vadasz A, Leibowitz H, Franzblau C: Development of a biopolymeric keratoprosthetic material. *Invest Ophthalmol Vis Sci* **29**(3), 393–400, 1988.

86 Dupont D, Gravagna P, Albinet P, Tayot JL, Romanet JP, Mouillon M, Eloy R:

Biocompatibility of human collagen type IV intracorneal implants. *Cornea* **8**(4), 251–258, 1989.

87 Beekhuis WH, McCarey BE, van Rij G, Waring GO III: Complications of hydrogel intracorneal lenses in monkeys. *Arch Ophthalmol* **105**, 116–122, 1987.

88 Jacob-LaBarre JT, Caldwell DR: Development of a new type of artificial cornea for treatment of endstage corneal diseases. In: *Progress in Biomedical Polymers*. Gebelein CG, Dunn RL (eds) Plenum Press, New York, 1990.

89 Thompson KP, Hanna KD, Gipson IK, Gravagna P, Warring GO III, Johnson-Wint B: Synthetic epikeratoplasty in rhesus monkeys with human type IV collagen. *Cornea* **12**(1), 35–45, 1993.

90 Crawford GJ, Constable IJ, Chirila TV, Vijayasekaran S, Thompson D: Tissue interaction with hydrogel sponges implanted in the rabbit cornea. *Cornea* **12**(4), 348–357, 1993.

91 Legeais JM, Rossi C, Renard G, Salvodelli M, D'Hermies F, Pouliquen YJ: A new fluorcarbon for keratoprosthesis. *Cornea* **11**, 538–545, 1992.

92 Crawford GJ, Chirila TV, Vijayasekaran S, Dalton PD, Constable IJ: Preliminary evaluation of a hydrogel core-and-skirt keratoprosthesis in the rabbit cornea. *J Refract Surg* **12**, 525–529, 1996.

93 Hicks C: AlphaCor cases: comparative outcomes. *Cornea* **22**(7), 583–590, 2003.

94 Chirila TV: An overview of the development of artificial corneas with porous skirts and the use of PHEMA for such an application. *Biomaterials* **22**(24), 3311–3317, 2001.

95 Myung D, Farooqui N, Waters D, Schaber S, Koh W, Carrasco M, Noolandi J, Frank CW, Ta CN: Glucose-permeable interpenetrating polymer network hydrogels for corneal implant applications: a pilot study. *Curr Eye Res* **33**(1), 29–43, 2008.

96 Myung D, Duhamel PE, Cochran JR, Noolandi J, Ta CN, Frank CW: Development of hydrogel-based keratoprostheses: a materials perspective. *Biotech Prog* **24**(3), 735–741, 2008.

97 Werblin, T: Eight years experience with Permalens intracorneal lenses in nonhuman primates. *Refract Corneal Surg* **8**(1), 12–22, 1992.

98 McDonald M: Assessment of the long-term corneal response to hydrogel intrastromal lenses implanted in monkey eyes for up to five years. *J Cataract Refract Surg* **19**(2), 213–222, 1993.

99 Sweeney DF, Vannas A, Hughes TC, Evans MD, McLean KM, Xie RZ, Pravin VK, Prakasam RK: Synthetic corneal inlays. *Clin Exp Optom* **91**(1), 56–66, 2008.

100 Gipson IK: Anatomy of the conjunctiva, cornea, and limbus. In: *The Cornea: Scientific Foundations and Clinical Practice*. 3rd edition, Chapter 1. Smolin G, Thoft R (eds). Little, Brown & Co., Boston/New York, 1994, p. 3.

101 Hanna C, O'Brien JE: Cell production and migration in the epithelial layer of the cornea. *Arch Ophthalmol* **64**, 536, 1960.

102 Gipson IK, Watanabe H, Zieske JD: Corneal wound healing and fibronectin. *Int Ophthalmol Clin* **33**, 149–163, 1993.

103 Pierschbacher MD, Ruoslahti E: Cell attachment activity of fibronectin can be duplicated by small synthetic fragments of the molecule. *Nature* **309**, 30, 1984.

104 Qin P, Kurpakus MA: The role of laminin-5 in TGF/EGF-mediated corneal epithelial cell motility. *Exp Eye Res* **66**, 569–579, 1998.

105 Gipson IK, Spurr-Michaud SJ, Tisdale AS: Anchoring fibrils form a complex network in human and rabbit cornea. *Invest Ophthalmol Vis Sci* **28**, 212–220, 1987.

106 Stepp MA: Corneal integrins and their functions. *Exp Eye Res* **83**, 3–15, 2006.

107 Zieske JD, Takahashi H, Hutcheon AEK, Dalbone AC: Activation of epidermal growth factor receptor during corneal epithelial migration. *Invest Ophthalmol Vis Sci* **41**, 1346–1355, 2000.

108 Grant M, Peng TK, Schultz GS, Adams JL, Shimizu RW: Effects of epidermal growth factor, and transforming growth factor-α on corneal cell chemotaxis. *Invest Ophthalmol Vis Sci* **33**(12), 3292–3301, 1992.

109 Wilson SE, Lloyd SA, He Y: Fibroblast growth factor-1 receptor messenger RNA expression in corneal cells. *Cornea* **12**(3):249–254, 1993.

110 Huang AJ, Tseng S: Corneal epithelial wound healing in the absence of limbal epithelium. *Invest Ophthalmol Vis Sci* **32**(1), 96–105, 1991.

111 Kikkawa Y, Yu H, Genersch E, Sanzen N, Sekiguchi K, Fassler R, Campbell K, Talts J, Ekblom P: Laminin isoforms differentially regulate adhesion, spreading, proliferation, and ERK activation of β1 integrin-null cells. *Exp Cell Res* **300**, 94–108, 2004.

112 Filenius S, Hormia M, Rissanen J, Burgeson R, Yamada Y, Araki-Sasaki K, Nakamura M, Virtanen I, Tervo T: Laminin synthesis and the adhesion characteristics of immortalized human corneal epithelial cells to laminin isoforms. Exp Eye Res **75**(1), 93–103, 2001.

113 Kao WW-Y, Funderburgh JL, Xia Y, Liu CY, Conrad GW: Focus on molecules: lumican. *Exp Eye Res* **82**, 3–4, 2006.

114 Filenius S, Tervo T, Virtanen I: Production of fibronectin and tenascin isoforms and their role in the adhesion of human immortalized corneal epithelial cells. *Invest Ophthalmol Vis Sci* **44**(8), 3317–3325, 2003.

115 Watanabe K, Nakagawa S, Nishida T: Stimulatory effects of fibronectin and EGF on migration of corneal epithelial cells. *Invest Ophthalmol Vis Sci* **28**, 205, 1987.

116 Tervo T, Sulonen J, Valtones S, Vannas A, Virtanen I: Distribution of fibronectin in human and rabbit corneas. *Exp Eye Res* **42**, 399–406, 1986.

117 Dee KC, Andersen TT, Bizios R: Osteoblast population migration characteristics on substrates modified with immobilized adhesive peptides. *Biomaterials* **20**, 221–227, 1999.

118 Mooradian DL, McCarthy JB, Skubitz APN, Cameron JD, Furcht LT: Characterization of FN-C/H-V, a novel synthetic peptide from fibronectin that promotes rabbit corneal epithelial cell adhesion, spreading and motility. *Invest Ophthalmol Vis Sci* **34**(1), 153–164, 1993.

119 Li F, Carlsson D, Lohmann C, Suuronen E, Vascotto S, Kobuch K, Sheardown H, Munger R, Nakamura M, Griffith M: Cellular and nerve regeneration within a biosynthetic extracellular matrix for corneal transplantation. *Proc Nat Acad Sci USA* **100**, 15346–15351, 2003.

120 Franco M, Nealey PF, Campbell S, Teixeira AI, Murphy CJ: Adhesion and proliferation of corneal epithelial cells on self-assembled monolayers. *J Biomed Mater Res* **52**, 261–269, 2000.

121 Hsiue GH, Lee SD, Wang CC, Shiue MH, Chang PC: pHEMA-modified silicone rubber film towards improving rabbit corneal epithelial cell attachment and growth. *Biomaterials* *14*, 591–597, 1993.

122 Hsiue GH, Lee SD, Wang CC, Shiue MH, Chang PC: Plasma-induced graft copolymerization of HEMA onto silicone rubber and TPX film improving rabbit corneal epithelial cell attachment and growth. *Biomaterials* **15**, 163–171, 1994.

123 Lee SD, Hsiue GH, Chang PC: Plasma-induced grafted polymerization of acrylic acid

and subsequent grafting of collagen onto polymer film as biomaterials. *Biomaterials* **17**, 1599–1608, 1996.

124 Latkany R, Tsuk A, Sheu M-S, Loh I-H, Trinkaus-Randall V: Plasma surface modification of artificial corneas for optimal epithelialization. *J Biomed Mater Res* **36**, 29–37, 1997.

125 Kobayashi H, Ikada Y: Covalent immobilization of proteins on to the surface of poly(vinyl alcohol) hydrogel. *Biomaterials* **12**, 747–751, 1991.

126 Kobayashi H, Ikada Y: Corneal cell adhesion and proliferation on hydrogel sheets bound with cell-adhesive proteins. *Curr Eye Res* **10**, 899–908, 1991.

127 Xie RZ, Sweeny DF, Baumer GJ, Johnson G, Griesser HJ, Steele JG: Effects of biologically modified surfaces of synthetic lenticules on corneal epithelialization in vivo. *Aust NZ J Ophthalmol* **25**(Suppl1), S46–S49, 1997.

128 Thiessen H, McLean K, Johnson G, Steele JG, Griesser HJ: Covalent immobilization of vitrogen to improve corneal epithelial tissue outgrafts and adhesion. In: *Transactions of the 25th Annual Meeting of the Society for Biomaterials*, Providence, RI, Volume 22, 1999, p. 450.

129 Evans MD, Xie RZ, Fabbri M, Madigan MC, Chaouk H, Beumer GJ, Meijs GF, Griesser HJ, Steele JG, Sweeney DF: Epithelialization of a synthetic polymer in the feline cornea: a preliminary study. *Invest Ophthalmol Vis Sci* **41**(7), 1674–1680, 2000.

130 Miyashita H, Shimmura S, Kobayashi H, Taguchi T, Asano-Kato N, Uchino Y, Kato M, Shimazaki J, Tanaka J, Tsubota K: Collagen-immobilized poly(vinyl alcohol) as an artificial cornea scaffold that supports a stratified corneal epithelium. *J Biomed Mater Res B Appl Biomater* **76**(1) 56–63, 2006.

131 Uchino Y, Shimmura S, Miyashita H, Taguchi T, Kobayashi H, Shimazaki J, Tanaka J, Tsubota K: Amniotic membrane immobilized poly(vinyl alcohol) hybrid polymer as an artificial cornea scaffold that supports a stratified and differentiated corneal epithelium. *J Biomed Maters Res B Appl Biomater* **81**(1) 201–206, 2007.

132 Rochefort JR, Jacob JT: Effect of surface active proteins and peptides on rabbit corneal epithelial cell growth. *Transactions of the Sixth World Biomaterials Congress*, Kamuela, Hawaii, Volume 1, 2000, p. 10.

133 Merrett K, Griffith CM, Deslandes Y, Pleizier G, Sheardown H: Adhesion of corneal epithelial cells to cell adhesion peptide modified pHEMA surfaces. *J Biomater Sci Polymer Edn* **12**, 647–671, 2001.

134 Goodman M, Bhumralkar M, Jefferson EA, Kwak J, Locardi E: Collagen mimetics. *Biopolymers* **47**, 127–142, 1998.

135 Johnson G, Jenkins M, McLean KM, Griesser HJ, Kwak J, Goodman M, Steele JG: Peptoid-containing collagen mimetics with cell binding activity. *J Biomed Mater Res* **51**, 612–624, 2000.

136 Steinert RF, Storie B, Smith P, McDonald M, van Rij G, Bores LD, Colin JP, Durrie DS, Kelley C, Price F Jr, Rostron C, Waring GO III, Nordan LT: Hydrogel intracorneal lenses in aphakic eyes. *Arch Ophthalmol* **114**, 135–141, 1996.

137 Parks RA, McCarey BE: Hydrogel keratophakia: Long-term morphology in the monkey model. *CLAO J* **17**(3), 216–222, 1991.

138 Werblin TP, Peiffer RL, Patel AS: Synthetic keratophakia for the correction of aphakia. *Ophthalmology* **94**, 926–934, 1987.

139 Evans MD, McLean KM, Hughes TC, Sweeney DF: A review of the development of a synthetic corneal onlay for refractive correction. *Biomaterials* **22**, 3319–3328, 2001.

140 Bi J, Downs JC, Jacob JT: Tethered protein/peptide-surface-modified hydrogels. *J Biomater Sci Polymer Edn* **15**(7), 905–916, 2004.

141 Jacob J, Bi J: Surface modifications for enhanced epithelialization. US Patent 6,689,165. Issued 2–10–04.

142 Jacob JT, Rochefort J, Bi J, Gebhardt BM: Corneal epithelial cell growth over tethered-protein/peptide surface-modified hydrogels. *J Biomed Mater Res Part B* **72B**, 198–205, 2005.

143 Wallace C, Jacob JT, Stoltz A, Bi J, Bundy K: Corneal epithelial adhesion strength to tethered-protein/peptide modified hydrogen surfaces. *J Biomed Mater Res* **72A**, 19–24, 2005.

144 Klenkler BJ, Griffith M, Becerril C, West-Mays JA, Sheardown H: EGF-grafted PDMS surfaces in artificial cornea applications. *Biomaterials* **26**(35), 7286–7296, 2005.

145 Sugawara T, Matsuda T: Synthesis of phenylazido-derivatized substances and photochemical surface modification to immobilize functional groups. *J Biomed Mater Res* **32**(2), 157–164, 1996.

146 Thissen H, Johnson G, Hartley PG, Kingshott P, Griesser HJ: Two-dimensional patterning of thin coatings for the control of tissue outgrowth. *Biomaterials* **27**, 35–47, 2006.

8

Reconstruction of the ocular surface using biomaterials

T. V. CHIRILA, L. W. HIRST, Z. BARNARD and
ZAINUDDIN, Queensland Eye Institute, Australia;
D. G. HARKIN, Queensland University of Technology,
Australia; I. R. SCHWAB, University of California,
Davis, USA

Abstract: This chapter discusses the effect on our vision of a large group of disorders, known as ocular surface disorders (OSDs), and presents the therapeutic strategies to reconstruct the afflicted ocular surface. If left untreated, OSDs lead to partial or total loss of eyesight. An overview of various treatment strategies is presented, with the emphasis on the development of the *ex vivo* expansion of corneal limbal epithelial cells (presumed to be stem or progenitor cells) and the creation of transplantable epithelial constructs. The use of naturally derived biomaterials (collagen, fibrin, etc.) or synthetic polymers (polylactides, thermoresponsive polymers, etc.) as substrata in these constructs is critically analyzed. Emphasis is placed on the substrata from silk fibroin, currently being developed by the authors.

Key words: ocular surface disorders, corneal limbal epithelial cells, epithelial constructs, naturally derived biomaterials as substrata, synthetic biomaterials as substrata.

8.1   Introduction

The quality of our vision is determined to a significant degree by the quality of the surface of our eyes, i.e. the ocular surface. A healthy, smooth and continuous ocular surface is essential for clear vision. The ocular surface is a complex entity that conceptually results from the functional integration of its anatomical components (conjunctival epithelium, corneoscleral limbus, corneal epithelium, tear film) with the adjacent structures (eyelid, eyelashes, lacrimal glands). Ultimately, the role of the ocular surface and adnexal tissues includes maintenance of corneal transparency, protection of the eye against external injury and infection, and comfort. The ocular surface is specialized to perform these functions. However, many acute, chronic or cicatrizing pathological conditions may lead to massive tissue destruction or trigger aggressive inflammatory responses from the ocular surface leading to irreversible scarring of the conjunctiva and opacification of the cornea. The spectrum of what is commonly covered by the term 'ocular surface disorders' (or 'diseases'), henceforth abbreviated as OSDs, is extensive, ranging from minor dry eye syndrome and blepharitis to potentially blinding conditions such as chemical and thermal injuries, or multiple surgeries. In an effort to classify the OSDs (Kruse, 2002), ten categories have been proposed, and more than 60 pathological conditions have been identified as OSDs, in addition to chemical, thermal, irradiation and mechanical injuries.

Of particular severity among OSDs are the limbal stem cell deficiency disorders. Epithelial corneal stem cells reside in the corneoscleral limbal region (Davanger and Evensen, 1971; Schermer *et al.*, 1986; Cotsarelis *et al.*, 1989; Dua and Azuara-Blanco, 2000; Kruse, 2002; Ang and Tan, 2004; Ahmad *et al.*, 2006), and it is well established that their depletion is associated with events that lead to visual impairment or total visual loss (Dua and Azuara-Blanco, 2000; Sangwan, 2002; Ang and Tan, 2004). Experiments in animals show that the more limbal epithelium that is damaged, the more the capacity of the ocular surface for healing is reduced. When more than half of the limbal tissue was removed, the re-epithelialization was slow and resulted in a dysfunctional (usually conjunctivalized) corneal epithelium (Chen and Tseng, 1991; Huang and Tseng, 1991). This is frequently accompanied by opacity of the stroma. Conjunctivalization is described as the movement of conjunctiva-like tissue across the normal barrier of the limbus and on to the corneal surface causing pain and loss of vision. Less severe injury may result in partial limbal stem cell deficiency, when conjunctivalization of the corneal surface may not be evident or there may only be partial replacement of the corneal epithelium by conjunctival epithelium. Severe limbal stem cell deficiency involves the entire corneal surface and is associated with congenital diseases (e.g. aniridia, ectodermal displasia) (Sugar, 2002), or can be caused by chemical or thermal burns (Kim and Khosla-Gupta, 2002), iatrogenic factors such as chronic use of certain topical medication or repeated surgeries of limbal region or conjunctiva (Schwartz and Holland, 2002), inherited or bacterial keratitis, and immunological disorders (e.g. Stevens–Johnson syndrome, cicatricial pemphigoid) (Tauber, 2002). Contact lens wear, especially associated with the use of cleaning solutions and preservatives, can also cause significant stem cell loss (Sendele *et al.*, 1983; Stenson, 1983; Bloomfield *et al.*, 1984; Jenkins *et al.*, 1993).

8.2   Treatment of ocular surface disorders

The management of limbal stem cell deficiency is complicated, and surgery has always been, by necessity, the treatment of choice. While minor to moderate limbal stem cell deficiency may be treated medically (i.e. through observation and medication) or by surgical procedures such as debridement or removal of conjunctival tissue, surgical replacement of diseased tissue and restoration of epithelial progenitor/stem cells are essential in the treatment of severe limbal stem cell deficiency. This requires transplantation of either autologous or allogeneic donor tissue. In the past, removal of abnormal epithelium (keratectomy) or penetrating or lamellar keratoplasty were the preferred surgical procedures, but it was soon realized that both have little chance of clinical success in the face of total limbal stem deficiency. Keratectomy was followed inevitably by re-conjunctivalization, and keratoplasty provided a stable ocular surface lasting only for as long as the donor epithelium was present, and inevitably the surface was later covered by conjunctival epithelium (Holland and Schwartz, 2002). Subsequently, the progress in ophthalmic microsurgery and in elucidating the biology of stem cells led to the current treatments of OSDs, but such evolution has occurred in stages. Thoft reported the first conjunctival transplantation to treat chemical burns (Thoft, 1977). He used autografts from the normal eye of the same patient. Although it is unlikely that conjunctival transplantation is followed by transdifferentiation into corneal epithelium, the conjunctival autografts are still used in the management of certain OSDs that are not necessarily associated with limbal stem cell loss, such as pterygium (Hirst, 2003). Thoft was also the first surgeon to perform transplantation of donor peripheral corneal limbal epithelium with a stromal carrier from cadaveric eyes to treat bilateral chemical burns and severe atopic keratoconjunctivitis (Thoft, 1984). Presumably, some stem/progenitor cells were harvested with the transplants in certain patients, which may explain the visual improvement in a small series of patients (Holland and Schwartz, 2002).

The advances in stem cell biology had a crucial impact on the treatment of severe OSDs (Holland and Schwartz, 2002; Kim *et al.*, 2003; Limb *et al.*, 2006; Boulton *et al.*, 2007; Revoltella *et al.*, 2007), especially after the anatomical localization of corneal stem cells was established. This achievement opened the era of 'cellular surgery', a term coined by some investigators (Kinoshita and Nakamura, 2005) based on the fact that in such surgical procedures the ocular surface's epithelial cells are harvested and expanded in an external environment prior to surgery. In the first clinical trial that applied this knowledge, conjunctival autografts were harvested deliberately to include cells from the corneal limbal region, and implanted in a series of 21 patients affected by some of the OSDs with the most devastating prognosis, such as chemical and thermal burns, keratopathy induced by contact lens wear and iatrogenic stem cell deficiency (Kenyon and Tseng, 1989). The outcome was successful: healing and surface stabilization occurred in almost all cases, and visual acuity was improved in 17 cases. The limbal autograft transplantation is restricted by the amount of tissue that can be removed from the patients' healthy contralateral eyes, as their healing can be seriously affected even when relatively small amounts of limbal epithelium are excised, and obviously it is not possible in cases of bilateral damage. Therefore, allograft transplantation techniques were also developed (Holland and Schwartz, 2002), where the limbal donor tissue was harvested from a living relative of the patient, or excised from cadaveric eyes. The transplantation of allogeneic tissue is restricted by the availability of suitable donor tissue and by immunological and biosafety concerns, and is generally associated with reduced clinical success because of the high rate of rejection. If this method of reconstruction of the ocular surface is to have any chance of success, it requires the administration of potent anti-rejection regimens, which can be associated with significant risks to the general health of the patient, especially considering that these treatments may be required for the rest of the patient's life.

Transplantation of human amniotic membrane (amnion) is another strategy for the management of OSDs, an important development to which some landmark reviews were dedicated (Tseng, 2002; John, 2003; Bouchard and John, 2004; Dua *et al.*, 2004). The amniotic membrane (AM) is the innermost layer of the placenta and one of the three foetal membranes. It consists of an epithelialized basement membrane resting on a relatively thick basement membrane and stroma. It has been used in the surgical reconstruction of a variety of tissues and organs since the beginning of the twentieth century. The first report on its use in the reconstruction of the ocular surface (conjunctiva) (de Rötth, 1940), was soon followed by reports on its transplantation in large series of patients with alkali burns (Sorsby and Symons, 1946; Sorsby *et al.*, 1947). After a long hiatus, the modern era of AM transplantation began in the early 1990s, when Battle and Perdomo in the Dominican Republic communicated its use for the treatment of conjunctival disorders including chemical burns (Battle and Perdomo, 1993). Soon after, Tseng and his collaborators published the use of AM for ocular surface reconstruction in an animal model (Kim and Tseng, 1995). Tseng's subsequent work in developing an adequate methodology for harvesting and preserving the membranes, as well as his further laboratory investigations and human clinical trials, provided a solid scientific and clinical foundation for the therapeutic use of AM in the management of some OSDs. It was also realized, however, that AM transplantation alone in patients with total limbal stem cell deficiency is unlikely to succeed. Consequently, limbal allografts and AM were transplanted in combination to enhance the clinical success in these cases (Tsubota *et al.*, 1996; Tseng *et al.*, 1998).

Some investigators believe that the success of AM transplantation relies on a series of processes potentially triggered by the presence of AM itself, including promotion of epithelialization, inhibition of conjunctival fibrosis, suppression of inflammatory cytokines and inhibition of protease activity (Kinoshita and Nakamura, 2005). According to a recent report (Connon *et al.*, 2006), transplanted AM can remain within the corneal tissue for long periods without being degraded and/or assimilated, but its persistence does not lead to inflammation, rejection or loss of transparency. Although the use of AM gained enormous popularity, as illustrated in over 500 reports published by the year 2006 (Maharajan *et al.*, 2007), there are some associated drawbacks that should not be ignored. In addition to its high cost, AM – as any human-derived tissue – is a potential vector for infectious diseases (Schwab *et al.*, 2006). Variation in donors and harvesting or processing methods makes a qualitative standardization of the AMs available to the surgeon almost impossible, and significant variability in the mechanical properties of the commercially available AM preparations has been reported (Chuck *et al.*, 2004). In conjunctival regeneration, the clinical success of AM transplantation is limited to several conjunctival defects (Hatton and Rubin, 2005). In many OSDs, the AM transplantation alone is not effective unless combined with transplantation of limbal epithelial stem cells or/and intraoperative topical use of mitomycin C (an anti-tumour antibiotic thought to reduce scar formation, but also with the potential for significant side effects). In addition, transplantation must be performed within days in the case of acute OSDs (e.g. burns) (Tseng, 2007). Finally, recent case studies (Maharajan *et al.*, 2007; Saw *et al.*, 2007) showed that in reality the AM transplantation can be associated with significant lack of clinical success.

8.3   *Ex vivo* expansion of ocular surface epithelial cells

Localization of corneal and conjunctival stem/progenitor cells on the ocular surface was a crucial step in the development of modern strategies to treat OSDs associated with limbal stem cell deficiency. Advances in our understanding of the role and composition of the extracellular matrix led to the next crucial event: the development of an *in vitro* procedure to grow and propagate these cells. A method was developed (Lindberg *et al.*, 1993) where the dissociated cells harvested from human corneal or conjunctival biopsies were serially co-cultured with γ-irradiated murine 3T3 fibroblasts (as feeder layers) in the presence of serum. This procedure made possible the creation of epithelial equivalent constructs, an alternative that is currently being investigated in many laboratories. Considering the problems encountered with the surgical approaches mentioned above, such a strategy has great promise (Nishida, 2003; Selvam *et al.*, 2006; Shortt *et al.*, 2007). An epithelial construct can be generated through the *ex vivo* expansion of human corneal limbal epithelial or conjunctival epithelial stem/progenitor cells. According to this strategy, a small tissue biopsy specimen is collected from the patient's contralateral normal eye, if healthy, and is then either cultured as an explant or dissociated into isolated cells, which are grown *in vitro* while placed on (or within) a substratum (carrier). The resulting tissue construct, either as an independent sheet or attached to the substratum (which ideally should be biodegradable), is then transplanted to the site where new tissue formation is required. If the contralateral eye is not healthy enough for harvest, allogeneic tissue acquired from donor eyes may be expanded *ex vivo* and then attached to a substratum in the same fashion.

It was a few years later that De Luca and colleagues in Italy published their landmark report (Pellegrini *et al.*, 1997) on the reconstruction of the damaged ocular surface in two patients using corneal limbal epithelial constructs expanded *in vitro*. Both patients (males) had severe alkali burns in one eye only, and the biopsies (1 mm^2) were taken from the healthy contralateral eyes. The dissociated cells were co-cultured with murine 3T3 feeder cells in a complex growth medium containing foetal bovine serum (FBS). In preliminary experiments included in this study, cells were harvested from three different regions of the ocular surface (cadaver or consenting donor), namely bulbar conjunctiva, central cornea and limbus, and grown as described above. It was found that only the limbal cells were able to generate a stratified construct. For the autologous transplantation, grafts were prepared from confluent cultures of about 2 million limbal cells each, which were released from the culture dish and mounted on petrolatum gauze or on a soft contact lens. In one patient, the gauze was removed immediately after grafting and then the cell layer was covered with a contact lens. In the other patient, the contact lens with the cell layer on the concave side was placed directly on the eye. A stable ocular surface was achieved in both patients and maintained 2 years after grafting. In one patient, a penetrating keratoplasty was performed later and visual acuity was improved. The other patient was satisfied with the significant improvement in comfort and refused keratoplasty, an understandable attitude considering his experience with three previous failed attempts. We should point out that in this instance the epithelial cell sheets were not attached to a substratum at the time of grafting on to the damaged ocular surface. While the cells were grown on commercial tissue culture plastic, the gauze and contact lens on to which they were mounted after culturing were purely designed to make manipulation of the cell sheets easier. Although substratum-free epithelial cell constructs were successful in these two patients, and the approach was used at least in one other instance by others (Daya *et al.*, 2005) (when the confluent cell sheet was mounted on nylon dressing prior to surgery and AM was used as a post-transplantation bandage), it is expected that the presence of a substratum (carrier) on which the limbal epithelial cells are not only grown and attached, but which is also transplanted together with the cell layer, would constitute a considerable surgical advantage. Consequently, the search for an adequate substratum in the creation of tissue-engineered constructs for the restoration of the ocular surface became part of the developing therapeutic strategies against OSDs and remains an ongoing interdisciplinary activity.

Although the conjunctival epithelial constructs have not been specifically mentioned in our exposition so far, there have been a significant number of reports on the transfer of conjunctival stem/progenitor epithelial cells as *in-vitro*-grown constructs. This work was excellently analysed in two recent reviews (Hatton and Rubin, 2005; Selvam *et al.*, 2006), hence we will not further expand on the subject. The localization of the stem/progenitor cells in the conjunctiva proved to be more ambiguous when compared with that in the cornea. Forniceal, palpebral and mucocutaneous regions were all proposed as zones with enriched content of stem/progenitor cells. The human conjunctival goblet cells with proliferative capacity are notoriously difficult to grow *in vitro* (Shatos *et al.*, 2003; Ang *et al.*, 2004). The clinical success of the transplantation of conjunctival epithelial constructs is limited owing to a tendency of these cells not to differentiate into the corneal epithelial phenotype; therefore, the limbal constructs are much more effective in the therapy of OSDs. An interesting approach was to co-culture limbal and conjunctival epithelial cells on AM and use the resulting constructs in human patients (Sangwan *et al.*, 2003).

8.4   Corneal equivalents as replacements or study models

We should mention here that the developmental work for tissue-engineered corneal limbal epithelial constructs differs in its approaches and aims from the development of artificial corneas (Chirila *et al.*, 1998; Duan *et al.*, 2006; Ruberti *et al.*, 2007; Sheardown and Griffith, 2008) or of tissue-engineered corneal equivalents (Griffith *et al.*, 1999; Schneider *et al.*, 1999; Germain *et al.*, 2000; Orwin and Hubel, 2000; Germain *et al.*, 2004; Duan *et al.*, 2006; Ruberti *et al.*, 2007; Sheardown and Griffith, 2008). The former are made from synthetic polymers and do not include biological components. While at least two models are US Food and Drug Administration (FDA)-approved for distribution and use, their implantation is generally associated with clinical complications. An artificial cornea is unsuitable for the reconstruction of the ocular surface, as its role is restricted to replacing an irreversibly damaged and opaque cornea where both the ocular surface and the underlying stroma and endothelium are damaged and there is no intent to induce a regenerative process. On the other hand, the tissue-engineered corneal equivalents as yet cannot fulfil the functional prerequisites to replace a damaged cornea, and their applications have been limited to *in vitro* studies. Although some experimental approaches are common to both epithelial constructs and corneal equivalents, the latter are confronted by some challenges that have so far prevented their clinical applications in human patients; such challenges include conservation of transparency, duplication of mechanical properties, reproduction of extracellular matrix components expression and of barrier–pump endothelial function, presence of neural elements and elimination of cell immortalization stage from the experimental protocols.

As a final remark, while both artificial corneas and tissue–engineered corneal equivalents are aiming at the total replacement of a dysfunctional cornea and should be used when other procedures for reconstruction have failed or are not practicable, the limbal or conjunctival epithelial constructs are intended to restore the integrity and function of damaged sectors of the ocular surfaces only. Ultimately, as the efficacy of stem cell transplantation procedures improves, the future need for the previous two alternatives may diminish (Mannis, 2002). This issue is not always understood, a situation that leads to publications where regrettably the two topics have been intermixed, resulting in significant confusion.

Some early research of corneal equivalents was not aimed at the treatment of OSDs, but contributed to a better understanding of corneal biology. The three-layer constructs were the first corneal equivalents to be reported (Minami et al., 1993), with the declared aim of producing an in vitro tool for investigating corneal pathophysiology. These equivalents were made by culturing bovine normal epithelial, stromal and endothelial cells in a matrix of collagen type I. The thickness of the final constructs was around 0.2 mm, and they had an epithelium stratified in four to five layers. In another development (Zieske et al., 1994), three-layer corneal equivalents were made as a tool to study the influence of endothelium on the differentiation of epithelial cells. They were prepared by casting a collagen gel containing animal or human keratocytes on the top of immortalized cultured murine corneal endothelial cells, and then seeding a suspension of animal or human epithelial cells on the top of the collagen layer. When such constructs were made without an endothelial layer, the epithelial cells did not express differentiation markers or basement membrane components. This is a fine example of using corneal equivalents to acquire further knowledge. One-layer constructs were made (Kahn et al., 1993) with the aim of providing an in vitro model for ocular toxicology studies. Human corneal epithelial cells immortalized by treatment with an SV40 hybrid virus were used in this study. The cells were able to synthesize corneal-specific keratins and to promote stratification, but many of the immortalized cell lines were still shedding free virus at the conclusion of experiments. Similar work was reported later by a Japanese group (Araki-Sasaki et al., 1995), who created one-layer constructs for biological studies by using epithelial cells immortalized with an SV40-adenovirus recombinant vector, which supposedly eliminated the shedding of the virus. The resulting epithelial constructs had properties similar to those of normal epithelium.

8.5   Naturally derived biomaterials as substrata for tissue-engineered epithelial constructs

Although – owing to its clinical success and popularity – AM was used as a substratum in the epithelial cell constructs soon after De Luca's report on substratum-free constructs, other materials were investigated for this purpose long before. In their quest to promote a suitable carrier, Tsai and Tseng cultured rabbit conjunctival epithelial cells on collagen type I or Matrigel™, and on a combination of these (Tsai and Tseng, 1988). It was found that both collagen and Matrigel™ promoted the growth and differentiation of the conjunctival cells leading to either monolayers (on collagen) or stratified sheets (on Matrigel™). Matrigel™ is a commercially available synthetic basement membrane derived from the Engelbreth–Holm–Swarm mouse sarcoma tumour cell line, and was developed by BD Biosciences (San Jose, CA, USA) based on research carried out in several laboratories of the National Institutes of Health (NIH) in Bethesda, MD, USA (Kleinman *et al.*, 1982; Kleinman *et al.*, 1986). Tsai later reported the culture of human conjunctival epithelial cells on collagen type I (Tsai *et al.*, 1994). When no other cells were included in the culture, the epithelial constructs were not stratified. In the presence of conjunctival fibroblasts or 3T3 cells, the constructs were multilayered and showed many characteristic epithelial features. We are not aware, however, of any therapeutic application of this research.

Other investigators also chose collagen as a substratum, but the approach was different. Animal (rabbit) corneal basal epithelial cells were obtained from biopsies and were cultured on crosslinked gelatine membranes or on the concave side of commercial collagen corneal shields (McCulley *et al.*, 1991). The collagen cornea shields (Willoughby *et al.*, 2002) contain mainly collagen type I and are manufactured from porcine sclera or bovine dermis. The shields are used for ocular surface protection following surgery or trauma, and for sustained administration of drugs. The degree of crosslinking, accomplished through ultraviolet (UV) light exposure, is variable and correlated to the intended duration of the device before dissolution. The mentioned study showed that following contact and 1 or 2 days of incubation, the cell layers grown on both substrata could be transferred on to rabbit denuded corneas or cryolathed stromal lenticules (both obtained from enucleated eyes). After removing the carriers, most of the cells remained attached to the stromal surface. In these experiments, the collagen shield was more suitable as a substratum in terms of growth rate and proliferation as compared with gelatin. The same concept was applied using primary cultures of human corneal epithelial cells, but the study was limited to collagen shields as substrata (He and McCulley, 1991). A variety of growth media were employed, and some of the collagen shields were coated with Matrigel™ or with collagen type IV. The coating enhanced cell attachment. However, the cells failed to reach confluence on the Matrigel™ layer, which is contrary to the results reported by Tsai and Tseng (see above). The multilayered cultures on the collagen type IV were successfully transferred on human denuded corneas (eye bank) through contact and 2–7 days of incubation. The adhesion was strong enough to withstand the removal of supporting collagen shields.

Although this procedure would presumably simplify surgery, it appears that other investigators did not pursue the concept. About a decade later, the same group repeated the experiments, this time using human corneal limbal epithelial cells or human amniotic cells seeded on collagen shields (He *et al.*, 1999). The substrata with cells were then transplanted *in vivo* on to the de-epithelialized corneas of 27 rabbits. For the first 2 days, the eyelids were kept sutured to maintain contact between cells and host stroma. The animals were monitored for 10 days. The procedure was successful in only ten eyes, as judged by the occurrence of re-epithelialization, formation of cell–substratum hemidesmosomes and confirmation of human-specific antigen presentation. This report suggested that the procedure of cell layers transplantation through cells–stroma contact is not exempted from failure and ultimately the surgery required may become as complex as in other cellular construct transplantations. However, the technique was recently resurrected as a procedure for transplantation of epithelial constructs (Di Girolamo *et al.*, 2007), with the difference that, instead of collagen shields, contact lenses made of synthetic polymers were proposed. Based on the observed occurrence of epithelial growth on the contact lenses used as bandages after pterygium surgery, two brands of 30-day continuous wear siloxane hydrogel contact lenses – Focus® Night & Day™ (CIBA Vision) and *Pure Vision*™ (Bausch & Lomb) – have been investigated as substrata for corneal limbal epithelial cells obtained from explants and cultured in autologous serum. The materials in the two contact lenses, known as 'lotrafilcon A' and 'balafilcon A', respectively, are quite different in structure and surface topography (Tighe, 2000; López-Alemany *et al.*, 2002). Cell growth, assessed through the analysis of morphology, proliferative capacity and cytokeratin profile, was seen only on lotrafilcon. Since commercial contact lenses are designed to resist epithelial adherence, the validity of this approach is doubtful.

Another proposed substratum material was a collagen–glycosaminoglycan (CG) copolymer, initially developed for skin regeneration (Yannas *et al.*, 1989). It is made by the coprecipitation of bovine collagen type I and shark cartilage chondroitin 6-sulfate. The material has been evaluated as a graft for the regeneration of experimentally injured rabbit conjunctiva (Hsu *et al.*, 2000). The grafts clearly inhibited scarring and induced the formation of a tissue resembling normal conjunctival stroma. However, no reports are available on the use of CG substrata for ocular surface reconstruction in human patients.

In Italy, De Luca's group continued their work and treated 18 human patients with limbal stem cell deficiency in one eye by grafting autologous limbal stem cells constructs (Rama *et al.*, 2001). This time, the cell from limbal biopsies were cultured on a layer of commercial fibrin sealant (Tissucol™, Baxter-Immuno, Austria), which was prepared by mixing solutions of thrombin and fibrinogen. The resulting fibrin is a biodegradable and biocompatible material, although there are biosafety issues associated with its use (Eyrich *et al.*, 2006). The grafts were implanted attached to the fibrin substratum. The restoration of the ocular surface was successful in 14 patients, where within 1 month the surface was covered with a transparent epithelium. The ocular surfaces were stable on follow-up between 1 and 2 years postoperatively, and three patients underwent successful penetrating keratoplasty about 1 year after the limbal transplantation. Schwab's group suggested new directions in the application of fibrin by growing human corneal limbal epithelial cells within a matrix of fibrin gel (Han *et al.*, 2002). In this study, both fibrinogen and thrombin components were prepared in a specialized machine, the CryoSeal FS System (ThermoGenesis Corp., Rancho Cordova, CA, USA). Cultured human corneal epithelial cells were added to the thrombin solution, and then mixed with the fibrinogen solution to form a fibrin gel with the cells embedded throughout. The cells proliferated within the gel matrix, showing normal growth kinetics. Despite all these promising results, there has been no subsequent use of fibrin reported in the literature with the exception of a recent animal study (Luengo Gimeno *et al.*, 2007). Severe limbal stem cell deficiency was experimentally induced in rabbit eyes by inflicting alkali burns in one eye, and limbal biopsies were harvested from the contralateral eye. Cells were grown on fibrin (Tissucol™) and the autografts were implanted about 3 weeks from the start of culture. The ocular surface was restored completely within 12 months, with a transparent, stratified epithelium covering the cornea. In the same study, for the first time platelet-rich plasma (PRP) was used as a substratum for limbal epithelial cells, and showed some advantages (e.g. elasticity and transparency) over fibrin. PRP is an autologous product consisting of a small volume of plasma containing a large number of platelets, which can be prepared from the blood of the patients, and is biodegradable and biocompatible. Its use in transplantations is increasingly advocated (Yazawa *et al.*, 2003; Luengo Gimeno *et al.*, 2006).

Although introduced slightly later than most of the materials discussed above, AM prevails as a substratum for *ex vivo* expanded epithelial stem/ progenitor cells. A thorough analysis of the human clinical trials that have used *ex vivo* expanded epithelial cells (Schwab *et al.*, 2006) indicated that of 20 studies (involving 275 patients) published between 1996 and 2005, AM was used in 16 studies as the substratum for cells, an estimate largely confirmed in a subsequently published review (Shortt *et al.*, 2007). The first reports on the use of AM as a substratum came from Schwab's team at the University of California at Davis (Schwab, 1999; Schwab *et al.*, 2000). In the first study (Schwab, 1999), 19 patients were involved. With the exception of 2 patients where sibling allogeneic limbal epithelial constructs were transplanted, all other patients received autologous constructs. A variety of substrata were used in the constructs including corneal stroma, collagen type I, soft contact lenses, collagen shields and AM; the latter was used in

7 cases. Surgical procedures were carried out between 1994 and 1998 and were followed up for durations between 2 and 24 months. At the time of reporting, 5 cases were unsuccessful, partially successful or undetermined. Only 1 unsuccessful outcome was reported with the AM. In a subsequent study (Schwab *et al.*, 2000), 14 patients received autologous or allogeneic grafts grown on AM, and were followed up for between 6 and 19 months. The treatment was successful in 10 patients. In these studies, successful clinical outcome was determined by restoration or improvement of patient's vision, re-epithelialization and non-recurrence of the original OSD. In a study carried out in Taiwan (Tsai *et al.*, 2000), 6 patients were treated with autologous limbal constructs on AM substratum, and monitored for 12–18 months. In all patients the vision improved and there were no recurrent problems.

Recently, sutureless AM transplantation has been developed and assessed in the rabbit eye, using adhesive materials instead of sutures. Either fibrin glue (Sekiyama *et al.*, 2007) or a novel 'chemically defined bioadhesive' (Takaoka *et al.*, 2008) have been evaluated as adhesives. The latter adhesive was prepared by the chemical reaction of aldehyde-functionalized dextran with ε-poly(L-lysine) (Nakajima *et al.*, 2007).

In spite of favourable clinical outcomes generally reported with AM as a substratum for the epithelial constructs, the procedure is affected by inherent difficulties in the growth and maintenance of the cells on AMs (Kinoshita and Nakamura, 2005), and by the drawbacks mentioned previously (see Section 8.2). In addition, some investigators obtained quite disappointing clinical results that led them with conclude that there is no advantage in using this procedure when compared with other limbal transplantation techniques or with transplantation of AM alone (Shimazaki *et al.*, 2002).

8.6   Synthetic biomaterials as substrata for tissue-engineered epithelial constructs

The first use of an artificial material in the reconstruction of the ocular surface should be rather regarded as a singular episode, as the material was not intended as a substratum for cellular constructs but as a substitute for the autologous mucosal membrane grafts in the reconstruction of the socket. Such membranes, harvested from the buccal or nasal regions, have been in occasional surgical use for the past four decades and they still have proponents, although their collection involves additional surgical procedures. In this study (Levin and Dutton, 1990), patients who lost an eye as a result of previous malignancies, cicatricial pemphigoid or congenital conditions, and could not maintain their artificial socket implants because of severe damage to conjunctiva, were treated by grafting 0.1-mm-thick sheets of polytetrafluoroethylene, supplied as Gore-Tex® (Gore & Associates, Flagstaff, AZ, USA). Within 2 weeks, the residual conjunctival epithelium grew beneath the Gore-Tex® membranes. In some instances, the polymer graft was removed to reveal complete epithelialization. Ultimately, being an opaque, hydrophobic and non-biodegradable material, polytetrafluoroethylene did not have any future in the field of ocular surface reconstruction.

Closer to our time, perhaps prompted by the drawbacks perceived with using AM, some investigators contemplated artificial substrata for the creation of limbal or conjunctival epithelial constructs. As shown below, a range of synthetic polymers were studied *in vitro* and in experimental animals, although not always with the purpose of creating limbal or conjunctival epithelial constructs.

As the epitome of biodegradable polymers, the lactone-based polymers, with the polylactides and polyglycolides as their prominent representatives, attracted some attention as potential substratum materials. In one study (Lee *et al.*, 2003), poly(lactide-*co*-glycolide) (PLGA) porous scaffolds were modified by treatment with collagen or hyaluronic acid, or mixed with particles of AM, or subjected to combinations of these treatments. *In vitro*, both corneal epithelial cells (commercial line) and human corneal stromal fibroblasts (obtained from biopsies) attached well to the scaffolds and proliferated throughout the cross-section. The PLGA scaffolds modified with collagen and hyaluronic acid were then used *in vivo* as grafts on rabbit eyes where conjunctival wounds were experimentally created. After 4 weeks, the wound contraction and scar formation were much less in the grafted than in the ungrafted eyes. In a more recent study (Zorlutuna *et al.*, 2006), a commercial polylactide (Resomer® LR 708) was combined with poly(3-hydroxybutyric acid-*co*-3-hydroxyvaleric acid), a natural biodegradable polymer. Membranes and porous scaffolds were both produced from this polymer mixture. The membranes were seeded with retinal pigment epithelial (RPE) cells, and the scaffolds were seeded with 3T3 fibroblasts. The RPE cells generated a stratified epithelium, while the 3T3 fibroblasts colonized the scaffolds and deposited neocollagen type I, prompting the authors to conclude that this polymer combination can function as a substratum material for corneal reconstruction, although is not clear why RPE cells were employed instead of corneal epithelial cells. Fibrous constructs made of another polymer from this class, poly(glycolic acid), were also reported as suitable scaffolds for the growing of corneal stromal cells (Hu *et al.*, 2005).

Another synthetic polymer investigated experimentally as a substratum for growing corneal cells was a polyurethane. In this study (Liliensiek *et al.*, 2006), a transparent polyurethane, commercially available as an optical adhesive (NOA61™, from Norland Products, Cranbury, NJ, USA), was modified by creating surface nanoscale topographic features. The attachment and growth of three types of human corneal cells (SV40-transformed epithelial cells, primary epithelial cells and primary fibroblast) were investigated in cultures. Topographic features (e.g. grooves, ridges) below 1 μm in size inhibited significantly the proliferation of all categories of cells. While this study may contribute to the vast field of research regarding the interactions between surface characteristics and cell attachment, it is of less relevance to epithelial constructs. The polymer in the study is available as a liquid that is curable by UV exposure and contains some toxic ingredients. As clearly indicated by the supplier (https://www.norlandprod.com/adhesives/NOA%20 61.html), such optical adhesives are strictly designed for binding 'to glass surfaces, metals, fiberglass and glass filled plastics', and prolonged contact with skin and contact with the eyes should be avoided. The investigators' assertion that this adhesive material has 'limited toxicity to corneal epithelial cells' is totally unsubstantiated and misleading; in fact, the optical adhesives do not have to be biocompatible as they are designated for use outside the body.

A research project was recently carried out in the laboratories of Singapore's National Eye Centre and Eye Research Institute, with the precisely defined aim of assessing a synthetic polymer, poly(ε-caprolactone) (PCL), as a potential substratum for conjunctival epithelial constructs (Ang *et al.*, 2006). PCL is a degradable material that is approved by the FDA for medical use. In the study, biaxially stretched PCL membranes were prepared to a thickness of around 6 μm. Some of the membranes were also treated chemically to enhance the hydrophilicity of their surface. Rabbit conjunctival epithelial cells were then cultured both as monolayers and as explants (the latter in a serum-free medium) on the PCL membranes, which successfully supported their attachment and proliferation leading to confluent stratified epithelial sheets. In parallel experiments it was found that the goblet cell densities on PCL and AM were not statistically different. Interestingly, the cell proliferation and stratification were greater on the PCL membranes with enhanced hydrophilicity. This finding is at odds with the well-documented trend of cells growing at interfaces of variable hydrophilicity: the more hydrophilic the surface, the fewer attached cells. It is also at odds with the principle of the strategy presented in the next section. The conjunctival epithelial constructs of this study were implanted subcutaneously in immune-deficient mice, and explanted after 1 week. The histopathological analysis revealed the formation of multilayered epithelia over the PCL membranes. There was no mention about the biodegradability of the PCL substrata, most likely because of the too short residence time. No evaluation in human eyes has yet been reported.

Poly(vinyl alcohol) (PVA) is a synthetic polymer that can be obtained with an enormous range of properties thanks to its indirect synthesis by the hydrolysis of poly(vinyl acetate), which allows variable degrees of hydrolysis and a variety of chemical and physical crosslinking methods. Being non-toxic and hydrophilic, with good mucoadhesive properties, PVA has received much attention as a biomaterial. In the early 1990s, Yoshito

Ikada's group at Kyoto University developed PVA hydrogels intended for artificial corneas (Chirila *et al.*, 2005). In order to promote epithelialization, the hydrogels' surface was modified by immobilization of extracellular matrix components (collagen, fibronectin or adhesion peptides). After successful *in vitro* corneal epithelial cell growth experiments, the collagen-immobilized PVA was used for *in vivo* experiments in rabbit corneas. Unfortunately, the placement on to the cornea and the implantation into the cornea were both associated with severe postoperative complications. PVA was abandoned as a keratoprosthetic material and the research group's interest was re-directed to polyurethanes (Chirila *et al.*, 2005). However, 15 years later, another team used collagen-immobilized PVA (henceforth COL-PVA), prepared following Ikada's methodology, as a substratum for cells (Miyashita *et al.*, 2006). Although this research was aimed at developing an epithelializable keratoprosthesis, it is worth mentioning it here since the cells seeded and grown on the PVA substratum were corneal limbal epithelial cells of either human or animal origin. The cells were cultured in the presence of 3T3 feeder cells, and they generated stratified epithelial layers displaying the characteristics of a corneal epithelium. The study also included the intralamellar grafting of epithelialized COL-PVA. While the grafts were easy to handle and suture, and showed mechanical properties similar to donor tissue grafts, 'the sutures became loose after a few days due to inflammation, causing the epithelium to detach from the polymer surface' (Miyashita *et al.*, 2006). In order to improve the outcome, the same team later developed a substratum where AM was glued to COL-PVA using a tissue adhesive based on citric acid (Uchino *et al.*, 2007). *In vitro*, rabbit limbal epithelial cells generated a stratified epithelium. In a comparative study *in vivo* using rabbits, AM-PVA and COL-PVA were implanted in pockets created on the cornea. All corneas transplanted with COL-PVA lost epithelium by 2 weeks, while those with AM-PVA showed partial or complete epithelialization in all eyes. Clearly, the better outcome was due entirely to the presence of AM, which probably would have happened even in the absence of PVA. However, it is difficult to fathom how an artificial cornea incorporating an AM can be made into a commercial product.

8.7   Strategies based on thermoresponsive polymers

8.7.1   The 'cell sheet engineering' approach

This approach is the result of work carried out over the last two decades by Teruo Okano's group at Tokyo Women's Medical University, and is based on the existence of polymers able to display thermoresponsitivity as they possess a so-called 'lower critical solution temperature (LCST)'. The phenomenon and substances displaying it, including polymers, have been known for a long time (Freeman and Rowlinson, 1960; Patterson, 1969; Taylor and Cerankowski, 1975). The most investigated polymer showing LCST is poly(N-isopropylacrylamide) (PIPAAm) (Heskins and Guillet, 1968; Fujishige et al., 1989; Kubota et al., 1990; Takata et al., 2002; Kara and Pekcan, 2003), which was also chosen by Okano for this application (Yamada et al., 1990; Okano et al., 1993; Okano et al., 1995; Nishida, 2003; Yang et al., 2006). In principle, at temperatures above 32 °C (which is the polymer's LCST), PIPAAm is hydrophobic and therefore can support the attachment, spreading and growth of cells. The hydrophobic behaviour is due to particularities in the structure of the polymer and to the hydrogen bond interactions between amide groups and water molecules. At temperatures above LCST, water is partially displaced from the macromolecular coil, the hydrogen bonds involving water are weakened and the hydrophobic interactions between polymer segments become dominant, resulting in a compact ('collapsed') conformation of the macromolecular chains that does not allow further water penetration. The routine cell incubation temperature (37 °C) is well above LCST, thus assuring normal growth of cells on the PIPAAm surfaces in their hydrophobic state. When the temperature is lowered below LCST, the polymer surface turns hydrophilic, as the hydrogen bonding between the hydrophilic segments and water molecules becomes dominant and leads to an extended conformation of the macromolecules. As soon as the surface turns hydrophilic and consequently swells in the aqueous medium to become hydrated, the cell sheet detaches completely because of the very poor propensity of cells in general to attach to hydrated surfaces. The confluent cell layer can be harvested as a single uninterrupted sheet; it was shown (Yamato et al., 2001) that normal cell–cell junctions and the extracellular matrix are maintained in the sheets obtained by this technique. Cell sheet engineering has been applied so far in ocular surface reconstruction and myocardial tissue engineering, as well as in alternative therapies such as endoscopic transplantation for treating cancers of the gastrointestinal tract, development of tracheal prostheses and healing enhancement after laser refractive surgery (Yang et al., 2006).

Application of the cell sheet engineering concept to the reconstruction of the ocular surface is a result of the collaboration between Nishida (at Osaka University Medical School) and Okano's team. In a preliminary study (Nishida et al., 2004a), human and rabbit corneal limbal epithelial cells were cultured on tissue culture dishes that were coated with a layer of PIPAAm by electron beam irradiation. Cells were cultured in the presence of 3T3 feeder cells (growth arrested with mitomycin C) at 37 °C for 2 weeks, and then harvested at 20 °C. Rabbit cell sheets were transplanted in rabbits with experimentally induced limbal stem cell deficiencies. The sheets were transferred while placed on poly(vinylidene difluoride) membranes, which were removed soon after grafting. For healing purposes, the operated corneas were covered with soft contact lenses. The animals were monitored for 6 months. Corneal transparency was restored and the grafts remained stable. There is a mention at the end of this study that four human patients were grafted with allogeneic or autologous limbal epithelial sheets, and grafts were stable after 2–6 months. Favourable results in rabbits were reported with sheets of oral mucosal epithelial cells (Hayashida *et al.*, 2005). Reconstruction of the ocular surface in four human patients using sheets of autologous oral mucosal epithelial cells was also reported (Nishida *et al.*, 2004b). Corneal transparency was restored and maintained over a mean follow-up period of 14 months. Visual acuity improved remarkably and the eyes were free of complications. It is worth mentioning that the cell sheet engineering approach was also used successfully by the same group to prepare sheets of human corneal endothelial cells (Ide *et al.*, 2006; Sumide *et al.*, 2006).

The cell sheet strategy offers some advantages over other procedures for the reconstruction of the ocular surface. For instance, cells can be harvested without using proteolytic enzymes. The avoidance of using biodegradable polymers as substrata which are transplanted together with the cell sheet is also regarded as an advantage (Yang *et al.*, 2006). However, there is still a need for a support in order to transfer the cell sheet on to the cornea. As for using oral mucosal epithelial cells, longer-term results in larger-groups are needed to prove the validity of the procedure, as this phenotype is unlikely to differentiate into the corneal phenotype.

8.7.2   Thermoresponsive gel matrix

The block copolymers of poly(*N*-isopropylacrylamide-*co*-butyl methacrylate) and poly(ethylene glycol) behave like thermoresponsive polymers able to undergo sol-gel transitions at ambient temperatures (Yoshioka *et al.*, 1994a; Yoshioka *et al.*, 1994b; Yoshioka *et al.*, 1994c). One such polymer, developed as Mebiol gel® (Mebiol Inc., Kanagawa, Japan), dissolves in water at temperatures below 20 °C to generate solutions but becomes hydrophobic at temperatures above 20 °C to form water-insoluble gels. It offers the possibility of embedding growing cells either by mixing them with the solution at low temperatures or by placing them on a solid gel substratum and then covering it with the solution. The temperature is then raised to the routine incubation value of 37 °C, when the matrix solidifies and the cells become embedded within it. A variety of cell types have been cultured successfully in a Mebiol gel® matrix, and recently the culture of human corneal limbal epithelial cells has also been reported (Sudha *et al.*, 2006). In this study, cells from donor tissue biopsies were grown between two plates of solidified gel. The cells proliferated profusely and by the tenth day migrated out of the gel matrix to form an external layer. Various assays indicated that the cells expressed presumed limbal stem cell association markers, transient amplifying cell markers and corneal differentiation markers. Mebiol gel® remains an interesting alternative as a substratum for limbal epithelial constructs, although the matrix is not biodegradable.

8.8 Preliminary evaluation of silk fibroin as a substratum for human limbal epithelial cells

8.8.1 Background

We have recently proposed and evaluated a silk protein as a potential substratum material in the development of limbal epithelial constructs (Chirila *et al.*, 2007; Chirila *et al.*, 2008). Silks are natural high-molecular-weight polypeptide composites belonging to the group of fibrous proteins – which also includes collagens, elastins, keratins and myosins – and are characterized by highly repetitive amino acid sequences leading to significant homogeneity of their secondary structure and remarkable mechanical properties and functional performance. Silks are produced mainly by the larvae of certain species in the class Insecta, including the order Lepidoptera (moths and butterflies), and by species in the class Arachnida, prominently the order Araneae (spiders). There is a great variation in the chemical composition, structure and properties of the silks between species. It was estimated (Kaplan *et al.*, 1994) that perhaps only 0.1% of the silks presently known have been characterized in any detail. However, the silk produced by the domesticated silkworm (*Bombyx mori*) has been widely investigated. Silkworm silk fibres are constituted of core fibrous proteins (fibroins), which are held together by coats of glue-like proteins (sericins). The secondary structure of fibroin consists in planar β-pleated sheets packed in an anti-parallel fashion (Marsh *et al.*, 1955). There has been an increasing interest in the use of silks, especially of silkworm silk, as biomaterials (Minoura *et al.*, 1990; Altman *et al.*, 2003; Gobin *et al.*, 2006; Wang *et al.*, 2006; Bettinger *et al.*, 2007; Hakimi *et al.*, 2007). Silkworm silk has a long record of use as surgical sutures, although these did elicit an inflammatory response in the eye (Moore and Aronson, 1969; Salthouse *et al.*, 1977; Soong and Kenyon, 1984; Altman *et al.*, 2003), which was attributed to the allergenic activity of sericins. By removing the sericin component, this problem is usually avoided (Santin *et al.*, 1999; Altman *et al.*, 2003; Panilaitis *et al.*, 2003; Meinel *et al.*, 2005), although there are some concerns (Kurosaki *et al.*, 1999) that in rare instances fibroin too may cause delayed hypersensitivity.

We have investigated the growth and morphology of human limbal epithelial cell cultures, established from donor tissue, after seeding on to *Bombyx mori* silk fibroin (BMSF) membranes. In our most recent study (Chirila *et al.*, 2008), the cells were cultured in the absence of feeder cells, and using a commercial serum-free culture medium. Comparison was made with cultures grown on tissue culture grade plastic. This was the first time that corneal limbal epithelial cells have been cultured on BMSF, although a significant number of other cell types have been grown on it, as recently reviewed (Wang *et al.*, 2006; Chirila *et al.*, 2008). BMSF proved to be a suitable substratum for the marrow mesenchymal stem cells in the tissue engineering of ligament, cartilage or bone (Wang *et al.*, 2006).

8.8.2   Experiments and results

The protocol to isolate fibroin from silk cocoons included the removal of sericin in hot sodium carbonate solutions, dissolution of raw fibroin in a concentrated solution of lithium bromide, filtration and dialysis against water. The membranes were obtained by the evaporation of water at room temperature, followed by stabilization with concentrated aqueous methanol. The resulting dry films of BMSF are remarkably transparent, smooth and easy to handle with forceps in a similar fashion to pieces of cellophane. Upon addition to the culture medium, the BMSF membranes remain flat and acquire a certain degree of flexibility.

Cultures of human limbal epithelial cells were established from donor corneoscleral rims discarded after routine keratoplasty. Primary cultures were grown in a commercial serum-free medium designed to promote growth of corneal epithelial progenitor cells (*PCT* Corneal Epithelium Medium, Chemicon Australia, Boronia, Victoria, Australia), referred to as CnT-20 medium. A quantitative comparison of the cell growth on BMSF and on tissue culture plastic was performed by seeding freshly passaged cells on to either substrate at a density of 3000 cells/cm^2. The total number of cells after 3 days in culture was counted in a phase-contrast fluorescent microscope, after staining the cell nuclei.

Despite some degree of variation between cell donors, the growth of cells on BMSF was found to be not significantly different from that displayed by the cells grown on tissue culture plastic (Fig. 8.1).

8.8.3   Discussion

We have demonstrated a similar growth of human corneal limbal epithelial cells on BMSF material and on tissue culture plastic. Importantly, this result was obtained under serum-free conditions thus encouraging the development of protocols that avoid the use of animal- or donor human-derived products. The transparency of BMSF membranes is an obvious advantage for a biomaterial targeted for the reconstruction of the ocular surface. Another advantage of using the BMSF membranes is the ability of fibroin to biodegrade slowly in a biological environment (Altman *et al.*, 2003; Wang *et al.*, 2008). Owing

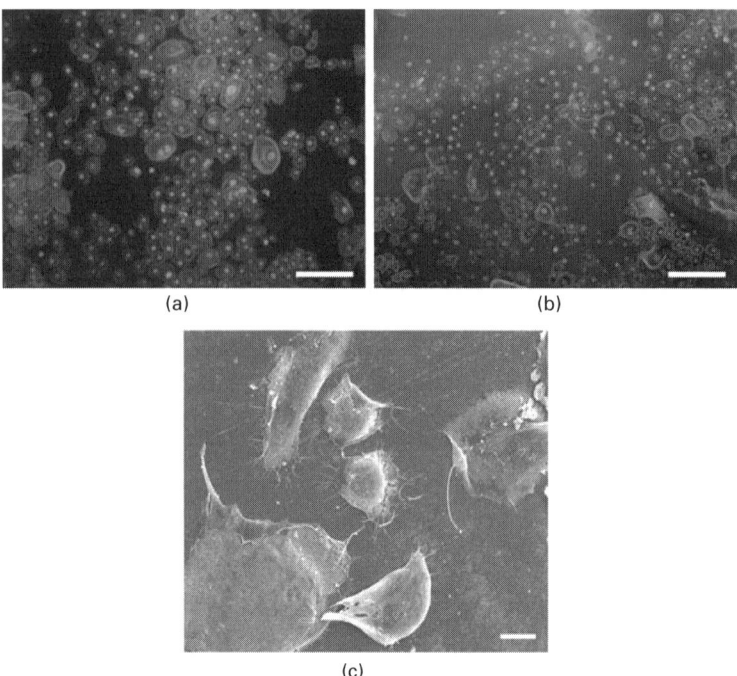

8.1 Cultures of human limbal epithelial cells grown on tissue culture plastic (a) and on BMSF membrane (b), originally stained with Hoechst 33324 nuclear dye and rhodamine phalloidin. Panel (c) shows a scanning electron microscope image of the cells after 3 days of growth on a BMSF membrane in a serum-free medium (CnT-20). Scale bars represent 200 μm (a), (b), and 10 μm (c).

to its defined chemical structure at the surface, BMSF can be modified to bind growth factors, defence peptides and other bioactive agents that may be beneficial in the incorporation and maintenance of the epithelial constructs. We believe that the BMSF membrane might therefore provide a valuable alternative to the AM. Nevertheless, a comparative study of cultures grown on BMSF and AM, including the identification of cellular phenotype, has yet to be performed.

The mechanism of cell attachment to BMSF in the absence of serum proteins remains an intriguing issue. Some studies (Minoura *et al.*, 1995a; Hakimi *et al.*, 2005) have shown that the adhesion of certain cells to BMSF was less than that observed on membranes made from the wild silkworm (*Antheraea pernyi*) silk fibroin. This was explained (Minoura *et al.*, 1995a) by the presence of the adhesion ligand peptide sequence arginine–glycine–aspartic acid (RGD) in the structure of wild silk fibroin, and it was tentatively suggested that the abundant presence of arginine alone in BMSF may be sufficient for imparting cell-adhesive properties. It was alternatively surmised (Minoura *et al.*, 1995b; Gotoh *et al.*, 1998) that such properties could also be a result of the electrostatic interactions between cell surface (with a net negative charge due to the glycocalyx) and the positively charged primary amine residues on the surface of BMSF. If this is the case, the cell adhesion to BMSF is a non-specific process. More recently, two peptide residues located near the N-terminus of the fibroin heavy chain that apparently enhanced the growth of fibroblasts were isolated from BMSF and identified as a decapeptide and an octapeptide (Yamada *et al.*, 2004). The assumption that these sequences may be hitherto unknown cell adhesion ligands has been neither substantiated nor confirmed so far.

8.9   Conclusions

OSDs have the potential to cause partial or complete limbal deficiency and result in pain and blindness. The search for a remedy to these diseases is vitally important, but such a remedy has not been forthcoming, despite an increased scientific emphasis for more than 30 years. Initially, this was because of the relative ignorance of the pathogenic processes. However, even with scientific investigation and understanding of the anatomical, physiological, and biochemical pathways of corneal limbal stem cells, progress in the search for these remedies has been slow and frustrating. Techniques for the *ex vivo* expansion and grafting of cultured epithelial sheets using cells harvested from the eye or even the oropharynx have not yet addressed the long-term needs of these patients. Perhaps this is because there has been little attention paid to the role of the stroma and its resident cells, which is immediately adjacent to the overlying epithelium. The extracellular matrix and its cellular components have a substantial, if poorly understood, effect on the regenerating epithelium. It is unlikely that an answer to the replacement of the surface lining will come without some acknowledgement of the importance of the underlying substratum. Communication between epithelial and stromal elements is vital for the normal function of the ocular surface and thus the grafting of healthy epithelial cells on to a damaged or diseased stroma is unlikely to produce successful outcomes. Whether the inner third lining of the cornea, the endothelium, will also – in the fullness of time – be shown to participate directly in the creation of a healthy ocular surface, remains to be seen.

Gazing into the crystal ball of medical science, one can only presume that the rehabilitation of the ocular surface will require a stable and mature epithelial layer together with stem/progenitor cells for replacing the constantly shed mature cells, and an active substratum. What the requirements of the substratum will be needs even more intense crystal gazing, but ultimately it will depend less on its composition and origin, i.e. either naturally derived materials or synthetic polymers, and more on its ability to support and activate an overlying epithelium with the necessary biochemical messages that promote, stabilize and characterize this epithelium. We believe that composite cultures of epithelial and stromal cells, including keratocytes and neuronal cells, will need to be developed in conjunction with new or modified biomaterials as substrata.

8.10   Acknowledgements

Support is acknowledged from the Prevent Blindness Foundation through Viertel's Vision, Queensland, Australia, and from Research to Prevent Blindness, New York, USA. We are grateful to Dr Edeline Wentrup-Byrne for her careful reading of the manuscript and for her helpful suggestions.

8.11   References

Ahmad S, Figueiredo F and Lako M (2006), 'Corneal epithelial cells: characterization, culture and transplantation', *Regen Med*, **1**, 29–44.
Altman G H, Diaz F, Jakuba C, Calabro T, Horan R L, Chen J, Lu H, Richmond J and Kaplan D L (2003), 'Silk-based biomaterials', *Biomaterials*, **24**, 401–416.
Ang L P K and Tan D T H (2004), 'Ocular surface stem cells and disease: current concepts and clinical applications', *Ann Acad Med Singapore*, **33**, 576–580.
Ang L P K, Tan D T H, Phan T T, Li J, Beuerman R and Lavker R M (2004), 'The in vitro and in vivo proliferative capacity of serum-free cultivated human conjunctival epithelial cells', *Curr Eye Res*, **28**, 307–317.
Ang L P K, Cheng Z Y, Beuerman R W, Teoh S H, Zhu X and Tan D T H (2006), 'The development of a serum-free derived bioengineered conjunctival epithelial equivalent using an ultrathin poly(ε-caprolactone) membrane substrate', *Invest Ophthalmol Vis Sci*, **47**, 105–112.
Araki-Sasaki K, Ohashi Y, Sasabe T, Hayashi K, Watanabe H, Tano Y and Handa H (1995), 'An SV40-immortalized human corneal epithelial cell line and its characterization', *Invest Ophthalmol Vis Sci*, **36**, 614–621.
Battle J F and Perdomo F J (1993), 'Conjunctival substitute with placental allotransplant', *Ophthalmology*, **100** (suppl iss 9), 107 (abstract 25).
Bettinger C J, Cyr K M, Matsumoto A, Langer R, Borenstein J T and Kaplan D L (2007), 'Silk fibroin microfluidic devices', *Adv Mater*, **19**, 2847–2850.
Bloomfield S E, Jakobiec F A and Theodore F H (1984), 'Contact lens induced keratopathy: a severe complication extending the spectrum of keratoconjunctivitis in contact lens wearers', *Ophthalmology*, **91**, 290–294.
Bouchard C S and John T (2004), 'Amniotic membrane transplantation in the management of severe ocular surface disease: indications and outcomes', *Ocul Surf*, **2**, 201–211.
Boulton M E, Albon J and Grant M B (2007), 'Stem cells in the eye', in Lanza R, Langer R and Vacanti J eds, *Principles of Tissue Engineering*, 3rd edn, Amsterdam, Elsevier, pp. 1011–1023.
Chen J J Y and Tseng S C G (1991), 'Abnormal corneal epithelial wound healing in partial-thickness removal of limbal epithelium', *Invest Ophthalmol Vis Sci*, **32**, 2219–2233.
Chirila T V, Hicks C R, Dalton P D, Vijayasekaran S, Lou X, Hong Y, Clayton A B,

Ziegelaar B W, Fitton J H, Platten S, Crawford G J and Constable I J (1998), 'Artificial cornea', *Prog Polym Sci*, **23**, 447–473.

Chirila T V, Chirila M, Ikada Y, Eguchi H and Shiota H (2005), 'A historical review of artificial cornea research in Japan', *Jpn J Ophthalmol*, **49**, S1–S13.

Chirila T, Barnard Z, Zainuddin and Harkin D (2007), 'Silk as substratum for cell attachment and proliferation', *Mater Sci Forum*, **561–565**, 1549–1552.

Chirila T V, Barnard Z, Zainuddin, Harkin D G, Schwab I R and Hirst L W (2008), 'Bombyx mori silk fibroin membranes as potential substrata for epithelial constructs used in the management of ocular surface disorders', *Tissue Eng A*, **14**, 1203–1211.

Chuck R S, Graff J M, Bryant M R and Sweet P M (2004), 'Biomechanical characterization of human amniotic membrane preparations for ocular surface reconstruction', *Ophthalmic Res*, **36**, 341–348.

Connon C J, Nakamura T, Quantock A J and Kinoshita S (2006), 'The persistence of transplanted amniotic membrane in corneal stroma', *Am J Ophthalmol*, **141**, 190–192.

Cotsarelis G, Cheng S-Z, Dong G, Sun T-T and Lavker R M (1989), 'Existence of slow-cycling limbal epithelial basal cells that can be preferentially stimulated to proliferate: Implications on epithelial stem cells', *Cell*, **57**, 201–209.

Davanger M and Evensen A (1971), 'Role of the pericorneal papillary structure in renewal of corneal epithelium', *Nature*, **229**, 560–561.

Daya S M, Watson A, Sharpe J R, Giledi O, Rowe A, Martin R and James S E (2005), 'Outcomes and DNA analysis of ex vivo expanded stem cell allograft for ocular surface reconstruction', *Ophthalmology*, **112**, 470–477.

de Rötth A (1940), 'Plastic repair of conjunctival defects with fetal membranes', *Arch Ophthalmol*, **23**, 522–525.

Di Girolamo N, Chui J, Wakefield D and Coroneo M T (2007), 'Cultured human ocular surface epithelium on therapeutic contact lens', *Br J Ophthalmol*, **91**, 459–464.

Dua H S and Azuara-Blanco A (2000), 'Limbal stem cells of the corneal epithelium', *Surv Ophthalmol*, **44**, 415–425.

Dua H S, Gomes J A P, King A J and Maharajan V S (2004), 'The amniotic membrane in ophthalmology', *Surv Ophthalmol*, **49**, 51–77.

Duan D, Klenkler B J and Sheardown H (2006), 'Progress in the development of a corneal replacement: keratoprostheses and tissue-engineered corneas', *Expert Rev Med Devices*, **3**, 59–72.

Eyrich D, Göpferich A and Blunk T (2006), 'Fibrin in tissue engineering', in Fisher J P ed., *Tissue Engineering*, New York, Springer, pp. 379–392.

Freeman P I and Rowlinson J S (1960), 'Lower critical points in polymer solutions', *Polymer*, **1**, 20–26.

Fujishige S, Kubota K and Ando I (1989), 'Phase transition of aqueous solutions of poly(*N*-isopropylacrylamide) and poly(*N*-isopropylmethacrylamide)', *J Phys Chem*, **93**, 3311–3313.

Germain L, Carrier P, Auger F A, Salesse C and Guérin S L (2000), 'Can we produce a human corneal equivalent by tissue engineering?', *Prog Ret Eye Res*, **19**, 497–527.

Germain L, Giasson C J, Carrier P, Guérin S L, Salesse C and Auger F A (2004), 'Tissue engineering of the cornea', in Wnek G E and Bowlin G L eds, *Encyclopedia of Biomaterials and Biomedical Engineering*, New York, Marcel Dekker Inc., pp. 1534–1544.

Gobin A S, Rhea R, Newman R A and Mathur A B (2006), 'Silk-fibroin-coated liposomes for long-term and targeted drug delivery', *Int J Nanomed*, **1**, 81–87.

Gotoh Y, Tsukada M and Minoura N (1998), 'Effect of the chemical modification of the arginyl residue in Bombyx mori silk fibroin on the attachment and growth of fibroblast cells', *J Biomed Mater Res*, **39**, 351–357.

Griffith M, Osborne R, Munger R, Xiong C, Doillon C J, Laycock N L C, Hakim M, Song Y and Watsky M A (1999), 'Functional human corneal equivalents constructed from cell lines', *Science*, **286**, 2169–2172.

Hakimi O, Grahn M F, Knight D P and Vadgama P (2005), 'Interaction of myofibroblasts with silk scaffolds', *Eur Cells Mater*, **10** (Suppl 2), 46.

Hakimi O, Knight D P, Vollrath F and Vadgama P (2007), 'Spider and mulberry silkworm silks as compatible biomaterials', *Composites B*, **38**, 324–337.

Han B, Schwab I R, Madsen T K and Isseroff R R (2002), 'A fibrin-based bioengineered ocular surface with human corneal epithelial stem cells', *Cornea*, **21**, 505–510.

Hatton M P and Rubin P A D (2005), 'Conjunctival regeneration', *Adv Biochem Eng Biotechnol*, **94**, 125–140.

Hayashida Y, Nishida K, Yamato M, Watanabe K, Maeda N, Watanabe H, Kikuchi A, Okano T and Tano Y (2005), 'Ocular surface reconstruction using autologous rabbit oral mucosal epithelial sheets fabricated ex vivo on a temperature-responsive culture surface', *Invest Ophthalmol Vis Sci*, **46**, 1632–1639.

He Y-G and McCulley J P (1991), 'Growing human corneal epithelium on collagen shield and subsequent transfer to denuded cornea in vitro', *Curr Eye Res*, **10**, 851–863.

He Y-G, Alizadeh H, Kinoshita K and McCulley J P (1999), 'Experimental transplantation of cultured human limbal and amniotic epithelial cells onto the corneal surface', *Cornea*, **18**, 570–579.

Heskins M and Guillet J E (1968), 'Solution properties of poly(*N*-isopropylacrylamide)', *J Macromol Sci A*, **2**, 1441–1455.

Hirst L W (2003), 'The treatment of pterygium', *Surv Ophthalmol*, **48**, 145–180.

Holland E J and Schwartz G S (2002), 'The evolution and classification of ocular surface transplantation', in Holland E J and Mannis M J eds, *Ocular Surface Disease: Medical and Surgical Management*, New York, Springer, pp. 149–157.

Hsu W-C, Spilker M H, Yannas I V and Rubin P A D (2000), 'Inhibition of conjunctival scarring and contraction by a porous collagen-glycosaminoglycan implant', *Invest Ophthalmol Vis Sci*, **41**, 2404–2411.

Hu X, Lui W, Cui L, Wang M and Cao Y (2005), 'Tissue engineering of nearly transparent corneal stroma', *Tissue Eng*, **11**, 1710–1717.

Huang A J W and Tseng S C G (1991), 'Corneal epithelial wound healing in the absence of limbal epithelium', *Invest Ophthalmol Vis Sci*, **32**, 96–105.

Ide T, Nishida K, Yamato M, Sumide T, Utsumi M, Nozaki T, Kikuchi A, Okano T and Tano Y (2006), 'Structural characterization of bioengineered human corneal endothelial cell sheets fabricated on temperature-responsive culture dishes', *Biomaterials*, **27**, 607–614.

Jenkins C, Tuft S, Liu C and Buckley R (1993), 'Limbal transplantation in the management of chronic contact-lens-associated epitheliopathy', *Eye*, **7**, 629–633.

John T (2003), 'Human amniotic membrane transplantation: Past, present, and future', *Ophthalmol Clin N Am*, **16**, 43–65.

Kahn C R, Young E, Lee I H and Rhim J S (1993), 'Human corneal epithelial primary cultures and cell lines with extended life span: in vitro model for ocular studies', *Invest Ophthalmol Vis Sci*, **34**, 3429–3441.

Kaplan D, Adams W W, Farmer B and Viney C (1994), 'Silk: biology, structure, properties, and genetics', in Kaplan D, Adams W W, Farmer B and Viney C eds, *Silk Polymers:*

Materials Science and Biotechnology, ACS Symposium Series 544, Washington, DC, American Chemical Society, pp. 2–16.

Kara S and Pekcan Ö (2003), 'Phase transitions of *N*-isopropylacrylamide gels prepared with various crosslinker contents', *Mater Chem Phys*, **80**, 555–559.

Kenyon K R and Tseng S C G (1989), 'Limbal autograft transplantation for ocular surface disorders', *Ophthalmology*, **96**, 709–723.

Kim J C and Tseng S C G (1995), 'Transplantation of preserved human amniotic membrane for surface reconstruction in severely damaged rabbit corneas', *Cornea*, **14**, 473–484.

Kim J Y, Djalilian A R, Schwartz G S and Holland E J (2003), 'Ocular surface reconstruction: limbal stem cell transplantation', *Ophthalmol Clin N Am*, **16**, 67–77.

Kim T and Khosla-Gupta B A (2002), 'Chemical and thermal injuries of the ocular surface', in Holland E J and Mannis M J eds, *Ocular Surface Disease: Medical and Surgical Management*, New York, Springer, pp. 100–112.

Kinoshita S and Nakamura T (2005), 'Corneal cells for regeneration', in Morser J and Nishikawa S I eds, *The Promises and Challenges of Regenerative Medicine*, Berlin, Springer–Verlag, pp. 63–83.

Kleinman H K, McGarvey M L, Liotta L A, Gehron Robey P and Tryggvason K (1982), 'Isolation and characterization of type IV procollagen, laminin, and heparan sulfate proteoglycan from the EHS sarcoma', *Biochemistry*, **21**, 6188–6193.

Kleinman H K, McGarvey M L, Hassell J R, Star V L, Cannon F B, Laurie G W and Martin G R (1986), 'Basement membrane complexes with biological activity', *Biochemistry*, **25**, 312–318.

Kruse F E (2002), 'Classification of ocular surface disease', in Holland E J and Mannis M J eds, *Ocular Surface Disease: Medical and Surgical Management*, New York, Springer, pp. 16–36.

Kubota K, Fujishige S and Ando I (1990), 'Single-chain transition of poly(*N*-isopropylacrylamide) in water', *J Phys Chem*, **94**, 5154–5158.

Kurosaki S, Otsuka H, Kunitomo M, Koyama M, Pawankar R and Matumoto K (1999), 'Fibroin allergy: IgE mediated hypersensitivity to silk suture materials', *J Nippon Med Sch*, **66**, 41–44.

Lee S Y, Oh J H, Kim J C, Young H K, Kim S H and Choi J W (2003), 'In vivo conjunctival reconstruction using modified PLGA grafts for decreased scar formation and contraction', *Biomaterials*, **24**, 5049–5059.

Levin P S and Dutton J J (1990), 'Polytef (polytetrafluoroethylene) alloplastic grafting as a substitute for mucous membrane', *Arch Ophthalmol*, **108**, 282–285.

Liliensiek S J, Campbell S, Nealey P F and Murphy C J (2006), 'The scale of substratum topographic features modulates proliferation of corneal epithelial cells and corneal fibroblats', *J Biomed Mater Res*, **79A**, 185–192.

Limb G A, Daniels J T, Cambrey A D, Secker G A, Shortt A J, Lawrence J M and Khaw P T (2006), 'Current prospects for adult stem cell-based therapies in ocular repair and regeneration', *Curr Eye Res*, **31**, 381–390.

Lindberg K, Brown M E, Chaves H V, Kenyon K R and Rheinwald J G (1993), 'In vitro propagation of human ocular surface epithelial cells for transplantation', *Invest Ophthalmol Vis Sci*, **34**, 2672–2679.

López-Alemany A, Compañ V and Refojo M F (2002), 'Porous structure of Purevision™ versus Focus® Night & Day™ and conventional hydrogel contact lenses', *J Biomed Mater Res (Appl Biomater)*, **63**, 319–325.

Luengo Gimeno F, Gatto S, Ferro J, Croxatto J O and Gallo J E (2006), 'Preparation of platelet-rich plasma as a tissue adhesive for experimental transplantation in rabbits', *Thromb J*, **4**, 18 (doi: 10.1186/1477–9560-4-18); http://www.thrombosisjournal.com/content/4/1/18.

Luengo Gimeno F, Lavigne V, Gatto S, Croxatto J O, Correa L and Gallo J E (2007), 'Advances in corneal stem-cell transplantation in rabbits with severe ocular alkali burns', *J Cataract Refract Surg*, **33**, 1958–1965.

Maharajan V S, Shanmuganathan V, Currie A, Hopkinson A, Powell-Richards A and Dua H S (2007), 'Amniotic membrane transplantation for ocular surface reconstruction: indications and outcomes', *Clin Exper Ophthalmol*, **35**, 140–147.

Mannis M J (2002), 'Prosthokeratoplasty in ocular surface disease', in Holland E J and Mannis M J eds, *Ocular Surface Disease: Medical and Surgical Management*, New York, Springer, pp. 263–268.

Marsh R E, Corey R B and Pauling L (1955), 'An investigation of the structure of silk fibroin', *Biochim Biophys Acta*, **16**, 1–34.

McCulley J P, He Y-G, Meyer D R, Moore M B and Li J (1991), 'In vitro transfer of rabbit corneal epithelium from carriers to denuded corneas or cryolathed lenticules', *Cornea*, **10**, 466–477.

Meinel L, Hofmann S, Karageorgiou V, Kirker-Head C, McCool J, Gronowicz G, Zichner L, Langer R, Vunjak-Novakovic G and Kaplan D L (2005), 'The inflammatory response to silk films in vitro and in vivo', *Biomaterials*, **26**, 147–155.

Minami Y, Sugihara H and Oono S (1993), 'Reconstruction of cornea in three-dimensional collagen gel matrix culture', *Invest Ophthalmol Vis Sci*, **34**, 2316–2324.

Minoura N, Tsukada M and Nagura M (1990), 'Physico-chemical properties of silk fibroin membrane as a biomaterial', *Biomaterials*, **11**, 430–434.

Minoura N, Aiba S, Higuchi M, Gotoh Y, Tsukada M and Imai Y (1995a), 'Attachment and growth of fibroblast cells on silk fibroin', *Biochem Biophys Res Commun*, **208**, 511–516.

Minoura N, Aiba S, Gotoh Y, Tsukada M and Imai Y (1995b), 'Attachment and growth of cultured fibroblast cells on silk protein matrices', *J Biomed Mater Res*, **29**, 1215–1221.

Miyashita H, Shimmura S, Kobayashi H, Taguchi T, Asano-Kato N, Uchino Y, Kato M, Shimazaki J, Tanaka J and Tsubota K (2006), 'Collagen-immobilized poly(vinyl alcohol) as an artificial cornea scaffold that supports a stratified corneal epithelium', *J Biomed Mater Res B: Appl Biomater*, **76B**, 56–63.

Moore T E and Aronson S B (1969), 'Suture reaction in the human cornea', *Arch Ophthalmol*, **82**, 575–579.

Nakajima N, Sugai H, Tsutsumi S and Hyon S-H (2007), 'Self-degradable bioadhesive', *Key Eng Mater*, **342–343**, 713–716.

Nishida K (2003), 'Tissue engineering of the cornea', *Cornea*, **22** (Suppl 1), 28–34.

Nishida K, Yamato M, Hayashida Y, Watanabe K, Maeda N, Watanabe H, Yamamoto K, Nagai S, Kikuchi A, Tano Y and Okano T (2004a), 'Functional bioengineered corneal epithelial sheet grafts from corneal stem cells expanded ex vivo on a temperature-responsive cell culture surface', *Transplantation*, **77**, 379–385.

Nishida K, Yamato M, Hayashida Y, Watanabe K, Yamamoto K, Adachi E, Nagai S, Kikuchi A, Maeda N, Watanabe H, Okano T and Tano Y (2004b), 'Corneal reconstruction with tissue-engineered cell sheets composed of autologous oral mucosal epithelium', *N Engl J Med*, **351**, 1187–1196.

Okano T, Yamada N, Sakai H and Sakurai Y (1993), 'A novel recovery system for cultured cells using plasma-treated polystyrene dishes grafted with poly(*N*-isopropylacrylamide)', *J Biomed Mater Res*, **27**, 1243–1251.

Okano T, Yamada N, Okuhara M, Sakai H and Sakurai Y (1995), 'Mechanism of cell detachment from temperature-modulated, hydrophilic–hydrophobic polymer surfaces', *Biomaterials*, **16**, 297–303.

Orwin E J and Hubel A (2000), 'In vitro culture characteristics of corneal epithelial, endothelial, and keratocyte cells in a native collagen matrix', *Tissue Eng*, **6**, 307–319.

Panilaitis B, Altman G H, Chen J, Jin H-J, Karageorgiou V and Kaplan D L (2003), 'Macrophage response to silk', *Biomaterials*, **24**, 3079–3085.

Patterson D (1969), 'Free volume and polymer solubility', *Macromolecules*, **2**, 672–677.

Pellegrini G, Traverso C E, Franzi A T, Zingirian M, Cancedda R and De Luca M (1997), 'Long-term restoration of damaged corneal surfaces with autologous cultivated corneal epithelium', *Lancet*, **349**, 990–993.

Rama P, Bonini S, Lambiase A, Golisano O, Paterna P, De Luca M and Pellegrini G (2001), 'Autologous fibrin-cultured limbal stem cells permanently restore the corneal surface of patients with total limbal stem cell deficiency', *Transplantation*, **72**, 1478–1485.

Revoltella R P, Papini S, Rosellini A and Michelini M (2007), 'Epithelial stem cells of the eye surface', *Cell Prolif*, **40**, 445–461.

Ruberti J W, Zieske J D and Trinkaus-Randall V (2007), 'Corneal-tissue replacement', in Lanza R, Langer R and Vacanti J eds, *Principles of Tissue Engineering*, 3rd edn, Amsterdam, Elsevier, pp. 1025–1047.

Salthouse T N, Matlaga B F and Wykoff M H (1977), 'Comparative tissue response to six suture materials in rabbit cornea, sclera, and ocular muscle', *Am J Ophthalmol*, **84**, 224–233.

Sangwan V S (2001), 'Limbal stem cells in health and disease', *Biosci Rep*, **21**, 385–405.

Sangwan V S, Vemuganti G K, Singh S and Balasubramanian D (2003), 'Successful reconstruction of damaged ocular outer surface in humans using limbal and conjunctival stem cell culture methods', *Biosci Rep*, **23**, 169–174.

Santin M, Motta A, Freddi G and Cannas M (1999), 'In vitro evaluation of the inflammatory potential of the silk fibroin', *J Biomed Mater Res*, **46**, 382–389.

Saw V P J, Minassian D, Dart J K G, Ramsay A, Henderson H, Poniatowski S, Warwick R M, Cabral S and AMTUG (2007), 'Amniotic membrane transplantation for ocular disease: a review of the first 233 cases from the UK user group', *Br J Ophthalmol*, **91**, 1042–1047.

Schermer A, Galvin S and Sun T-T (1986), 'Differentiation-related expression of a major 64K corneal keratin in vivo and in culture suggests limbal location of corneal epithelial stem cells', *J Cell Biol*, **103**, 49–62.

Schneider A I, Maier-Reif K and Graeve T (1999), 'Constructing an in vitro cornea from cultures of the three specific corneal cell types', *In Vitro Cell Develop Biol – Animal*, **35**, 515–526.

Schwab I R (1999), 'Cultured corneal epithelia for ocular surface disease', *Trans Am Ophthalmol Soc*, **97**, 891–986.

Schwab I R, Reyes M and Isseroff R R (2000), 'Successful transplantation of bioengineered tissue replacements in patients with ocular surface disease', *Cornea*, **19**, 421–426.

Schwab I R, Johnson N T and Harkin D G (2006), 'Inherent risks associated with manufacture of bioengineered ocular surface tissue', *Arch Ophthalmol*, **124**, 1734–1740.

Schwartz G S and Holland E J (2002), 'Iatrogenic limbal stem deficiency', in Holland E J and Mannis M J eds, *Ocular Surface Disease: Medical and Surgical Management*, New York, Springer, pp. 128–133.

Sekiyama E, Nakamura T, Kurihara E, Cooper L J, Fullwood N J, Takaoka M, Hamuro J and Kinoshita S (2007), 'Novel sutureless transplantation of bioadhesive-coated, freeze-dried amniotic membrane for ocular surface reconstruction', *Invest Ophthalmol Vis Sci*, **48**, 1528–1534.

Selvam S, Thomas P B and Yiu S C (2006), 'Tissue engineering: current and future approaches to ocular surface reconstruction', *Ocul Surf*, **4**, 120–136.

Sendele D D, Kenyon K R, Mobilia E F, Rosenthal P, Steinert R and Hanninen L A (1983), 'Superior limbic keratoconjunctivitis in contact lens wearers', *Ophthalmology*, **90**, 616–622.

Shatos M A, Ríos J D, Horikawa Y, Hodges R R, Chang E L, Bernardino C R, Rubin P A D and Dartt D A (2003), 'Isolation and characterization of cultured human conjunctival goblet cells', *Invest Ophthalmol Vis Sci*, **44**, 2477–2486.

Sheardown H and Griffith M (2008), 'Regenerative medicine in the cornea', in Atala A, Lanza R, Thomson J A and Nerem R M eds, *Principles of Regenerative Medicine*, Amsterdam, Elsevier, pp. 1060–1071.

Shimazaki J, Aiba M, Goto E, Kato N, Shimmura S and Tsubota K (2002), 'Transplantation of human limbal epithelium cultivated on amniotic membrane for the treatment of severe ocular surface disorders', *Ophthalmology*, **109**, 1285–1290.

Shortt A J, Secker G A, Notara M D, Limb G A, Khaw P T, Tuft S J and Daniels J T (2007), 'Transplantation of ex vivo cultured limbal epithelial stem cells: a review of techniques and clinical results', *Surv Ophthalmol*, **52**, 483–502.

Soong H K and Kenyon K R (1984), 'Adverse reactions to virgin silk sutures in cataract surgery', *Ophthalmology*, **91**, 479–483.

Sorsby A and Symons H M (1946), 'Amniotic membrane grafts in caustic burns of the eye (Burns of the second degree)', *Br J Ophthalmol*, **30**, 337–345.

Sorsby A, Haythorne J and Reed H (1947), 'Further experience with amniotic membrane grafts in caustic burns of the eye', *Br J Ophthalmol*, **31**, 409–418.

Stenson S (1983), 'Superior limbic keratoconjunctivitis associated with soft contact lens wear', *Arch Ophthalmol*, **101**, 402–404.

Sudha B, Madhavan H N, Sitalakshmi G, Malathi J, Krishnakumar S, Mori Y, Yoshioka H and Abraham S (2006), 'Cultivation of human corneal limbal stem cells in Mebiol gel® – A thermo-reversible gelation polymer', *Indian J Med Res*, **124**, 655–664.

Sugar J (2002), 'Congenital stem cell deficiency', in Holland E J and Mannis M J eds, *Ocular Surface Disease: Medical and Surgical Management*, New York, Springer, pp. 93–99.

Sumide T, Nishida K, Yamato M, Ide T, Hayashida Y, Watanabe K, Yang J, Kohno C, Kikuchi A, Maeda N, Watanabe H, Okano T and Tano Y (2006), 'Functional human corneal endothelial cell sheets harvested from temperature-responsive culture surfaces', *FASEB J*, **20**, 392–394.

Takaoka M, Nakamura T, Sugai H, Bentley A J, Nakajima N, Fullwood N J, Yokoi N, Hyon S-H and Knoshita S (2008), 'Sutureless amniotic membrane transplantation for ocular surface reconstruction with a chemically defined bioadhesive', *Biomaterials*, **29**, 2923–2931.

Takata S, Suzuki K, Norisuye T and Shibayama M (2002), 'Dependence of shrinking kinetics of poly(N-isopropylacrylamide) gels on preparation temperature', *Polymer*, **43**, 3101–3107.

Tauber J (2002), 'Autoimmune diseases affecting the ocular surface', in Holland E J and Mannis M J eds, *Ocular Surface Disease: Medical and Surgical Management*, New York, Springer, pp. 113–127.

Taylor L D and Cerankowski L D (1975), 'Preparation of films exhibiting a balanced temperature dependence to permeation by aqueous solutions – A study of lower consolute behavior', *J Polym Sci Polym Chem Ed*, **13**, 2551–2570.

Thoft R A (1977), 'Conjunctival transplantation', *Arch Ophthalmol*, **95**, 1425–1427.

Thoft R A (1984), 'Keratoepithelioplasty', *Am J Ophthalmol*, **97**, 1–6.

Tighe B (2000), 'Silicone hydrogel materials – how do they work?', in Sweeney D ed., *Silicone Hydrogels: The Rebirth of Continuous Wear Contact Lenses*, Oxford, Butterworth-Heinemann, pp. 1–21.

Tsai R J-F and Tseng S C G (1988), 'Substrate modulation of cultured rabbit conjunctival epithelial cell differentiation and morphology', *Invest Ophthalmol Vis Sci*, **29**, 1565–1576.

Tsai R J-F, Ho Y-S and Chen J-K (1994), 'The effects of fibroblasts on the growth and differentiation of human bulbar conjunctival epithelial cells in an in vitro conjunctival equivalent', *Invest Ophthalmol Vis Sci*, **35**, 2865–2875.

Tsai R J-F, Li L-M and Chen J-K (2000), 'Reconstruction of damaged corneas by transplantation of autologous limbal epithelial cells', *N Engl J Med*, **343**, 86–93.

Tseng S C G (2002), 'Amniotic membrane transplantation for ocular surface reconstruction', *Biosci Rep*, **21**, 481–489.

Tseng S C G (2007), 'Editorial: Evolution of amniotic membrane transplantation', *Clin Exper Ophthalmol*, **35**, 109–110.

Tseng S C G, Prabhasawat P, Barton K, Gray T and Meller D (1998), 'Amniotic membrane transplantation with or without limbal allografts for corneal surface reconstruction in patients with limbal stem cell deficiency', *Arch Ophthalmol*, **116**, 431–441.

Tsubota K, Satake Y, Ohyama M, Toda I, Takano Y, Ono M, Shinozaki N and Shimazaki J (1996), 'Surgical reconstruction of the ocular surface in advanced ocular cicatricial pemphigoid and Stevens–Johnson syndrome', *Am J Ophthalmol*, **122**, 38–52.

Uchino Y, Shimmura S, Miyashita H, Taguchi T, Kobayashi H, Shimazaki J, Tanaka J and Tsubota K (2007), 'Amniotic membrane immobilized poly(vinyl alcohol) hybrid polymer as an artificial cornea scaffold that supports a stratified and differentiated corneal epithelium', *J Biomed Mater Res B: Appl Biomater*, **81B**, 201–206.

Wang Y, Kim H-J, Vunjak-Novakovic G and Kaplan D L (2006), 'Stem cell-based tissue engineering with silk biomaterials', *Biomaterials*, **27**, 6064–6082.

Wang Y, Rudym D D, Walsh A, Abrahamsen L, Kim H-J, Kim H S, Kirker-Head C and Kaplan D L (2008), 'In vivo degradation of three-dimensional silk fibroin scaffolds', *Biomaterials*, **29**, 3415–3428.

Willoughby C E, Batterbury M and Kaye S B (2002), 'Collagen corneal shields', *Surv Ophthalmol*, **47**, 174–182.

Yamada H, Igarashi Y, Takasu Y, Saito H and Tsubouchi K (2004), 'Identification of fibroin-derived peptides enhancing the proliferation of cultured human skin fibroblasts', *Biomaterials*, **25**, 467–472.

Yamada N, Okano T, Sakai H, Karikusa F, Sawaski Y and Sakurai Y (1990), 'Thermo–responsive polymeric surfaces; control of attachment and detachment of cultured cells', *Makromol Chem Rapid Commun*, **11**, 571–576.

Yamato M, Utsumi M, Kushida A, Konno C, Kikuchi A and Okano T (2001), 'Thermo-responsive culture dishes allow the intact harvest of multilayered keratinocyte sheets without dispase by reducing temperature', *Tissue Eng*, **7**, 473–480.

Yang J, Yamato M, Nishida K, Ohki T, Kanzaki M, Sekine H, Shimizu T and Okano T (2006), 'Cell delivery in regenerative medicine: the cell sheet engineering approach', *J Controlled Release*, **116**, 193–203.

Yannas I V, Lee E, Orgill D P, Skrabut E M and Murphy G F (1989), 'Synthesis and characterization of a model extracellular matrix that induces partial regeneration of adult mammalian skin', *Proc Natl Acad Sci USA*, **86**, 933–937.

Yazawa M, Ogata H, Nakajima T, Mori T, Watanabe N and Handa M (2003), 'Basic studies on the clinical applications of platelet-rich plasma', *Cell Transplant*, **12**, 509–518.

Yoshioka H, Mikami M, Mori Y and Tsuchida E (1994a), 'A synthetic hydrogel with thermoreversible gelation. I. Preparation and rheological properties', *J Macromol Sci A*, **31**, 113–120.

Yoshioka H, Mikami M, Mori Y and Tsuchida E (1994b), 'A synthetic hydrogel with thermoreversible gelation. II. Effects of added salts', *J Macromol Sci A*, **31**, 121–125.

Yoshioka H, Mori Y and Cushman J A (1994c), 'A synthetic hydrogel with thermoreversible gelation. III. An NMR study of the sol-gel transition', *Polym Adv Technol*, **5**, 122–127.

Zieske J D, Mason V S, Wasson M E, Meunier S F, Nolte C J M, Fukai N, Olsen B R and Parenteau N L (1994), 'Basement membrane assembly and differentiation of cultured corneal cells: importance of culture environment and endothelial cell interaction', *Exper Cell Res*, **214**, 621–633.

Zorlutuna P, Tezcaner A, Kıyat I, Aydınlı A and Hasırcı V (2006), 'Cornea engineering on polyester carriers', *J Biomed Mater Res*, **79A**, 104–113.

9

Tissue engineering of the lens: fundamentals

A. GWON, University of California, Irvine, USA

Abstract: This chapter discusses the current state of tissue engineering of the lens, including both development *in vitro* for implantation *in vivo* and spontaneous regeneration *in vivo*. It goes on to discuss the primary requirements for *in vivo* lens regeneration and the use of biodegradable and non-degradable scaffolds to enhance the process. It addresses the need for a tissue-engineered alternative for the treatment of cataract and presbyopia, and the potential application in humans.

Key words: lens regeneration, tissue engineering of the lens, lens transdifferentiation, lens refilling, biodegradable polymers.

9.1   Introduction

Cataract is the leading cause of blindness worldwide affecting approximately 100 million eyes. While there is no proven medical treatment to prevent formation or progression of age-related cataract, cataract surgery is very successful in restoring functional vision with approximately 10 million cataract operations performed each year (Foster, 2000). The major challenge in modern-day cataract and presbyopia surgery is the inability to restore the natural accommodating properties of the lens. Tissue engineering has the potential to restore all the functional properties of the lens, including accommodation.

Research in tissue engineering of the lens incorporates both the *in vitro* engineering of a lens for implantation *in vivo* and the *in vivo* regeneration of the lens. In applying these techniques to the lens, the goal is to regenerate a lens that would have all the properties of the natural lens including transparency, focusing power, spectral transmission and accommodative ability.

9.2   *In vitro* engineering of the lens

Wolffian regeneration of the ocular lens has been described in the newt and *Xenopus laevis*, and it has been suggested that this process could allow the *in vitro* growth of ocular lens tissue for implantation. Wolffian regeneration is actually an example of lens transdifferentiation from another ocular tissue and occurs after total removal of the lens with its capsule. It has also been reported to occur in salamanders and in some adult fish. In the adult newt, lens regeneration begins with proliferation and dedifferentiation of dorsal iris pigment epithelial cells (PECs). Dedifferentiation initiates cell-cycle re-entry and, at approximately 10 days post-lensectomy, a lens vesicle is formed from the depigmented dorsal PECs. The internal layer of the lens vesicle thickens and synthesis of lens crystallins (markers of lens differentiation) begins. As PEC proliferation and depigmentation subsides, lens fiber differentiation proceeds. PECs from the whole eye of any species, including humans, are capable of transdifferentiation into lens cells under certain conditions. The exact molecular mechanisms involved in the spatial regulation of newt lens regeneration are unknown, but the presence of Hox genes, pax-6, fibroblast growth factors (FGFs), fibroblast growth factor receptors (FGFRs), retinoic acid receptors (RARs) and prox-1 has been demonstrated in the lens vesicle and regenerating lens of the newt, particularly pax-6, prox-1 and FGFR-1 (Del Rio-Tsonis and Tsonis, 2003).

In *X. laevis* and a related species, *X. tropicalis*, the lens can transdifferentiate from the inner layer of the outer cornea in the young animal. The factors responsible for this type of transdifferentiation reside in the neural retina, accumulate in the vitreous and are only available to the cornea when the lens is removed. When the outer cornea is cultured, *in vitro* transdifferentiation can be induced by the presence of FGF-1. Other genes expressed in cornea-to-lens transdifferentiation include pax-6, otx-2 and sox-3 (Del Rio-Tsonis and Tsonis, 2003; Tsonis and Rio-Tsonis, 2004; Tsonis, 2006).

The possibility of engineering the lens *in vitro* for implantation *in vivo* has been suggested by Tsonis (2006) and is supported by studies on transdifferentiation. While lens regeneration normally occurs only from the dorsal iris by transdifferentiation of iris PECs, Tsonis was able to identify several factors necessary for lens induction by focusing on the key differences in dorsal and ventral iris cells. Using six-3 and retinoic acid, he was able to accomplish transgenesis of the ventral iris. Six-3 is a major eye development regulator and collaborates with pax-6. He was also able to do the same by inhibition of bone morphogenic protein (BMP), which lies upstream of the pax-6/six-3 loop. The ability to induce lens formation from the ventral iris cells using known regulatory factors is a major contribution to the field of lens induction and may have relevance in efforts to induce PEC transdifferentiation *in vitro*. The capacity of PECs for *in vitro* transdifferentiation is widespread in the animal kingdom and has been reported for elderly humans under certain conditions. Both aged human cells and embryonic stem cells can transdifferentiate into lentoids, amorphous structures containing lens fibers but without a firm lens structure surrounded by epithelium. However, in the newt, the PECs can be reaggregated *in vitro* and implanted in the eye and shown to transdifferentiate into lens tissue with anterior-to-posterior polarity (Ito *et al.*, 1999). Tsonis suggests that it is then possible that *in vitro* aggregated PECs can build a perfect lens when implanted *in vivo*. It is possible that the same PECs can be grown on a suitable scaffold *in vitro* for implantation *in vivo* (Tsonis, 2006).

If a lens substitute can be engineered *in vitro*, it must then be implanted into the human eye. This may present some considerable challenges. The delicate nature of the zonules makes fixation of any lens tissue difficult, as demonstrated in studies performed by Van Alphen. He attempted transplantation of homografts from young rabbits and monkey heterografts into rabbits. The grafts were placed posterior to the iris but not fixated. Many of the transplants extruded, others turned cloudy within 5 days. Still, some of the homografts remained clear for up to 18 months, although they eventually became cloudy and the eye developed iritis. The more successful heterografts became cloudy in 10 days and were associated with severe anterior segment inflammation (Van Alphen, 1959). Thus, merely placing a lens within the posterior segment can be associated with cataract formation and lens extrusion. For successful implantation of a tissue-engineered lens, some method of fixation to the zonular/ciliary body complex would need to be developed for the lens to remain clear and be able to achieve accommodation.

In summary, the study of lens transdifferentiation has provided information on the molecular mechanisms involved in creating a lens and has the potential for creating substitute lenses for implantation *in vivo*. However, the challenge of implantation of a fairly large lens and its fixation within the eye has yet to be addressed.

9.3   *In vivo* lens regeneration

9.3.1   Lens stem cells

Another approach to tissue engineering a replacement for the ocular lens is the use of stem cells. Stem cells are characterized as relatively undifferentiated cells that have the capacity to self-renew and to generate one or more daughter cells. In the adult, stem cells will continually replenish lost cells in normal or damaged tissue. They have the potential to restore tissue lost by disease in many parts of the body.

Much of the work on stem cells in the eye has centered on the role of limbal stem cells in the maintenance of corneal epithelium and the identification of progenitor cells in the retina and ocular vasculature. Very little is known about lens epithelial stem cells. The slow cycling nature of lens epithelial cells and their ability to terminally differentiate into fiber cells are suggestive of a stem cell lineage (Zhou *et al.*, 2006; Remington and Meyer, 2007). True identification of lens cells as stem cells has been impeded by the lack of a definitive marker for ocular stem cells (Boulton and Albon, 2004). However, since stem cells generate tumors and the lens does not naturally develop tumors (although Mahon was able to induce a cancerous growth in the lens of transgenic mice (Mahon et al., 1987)), it has been suggested that lens stem cells may not be present within the capsule and may in fact reside outside it in the nearby ciliary body (Zhou et al., 2006; Remington and Meyer, 2007).

The ability of embryonic stem cells to produce a lens was reported by Ooto, who showed that primate embryonic stem cells could differentiate into lentoids that expressed αA-crystallin and pax-6 and increased in number with increasing FGF-2 concentration (Ooto et al., 2003). Whether such stem cells would have utility in speeding the process of lens differentiation in vivo has yet to be explored.

9.3.2   Lens epithelial cell regeneration

Like all epithelial cells throughout the body, the lens epithelium has a natural ability to replenish itself when injured and, in so doing, can regenerate the lens. The process is initiated by lens epithelial cell proliferation and migration over the lens capsule/basement membrane prior to undergoing lens fiber differentiation. Lens fiber differentiation is known to depend on a number of factors including suppression of Src family kinase activity and coordinated activity of many molecules, such as cyclin-dependent kinase (CDK) inhibitors p27 and p57, and Rb proteins (Menko, 2002). Among the most studied growth factors, FGF, insulin-like growth factor (IGF) (also known as lentropin) and BMP have been implicated as being important in lens epithelial cell differentiation (Beebe et al., 1980; Beebe et al. 1987; Chamberlain and McAvoy, 1987; Lang, 1999; Gwon, 2006).

Modern-day extracapsular cataract and/or lens extraction (ECCE) surgery, which leaves behind the cells that contribute to secondary opacification of the posterior capsule (PCO), provides the cells for creation of a new lens. While most investigators have utilized a rabbit model, lens regeneration has also been demonstrated in mice (Lois et al., 2003; Lois et al., 2005; Medvedovic et al., 2006), dogs (de Landau, 1838 (as cited in Randolph, 1900); Milliot, 1872), cows (de Landau, 1838), sheep (Milliot, 1872), cats (Milliot, 1872; Gwon et al., 1993b), guinea pigs (Milliot, 1872), primates (Agarwal et al., 1964) and humans (Gunn, 1888; Becker, 1900 (as cited in Randolph, 1900). In general, the rate of regeneration is inversely related to the age of the animal (Milliot, 1872; Gwon et al., 1992) and the lens has the ability to regenerate two or three times after repeated extraction (Middlemore, 1832; Loewenhardt,1841). Lens regeneration has been shown to occur at a slower rate and with less clarity after cataract removal (Sikharulidze, 1956; Chanturishvili, 1958; Stewart, 1960; Gwon et al., 1993b; Gwon, 2006).

The current ECCE surgical techniques typically require a 5–6 mm anterior continuous curvilinear capsulorrhexis (CCC). Without an intact anterior capsule, the residual anterior lens epithelial cells migrate and undergo myoblastic transformation contributing to wrinkling of the posterior capsule and visual distortion (Fagerholm and Philipson, 1981; McDonnell *et al.*, 1983; Cobo *et al.*, 1984; McDonnell *et al.*, 1984; Jacob *et al.*, 1987; Apple *et al.*, 1992; Auffarth *et al.*, 1995). As first reported by Cocteau and D'Etoille, the residual lens epithelial cells that contribute to secondary cataract formation regenerate and differentiate more normally if the integrity of the lens capsule is restored following endocapsular lens extraction in rabbits (Cocteau and D'Etoille, 1827; Gwon, 2006).

9.3.3   Restoring lens capsule integrity

The lens capsule provides a structural framework within which the regenerated lens takes its form. It may be considered as an external scaffold. As prior investigators have shown, it must be fully restored for the epithelium to regenerate into a lens (Cocteau and D'Etoille, 1827; Mayer, 1832; Middlemore, 1832; Textor, 1842 (as cited in Randolph, 1900); Milliot, 1872). Mayer showed that lens regeneration requires an intact anterior capsule and that the regenerative process begins in the periphery of the capsule and progresses centrally toward the site of the anterior incision (Mayer, 1832). His work was later confirmed by Milliot (1872). Middlemore demonstrated that successful lens regeneration required an intact posterior capsule and Textor showed that the form of the regenerated lens depended on the lesion of the capsule and the manner in which it had cicatrized (Middlemore, 1832; Textor, 1842 (as cited in Randolph, 1900)). A century later, Bito and co-workers suggested that physical forces exerted on the lens may affect the rate of lens cell proliferation and the distribution of dividing cells in the lens (Bito *et al.*, 1965). Other researchers showed, by histological analyses of regenerating lenses, that a taut capsule supports more normal cell growth and lens fiber differentiation while abnormal myofibroblastic proliferation occurred in areas of capsule wrinkling (Coulombre and Coulombre, 1971; Gwon *et al.*, 1990).

By performing endocapsular lens extraction through a 1–2 mm CCC, most of the capsule is retained and the anterior capsulotomy can be readily sealed by various techniques (Gindi *et al.*, 1985; Gwon *et al.*, 1993a; Koopmans *et al.*, 2003; Koopmans, 2006). Anterior chamber fibrin formation is routinely seen following cataract/lens surgery in rabbits and to a lesser extent in humans. This fibrin may seal the capsulotomy to form a linear scar allowing regeneration of a spherical lens. More often, the capsulotomy will remain open or seal the anterior to the posterior capsule resulting in a 'donut-shaped lens regenerate' (Fig. 9.1) (Gwon *et al.*, 1993a). As with other surgical wounds, it is apparent that a suitable means for sealing the anterior capsulotomy and restoring the continuity of the anterior capsule might be of benefit in normalizing the shape of the regenerated lens.

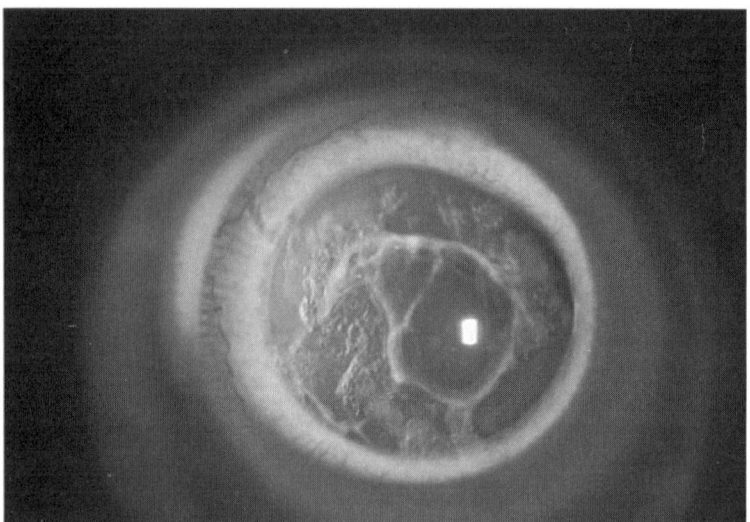

9.1 'Donut-shape' regenerated lens – no regeneration in areas of adhesions between anterior and posterior capsule.

Normal lens wound healing proceeds in two stages. In the first stage, semi-differentiated epithelial cells proliferate and migrate to form a plug in the wound (scar tissue). The lens epithelium tends to stick to the capsule and the epithelium outside the margins of the wound is broken down. The breakdown of the blood–aqueous barrier leads to anterior chamber inflammation. The presence of cytokines and fibrin in the anterior chamber may help seal a small tear in the lens capsule. In the second stage, lens epithelial cells proliferate under the scar tissue to form a monolayer. From this monolayer a new capsule is laid down (Fagerholm, 1982).

In an effort to promote lens healing, Bushman used human fibrinogen concentrate to seal traumatic anterior capsule perforations and prevent traumatic cataract formation, but the results were inconsistent (Buschmann, 1987; Buschmann, *et al.*, 1987; Buschmann, 1990). Gwon and co-workers have had more success using a collagen patch made from bovine type I collagen to seal the anterior capsulotomy. The capsule tear is thus bridged and the collagen patch serves as the basement membrane for epithelial cells to migrate across the wound. The reformed lens capsule provides a structural support for the more normal regeneration of the residual lens epithelia and a more consistently spherical lens (Fig. 9.2) (Gwon *et al.*, 1993a). An alternative approach is to use a silicone plug as reported by Koopmans (Koopmans *et al.*, 2003; Koopmans *et al.*, 2006). However, even with capsule closure, adherence of the anterior and posterior capsule may occur and limit lens reformation (Middlemore, 1832; Milliot, 1872; Gwon, 2006). Thus, an

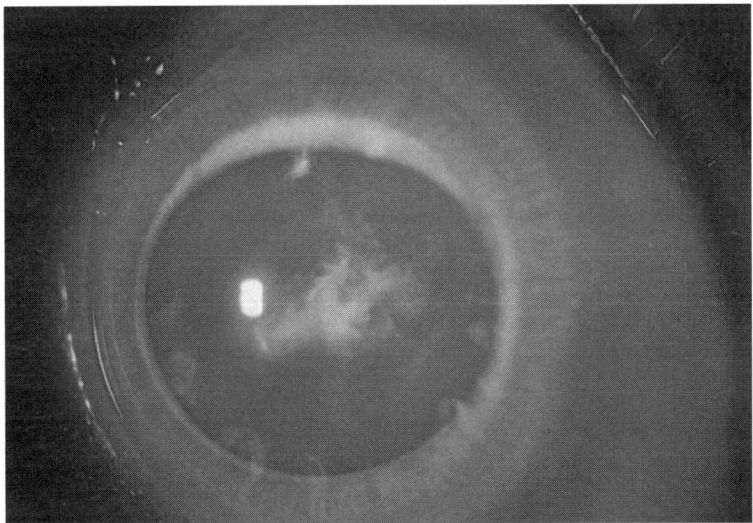

9.2 Spherical lens – lens regenerate is spherical following closure of the anterior capsulotomy. Nucleus has poor clarity with a 'star-shaped' appearance. The cortex has good structure and clarity.

internal scaffold to maintain capsule tautness and separation of the anterior and posterior capsule is necessary.

9.3.4   Controlling lens epithelial proliferation and differentiation

In mammals, the lens vesicle is formed during embryological development by invagination of the lens placode, which is induced from surface ectoderm by signals from the retina primordium. Some ectodermal cells remain inside the lens vesicle after invagination and closure, possibly acting as a scaffold for the initial orientation of lens fibers. These cells eventually cytolyse and disappear. Initially, epithelial cells proliferate along the anterior and posterior capsule, followed by elongation of the posterior epithelial cells, anterior migration and eventual loss of fiber nuclei, and differentiation into lens fibers at the equatorial zone. The lens fibers form the fetal lens nucleus and are gradually compacted as differentiation proceeds from the equator of the maturing lens. In the regenerating lens provided with an intact capsular bag, lens fiber differentiation also begins with formation of a monolayer of epithelium across the anterior and posterior capsule, followed by elongation of the posterior epithelial cells, anterior migration of fiber nuclei and loss of nuclei. Subsequently, these lens fibers form the nucleus, and are gradually compacted as differentiation proceeds from the lens equator (Piatigorsky, 1981; Gwon, 2006). The regenerated lenses have been shown to contain all three major crystallins – alpha, beta and gamma – in proportions similar to fetal or normal lenses (Gwon et al., 1989).

However, the rate of lens differentiation during regeneration may vary in the different parts of the capsule bag resulting in abnormal alignment of the earliest regenerating lens fibers (Gwon et al., 1990). In order to synchronize the regenerative process, it is desirable to delay lens differentiation until the entire capsule is covered by a confluent monolayer of lens epithelium. Ideally, one would aim to replicate the embryological environment by creating a scaffold of amniotic fluid or similar constituents normally present during lens invagination in embryogenesis. An initial attempt by Sikharulidze showed the rate of regeneration and the quality of the regenerated lens material was improved if a fragment of partially cytolyzed fetal tissue was inserted within the capsule at the time of lens evacuation (Sikharulidze, 1956). Subsequently, Stewart demonstrated that the regenerated lens had an optical density (refractive power) similar to that of the normal crystallin lens when fetal tissue had been implanted, i.e. 5–10 diopters in the 6-month-old rabbit (Stewart and Espinasse, 1959; Stewart, 1960). Other investigators had mixed results using cytolized ectodermal tissue (Chanturishvili, 1958; Binder et al., 1962; Petit, 1963; Agarwal, 1964; Angra et al., 1973). A review of their work can be found in a paper by Gwon (Gwon, 2006).

9.4   Scaffolds

Tissue engineering techniques generally require the use of a porous bioresorbable scaffold to serve as a three-dimensional template for initial cell attachment and subsequent tissue formation both in vitro and in vivo (Hutmacher et al., 2001). The porosity of the scaffold often serves to allow the flow of nutrients and in some cases can control the integration of cells within its matrix.

The ocular lens is a crystalline, transparent biconvex structure whose sole function is to transmit and refract light on the retina. As an organ, the lens is unique in its derivation from one cell type, in its retention throughout life of all cells that are ever produced, in having no blood or nerve supply and in synthesizing unique proteins (Rafferty, 1985). Since the lens is avascular, its pathology is simpler than most other tissues and primary inflammatory processes do not occur (Duke-Elder, 1969a). Thus, scaffolds for lens engineering have specific requirements. Foremost is the need for transparency to support visual function in the postoperative period. It must be biocompatible with the lens epithelium and capsule. Immunogenic processes are not a major concern as the closed capsule is a barrier to inflammatory processes. The avascularity of the lens may be beneficial in limiting cellular infiltration but may also limit the ability to degrade a bioresorbable scaffold. Matching the lens differentiation rate with the degradation and resorption rate of the scaffold is perhaps the biggest challenge to successful regeneration of an optically clear lens. Alternatively, a non-degradable scaffold can offer transparency and refractive ability that can be retained within the surrounding regenerating lens tissue. Both biodegradable and non-degradable scaffolds have been evaluated in the rabbit lens regeneration model.

9.4.1   Biodegradable scaffolds

Tissue-engineered biodegradable scaffolds have been developed as a three-dimensional template for initial cell attachment and subsequent tissue formation for both *in vitro* and *in vivo* applications. As outlined by Hutmacher, the ideal scaffold should have the following characteristics: (a) be porous for cell growth and transport of nutrients and metabolic waste; (b) be biocompatible and bioresorbable with controllable degradation and a resorption rate to match tissue replacement; (c) have suitable surface chemistry for cell attachment, proliferation and differentiation; (d) have mechanical properties to match the tissue site; and (e) have a reproducible process for fabrication. Thus, many of the biodegradable scaffolds that have been utilized contain natural polymers such as collagen and glycosaminoglycans as components (Hutmacher *et al.*, 2001).

Natural biological materials have several advantages and disadvantages over synthetic materials. Because they are identical or similar to substances already found in the body, the likelihood of toxicity or chronic inflammation may be reduced. They generally have inherent biological activity, which can be utilized for cell signaling. They are susceptible to naturally occurring enzymes and are thus biodegradable. They have the disadvantage of being frequently immunogenic and are difficult to manipulate or process. Some of the more commonly studied natural materials for tissue engineering are collagen, elastin, hyaluronic acid (HA), agarose, alginate, chitosan and fibrin gels (Mann, 2003). Of these, HA is the only optically clear material that can maintain its clarity in the lens capsule bag.

Hyaluronic acid

HA is particularly attractive as a scaffold in lens engineering because of its long history of biocompatibility and use in the eye. It is a naturally occurring glycosaminoglycan distributed widely in the extracellular matrix throughout the body and contributes significantly to cell proliferation and migration. It is soluble and interacts with binding proteins, proteoglycans and growth factors. It actively contributes to the regulation of water balance (Hutmacher *et al.*, 2001). As mentioned, it can retain its clarity in the lens capsule bag. It is found in high concentrations in the developing fetus and is implicated in the fetal ability to heal without scarring (Longaker *et al.*, 1989; Longaker *et al.*, 1990; Longaker and Adzick, 1991; Longaker *et al.*, 1991; Mast *et al.*, 1991). HA is naturally broken down by hyaluronidase and is readily available as a viscosurgical tool for ocular surgery.

In a series of unpublished studies, various HA-based products have been evaluated for their ability to enhance the regenerative process in the rabbit lens. Of these, the cohesive HA, Healon® Ophthalmic Viscosurgical Device (OVD) (Advanced Medical Optics, Santa Ana, CA, USA), has given the most consistent results to date. When Healon® OVD was given at doses of 0.05–0.1 ml, the capsule bag remained distended during the regenerative process. New lens regrowth filling 5–20% of the capsule bag was first noted at days 19–21 and generally filled the capsule bag by 41–54 days. In some eyes the capsule bag flattened by 1 week indicating early dissolution of HA and resulting in some abnormally shaped lens regenerates. In eyes where the capsule bag remained distended during the regenerative process the lenses were spherical with abnormal early growth resulting in an irregular star-shaped nucleus and fairly good cortical structure and clarity (Fig. 9.2). The abnormal nucleus has been partially attributed to variations in the maturation process in different parts of the capsule bag in the early stages of regeneration.

Cross-linked hyaluronic acid

In the search for a longer-lasting scaffold to maintain the tautness of the capsule and control the proliferative process in the lens capsule, a cross-linked HA gel was evaluated. The HA gel products tested were Restylane® and Perlane® (Q-Med Scandinavia, Inc., Princeton, NJ, USA). They were chosen because of their ability to degrade slowly over a 6- to 12-month period when injected intradermally for soft tissue augmentation (Duranti *et al.*, 1998). However, when injected into the capsule bag at the time of lens removal, we saw no evidence of degradation of either cross-linked HA gel over a 12-month period. Instead the cross-linked HA gel became compacted in a spherical ball-like nucleus in the center of the regenerating tissue. However, the regenerative process was synchronized for 360° around the cross-linked HA. Early lens regrowth was inversely related to the amount of cross-linked HA injected and could be seen at 8–12 days with a dose of 0.025–0.05 ml and at 3 weeks with a dose of 0.1 ml. As time progressed, the regenerated lenses were spherical and the regenerated lens cortical structure was clear with normal lens fiber alignment around the spherical compacted residual HA material (Fig. 9.3) (Gwon and Gruber, 2005).

The ability of the regenerating lens to dissolve a cohesive or dispersive HA and not a cross-linked HA has yet to be explained. It may be that, once lens fiber differentiation has occurred, hyaluronidase is unavailable to breakdown exogenous cross-linked HA used in these studies. HA and its metabolism by hyaluronidase has been studied in various tissues. In these

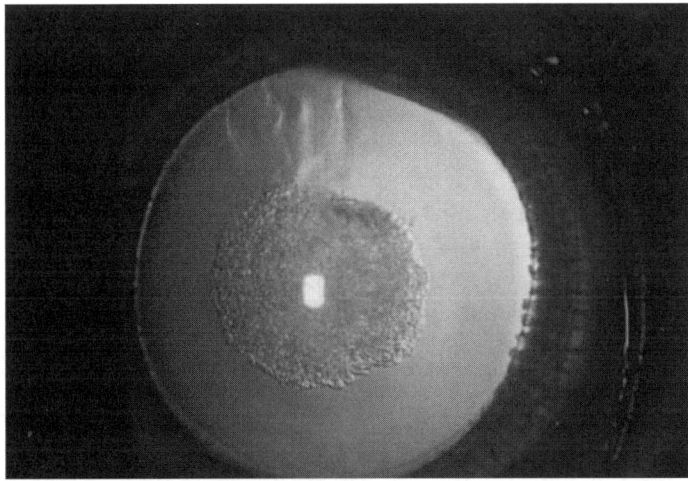

9.3 Synchronized lens regeneration – regenerated lens is spherical with clear normal cortex surrounding spherical nucleus of compacted cross-linked HA (7 months postoperative).

studies, undifferentiated, rapidly proliferating cells have high HA levels. It is thought that hyaluronidase may mediate the process by which cells lose their HA matrix and slow proliferation before differentiation can commence (Stern, 2004).

Hyaluronidase

While the cross-linked HA failed to dissolve over time, it provided a means to understand the residence time desired for a biodegradable scaffold. By providing hyaluronidase at various times during the postoperative period following implantation of a cross-linked HA, we were able to study the regenerative process with a biodegradable scaffold. When hyaluronidase was given intravitreally at 0, 3, 5, 7, 9 and 10 days postoperatively, limited lens regeneration was observed as early as 2–4 weeks post-operation. Full lens regrowth was seen by days 42–67 in the 0, 3, 5 and 10 day groups and by day 109 in the 7 and 9 day groups. Regenerated lens clarity was greatest in the 0, 3 and 5 day groups compared with the 7, 9 and 10 day groups (Gwon and Gruber, 2008). While a clear lens regenerate has not been established in the rabbit model, these initial studies suggest that a gradual dissolution of the HA scaffold over a 2- to 4-week time period improves the clarity and structure of the lens regenerate.

In an alternative method of addressing small opacities and residual scaffold material, an attempt was made to treat one regenerated lens with focal photocoagulation. Focal photocoagulation provided limited removal of retained HA and possibly some lens tissue (Gwon, 2005; Gwon and Gruber, 2005; Gwon, 2007; Gwon and Gruber, 2007a; Gwon and Gruber, 2007b).

In summary, lens regeneration following endocapsular lens/cataract extraction in the rabbit may be enhanced by providing a suitable internal and external scaffold. The external scaffold, i.e. lens capsule, can be sealed by placement of a collagen/silicone patch or fibrin adhesive after lens/cataract extraction through a small, approximately 1–2 mm, capsulotomy. The ideal internal scaffold has yet to be designed. However, the data suggest that HA provides a good biodegradable scaffold that can be modified for optimum retention/dissolution time to enhance the alignment of the earliest regenerating lens epithelium.

9.4.2   Non-degradable scaffolds

Synthetic non-degradable scaffolds for tissue engineering may offer some advantages over natural degradable biomaterials. They can typically be reproducibly and reliably manufactured. They can be tailored for specific application and sterilization is often easier (Mann, 2003; Dvir et al., 2005).

In comparison to scaffolds for replacement of other body tissues, the ocular environment has additional, specific requirements for a non-degradable scaffold. In addition to being biocompatible with the lens epithelium and capsule, it must be transparent and have the spectral transmission and refractive properties of the natural lens. By correcting for a patient's aphakia and refractive error, it should permit a quicker postoperative recovery time and restoration of functional vision. In order to limit any visual distortion related to the interface between the synthetic polymer and the naturally regenerating lens tissue, it should ideally have the same refractive index as the natural lens.

Foldable lens

The concept of providing an internal scaffold for the lens epithelium by implantation of a semi-permeable synthetic foldable lens was suggested by Gwon and co-workers in 1998. In that study, an Acuvue® (etafilcon A, 58% H_2O, Vistakon, Jacksonville, FL, USA) contact lens was modified for intralenticular implantation in the capsule bag in the rabbit. While lens epithelial proliferation and differentiation occurred around the synthetic polymer, the regenerated lens anterior and peripheral to the implant was clear with excellent structure, while the posterior regenerated lens structure was poor, except in one eye. In that one eye, lens differentiation was seen anterior and posterior to the intralenticular implant forming two lenses within the capsule bag. Lens structure and clarity were excellent permitting a good view of retinal structures (Gwon et al., 1998). It is unknown why the posterior regenerating lens tissue was opaque. It may be that the intralenticular lens blocked transport of nutrients from the anterior lens epithelium necessary for the posterior differentiating fibers and/or blocked the metabolic waste products from being released.

Injectable lens

The difficulty of implanting a foldable lens through a 1–2 mm capsulorrhexis has led many investigators to pursue an injectable polymer for lens refilling. The concept of injecting a synthetic polymer to replace the natural or cataractous crystalline lens was first suggested in 1964 by Kessler (Kessler, 1964; Kessler, 1966; Kessler, 1975). Since that time numerous investigators have worked on developing a suitable polymer that would have the flexibility of the natural lens and be capable of restoring accommodation in the presbyopic and/or cataractous eye. These polymers are generally transparent and liquid for easy injection into the capsule bag through a small, 1–2 mm capsulotomy. Once in the capsule bag, they polymerize to create a lens that conforms to the shape of the bag. Investigators have used: silicone polymers of low modulus, such as polydimethylsiloxane; or hydrogels – including poly(1-hydroxy-1,3-propandiol), polyether (such as poly(ethylene glycol) (PEG)), polyalcohol, poly(vinyl pyrrolidone) (PVP) and poly (acryl amide) hydrogels (Agarwal et al., 1967a,b; Parel et al., 1981, 1986; Haefliger et al., 1987; Deacon, 1988; Hettlich et al., 1994; Nishi et al., 1998b; deGroot et al., 2001; Han et al., 2003; Koopmans et al., 2003; Wong et al., 2007; Aliyar et al., 2005; Kwon et al., 2005; Yoo et al., 2007). Recent reviews by Norrby and Yoo discuss the current state of injectable polymers for lens refilling (Norrby, 2005; Yoo et al., 2007).

To date, advances with lens refilling have had moderate success with limited accommodation shown in primate models. Primary failure has been linked to the development of scarring and folds in the lens capsule, epithelial cell proliferation and secondary (PCO). While most investigators have regarded the development of PCO as a hindrance to the development of an injectable accommodating lens (Agarwal et al., 1967a,b; Parel et al., 1981, 1986; Hettlich et al., 1994; Haefliger et al., 1987; Nishi et al., 1998b; deGroot et al., 2001; Han et al., 2003; Koopmans et al., 2003; Aliyar et al., 2005; Kwon et al., 2005; Wong et al., 2007), it is also possible that the residual lens epithelium may be encouraged to regenerate and differentiate around a synthetic polymer and develop a tissue-engineered lens.

In a study by Gwon, coating the capsule bag with HA prior to injection of a silicone polymer in rabbits resulted in less capsule fibrosis and a clear regenerative tissue surrounding the silicone polymer anteriorly and peripherally and slightly opaque tissue posterior to the synthetic scaffold. Lens regeneration was observed as early as 15 days postoperatively. Thus, if the clarity of the posterior regenerating tissue could be improved, an injectable synthetic polymer has the potential to offer restoration of good functional vision in the adult (Gwon, 2007; Gwon and Gruber, 2007a,b; A. Gwon, L. Gruber, S. Norrby, T. Terwee, H. Weber and S.A. Koopmans, unpublished observations, 2008). It is well known that silicone intraocular lenses are associated with more capsular fibrosis than acrylic polymers. Whether the HA provided a barrier between the silicone polymer and the capsule or had a molecular role in inhibiting capsular fibrosis are yet to be discerned.

9.5   Potential human application

The first evidence of the regenerative ability of the natural lens in humans was reported by Sommering in 1828 (Duke-Elder, 1969b) when he observed the development of a ring-like transparent mass in the lens capsule following extracapsular lens extraction in humans. The so-called 'Elschnig pearls/ Sommering ring' formation and PCO continue to be common complications of modern extracapsular cataract surgery, yet may provide the necessary initial cells for engineering a replacement lens.

Further evidence of the regenerative ability of the human lens is provided in a report by Marcus Gunn. He observed the growth of new lens fibers in an adult after spontaneous absorption of a traumatic cataract sustained in early life (Gunn, 1888). Subsequently, Randolph reported that Becker had noted a transparent new formation in an 80-year-old female patient at the site of the crystalline lens, which had been removed 11 years previously (Randolph, 1900).

9.6   Conclusions

Tissue engineering has the potential to restore all the functional properties of the lens, including accommodation, as the regenerating process is initiated with reformation of the fetal lens and recreation of a young flexible lens. With minimal modification of current surgical techniques it is possible to restore the lens capsule and the residual lens epithelial cells left in the capsule bag can be directed to grow with the well-defined spatial order of the natural lens (Fig. 9.4).

While the insertion of a biodegradable HA-based scaffold has improved the structure of the regenerating lens, the alignment of the earliest regenerating lens fibers and the optimum balance between regenerating fibers and degradation of the scaffold remain a challenge. A further understanding of the molecular role of HA and the mechanical properties affecting the regenerative process is the subject of ongoing research.

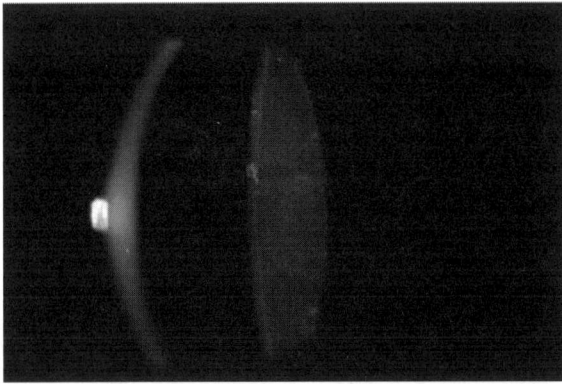

9.4 Spherical regenerated lens with good structure and clarity after dissolution of HA scaffold (2 months postoperative).

Because of time requirements for age-related cytogenesis rates, it is anticipated that the use of a biodegradable scaffold for the treatment of cataract/refractive errors would be more applicable to the pediatric population and might entail the use of serial spectacles and/or contact lenses during the regenerative process. It may also be possible to accelerate the regenerative process in adults by molecular or cellular means.

Alternatively, the natural regenerating lens tissue may be directed to grow in the concentric pattern of the normal lens around a suitably flexible and biocompatible synthetic polymeric scaffold with refractive properties that would be suitable for treatment of cataract and refractive errors and provide true accommodation and correction of presbyopia in the adult.

9.7   Future trends

The current trend in cataract surgery is toward minimally invasive techniques that will restore accommodation in both the cataract and presbyopic patient. Tissue engineering of the lens can be accomplished through the design of new materials to control the regenerative process or through molecular stimulation of the spontaneously regenerating lens. In the former instance, work with synthetic refractive polymers shows great promise. The latter approach provides a basic understanding of the genes and molecular mechanisms involved which could potentially lead to a non-engineered approach to regenerating the lens *in vivo*.

The ultimate goal of these approaches will be to restore all the natural properties and functions of the lens, including transparency, focusing power, spectral transmission and accommodative ability.

9.8   Acknowledgements

The author wishes to thank the following: Brad Gray and Lawrence Gruber for their invaluable assistance in manuscript and laboratory support; Carolyn Bates, Shelley Buchen, John Lally and Jim Deacon for their advice and support; Jane Rady and the late Irving H. Leopold for their support and encouragement; and numerous colleagues and friends who have contributed their research efforts and expertise in the area.

9.9   References

Agarwal LP, Angra SK, Khosla PK, Tandon HD (1964) Lens regeneration in mammals. I – Rabbits. *Orient Arch Ophthalmol* **2**:1–17.

Agarwal LP, Narsimhan EC, Mohan M (1967a) Experimental lens refilling – I. *Orient Arch Ophthalmol* **5**:205–212.

Agarwal LP, Narsimhan EC, Mohan M (1967b) Experimental lens refilling – II. *Orient Arch Ophthalmol* **5**:278–280.

Aliyar HA, Hamilton PD, Ravi N (2005) Refilling of ocular lens capsule with copolymeric hydrogel containing reversible disulfide. *Biomacromolecules* **6**:204–211.

Angra SK, Agarwal LP, Khosla PK (1973) Lens regeneration in mammals-I. *East Arch Ophthalmol* **1**:214–224.

Apple DJ, Solomon KD, Tetz MR, Assia EI, Holland EY, Legler UFC, Tsai JC, Casteneda VE, Hoggatt JP, Kostick AMP (1992) Posterior capsule opacification. *Surv Ophthalmol* **37**:73–116.

Auffarth GU, Wesendahl TA, Assia EI, Apple DJ (1995) Pathophysiology of modern capsular surgery. In Steinert RF (Ed.): *Cataract Surgery: Technique, Complications, and Managment*. Philadelphia, PA, USA, W.B. Saunders, pp. 314–324

Beebe DC, Feagans DE, Jebens HA (1980) Lentropin: a factor in vitreous humor which promotes lens fiber cell differentiation. *Proc Natl Acad Sci USA* **77**(1):490–493.

Beebe DC, Silver MH, Belcher KS, Van Wyk JJ, Svoboda ME, Zelenka PS (1987) Lentropin, a protein that controls lens fiber formation, is related functionally and immunologically to the insulin-like growth factors. *Proc Natl Acad Sci USA* **84**:2327–2330.

Binder HF, Binder RF, Wells AH, Katz RL (1962) Influence of embryonic implants upon lens regeneration in rabbits. *Br J Ophthalmol* **46**:416–421.

Bito LZ, Davidson H, Snider N (1965) The effects of autonomic drugs on mitosis and DNA synthesis in the lens epithelium and on the composition of the aqueous humour. *Exp Eye Res* **4**:54–61.

Boulton M, Albon J (2004) Stem cells in the eye. Review. *Int J Biochem Cell Biol* **36**:643–657.

Buschmann W (1987) Microsurgical treatment of lens capsule perforations Part II: experimental research. *Ophthalmic Surg* **18**(4):276–282.

Buschmann W (1990) Erhaltung verletzer Linsen durch mikrochirurgische Versorgung der Kapselwunden. *Klin Mbl Augenheilk* **196**:329–333.

Buschmann W, Gehrig OM, Vogt E, Raab H, Römer M (1987) Microsurgical treatment of lens capsule perforations Part I: experimental research. *Ophthalmic Surg* **18**(10):731–737.

Chamberlain CG and McAvoy JW (1987) Evidence that fibroblast growth factor promotes lens fiber differentiation. *Curr Eye Res* **6**:1165.

Chanturishvili P (1958) The role of the ectoderm in the development of the crystallin lens. *Trans Ophthalmol Soc UK* **78**:411–438.

Cobo LM, Ohsawa E, Chandler D, Arguello R, George G (1984) Pathogenesis of capsular opacification after extracapsular cataract extraction, an animal model. *Ophthalmology* **91**:857–863.

Cocteau MM, D'Etoille L (1827) Reproduction du crystallin [Experiments relative to the reproduction of the lens]. *J Physiol Exp (Paris)* **7**:30–744.

Coulombre JL, Coulombre AJ (1971) Lens development: V. Histological analysis of the mechanism of lens reconstitution from implants of lens epithelium. *J Exp Zool* **176**:15–24.

Deacon J (1988) Development of an injectable intraocular lens. MSc Thesis, Department of Bioengineering University of Utah.

de Groot JH, van Beijma FJ, Haitjema HJ, Dillingham KA, Hodd KA, Koopmans SA, Norrby S (2001) Injectable intraocular lens materials based upon hydrogels. *Biomacromolecules* **2**(3):628–634.

Del Rio-Tsonis KD, Tsonis PA (2003) Eye regeneration at the molecular age. *Dev Dyn* **226**:211–224.

Duke-Elder S (Ed.) (1969a) Chapter I in *System of Ophthalmology*, Vol. XI, *Diseases of the Lens and Vitreous: Glaucoma and Hypotony*, London, Henry Kimpton, pp. 3–18.

Duke-Elder S (Ed.) (1969b) Chapter V in *System of ophthalmology*, Vol. XI, *Diseases of the Lens and Vitreous: Glaucoma and Hypotony*, London, Henry Kimpton, pp. 233–243.

Duranti F, Salti G, Bovani B, Calandra M, Rosati ML (1998) Injectable hyaluronic acid gel for soft tissue augmentation. *Dermatol Surg* **24**(12):1317–1325.

Dvir T, Ysur-Gang O, Cohen S (2005) Designer scaffold for tissue engineering and regeneration. *Israel J Chem* **45**:487–494.

Fagerholm PP, Philipson BT (1981) Human lens epithelium in normal and cataractous lenses. *Invest Ophthalmol Vis Sci* **21**:408–414.

Fagerholm PPP (1982) The response of the lens to trauma. *Trans Ophthalmol Soc UK* **102**:369–374.

Foster A (2000) VISION 2020 – the cataract challenge. *J Comm Eye Health* **13**(34):17–19.

Gindi JJ, Wan WL, Schanzlin DJ (1985) Endocapsular cataract surgery-1. Surgical technique. *Cataract, Int J Cataract Surg* **2**:5–10.

Gunn, M (1888) Growth of new lens fibers after spontaneous absorption of traumatic cataract. *Trans Ophthalmol Soc UK* **8**:126.

Gwon AE (2005) Controlled ocular lens regeneration. US Patent 6,945,971, issued September 20, 2005.

Gwon A (2006) Lens regeneration in mammals: a review. *Surv Ophthalmol* **51**:51–62.

Gwon AE (2007) Controlled ocular lens regeneration. US Patent 7,278,990, issued October 9, 2007.

Gwon A, Gruber L (2005) Tissue engineering of the Lens. In *ARVO 2005 Annual Meeting*, Ft Lauderdale, FL, Abstract 2871.

Gwon A, Gruber L (2006) Modulating lens regeneration. In *ARVO 2006 Annual Meeting*, Ft Lauderdale, FL, Abstract 1997.

Gwon A, Gruber L (2007a) Lens regeneration with an injectable polymeric Scaffold. In *ARVO 2007 Annual Meeting*, Ft Lauderdale, FL, Abstract 5434.

Gwon A, Gruber L (2007b) Engineering of the crystallin lens. In *Proceedings of the 7th International Conference on Hyaluron, International Society for the Hyaluroa Sciences (ISHAS)*, Charleston, SC.

Gwon A, Gruber L (2008) Modification of a hyaluronic acid scaffold for lens engineering. In *ARVO 2008 Annual Meeting*, Ft Lauderdale, FL, Abstract# 3732.

Gwon A, Kuszak J, Gruber L (1998) Intralenticular implant study in pigmented rabbits: opacity lensmeter assessment. *J Cataract Refract Surg* **25**:268–277.

Gwon A, Enomoto H, Horowitz J, Garner M (1989) Induction of de novo synthesis of crystalline lenses in aphakic rabbits. *Exp Eye Res* **49**:913–926.

Gwon AE, Gruber L, Mundwiler K (1990) A histologic study of lens regeneration in aphakic rabbits. *Invest Ophthalmol Vis Sci* **31**(3):540–547.

Gwon AE, Jones RL, Gruber LJ, Mantras C (1992) Lens regeneration in rabbits measured by image analysis. *Invest Ophthalmol Vis Sci* **33**:201–205.

Gwon A, Mantras C, Gruber L (1993a) Restoring lens capsule integrity enhances lens regeneration in New Zealand albino rabbits and cats. *J Cataract Refract Surg* **19**:735–746.

Gwon A, Mantras C, Gruber L, Cunanan C (1993b) Lens regeneration in NZA rabbits following endocapsular cataract extraction. *Invest Ophthalmol* **34**:2124–2129.

Haefliger E, Parel J-M, Fantes F, Norton EWD, Anderson DR, Forster RK, Hernadez E, Feuer WJ (1987) Accommodation of an endocapsular silicone lens (Phaco-Ersatz) in the nonhuman primate. *Ophthalmology* **94**:471–477.

Han YK, Kwon JW, Kim JS, Cho CS, Wee WR, Lee JH (2003) In vitro and in vivo study of lens refilling with poloxamer hydrogel. *Br J Ophthalmol* **87**:1399–1402.

Hettlich H-J, Lucke K, Asiyo-Vogel MN, Schulte M, Vogel A (1994) Lens refilling and endocapsular polymerization of an injectable intraocular lens: In vitro and in vivo study of potential risks and benefits. *J Cataract Refract Surg* **20**:115–123.

Hutmacher DW, Goh JCH, Teoh SH (2001) An introduction to biodegradable materials for tissue engineering applications. *Ann Acad Med Singapore* **30**:183–191.

Ito M, Hayashi T, Kuroiwa A, Okamoto M (1999) Lens formation by pigmented epithelial cell reaggregate from dorsal iris implanted into limb blastema in the adult newt. *Dev Growth Differ* **41**:429–440.

Jacob TJC (1987) Human lens epithelial cells in culture: a quantitative evaluation of growth rate and proliferative capacity. *Exp Eye Res* **45**:93–104.

Kessler J (1964) Experiments in refilling the lens. *Arch Ophthalmol* **71**:412–417.

Kessler J (1966) Refilling the rabbit lens. Further experiments. *Arch Ophthalmol* **76**:596–598.

Kessler J (1975) Lens refilling and regrowth of lens substance in the rabbit eye. *Ann Ophthalmol* **7**:1059–1062.

Koopmans SA, Terwee T, Barkhof J, Haitjema HJ, Kooijman AC (2003) Polymer refilling of presbyopic human lenses in vitro restores the ability to undergo accommodative changes. *Invest Ophthalmol Vis Sci* **44**(1):250–257.

Koopmans SA, Terwee T, Glasser A, Wendt M, Vilupuru AS, van Kooten TG, Norrby S, Haitjema HJ, Kooijman AC (2006) Accommodative lens refilling in rhesus monkeys. *Invest Ophthalmol Vis Sci* **47**(7):2976–2984.

Kwon JW, Han YK, Lee WJ, Cho CS, Paik SJ, Cho DI, Lee JH, Wee WR (2005) Biocompatibility of poloxamer hydrogel as an injectable intraocular lens – A pilot study. *J Cataract Refract Surg* **31**:607–613.

Lang RA (1999) Which factor stimulate lens fiber cell differentiation in vivo? *Invest Ophthalmol Vis Sci* **40**(13):3075–3077.

Loewenhardt (1841) Einige Versuche um die Regeneration der Krystallinse. *Neune Notizen von Froriep* **19**:344.

Lois N, Dawson R, McKinnon AD, Forrester JV (2003) A new model of posterior capsule opacification in rodents. *Invest Ophthalmol Vis Sci* **44**:3450–3457.

Lois N, Taylor J, McKinnon AD, Forrester JV (2005) Posterior capsule opacification in mice. *Arch Ophthalmol* **123**:71–77.

Longaker MT, Adzick NS, Hall JL, Stair SE, Crombleholme TM, Duncan BW, Bradley SM, Harrison MR, Stern R (1990) Studies in fetal wound healing, VII. Fetal wound healing may be modulated by hyaluronic acid stimulating activity in amniotic fluid. *J Pediatric Surg* **25**(4):430–433.

Longaker MT, Adzick NS (1991) The biology of fetal wound healing: A review. Fetal Treatment Program, University of California, San Francisco 94143-0506. *Plast Reconstr Surg* **87**(4):788–798.

Longaker MT, Chiu ES, Harrison MR, Crombleholme TM, Langer JC, Duncan BW, Adzick NS, Verrier ED, Stern R (1989) Studies in fetal wound healing: IV. Hyaluronic acid-stimulating activity distinguishes fetal wound fluid from adult wound fluid. Fetal Treatment Program, University of California, San Francisco 94143-0506. *Ann Surg* **210**(3):667–672.

Longaker MT, Chiu ES, Adzick NS, Stern M, Harrison MR, Stern R (1991) Studies in fetal wound healing: V. A prolonged presence of hyaluronic acid characterizes fetal wound fluid. Fetal Treatment Program, University of California, San Francisco 94143-0506. *Ann Surg* **213**(4):292–296.

Mahon KA, Chepelinsky AB, Khillan JS, Overbeek PA, Piatigorsky J, Westphal H (1987) Oncogenesis of the lens in transgenic mice. *Science* **235**(4796):1622–1628.

Mann BK (2003) Biologic gels in tissue engineering. *Clin Plastic Surg* **30**:601–609.

Mast BA, Flood LC, Haynes JH, DePalma RL, Cohen IK, Diegelman RF, Krummel TM (1991) Hyaluronic acid is a major component of the matrix of fetal rabbit skin and wounds: implications for healing by regeneration. Division of Pediatric Surgery, Medical College of Virginia, Virginia Commonwealth University, Richmond, VA. *Matrix (Germany)* **11**(1):63–68.

Mayer (1832) Uber die reproduktion der Krystallinse. *J Chirurgie Augenheilkunde (Berlin, von Graefe und Walther)* **17**:524.

McDonnell P, Zarbin M, Green W (1983) Posterior capsule opacification in pseudophakic eyes. *Ophthalmology* **90**:1548–1553.

McDonnell PJ, Stark WJ, Green RG (1984) Posterior capsular opacification: a specular microscopic study. *Ophthalmology* **9**(7):853–856.

Medvedovic M, Tomlinson CR, Call MK, Grogg M, Tsonis PA (2006) Gene expression and discovery during lens regeneration in mouse: regulation of epithelial to mesenchymal transition and lens differentiation. *Molecular Vis* **12**:422–440.

Menko AS (2002) Lens epithelial cell differentiation. *Exp Eye Res* **75**:485–490. doi: 10.1006/exer.2002.2057, available online at http://www.idealibrary.com.

Middlemore R (1832) On the reproduction of the crystalline lens. *Lond Med Gaz* **10**:344–348.

Milliot B (1872) De la regeneration du crystallin chez quelques mammiferes. *J Anatomie Physiologie (Paris)* **8**:1.

Nishi O, Nishi K, Sakanishi K (1998a) Inhibition of migrating lens epithelial cells at the capsular bend created by the rectangular optic edge of a posterior chamber intraocular lens. *Ophthalmic Surg Lasers* **29**:587–594.

Nishi O, Nishi K, Mano C, Ichihara M, Honda T (1998b) Lens refilling with injectable silicone in rabbit eyes. *J Cataract Refract Surg* **24**:975–982.

Norrby S (2005) Injectable polymer. In *Refractive Lens Surgery*, Berlin Heidelberg, Springer, pp. 173–186.

Ooto S, Hauta M, Honda Y, Kawasaki H, Sasai Y, Takabashi M (2003) Induction of the differentiation of lentoids from primate embryonic stem cells. *Invest Ophthalmol Vis Sci* **44**:2689–2693.

Parel J-M, Treffers WF, Gelender H, Norton EWD (1981) Phaco-Ersatz: a new approach to cataract surgery. *Ophthalmology* **88**(9), Suppl:95.

Parel J-M, Gelender H, Trefers WF, Norton EWD (1986) Phaco-Ersatz: cataract surgery designed to preserve accommodation. *Graefe's Arch Clin Exp Ophthalmol* **224**:165–173.

Petit T (1963) A study of lens regeneration in the rabbit. *Invest Ophthalmol Vis Sci* **2**:243–251.

Piatigorsky J (1981) Lens differentiation in vertebrates, a review of cellular and molecular features. *Differentiation* **19**:134–153.

Rafferty NS (1985) Lens morphology. In *The Ocular Lens*, Maisel H. (Ed.), New York and Basel, Marcel Dekker, Inc. Chapter 1, pp. 1–60.

Randolph RL (1900) The regeneration of the crystalline lens: An experimental study. *Johns Hopkins Hospital Rep* **9**:237.

Remington SG, Meyer RA (2007), Lens stem cells reside outside the lens capsule: an hypothesis. *Theor Biol Med Model* **4**:22.

Sikharulidze TA (1956) Exchange of crystallin lens in rabbits by embryonic skin ectoderm. *Bull Acad Sci Georg S.S.R.* **14**:337.

Stern R (2004) Mammalian hyaluronidases. In *Hyaluronan Today*, Vincent C (Ed.), Hascall/Masaki, Yanagishita, http://www.glycoforum.gr.jp/science/hyaluronan/hyaluronanE.html.

Stewart DS (1960) Further observations on regenerated crystalline lenses in rabbits, with special reference to their refractive qualities. *Trans Ophthalmol Soc UK* **80**:357.

Stewart DS, 'Espinasse PG (1959) Regeneration of the lens of the eye in the rabbit. *Nature* **183**:1815.

Tsonis PA, Rio-Tsonis KD (2004) Lens and retina regeneration: transdifferentiation, stem cells, and clinical applications. *Curr Eye Res* **78**:161–172.

Tsonis PA (2006) How to build and rebuild a lens. *J Anat* **209**:433–437.

Van Alphen GWHM (1959) Transplantation of the lens. *Arch Ophthalmol* **61**:115–126.

Wong KH, Koopmans SA, Terwee T, Kooijman AC (2007) Changes in spherical aberration after lens refilling with silicone oil. *Invest Ophthalmol Vis Sci* **48**:1261–1267.

Yoo MK, Choi YJ, Lee JH, Wee WR, Cho CS (2007) Injectable intraocular lens using hydrogels. *J Drug Deliv Sci Tech* **17**:81–85.

Zhou M, Leiberman J, Xu J, Lavker RM (2006). A hierarchy of proliferative cells exists in mouse lens epithelium: Implications for lens maintenance. *Invest Ophthalmol Vis Sci* **47**:2997–3003.

10

Bioinspired biomaterials for soft contact lenses

T. GODA, T. SHIMIZU and K. ISHIHARA,
The University of Tokyo, Japan

Abstract: This chapter describes representative bioinspired biomaterials, synthetic phospholipid polymers, for use as soft contact lens materials with advanced biocompatibility. The chapter first reviews how the phospholipid polymer was inspired from natural phospholipids in the cell membrane in order to develop biocompatible materials and why the phospholipid polymer shows superior biocompatibility from the physicochemical and biological viewpoints. The chapter then describes the application of materials containing the phospholipid polymer in daily-wear, daily-disposable, extended-wear, and continuous-wear soft contact lenses with enhanced protein repellency, water wettability, and biocompatibility.

Key words: phospholipid polymer, bioinertness, silicone hydrogel, oxygen permeability, water wettability.

10.1　Introduction

In many recent clinical trials of artificial materials, very few candidates turned out to be compatible with living organisms and tissues. That is, the living body rejects most of the naturally occurring and synthetically delivered artificial materials by inducing acute biological reactions such as inflammation, immune responses, and blood coagulation; or by producing toxicity, unfavorable deterioration, or corrosion of the materials themselves (Ratner *et al.*, 2004). Besides being biologically compatible, biomaterials must meet several physicochemical requirements for therapeutic use in specific clinical situations. As for soft contact lenses, for example, the fundamental requirements of the candidate material are that they must possess optical properties suitable for vision correction. Hence, it is difficult to develop biomaterials that meet both biological and physicochemical requirements. Therefore, biologically inspired or biomimetic materials that mimic molecular designs, functionality, or nanostructures found in nature have been developed for successful therapeutic application (Shin *et al.*, 2003). Hereafter, we discuss the use of a representative bioinspired material, the phospholipid polymer, as soft contact lens material. The natural properties of the phospholipid polymer make it capable of mediating mild interaction with biomolecules and cell membrane surfaces to prevent undesired biological reactions inside

263

the living body. The bioinertness of this material may be of great use for the development of a soft contact lens material with superior biocompatibility. With the increase in the popularity of contact lenses in the world, great interest has been generated in the potential complications of contact lens usage and in the means to reduce the frequency and severity of such complications. For example, the risk of infectious complications associated with the frequent use of contact lenses results in the pathophysiologic changes that predispose the eye to microbial invasion and replication (Stapleton *et al.*, 2007). *Pseudomonas aeruginosa* and *Staphylococcus epidermidis* are major causative agents of infectious keratitis in patients using soft contact lenses (Ladage *et al.*, 2004). Adhesion of these bacteria to soft contact lenses is influenced by lens surface properties because the adhesion originates in adhesive protein in the extracellular matrices produced by the bacteria themselves. Therefore, the bioinertness of the contact lens material impairs the susceptibility to biofilm formation. In addition, the phospholipid polymer exhibits a good processability, which further justifies its use in the manufacture of soft contact lenses. Introduction of the phospholipid polymer into an appropriate material by means of a wide variety of chemical methods facilitates the regulation of the physicochemical properties required for soft contact lenses.

10.2   Bioinspired phospholipid polymer

As described above, biocompatibility is a key criterion for the preparation of biomaterials. Generally, non-specific protein adsorption on to a biomaterial triggers a series of biological cascade reactions (Colman and Schmaier, 1997). The bioinert natural cell membrane surface is the best example of a material capable of preventing non-specific protein adsorption. A cell membrane as a self-assembly with a bilayer structure is organized by amphiphilic phospholipids as a unit in association with membrane proteins, glycoproteins, and glycolipids (Singer and Nicolson, 1972). Of these, phosphatidylcholine is the main component of the phospholipids in the human erythrocyte cell membrane. This compound is composed of a hydrophilic phosphorylcholine headgroup and two hydrophobic long alkyl-chain tails. The hydrophilic headgroup is oriented in the outer leaflet of the erythrocyte, which is believed to prevent non-specific protein adsorption on to the cell membrane. Applying the natural cell membrane itself directly to the biomaterial surface, however, is a problem because the cell membrane cannot be stably immobilized on a material surface for a specific duration because of the weak interaction of the membrane with the material surface and because of the membrane's self-assembled structure. Furthermore, covalent bonding between the phospholipid molecules is not possible because of their lack of chemical reactivity. This obstacle has been overcome by a chemical innovation. Inspired by the molecular structure of the headgroup in the phosphatidylcholine, a new compound named

2-methacryloyloxyethyl phosphorylcholine (MPC) was synthesized with the aim of conferring biocompatibility to a material by the stable introduction of the phosphorylcholine headgroup into an artificial material by chemical reactions (Ishihara *et al.*, 1990a) (see Fig. 10.1). Since MPC is a monomeric methacrylate possessing a phosphorylcholine headgroup in the side chain, the bioinspired headgroup can be easily attached to any polymer via conventional polymerization techniques by using suitable monomeric compounds (Iwasaki and Ishihara, 2005). Polymers prepared in this way are called 'phospholipid polymers' or 'MPC polymers'. A wide variety of organic, ceramic, metallic, and composite materials containing a phospholipid polymer have been investigated for clinical application. Previous results indicated that the phospholipid polymer strongly prevents non-specific adsorption of biomolecules under biological environments. In addition, the phospholipid polymer confers water wettability and lubricity to a material surface (Ho *et al.*, 2003). The formation of a hydrated layer around the headgroup markedly reduces friction by fluid lubrication mechanisms and provides excellent wettability at the interface. These key performances of the phospholipid polymer mainly originate in hydrophilicity and electroneutrality due to the zwitterionic structure of the headgroup. In particular, the zwitterionic headgroup has a very minor effect on the structure of the hydrogen-bonding network of water molecules that endow resistance to non-specific adsorption of biomolecules (Ishihara *et al.*, 1998; Kitano *et al.*, 2003). Moreover, the phospholipid polymer does not attract biomolecules with local charges because of the electroneutrality

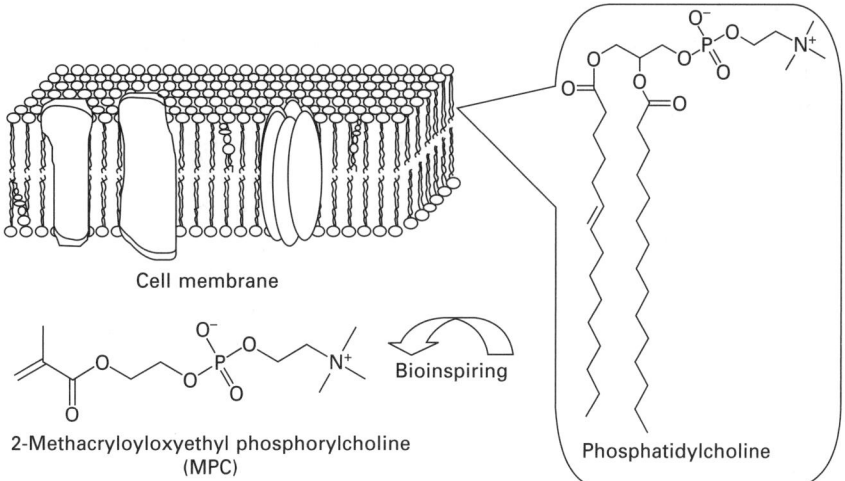

Cell membrane

Bioinspiring

2-Methacryloyloxyethyl phosphorylcholine
(MPC)

Phosphatidylcholine

10.1 Molecular design of MPC as a main component of synthetic phospholipid polymers. The chemical structure of MPC is close to that of phosphatidylcholine. Phospholipid polymers provide biocompatibility by forming stable cell membrane-like interfaces.

of the headgroup due to intramolecular salt formation (Xu *et al.*, 2007). The electroneutrality of the phosphorylcholine group may also stabilize the dimensions and solubility of poly(MPC) regardless of the ionic strength in the aqueous media (Matsuda *et al.*, 2006). In the following section, we describe the use of the bioinspired phospholipid polymer for enhancement of biocompatibility and wettability; these factors being strongly related to comfort issues of soft contact lenses.

10.3 Requirements for biocompatible soft contact lenses

Before describing the applications of the phospholipid polymer for soft contact lenses, let us review the conditions necessary for designing soft contact lens materials. The candidate polymer must satisfy the following requirements: the material must be transparent with suitable optical properties such as transparency and sphere power availability, must possess chemical and thermal stability, and must exhibit a high tensile and tear strength for lens-handling durability. In addition, since the material is directly in touch with the corneal epithelium, the material should be wettable to allow coverage with tear film, biocompatible, protein adsorption-resistive, electrolyte permeable, and oxygen permeable so as to avoid insult to the eye tissue. The potential hydrophobicity of a material increases the risk of dehydration of the lens as well as excessive lipid deposition. Protein adsorption on lenses concurrently decreases visual acuity, makes the lenses uncomfortable, and also reduces the wear lifetime. The contact lenses should transmit as much oxygen from the atmosphere into corneal tissues as in a no-lens situation (at least 87 barrer/mm) because, owing to the lack of blood circulation in transparent cornea, insufficient oxygen transport through the lens causes corneal edema resulting in a number of adverse physiological responses, such as excessive corneal swelling in overnight wear (Harvitt and Bonanno, 1999). Finally, from the manufacturer's viewpoint, the material must be suitable for bulk polymerization and for manufacture using current production techniques.

The importance of the irreversible interaction of tear components with soft contact lenses has long been recognized. Two of the most significant variables in the development of lens biofouling are duration of wear and individual patient tear chemistry. The wear period is now much more carefully controlled with the advent of daily-wear disposable soft contact lenses. However, the development of materials with enhanced antibiofouling properties needs further improvement. The contributions of the material's surface to the inflammatory response is becoming increasingly important with the advent of continuous-wear and long-term-wear soft contact lenses, as previously mentioned in the Introduction. Adhesions and activations of neutrophils are affected by surface characteristics which, in turn, influence the inflammatory response to the lens. Bacterial adhesion to soft contact lens materials is the first stage in contact lens-associated microbial keratitis, which may ultimately lead to corneal ulceration. The candidate materials should possess protein adsorption resistance, biocompatibility, and tear wettability as well as bulk polymer characteristics for continuous and extended wear. Thus, the use of a bioinspired phospholipid polymer is one of the effective ways to enhance the antifouling properties and biocompatibility of the lens. Recently, soft contact lenses have been developed mainly for use as daily, daily disposable, extended, and continuous wear. The phospholipid polymer has succeeded in enhancing the overall biocompatibility of all types of soft contact lenses, as described in the following sections.

10.4   Phospholipid polymer for daily-wear soft contact lenses

Daily-wear soft contact lenses with routine maintenance have a longer history of use than the other types of lenses. They have been available since the development of poly(2-hydroxyethyl methacrylate) (poly(HEMA)) hydrogels as a soft contact lens material (Wichterle and Lim, 1960). The hydrogel contains 38% water, has reasonable wettability, and offers the wearer comfort. Various types of derivative hydrogels containing different hydrophilic monomer units – such as methacrylic acid, N-vinylpyrrolidinone (NVP), and glyceryl methacrylate – have been developed with increased water content, subsequent oxygen permeability, and surface water wettability. Many attempts have focused on the enhancement of oxygen transport by either using a hydrophilic polymer or by making the hydrogel lens thinner. However, these hydrogels did not generate ideal results because of the induction of mechanical weakness and a tendency to adsorb tear proteins and lipids. For example, US Food and Drug Administration (FDA) II Group materials that contain NVP tend to adsorb more lipids than other conventional soft contact lens materials (Jones et al., 1997). Spoliation occurs more easily for materials with higher water content, not because of the water content itself, but because of the presence of NVP. In addition, soft contact lenses with relatively high water content tend to increase the occurrence of bacterial adhesion (Dang et al., 2003). In the case of ionic materials, e.g. methacrylic acid which is commonly introduced to elevate the oxygen permeability, lysozyme – a major protein of the tear fluid working as an enzyme that damages the bacterial cell wall by catalyzing hydrolysis of peptidoglycan and chitodextrins – is extensively adsorbed on materials that contain carboxylate groups (Keith et al., 2003). Lysozyme adsorption should originate in the electrostatic attraction between the negatively charged methacrylic acid and the positively charged lysozyme. Although it has been reported that the adsorbed lysozyme on the lens does not generate an adverse clinical reaction owing to the enzyme's antibacterial effects, the electrostatically attached lysozyme on the lens surface may not be as effective for its original function as an enzyme. Furthermore, the adsorbed lysozyme has to be completely washed away once the contact lenses are removed from the eyes because it may cause bacterial contamination of the lenses. Such a routine is not only a great inconvenience for wearers, but may also increase the potential risk of infectious eye diseases such as microbial keratitis.

Phospholipid polymers have been introduced into conventional soft contact lens material. The US company CooperVision produces a soft contact lens material containing MPC units (Proclear®, omafilcon A) that is categorized in the FDA II Group (Fig. 10.2). This hydrogel is made of a cross-linked random copolymer of HEMA and MPC (Taddei *et al.*, 2005). The water content and oxygen permeability of this hydrogel are 62% and 33 barrers, respectively. Researchers discovered that good mechanical characteristics were obtained while still achieving moderate oxygen permeability that maintained corneal health during wear. Poly(HEMA-co-MPC) hydrogel soft contact lenses offer a high level of bioinertness due to a poor adhesion of the eukaryotic cells of the corneal epithelium to the bioinspired surface. The anti-adhesive ability also impairs susceptibility to bacterial attachment and biofilm formation on soft contact lenses. Soft contact lenses made of omafilcon A were less susceptible to biofilm formation by *S. epidermidis* or *P. aeruginosa* in *in vitro* experiments (Selan *et al.*, 2009). An increase in the antibiotic susceptibility of bacterial clusters is associated with diminished bacterial adhesion. The enhancement of the anti-adhesion property against biomolecules and cells should result in superior protein adsorption resistance of the MPC unit due to the creation of a cell membrane analogous interface

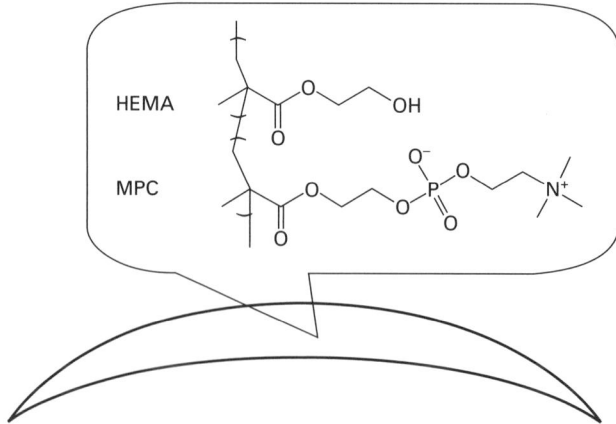

10.2 Chemical structure of Proclear® soft contact lens (omafilcon A). The bulk material is a cross-linked copolymer hydrogel of HEMA and MPC.

on the soft contact lens surface. Reduced susceptibility of the phospholipid polymer to biofilm formation is noteworthy. Indeed, removal of bacterial biofilm is difficult using drug therapy and existing lens-disinfectant systems because of antibiotic-resistant bacteria. The advantages of the introduction of the phosphorylcholine headgroup into the material by chemical methods may translate into more effective disinfection, leading to reduced risk of contact lens-related eye infections for patients who use extended-wear soft contact lenses. Furthermore, omafilcon A is as good at relieving dry eye symptoms as soft contacts lenses with higher water contents such as hioxifilcon G72-HW, which has a water content of 72% due to the advanced water wettability of the lenses induced by the MPC moiety (Riley *et al.*, 2005). This water-retentive effect of the phospholipid polymer is quite important because dryness symptoms, especially reports of increasing dryness late in the day, have been cited in a number of studies as a reason for discontinuing or limiting lens wear.

10.5   Phospholipid polymer for daily-disposable soft contact lenses

Daily-disposable lenses do not need lens treatment after removal from the eyes and thus there is less risk of infectious diseases. The simplicity in handling procedures and reasonable price have brought great commercial success for daily-disposable lens manufacturers in recent years. However, a significant number of people suffer from dry eye symptoms due to tear film break-up on the surface of the soft contact lenses. One strategy to improve wear comfort in a cost-effective way is the deposition or immobilization of hydrophilic polymers as wetting agents on daily-disposable soft contact lenses. For example, Johnson & Johnson brought out Acuvue® Moist™ for such a purpose. Although the bulk properties of the lenses remain the same as those of previous lenses manufactured from etafilcon A, the new lenses are formulated with a hydrophilic polymer, poly(NVP), which is immobilized in the matrix of etafilcon A to form an interpenetrating polymer network (IPN) or semi-IPN structures, and is not released from the lens during wear. The coverage of the lens surface with the hydrophilic polymer in turn shows a 55% reduction in friction relative to the unmodified material when taken straight from the packaging solution (Ross *et al.*, 2007). This should lead to an improvement in the overall comfort of the lenses. CIBA developed the Focus Dailies™ contact lens, which is made of nelfilcon A with the deposition of poly(vinyl alcohol) (PVA) by soaking in a PVA solution (Peterson *et al.*, 2006). In this case, the hydrophilic polymer is released from the lenses during wear and thus produces a 25% reduction in friction on the lens surface compared with the original lenses. Similarly, CooperVision produced the One Day Aquair Evolution™ contact lens for the Japanese market. It is made of ocufilcon D with the deposition of MPC-containing polymers on the surface (Fig. 10.3). This polymer is a random copolymer of MPC and *n*-butyl methacrylate (BMA) and functions as a wetting agent. This amphiphilic type of phospholipid polymer has the commercial name Lipidure® (NOF Co., Tokyo, Japan) and demonstrates a better moisture-retaining capability than hyaluronic acid (Shaku *et al.*, 1997). This polymer physically attaches on the lens surface via hydrophobic interaction of the BMA units, and prevents the significant frequency and intensity of dryness and discomfort-related symptoms experienced by patients during soft contact lens wear. We independently synthesized another phospholipid polymer composed of MPC and methacryloyloxyethyl trimethylammonium chloride (MTAC) for electrostatic attachment of the cationic polymer on anionic etafilcon A to produce protein adsorption-resistant, hydrophilic, and comfortable to wear soft contact lenses (Shimizu *et al.*, 2008). Poly(MPC-co-MTAC) showed stronger binding with etafilcon A compared with the amphiphilic phospholipid polymer with etafilcon A, because it is not only attached on the surface but is also retained within the matrix of the soft contact lens, assuring the controlled release of the polymer that will lead to extended comfort for patients. The amount of lysozyme adsorption on the surface of this contact lens material showed a 20% reduction due to the protein adsorption resistance of the attached poly(MPC-co-MTAC).

10.6   Phospholipid polymer for continuous-wear soft contact lenses

A recent innovation in the field of soft contact lens materials was the development of silicone hydrogels that achieved continuous wear with a sufficient oxygen supply to the cornea through the lens (Nicolson and

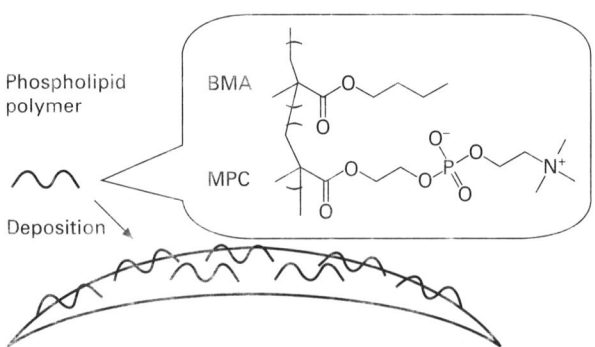

10.3 Illustration of the physical deposition of the phospholipid polymer (Lipidure®) as a wetting agent on One Day Aquair Evolution™ soft contact lens (ocufilcon D).

Vogt, 2001). Now, silicone hydrogel soft contact lenses are increasing in popularity with practitioners and patients for use as extended-daily-wear or continuous-wear lenses. The silicone polymers are well known for their high oxygen permeability compared with conventional polymers. The bulkiness of the siloxane group and high polymer chain mobility induce the high oxygen permeability of these materials. The silicone hydrogels are made of high oxygen permeable poly(dimethyl siloxane) (PDMS)-based macromers combined with various hydrophilic monomers to improve the rubbery characteristic and to increase the surface hydrophilicity of silicone. Additionally, silicone hydrogel materials can permeate some electrolytes dissolved in the tear fluid through the water phase in the hydrogel. Phase separation of silicone components and hydrophilic polymers in their bulk composition balances both the oxygen and electrolyte permeations (Tighe, 2004). Various approaches have been adopted by several manufacturers to produce silicone hydrogels with good mechanical properties, varied water content, and oxygen permeabilities. However, the problem with soft contact lens application is that the siloxane component tends to concentrate on the surface of the hydrogel, which creates a hydrophobic and biofouling surface. It has been found that the low surface energy of the native silicone hydrogels is vulnerable to adherent bacteria and cells. In other cases, the residual silicone oil from the retinal detachment treatment can also increase the incidence of endophthalmitis. Studies have shown that hydrophobic surfaces probably facilitate bacterial colonization and biofilm production, while hydrophilic surfaces seemed to be useful in limiting bacterial adherence and colonization (Kunz et al., 1999). Hence, the surface modification of silicone hydrogels is a promising approach for decreasing the incidence of endophthalmitis and improving biocompatibility. Surface modification techniques such as gas plasma treatment and graft polymerization of hydrophilic monomers on the lens surface have also been applied (Tighe, 2004). Both PureVision™ (balafilcon A, Bausch & Lomb) and Focus Night & Day™ (lotrafilcon A, CIBA Vision) are treated using gas plasma techniques. The difference between these two products is that Bausch & Lomb have opted for plasma oxidation, whereas CIBA Vision has chosen to apply a plasma coating. In the former case, glassy islands are produced on the surface and in the latter case the coating is produced by a 25-nm-thick, dense, high-refractive-index coating. The dynamic contact angle results indicate that the two types of lenses have a very similar receding contact angle (θ_R) but different advancing contact angles (θ_A). Focus Night & Day™ lenses are appreciably more wettable than PureVision™ lenses; the former lenses have a θ_A of 80° with a relatively low level of hysteresis of 35° and no significant change after 10 days of spoliation. PureVision™ lenses have a higher θ_A of 103° and a high level of hysteresis of 65°, with a slight increase in these values after 10 days of *in vitro* spoliation. One of the advantages of these plasma-treated methods is that lens manufacturers are united in their efforts to endow wettability using simple methods. However, the hydrophilic nature of oxidized silicone is only temporary since the migration of PDMS chains leads to recovery of the native hydrophobic state.

Surface modification of silicone hydrogels with a bioinspired phospholipid polymer has been conducted in several ways (Willis *et al.*, 2001). It is better to bind MPC covalently to the silicone hydrogel surface since physically adsorbed coatings may have the disadvantage of detachment during practical use. Recently, as a model case, we conducted graft polymerization of MPC on the PDMS surface using photo-induced radical polymerization techniques (Goda *et al.*, 2006). This modification method fits existing contact lens manufacturing processes where the graft polymerization is efficiently initiated by irradiation of ultraviolet (UV) rays in the MPC aqueous solution. In addition, the grafted polymer directly binds to the substrate via covalent bonding, which is chemically more stable than the plasma oxidized groups on the PDMS outermost surface (Fig. 10.4). This technique remarkably improved surface wettability and protein adsorption resistance. Dynamic water contact angles on the PDMS decreased from 117° to 60° in θ_A and from 81° to 34° in θ_R after the surface modification, and the amount of protein adsorption was reduced to less than 50% compared with the original surface, while the oxygen permeability of the modified PDMS membrane was maintained at more than 99% relative to that of non-treated PDMS. Another strategy to bind MPC chemically on the surface of silicone hydrogel lenses is to use an air plasma treatment (Huang *et al.*, 2007). The process is carried out in a cylindrical glow discharge chamber under low air pressure with specific applied power and radiofrequency. After pretreatment with air plasma, the hydrogel is soaked in a concentrated MPC aqueous solution and then put into the discharge chamber to be treated with air plasma again. The water

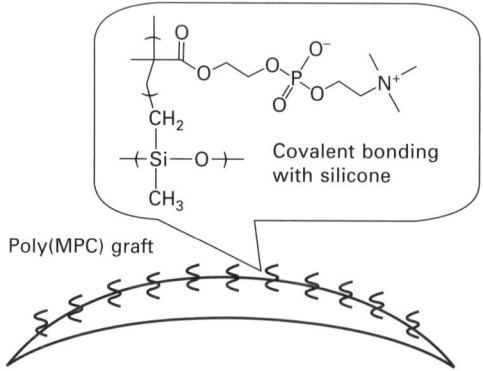

10.4 Illustration of the surface modification of PDMS by photo-initiated grafting with poly(MPC).

contact angle decreased from 108° to 36° after the treatment. The reduction in the amount of bacterial adhesion on the treated surface was 60%. The results suggest that silicone hydrogel treated with MPC by the air plasma technique may be useful for contact lens applications.

10.7   New developments

In designing a polymer hydrogel for advanced soft contact lens material with suitable bulk properties and biocompatibility, we should consider strategies not only to acquire sufficient oxygen transport and electrolyte permeability, render good mechanical properties, and form a homogeneous network structure as an optical material, but also to endow water wettability, protein adsorption resistance, and overall biocompatibility from the viewpoint of polymer chemistry and materials science. One known way to design soft contact lenses for extended and continuous wear is to add silicone-containing monomers to the hydrogel syntheses. Bulk phase morphology between the polysiloxane and a hydrophilic polymer is the crucial factor for determining oxygen permeability. A model analysis evaluation of phase-separated systems can predict that a complete phase separation (least amount of interphase regions) is essential for obtaining the high oxygen permeability that is theoretically achievable. In other words, a hydrogel forming a well-dispersed or miscible phase of polysiloxane exhibits low oxygen permeability, being far below the theoretical maximum value of a perfectly phase-separated silicone hydrogel (Nicolson and Vogt, 2001). Therefore, the main issue is how to organize a hybrid material made of silicone hydrogel and a hydrophilic polymer. Previous approaches to obtain hydrogels with high oxygen permeability were mainly based on the synthesis of biphasic materials, essentially represented by block-copolymers including polysiloxane and a hydrophilic polymer. However, the existing process for producing these biphasic materials is quite expensive and complicated in view of the necessity of performing a surface plasma treatment at the last stage of manufacturing. As an alternative method for bulk modification, a biphasic silicone preparation based on IPN formation has recently been developed for ophthalmologic materials (Chekina et al., 2006). The physical entanglements of the polymer chains improve both the bulk and surface stability of the material. The IPN structure is able to combine different polymer properties, while at the same time minimizing any incompatibility effects. Therefore, this approach avoids the need to synthesize new compounds or to make surface treatments. In 2004, intrinsically wettable silicone hydrogel lens materials such as Acuvue® Advance® (galyfilcon A, Johnson & Johnson) and Acuvue® Oasys® (senofilcon A, Johnson & Johnson) were released. These lenses incorporate poly(NVP) as a wetting agent via IPN and thus require no surface treatment. They show higher oxygen permeability with higher water content than previous silicone hydrogel lenses as well as correspondingly lower modulus related to the higher water content. Quite recently, a new type of wettable silicone hydrogel lens has been marketed. Biofinity® (comfilcon A, CooperVision) and Avaira™ (enfilcon A, CooperVision) do not have surface coating and an intrinsic wetting agent. Still, they display both high oxygen permeability and water content. For example, Biofinity® has an oxgen permeability of 128 barrer for a water content of 48%. As an alternative to surface treatment or use of a polymeric wetting agent IPN, high surface energy molds have been used in the manufacturing process to encourage the orientation of the polar components on the lens surface. Silicone hydrogel soft contact lenses with ophthalmically acceptable surface wettability can be produced using polar resin molds made of ethylene–vinyl alcohol copolymer or PVA resins instead of non-polar ones (Chen *et al.*, 2008).

A silicone hydrogel comprising the phospholipid polymer as a wetting agent was developed via sequential IPN techniques (Shimizu *et al.*, 2009) (Fig. 10.5). The cross-linked silicone polymer as the first network was prepared from methyl *bis*(trimethylsilyloxy)silylpropyl glycerol methacrylate (SiGMA). The SiGMA is a silicone-functionalized glycerol methacrylate that contains a pendant hydroxyl group in the middle of the molecule and is effective for copolymerizing with a hydrophilic monomer due to the enhanced compatibility. The hydrophilic second network was then prepared by polymerization of MPC with a cross-linker to endow the silicone hydrogel with water wettability, protein adsorption resistance, and biocompatibility. The IPN structure is suitable for combining polymers with different polarities without forming inhomogeneous compounds or microscopic phase separation in the bulk. In addition, the physical and topological entanglements of the two independently cross-linked polymers in the IPN generate a stable three-dimensional structure at a state of forced miscibility. This IPN hydrogel is

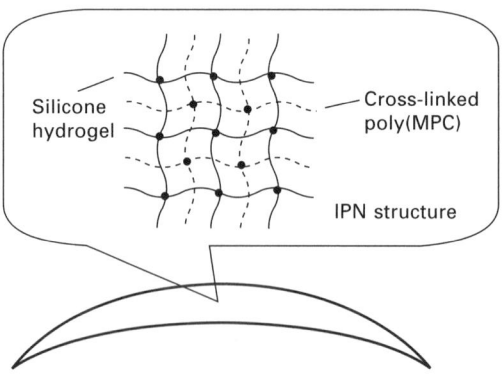

10.5 Illustration of a silicone hydrogel lens containing cross-linked poly(MPC) IPN as a wetting agent.

prepared by the following three steps. (a) A cross-linked poly(SiGMA) hydrogel is synthesized by UV irradiation with a cross-linker and photosensitizer. (b) The purified poly(SiGMA) hydrogel is then immersed in a solution of MPC in isopropanol to become fully swollen. (c) The cross-linked poly(MPC) network is then formed in the silicone hydrogel by the same method as the formation of the first network. The obtained hybrid material with a water content of 41% shows extreme hydrophilicity, and its superior protein adsorption resistance originates in the second poly(MPC) network on the surface, together with optical transparency, flexibility, and oxygen permeability (111 barrer) derived from the first poly(SiGMA) network. Notably, the water contact angle on the IPN hydrogel surface is measured to be 0° by the captive bubble technique. Surface analysis indicates that such an extremely hydrophilic surface of the IPN hydrogel is achieved by the enrichment of the MPC unit on the outermost surface. The amount of protein adsorption on the IPN hydrogel is 28% of that on the poly(SiGMA) hydrogel. The IPN hydrogel may be a strong candidate for use with continuous-wear soft contact lens materials, showing advanced wear comfort and biocompatibility.

10.8   Conclusions

In this chapter we described the application of a bioinspired phospholipid polymer for enhancement of the biocompatibility of daily, daily-disposable, extended-wear or continuous-wear soft contact lenses in various ways. As a result of the development of MPC as a main constituent showing biocompatibility in the artificially synthesized phospholipid polymer, various chemical methods can be used to introduce a bioinspired phospholipid polymer into a wide variety of soft contact lens materials. The phospholipid polymer not only reduces the frequency of eye dryness symptoms because of its hydrophilic and water-retentive nature, but also reduces susceptibility to biofilm formation followed by non-specific protein adsorption prevention. These properties of the phospholipid polymer favorably decrease the potential risk of endophthalmitis related to contact lens wear.

10.9   Future trends

Advances in materials suitable for the high-volume, low-cost production necessary for today's daily-disposable lenses market will continue. By replacing soft contact lenses more often, patients can avoid potential risks associated with deposits, including reduced visual acuity, lens comfort, and wettability. Most companies are now introducing the next generation of daily-disposable lenses that are expected to offer better comfort and vision than their predecessors. Many more lenses are also now starting to be marketed specifically to help wearers who suffer from dryness symptoms. In the past, the lenses available had in a restricted range of properties, which limited the type and number of patients who might benefit. Thanks to the development of new lens materials, a wide variety of patients with dryness symptoms can now wear the new, more comfortable lenses.

Macroscopically, the market will polarize into continuous wear and daily-disposable wear, driven by wearers seeking better oxygen supply, biocompatibility, and wear comfort at reasonable prices. At the same time, the development of diverse soft contact lenses will result in unlimited numbers and types of patients who might benefit, by providing such patients with the most suitable lenses. The use of a phospholipid polymer for soft contact lenses in an effective way will help the material to elevate overall biocompatibility.

10.10   Sources of further information and advice

The MPC as a base component of phospholipid polymers is now prepared on an industrial scale by NOF Co. (Tokyo, Japan) based on our results (Ishihara *et al.*, 1990a). The fundamental biological data of phospholipid polymers have been reported in the literature (Ishihara *et al.*, 1990b, 1991, 1992; Defife *et al.*, 1995; Ueda *et al.*, 1995; Sakaki *et al.*, 1999; Sawada *et al.*, 2003, 2006). The phospholipid polymer is developed not only for soft contact lenses, but also for other biomedical applications. For example, one of the most successful applications is in artificial joints (Moro *et al.*, 2004). Nanoscaled grafting of the poly(MPC) on to the cross-linked polyethylene surface provides good lubricity, wear resistance, and biocompatibility in biological environments (Kyomoto *et al.*, 2007). Such excellent functions of the modified surface could avoid the activation of cell systems by the wear particles, thus entirely preventing periprosthetic osteolysis and subsequent aseptic loosening. In addition, prevention of non-specific protein adsorption is very useful for the reduction of noise intensity in biosensors and for enhancing affinity in enzyme-linked immuno-sorbent assays (Goto *et al.*, 2008).

10.11   References

Chekina N, Pavlyuchenko V, Danilichev V, Ushakov N, Novikov S and Ivanchev S (2006), 'A new polymeric silicone hydrogel for medical applications: synthesis and properties', *Polym Adv Technol*, **17**, 872–877. DOI: 10.1002/pat.820.

Chen C, Hong Y and Manesis N (2008), 'Wettable silicone hydrogel contact lenses and related compositions and methods', US Patent Application 20080048350.

Colman R and Schmaier A (1997), 'Contact system: a vascular biology modulator with anticoagulant, profibrinolytic, antiadhesive, and proinflammatory attributes', *Blood*, **90**, 3819–3843.

Dang Y, Rao A, Kastl P, Blake R, Schurr M and Blake D (2003), 'Quantifying *Pseudomonas aeruginosa* adhesion to contact lenses', *Eye Contact Lens*, **29**, 65–68.

Defife K, Yun J, Azeez A, Stack S, Ishihara K, Nakabayashi N, Colton E and Anderson J (1995), 'Adhesion and cytokine production by monocytes on poly(2-methacryloyloxyethyl phosphorylcholine-co-alkyl methacrylate)-coated polymers', *J Biomed Mater Res*, **29**, 431–439. DOI: 10.1002/jbm.820290403.

Goda T, Konno T, Takai M, Moro T and Ishihara K (2006), 'Biomimetic phosphorylcholine polymer grafting from polydimethylsiloxane surface using photo-induced polymerization', *Biomaterials*, **27**, 5151–5160. DOI: 10.1016/j.biomaterials.2006.05.046.

Goto Y, Matsuno R, Konno T, Takai M and Ishihara K (2008), 'Polymer nanoparticles covered with phosphorylcholine groups and immobilized with antibody for high-affinity separation of proteins', *Biomacromolecules*, **9**, 828–833. DOI: 10.1021/bm701161d.

Harvitt D and Bonanno J (1999), 'Re-evaluation of the oxygen diffusion model for predicting minimum contact lens Dk/t values needed to avoid corneal anoxia', *Optom Vis Sci*, **76**, 712–719.

Ho S, Nakabayashi N, Iwasaki Y, Boland T and LaBerge M (2003), 'Frictional properties of poly(MPC-co-BMA) phospholipid polymer for catheter applications', *Biomaterials*, **24**, 5121–5129. DOI: 10.1016/S0142-9612(03)00450-2.

Huang X, Yao K, Zhang H, Huang H and Xu Z (2007), 'Surface modification of silicone intraocular lens by 2-methacryloyloxyethyl phosphoryl-choline binding to reduce *Staphylococcus epidermidis* adherence', *Clin Exper Ophthalmol*, **35**, 462–467. DOI: 10.1111/j.1442-9071.2007.01516.x.

Ishihara K, Ueda T and Nakabayashi N (1990a), 'Preparation of phospholipid polylners and their properties as polymer hydrogel membranes', *Polym J*, **22**, 355–360.

Ishihara K, Aragaki R, Ueda T, Watanabe A and Nakabayashi N (1990b), 'Reduced thrombogenicity of polymers having phospholipid polar groups', *J Biomed Mater Res*, **24**, 1069–1077. DOI: 10.1002/jbm.820240809.

Ishihara K, Ziats N, Tierney B, Nakabayashi N and Anderson J (1991), 'Protein adsorption from human plasma is reduced on phospholipid polymers', *J Biomed Mater Res*, **25**, 1397–1407. DOI: 10.1002/jbm.820251107.

Ishihara K, Oshida H, Endo Y, Ueda T, Watanabe A and Nakabayashi N (1992), 'Hemocompatibility of human whole blood on polymers with a phospholipid polar group and its mechanism', *J Biomed Mater Res*, **26**, 1543–1552. DOI: 10.1002/jbm.820261202.

Ishihara K, Nomura H, Mihara T, Kurita K, Iwasaki Y and Nakabayashi N (1998), 'Why do phospholipid polymers reduce protein adsorption?', *J Biomed Mater Res*, **39**, 323–330. DOI: 10.1002/(SICI)1097-4636(199802)39:2<323::AID-JBM21>3.0.CO;2-C.

Iwasaki Y and Ishihara K (2005), 'Phosphorylcholine-containing polymers for biomedical applications', *Anal Bioanal Chem*, **381**, 534–546. DOI: 10.1007/s00216-004-2805-9.

Jones L, Evans K, Sariri R, Franklin V and Tighe B (1997), 'Lipid and protein deposition of N-vinyl pyrrolidone-containing group II and group IV frequent replacement contact lenses', *CLAO J*, **23**, 122–126.

Keith D, Christensen M, Barry J and Stein J (2003), 'Determination of the lysozyme deposit curve in soft contact lenses', *Eye Contact Lens*, **29**, 79–82.

Kitano H, Imai M, Mori T, Gemmei-Ide M, Yokoyama Y and Ishihara K (2003), 'Structure of water in the vicinity of phospholipid analogue copolymers as studied by vibrational spectroscopy', *Langmuir*, **19**, 10260–10266. DOI: 10.1021/la0349673.

Kunz R, Anders C, Heinrich L and Gersonde K (1999), 'Investigation into the mechanism of bacterial adhesion to hydrogel-coated surfaces', *J Mater Sci Mater Med*, **10**, 649–652. DOI: 10.1023/A:1008943909728.

Kyomoto M, Moro T, Konno T, Takadama H, Yamawaki N, Kawaguchi H, Takatori Y, Nakamura K and Ishihara K (2007), 'Enhanced wear resistance of modified cross-linked polyethylene by grafting with poly(2-methacryloyloxyethyl phosphorylcholine)', *J Biomed Mater Res A*, **82**, 10–17. DOI: 10.1002/jbm.a.31134.

Ladage P, Yamamoto N, Robertson D, Jester J, Petroll W and Cavanagh H (2004), '*Pseudomonas aeruginosa* corneal binding after 24-hour orthokeratology lens wear', *Eye Contact Lens*, **30**, 173–178.

Matsuda Y, Kobayashi M, Annaka M, Ishihara K and Takahara, A (2006), 'Dimension of poly(2-methacryloyloxyethyl phosphorylcholine) in aqueous solutions with various ionic strength', *Chem Lett*, **35**, 1310–1311. DOI: 10.1246/cl.2006.1310.

Moro T, Takatori Y, Ishihara K, Konno T, Takigawa Y, Matsushita T, Chung U-I, Nakamura K and Kawaguchi H (2004), 'Surface grafting of artificial joints with a biocompatible polymer for preventing periprosthetic osteolysis', *Nat Mater*, **3**, 829–836. DOI: 10.1038/nmat1233.

Nicolson P and Vogt J (2001), 'Soft contact lens polymers: an evolution', *Biomaterials*, **22**, 3273–3283. DOI: 10.1016/S0142-9612(01)00165-X.

Peterson R, Wolffsohn J, Nick J, Winterton L and Lally J (2006), 'Clinical performance of daily disposable soft contact lenses using sustained release technology', *Cont Lens Anterior Eye*, **29**, 127–134. DOI: 10.1016/j.clae.2006.03.004.

Ratner B D, Hoffman A S, Schoen F J and Lemons J E eds (2004), *Biomaterials Science*, 2nd edn, Amsterdam, Elsevier.

Riley C, Chalmers R and Pence N (2005), 'The impact of lens choice in the relief of contact lens related symptoms and ocular surface findings', *Cont Lens Anterior Eye*, **28**, 13–19. DOI: 10.1016/j.clae.2004.09.002.

Ross G, Mann A, Franklin V and Tighe B (2007), 'Disclosure – the true story of daily disposable lens surfaces', In 31st BCLA Clinical Conference and Exhibition, 31 May-3 June, Manchester, UK, p. 122.

Sakaki S, Nakabayashi N and Ishihara K (1999), 'Stabilization of an antibody conjugated with enzyme by 2-methacryloyloxyethyl phosphorylcholine copolymer in enzyme-linked immunosorbent assay', *J Biomed Mater Res A*, **47**, 523–528. DOI: 10.1002/(SICI)1097-4636(19991215)47:4<523::AID-JBM8>3.0.CO;2-J.

Sawada S, Sakaki S, Iwasaki Y, Nakabayashi N and Ishihara K (2003), 'Suppression of the inflammatory response from adherent cells on phospholipid polymers', *J Biomed Mater Res A*, **64**, 411–416. DOI: 10.1002/jbm.a.10433.

Sawada S, Iwasaki Y, Nakabayashi N and Ishihara K (2006), 'Stress response of adherent cells on a polymer blend surface composed of a segmented polyurethane and MPC copolymers', *J Biomed Mater Res A*, **79**, 476–484. DOI: 10.1002/jbm.a.30820.

Selan L, Palma S, Scoarughi G, Papa R, Veeh R, Clemente D and Artini M (2009), 'Phosphorylcholine impairs susceptibility to biofilm formation of hydrogel contact lenses', *Am J Ophthalmol*, **147**, 134–139. DOI: 10.1016/j.ajo.2008.07.032.

Shaku M, Kuroda H, Oba A, Okura S, Ishihara K and Nakabayashi N (1997), 'Enhancing stratum corneum functions with a bifunctional phospholipid polymer', *Cosmet Toiletries*, **112**, 65–76.

Shimizu T, Goda T, Konno T, Takai M and Ishihara K (2008), 'Improved protein adsorption on soft contact lenses treated with phospholipid polymers', In *8th World Biomaterials Congress*, 28 May–1 June 2008, Amsterdam, The Netherlands, abstract P-Sat-I-565, p. 2249.

Shimizu T, Konno T, Takai M and Ishihara K (2009), 'Super hydrophilic surface realized by IPN structure of silicone hydrogel', In *Proceedings of IUMRS-ICA, Symposium K*, 9–13 December 2008, Nagoya, Japan, KO-10 (in Press).

Shin H, Jo S and Mikos A (2003), 'Biomimetic materials for tissue engineering', *Biomaterials*, **24**, 4353–4364. DOI: 10.1016/S0142-9612(03)00339-9.

Singer S and Nicolson G (1972), 'The fluid mosaic model of the structure of cell membranes', *Science*, **175**, 720–731.

Stapleton F, Keay L, Jalbert I and Cole N (2007), 'The epidemiology of contact lens related infiltrates', *Optom Vis Sci*, **84**, 257–272.

Taddei P, Balducci F, Simoni R and Monti P (2005), 'Raman, IR and thermal study of a new highly biocompatible phosphorylcholine-based contact lens', *J Mol Struct*, **744–747**, 507–514. DOI: 10.1016/j.molstruc.2004.10.118.

Tighe B (2004), 'Silicone hydrogels: structure, properties and behaviour' In Sweeney D ed., *Silicone Hydrogels – Continuous-Wear Contact Lenses*, 2nd edn, Oxford, Butterworth-Heinemann, pp. 1–27.

Ueda T, Ishihara K and Nakabayashi N (1995), 'Adsorption–desorption of proteins on phospholipid polymer surfaces evaluated by dynamic contact angle measurement', *J Biomed Mater Res*, **29**, 381–387. DOI: 10.1002/jbm.820290313.

Wichterle O and Lim D (1960), 'Hydrophilic gels for biological use', *Nature*, **185**, 117–118. DOI: 10.1038/185117a0.

Willis S, Court J, Redman R, Wang J, Leppard S, O'Byrne V, Small S, Lewis A, Jones S and Stratford P (2001), 'A novel phosphorylcholine-coated contact lens for extended wear use', *Biomaterials*, **22**, 3261–3272. DOI: 10.1016/S0142-9612(01)00164-8.

Xu Y, Takai M, Konno T and Ishihara K (2007), 'Microfluidic flow control on charged phospholipid polymer interface', *Lab Chip*, **7**, 199–206. DOI: 10.1039/b616851p.

11

Contact lenses: the search for superior oxygen permeability

N. EFRON, Queensland University of Technology, Australia;
P. B. MORGAN and C. MALDONADO-CODINA,
The University of Manchester, UK; N. A. BRENNAN,
Brennan Consultants Pty Ltd, Australia

Abstract: Although contact lenses were invented over 120 years ago, it is only in the past decade that a solution has been found to the problem of allowing sufficient atmospheric oxygen to permeate the lens and reach the underlying ocular tissues so as to allow normal corneal function and avoid hypoxic complications. That solution is 'silicone hydrogel' materials, which were introduced into the market in 1998 and have been measured to have oxygen permeability values ranging from 60 to 140 barrer; this compares with 0 barrer for both glass (used from 1889 to 1938) and Perspex (used from 1938 to 1972), and <35 barrer for hydrogel lenses (used from 1972 to 1998). There is essentially no difference between the various types of silicone hydrogel lenses with respect to the oxygen flux that reaches the eye through the lens, which is sufficient for normal metabolic function.

Key words: contact lenses, silicone hydrogels, oxygen transmissibility, cornea, oxygen flux.

11.1   Introduction

11.1.1 Historical note

Most people are surprised to learn that contact lenses were invented over 120 years ago – on 1 February, 1889, to be precise. On this day a 25-year-old medical student named August Müller (1864–1949) submitted the results of his final year project, entitled 'Brillengläser und Hornhautlinsen' ('spectacle lenses and cornea-lenses'), to the University of Kiel in Germany (Pearson and Efron, 1989). As can be seen from Fig. 11.1, Müller wore spectacles to correct high myopia. In what must have been perceived as a bold and perhaps dangerous experiment, Müller fitted himself with large, thick glass contact lenses (known as 'haptic' lenses); however, he was only able to wear them for half an hour, and provided the following graphic description of his experience (Pearson and Efron, 1989):

> Gradually, about a quarter of an hour after insertion, a sensation of pressure and burning appeared, which could not be localised exactly. After a further quarter of an hour, the sensation became so agonising that I had to remove

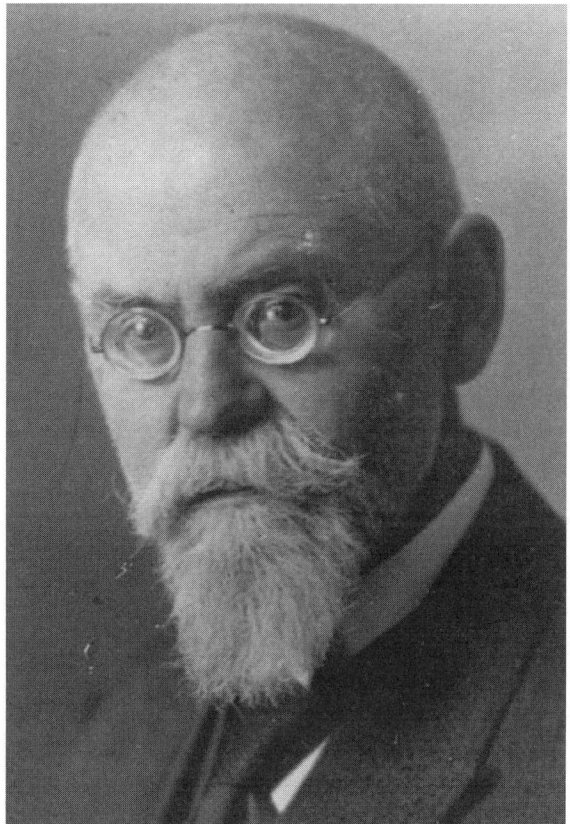

11.1 August Müller (here aged 66 years), the first person to fit contact lenses for the correction of myopia.

the lenses. Upon their removal, the violent pain immediately stopped and a short while after I could use the eyes again.

Müller was so disappointed with the results of his experiments that he gave up the idea of becoming an eye specialist and went on to practise as an orthopaedic surgeon.

This pioneering work signalled the beginning of the battle to develop contact lenses that could be worn comfortably and continually for many hours. As it turned out, Müller was entirely correct in ascribing the failure of his own lens-wearing experiments to '... a disturbance of nourishment of corneal tissue'. Unlike all other tissues in the body, the cornea does not contain blood vessels (so that it can remain optically transparent); therefore, in order to respire normally, it must obtain oxygen directly from, and eliminate carbon dioxide directly to, the atmosphere. Although he did not know it at the time, Müller's haptic lenses prevented this necessary exchange of respiratory gases.

Up until 1938, all contact lenses were made of glass. Although glass is impermeable to oxygen, clinicians managed to circumvent this problem to some extent by introducing fenestrations (small holes) in the lens periphery to facilitate a limited tear exchange (and consequent gaseous exchange). After 1938, contact lenses began to be manufactured in clear plastic (Perspex – poly(methyl methacrylate) or PMMA). PMMA had the advantages of being lighter and more durable (less likely to shatter), and it was easier to manufacture lenses using lathing and moulding technology. However, PMMA is also impermeable to oxygen, and strategies still had to be employed to facilitate corneal oxygenation during lens wear, such as the introduction of fenestrations and fitting smaller 'corneal lenses' that moved around on the cornea during blinking and enhanced tear and gaseous exchange beneath the lens.

Possibly the greatest understatement that can be found in the literature pertaining to contact lens development is the final sentence of a paper entitled 'Hydrophilic gels for biological use', published in *Nature* on January 9, 1960, by Wichterle and Lim (1960), which reads: 'Promising results have also been obtained in experiments in other cases, for example, in manufacturing contact lenses, arteries, etc.' This is the only mention in that paper, and the first mention in the scientific literature, of the possibility of manufacturing contact lenses from hydrophilic materials.

Initial attempts by Wichterle to produce soft lenses from poly(2-hydroxyethyl methacrylate) (PHEMA), and manufactured using cast moulding, met with limited success. Unable to attract support from the Institute of Macromolecular Research in Czechoslovakia (now The Czech Republic) where he worked, and indeed discouraged by his superiors, Wichterle was forced to conduct further secret experiments in his own home. Working with a children's mechanical construction kit, Wichterle developed the spin-casting technique and eventually managed to persuade his peers to conduct further trials at the Institute. He claims to have produced 'the first suitable contact lenses' in late 1961 (Wichterle, 1978), which presumably approximates to the first occasion when a soft lens was actually worn on a human eye. The patent to develop soft contact lenses was subsequently acquired by Bausch & Lomb in the USA, who introduced soft lenses commercially into the world market in 1972.

Lenses manufactured from PHEMA were an immediate market success, primarily by virtue of their superior comfort and enhanced biocompatibility. However, clinical experience and laboratory studies indicated that the poor physiological response of the anterior eye during wear of the early thick PHEMA lenses could be improved by making soft lenses more permeable to oxygen – specifically, by making them thinner and of a higher water content.

11.1.2 Physiological considerations

If a contact lens blocks off the normal oxygen supply, the corneal epithelium will become hypoxic and will begin to respire anaerobically. This leads to a build-up of lactic acid, which diffuses into the corneal stroma, creating an osmotic force that draws in water (Klyce, 1981). The cornea then develops oedema and becomes less transparent, and the eye becomes uncomfortable. Carbon dioxide that is prevented by a contact lens from escaping from the corneal surface dissolves in the tears forming carbonic acid (Efron and Ang, 1990). The resulting acidosis compromises the physiological integrity of the cornea to a small extent, but the effects of hypoxia are far more critical. Other adverse hypoxic effects of contact lenses can include epithelial microcysts, epithelial thinning, stromal neovascularization, long-term stromal thinning, corneal warpage and endothelial polymegethism and pleomorphism (Efron, 2004).

The solution to the problem of hypoxia is to design contact lenses that maximize corneal oxygenation during lens wear. During the last quarter of the twentieth century, the majority of contact lenses fitted were made of soft hydrophilic materials. These lenses are fitted in such a way that they completely cover the cornea; therefore, the only option for preventing hypoxia is to use soft materials that are permeable to oxygen.

The ease with which oxygen can diffuse through a contact lens (defined by the term 'oxygen transmissibility', or Dk/t) is a function of the oxygen permeability (Dk) of the hydrogel material from which the lens is made and the thickness of the lens (a more complete definition of these terms is provided later in this chapter). A thinner lens provides less resistance to oxygen flow; however, nothing much can be done about lens thickness, because a lens must have a certain thickness profile to achieve the desired optical power for vision correction. Furthermore, if a lens is made too thin, it will fall apart. This leaves material Dk as the only variable. Hydrogel materials have water contents ranging from 35% to 75%. The higher the water content, the greater is the Dk – but higher water content materials tend to be more fragile.

During the waking hours, the cornea receives enough oxygen to avoid excessive oedema. There is a small but significant minority of patients who need or desire to sleep in lenses, but it is here that we encounter another problem that is best expressed as a paradox: even if it was possible to make an extremely thin contact lens out of 100% water, this would still not be sufficient to prevent corneal oedema during sleep. Slightly increased levels of corneal oedema are not dangerous in the short term (Efron, 2004); indeed, even in non-lens-wearers the cornea experiences low levels of oedema during sleep. Nevertheless, many changes can be observed in the cornea in association with chronic low level hypoxia and oedema, such as epithelial weakening, limbal vascular ingrowth, endothelial polymegethism and stromal thinning (Efron, 2004).

Perhaps the most critical of these chronic changes is a structural and metabolic weakening of the corneal epithelium. An intact epithelium provides a vital defence against invasion by potentially pathogenic micro-organisms, which could either enter the eye by chance or, in a lens wearer, via contaminated fingers and/or contact lens storage solutions (Fleiszig, 2006). The introduction of disposable lenses in the 1980s largely solved problems relating to the build-up of lens deposits; however, because the disposable lenses introduced at that time were still made of hydrogel materials, their capacity to minimize hypoxic effects such as oedema were just the same as non-disposable lenses.

As mentioned above, most lens wearers choose to sleep in contact lenses (a practice known clinically as 'extended wear') because of the increased convenience; however, this introduces a greater physiological challenge to the eye than conventional daily 'open-eye' lens wear. During sleep, the atmosphere is replaced by the closed eyelid. Under these conditions, oxygen is derived from the capillary plexus of the palpebral conjunctiva – the vascularized tissue that lines the posterior surface of the eyelid. The oxygen tension in these vessels is 55 mmHg, which is about one-third of the oxygen tension in the atmosphere (about 155 mmHg at standard temperature and pressure at sea level) (Efron and Carney, 1979).

11.1.3 Silicone elastomer contact lenses

It had long been known in the contact lens industry that the physiological problems caused by conventional hydrogel lenses could potentially be overcome by making contact lenses from silicone rubber, which forms a unique category among contact lens materials. Silicone rubber is an optically transparent elastomer that has an extremely high permeability to oxygen and carbon dioxide and therefore provides minimal interference to corneal respiration; however, it is difficult to manufacture and its surface is hydrophobic and must be treated to allow comfortable wear. There was some patent activity in respect of attempts to manufacture clinically viable lenses from this material in the mid 1960s to early 1970s, and Mandell (1988) claims to have personally observed ten patients who were wearing such lenses in 1965, noting very poor clinical results.

A silicone elastomer contact lens is a 'soft lens' in terms of its physical behaviour and lenses are fabricated from this material in the form of a soft lens. Unlike all other soft lens materials, silicone elastomer does not contain water and in this respect is analogous to a hard lens material. The considerable difficulties involved in enhancing surface wettability severely limited the clinical application of this lens, and an alternative approach was required.

11.2   Silicone hydrogel contact lenses

11.2.1 Background

The allure of a contact lens made from a material with a phenomenally high oxygen performance never escaped the contact lens industry. The development of such a lens would be critical to solving the hypoxic lens-related problems outlined above. Polymer scientists in the contact lens industry had long recognized that many of the problems associated with silicone elastomers for contact lens fabrication could be theoretically overcome by creating a silicone–hydrogel hybrid.

The patent literature shows that combining silicone with conventional hydrogel monomers has been a goal for polymer scientists since the late 1970s. The greatest obstacle to this approach, however, is that silicone is hydrophobic and poorly miscible with hydrophilic monomers, resulting in opaque, phase-separated materials. In order to solve this problem, two main approaches have been utilized (Tighe 2004). The first approach involves the insertion of polar groups into the section of a siloxymethacrylate monomer known as tris(trimethylsiloxy)methacryloxy propylsilane (TRIS), at the point of the arrow in Fig. 11.2, in order to aid its miscibility with hydrophilic monomers (Tanaka *et al.*, 1979; Künzler & Ozark, 1994). The second approach is that of utilizing macromers. Macromers are large monomers formed by preassembly of structural units that are designed to bestow particular properties on the final polymer (Tighe, 2004).

11.2 Molecular structure of key components of silicone-based contact lens materials. PDMS, polydimethylsiloxane; TRIS, tris (trimethyl-siloxy) methacryloxy propylysilane; TPVC, tris(trimethylsiloxysilyl) propylvinyl carbamate.

11.2.2 Market introduction

The first two silicone hydrogels were launched in the late 1990s – the balafilcon A lens (Bausch & Lomb) and the lotrafilcon A lens (CIBA Vision). Both were licensed for 30 days of continuous wear. The balafilcon A lens has an equilibrium water content (EWC) of 36% and a Dk/t of 110 barrer/cm (at –3.00D). The balafilcon A material is formulated by copolymerizing a carbamate-substituted TRIS-based material known as tris(trimethyl siloxysilyl) propylvinyl carbamate (TPVC) (Fig. 11.2) with N-vinylpyrrolidone (NVP).

The lotrafilcon A lens has an EWC of 24% and a Dk/t of 175 barrer/cm (at –3.00D). Tighe (2004) describes the lens as being a fluoroether macromer copolymerized with TRIS and DMA (N,N-dimethyl acrylamide) in the presence of a diluent. Its biphasic (two-channel) structure means that oxygen and water permeability channels are not reliant on each other. The silicone-containing phase allows passage of oxygen while the water phase primarily allows the lens to move.

Both of these lenses would be unsuitable for wear without further treatment due to the fact that the resultant material surfaces are very hydrophobic. In order to overcome this problem, both lenses are surface-treated using gas plasma techniques. High energy gases or gas mixtures (the plasma) are used to modify the lens surface properties without changing the bulk properties. The result for the balafilcon lens is that surface wettability is gained via plasma oxidation, which produces glassy silicate islands on the lens surface (Maldonado-Codina et al., 2004a; Maldonado-Codina and Efron, 2005).

The lotrafilcon lens is coated with a dense 25-nm-thick coating. Both resultant surfaces have low molecular mobility, which minimizes the migration of hydrophobic silicone groups to the surface. However, despite these surface modifications, wettability problems with these lenses have been reported (Maldonado-Codina and Morgan, 2007). It is generally accepted that these lenses have inferior wettability compared with conventional hydrogels; this occurs as a result of the hydrophobic interaction of silicone with the tear film.

Another important difference between these materials and conventional hydrogels is the fact that they have significantly greater elastic moduli, i.e. they are 'stiffer'. Such mechanical characteristics mean that the lenses are easy to handle but they have also been implicated in the aetiology of a number of clinical complications (Dumbleton, 2003). These include higher incidences of superficial epithelial arcuate lesions, mucin balls and localized contact lens papillary conjunctivitis, especially with continuous wear of these lenses (Skotnitsky et al., 2002). The stiffness of the material may contribute to the mechanical irritation of the lens rubbing against the conjunctiva of the upper eyelid, producing a localized response.

The design of the lens, and in particular the edges, may have an impact on ocular compatibility. It has also been suggested that the design of the lens edge in conjunction with the mechanical properties of silicone hydrogel lenses may be responsible for increased conjunctival staining and conjunctival epithelial flaps observed with these lenses (Loftstrom & Kruse, 2005). A knife-point edge or chisel-shaped edge may cause more conjunctival staining and flap formation than a round edge by 'carving' into the conjunctival tissue. It has been proposed that certain edge designs incorporating localized increases in posterior edge lift, reduced peripheral thickness or peripheral channels may reduce the pressure on the conjunctiva (Weidemann and Lakkis, 2005).

11.2.3 'Second-generation' lenses

In an attempt to improve on the problems encountered with the early silicone hydrogels, manufacturers have engaged in a programme of research aimed at manufacturing silicone hydrogel lenses with improved mechanical and surface characteristics. This has resulted in the gradual emergence of 'second-generation' silicone hydrogel lenses such as galyfilcon A, senofilcon A, narafilcon A, enfilcon A, comfilcon A and Clariti. Table 11.1 compares the properties of all the silicone hydrogel lenses currently on the market.

The main advantage of these second-generation silicone hydrogels, compared with the early silicone hydrogels, is that they have increased water contents and reduced moduli, and they do not need to be surface treated. The mechanical and surface properties can be thought of as being 'in between' those of conventional hydrogels and the early silicone hydrogels. Recent clinical work indicates that there may be a lower incidence of contact lens-induced papillary conjunctivitis with these lenses (Maldonado-Codina et al., 2004b).

Some of the lenses in Table 11.1 are based on materials containing TRIS-like components. The Johnson & Johnson products – galyfilcon A, senofilcon A and narafilcon A – are based on Tanaka's original patent (Tanaka et al., 1979), following its expiration after 25 years, using a modified TRIS molecule, a silicone macromer and hydrophilic monomers such as 2-hydroxyethyl methacrylate and N,N-dimethylacrylamide. Alcohol is used as a solvent to aid the miscibility of these ingredients and is then extracted following polymerization. High molecular weight poly(N-vinylpyrrolidone) (PVP) is the internal wetting agent ('Hydraclear') used in these lenses, which is entangled and therefore 'entrapped' within the lens matrix. It is this that allows the lenses to be manufactured without requiring a surface treatment (Maiden et al., 2002; McCabe et al., 2004). The PVP essentially works by shielding the silicone from the tear film at the lens interface.

The CooperVision products – comfilcon A and enfilcon A – are not based on TRIS chemistry. They are composed solely of silicon-containing macromers

Table 11.1 Properties of currently available silicone hydrogel contact lenses

	Focus Night & Day	Pure Vision	Acuvue Advance	Air Optix	Acuvue Oasys	Biofinity	PremiO	Avaira	Clariti	TruEye
Manufacturer	CIBA Vision	Bausch & Lomb	Johnson & Johnson	CIBA Vision	Johnson & Johnson	Cooper Vision	Menicon	Cooper Vision	Sauflon	Johnson & Johnson
Year entered market	1999	1999	2003	2004	2005	2006	2007	2008	2008	2008
USAN[a]	Lotrafilcon A	Balafilcon A	Galyfilcon A	Lotrafilcon B	Senofilcon A	Comfilcon A	Asmofilcon A	Enfilcon A	(Not in USA)	Narafilcon A
Water content (%)	24	36	47	33	38	48	40	46	58	46
Modulus (MPa)	1.52	1.50	0.43	1.00	0.72	0.75	0.91	0.50	0.50	0.66
Surface treatment	Plasma coating	Plasma oxidation	None (internal wetting agent, PVP)	Plasma coating	None (internal wetting agent, PVP)	None (internal wetting agent, undisclosed)	Plasma treatment	None (internal wetting agent, undisclosed)	None (wetting process undisclosed)	None (internal wetting agent, PVP)
Principal monomers	DMA, TRIS, siloxane monomer	NVP, TPVC, NCVE, PBVC	MPDMS, DMA, HEMA, EGDMA, siloxane macromer, PVP	DMA, TRIS, siloxane monomer	MPDMS, DMA, HEMA, siloxane macromer, TEGDMA, PVP	NVP, VMA, IBM, TAIC, M3U, FM0411M, HOB	SIMA, SIA, DMA, pyrrolidone derivative	NVP, VMA, IBM, TAIC, M3U, FM0411M, HOB	Not disclosed	MPDMS, DMA, HEMA, siloxane macromer, TEGDMA, PVP

[a] United States Adopted Name.
[b] Manufacturer-reported values.

Abbreviations: PVP, polyvinyl pyrrolidone, MPDMS: monofunctional polydimethylsiloxane; DMA, N,N-dimethylacrylamide; HEMA, hydroxyethyl methacrylate; EGDMA, ethyleneglycol dimethacrylate; TEGDMA, tetraethyleneglycol dimethacrylate; TRIS, trimethyl siloxysilyl; NVP, N-vinyl pyrrolidone, TPVC, tris-(trimethyl siloxysilyl) propylvinyl carbamate; NCVE, N-carboxyvinyl ester; PBVC, poly(dimethylsiloxy) di(silylbutanol) bis(vinyl carbamate); VMA, N-vinyl-N-methylacetamide; IBM, isobornyl methacrylate; TAIC, 1,3,5-triallyl-1,3,5-triazine-2,4,6($1H,3H,5H$)-trione; M3U, bis(methacryloyloxyethyl iminocarboxy ethyloxypropyl)-poly(dimethylsiloxane)-poly(trifluoropropylmethylsiloxane)-poly(methoxy-poly(ethyleneglycol) propylmethylsiloxane); FM0411M, methacryloyloxyethyl iminocarboxyethyloxypropyl-poly(dimethylsiloxy)-butyldimethylsilane; HOB, 2-hydroxybutyl methacrylate; SIMA, siloxanyl methacrylate; SIA, siloxanyl acrylate.

and require no surface treatment or wetting agent. The patents surrounding these materials refer to a monofunctional macromer (i.e. the monomer contains only one double bond, which takes part in the polymerization process) being combined with another rubber-like siloxy macromer. This results in materials with much longer chains (higher molecular weight) compared with the other silicone hydrogels (Iwata *et al.*, 2005; Iwata *et al.*, 2006). The patents also discuss other hydrophilic monomers which are presumably the key to why these materials do not need to be surface treated. The material chemistry of the CooperVision lenses provides a higher than expected *Dk/t* for its water content. The introduction of these second-generation lenses has also resulted in a significant rise in the number of silicone hydrogel lenses being prescribed world-wide, primarily on a daily-wear basis (Morgan *et al.*, 2009b) (Fig. 11.3).

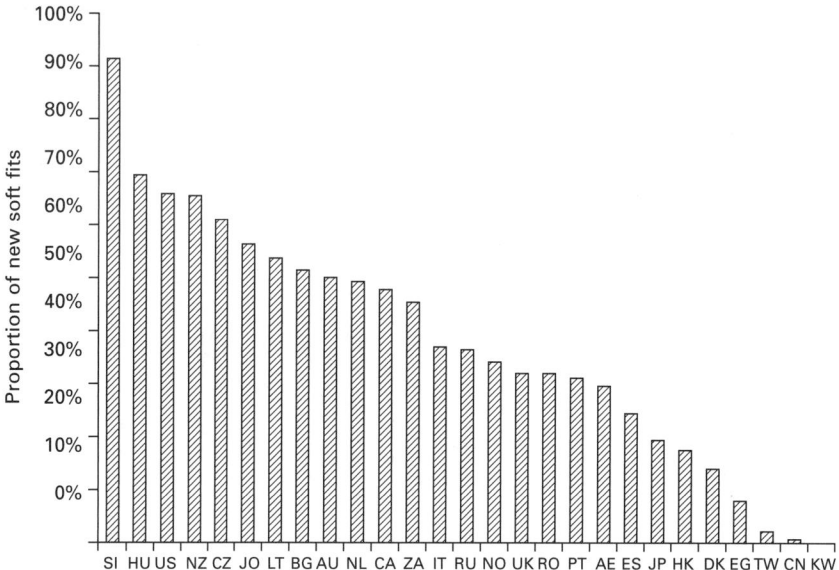

11.3 Percentage of silicone hydrogel contact lenses fitted, in relation to all soft lenses fitted, in 27 nations in 2008. Country codes: AE, United Arab Emirates; AU, Australia; BG, Bulgaria; CA, Canada; CN, China; CZ, Czech Republic; DK, Denmark; EG, Egypt; ES, Spain; HK, Hong Kong; HU, Hungary; IT, Italy; JO, Jordan; JP, Japan; KW, Kuwait; LT, Lithuania; NL, Netherlands; NO, Norway; NZ, New Zealand; PT, Portugal; RO, Romania; RU, Russia; SI, Slovenia; TW, Taiwan; UK, United Kingdom; US, United States; ZA, South Africa. Data from Morgan *et al.* (2009b).

11.3 Oxygen performance of silicone hydrogel lenses

11.3.1 Definitions

Dk is a property of the contact lens material itself, where *D* is the diffusivity and *k* is the solubility of the material. The diffusivity is a measure of how quickly oxygen can move through a material while the solubility is a measure of how much oxygen the material can hold. The *Dk* of a hydrogel will vary with temperature. *Dk* is essentially governed by the EWC in conventional hydrogels. This relationship is based on the ability of oxygen to pass through the water rather than through the material itself. The relationship between EWC and *Dk* has been found to be (Morgan & Efron, 1998):

$$Dk = 1.67\,e^{0.0397\text{EWC}}$$

where *e* is the natural logarithm (Fig. 11.4).

In order to calculate the amount of oxygen that will move from the anterior to the posterior surface of a lens, the *Dk* is divided by the thickness of the lens (*t*). The units of *Dk* have been traditionally known as 'Fatt units' (after Professor Irving Fatt who carried out much of the early work on the *Dk* of contact lens materials) or 'barrer', whereby:

$$Dk \text{ (barrer)} = 10^{-11} \text{ (cm}^2 \times \text{mlO}_2\text{)/(s} \times \text{ml} \times \text{mmHg)}$$

$$Dk/t \text{ (barrer/cm)} = 10^{-9} \text{ (cm} \times \text{mlO}_2\text{)/(s} \times \text{ml} \times \text{mmHg)}$$

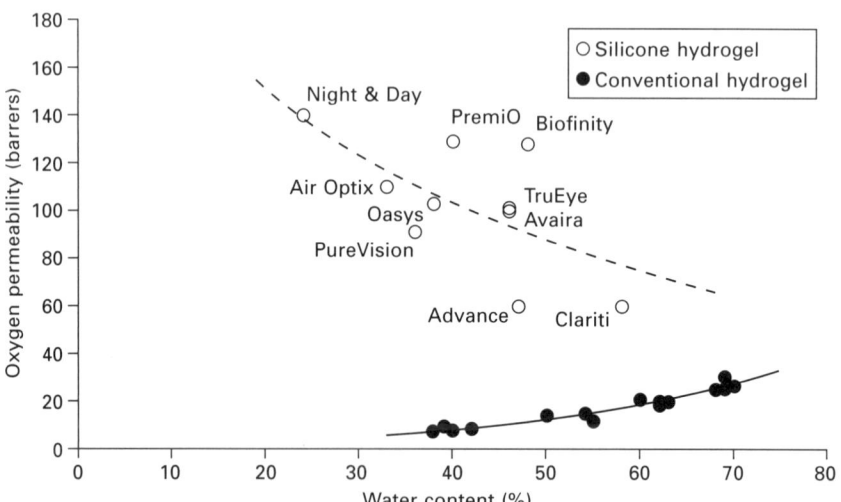

11.4 Relation between *Dk* versus water content for conventional hydrogel and silicone hydrogel contact lenses.

However, the SI unit for pressure is the pascal (Pa). Because the unit mmHg is now becoming obsolete internationally, it is being advocated that the closest accepted metric unit of pressure – 100 Pa, or hectopascal (hPa) – should replace mmHg (ISO, 2006a). The new units are referred to as 'Dk units' in this latest British and International Standard. When hPa is used, Dk and Dk/t values are quoted as below:

$$(Dk) \text{ in 'Dk units'} = 10^{-11} \text{ (cm}^2 \times \text{mlO}_2)/(\text{s} \times \text{ml} \times \text{hPa})$$

$$(Dk/t) \text{ in '}Dk/t \text{ units'} = 10^{-9} \text{ (cm} \times \text{mlO}_2)/(\text{s} \times \text{ml} \times \text{hPa})$$

The difficulty here is that converting from the traditional barrer or Fatt units to ISO units involves multiplying Dk or Dk/t by the constant 0.75. Thus, for example, a lens quoted with a traditional Dk/t of 40 units will have a revised ISO Dk/t of 30 units. It is understandable that such a 'downsizing' will be resisted by contact lens manufacturers, because higher numeric Dk/t values are perceived clinically as being 'superior' when evaluating the oxygen performance of contact lenses with Dk values less than 35 barrer. Since virtually all of the relevant literature still uses non-SI units for citing Dk and Dk/t values, 'barrer' units will be cited in this chapter.

11.3.2 Measurements on silicone hydrogel lenses

Although the manufacturers of silicone hydrogel contact lenses have published values of Dk relating to their products, the precise methodology used in determining these values is not readily available. A number of authors have therefore sought to derive independent estimates of the Dk of commercially available products. Three methods have been described for the measurement of contact lens Dk (Brennan et al., 1987). The polarographic (or 'Fatt') method (ISO 9913-1 Part 1 (ISO, 1996a)) involves placing a contact lens on a polarographic oxygen sensor and measuring the rate at which oxygen passes through the material from the atmosphere to the sensor electrodes. In the coulometric technique (ISO 9913-1 Part 2 (ISO, 1996b), an oxygen-free carrier gas passes over one side of the lens and transfers oxygen that has passed through it to an electrolytic fuel cell where a quantitative decomposition occurs. The gas-to-gas, or 'volumetric', method (Mizutani et al., 1992) involves mounting a lens material specimen between two fixed-volume chambers, one of which is pressurized with 100% oxygen up to several atmospheres greater than the second chamber. Oxygen passing through the lens in response to this pressure gradient is detected as a pressure increase in the second chamber. Most Dk data reported in the ophthalmic literature have been conducted using the polarographic or coulometric techniques.

Here we shall review the work of six groups of researchers (Alvord et al., 1998; Morgan et al., 2001; Compan et al., 2002; Young and Benjamin,

2003; Efron *et al.*, 2007; Chhabra *et al.*, 2007) who have so far published estimates of the *Dk* of commercially available silicone hydrogel contact lenses. The two silicone hydrogel lenses that were introduced into the market in 1998 – lotrafilcon A and balafilcon A – were the only lenses on the market until 2003, at which time other products began to appear. Thus, the earlier studies of Alvod *et al.* (1998), Morgan *et al.* (2001), Compan *et al.* (2002) and Young and Benjamin (2003) only considered one or both of these lenses.

All of the authors of these studies have noted that the high *Dk* of silicone hydrogels places these materials outside the applicability of both the polarographic ISO standard and coulometric ISO draft standards for contact lens *Dk* determination, which were designed for measuring the oxygen performance of low-*Dk* conventional hydrogels. As such, various adaptations and refinements to existing methodology have had to be adopted to make these determinations.

Determinations pre-2004

The *Dk* of lotrafilcon A lenses was determined by Alvord *et al.* (1998) and Morgan *et al.* (2001). Alvord *et al.* (1998) adapted the standard coulometric method. Lenses with a thickness (*t*) ranging from 30 μm to over 300 μm were measured in a liquid-to-gas and a gas-to-gas configuration in an effort to combine features of the ISO standards to yield a valid measurement of the intrinsic material *Dk*. Different results were obtained, which depended upon factors such as whether or not a water overlay was used, whether liquid-to-gas or gas-to-gas procedures were adopted and stirring speed (Table 11.2).

Morgan *et al.* (2001) modified equipment for both polarographic and coulometric methods that included front surface masking to eliminate the 'edge effect'. They used these two techniques to measure the *Dk* of lotrafilcon A (Table 11.2). The coulometric technique yielded typical standard errors of <10%. They concluded that the coulometric method is preferable for the measurement of contact lens materials with *Dk* > 70 barrer.

Compan *et al.* (2002) and Young and Benjamin (2003) measured the *Dk* of lotrafilcon A and balafilcon A. Whereas Compan *et al.* (2002) used the so-called 'stacking procedure' (see below for a complete description of this technique), Young and Benjamin (2003) used conventional polarographic methodology to measure lenses of various power and thus differing thickness profiles. This is in essence a variation on the stacking technique, in that it is an alternative strategy for measuring oxygen flow through differing thicknesses of the same material (Table 11.2).

Source	Technique	Focus Night & Day	PureVision	Acuvue Advance	Air Optix	Acuvue Oasys	Biofinity	PremiO	Avaira	Clariti	TruEye
Manufacturer[a]	Various (see text)	140	91	60	110	103	128	129	100	60	100
Alvord et al., 1998[b]	Coulometric (various conditions)	140 ± 2 150 ± 5 170 ± 2									
Morgan et al., 2001	Polarographic Coulometric	168.53[a] 154.69[c]									
Compan et al., 2002[d]	Polarographic	141 ± 5	107 ± 4								
Young and Benjamin, 2003	Polarographic (repeated)	176.1[g] 190.2[h]	111.3[e] 102.2[f]								
Efron et al., 2007[b]	Polarographic	162.0 ± 9.8	75.9 ± 6.6	75.2 ± 9.8	80.5 ± 4.9	107.4 ± 7.4					
Chaabra et al., 2007[d]	Polarographic	181 ± 17	108 ± 5	72.3 ± 3	120 ± 6	100 ± 4	126 ± 4				

[a] No error estimates given.
[b] Error given as mean ± standard error.
[c] Error given as: +SEM, 3.79; –SEM, 3.62.
[d] Error estimates not defined.
[e] Error given as 95% confidence interval (CI): 103.6–120.3.
[f] Error given as 95% CI: 90.5–116.7.
[g] Error given as 95% CI: 165.1–188.7.
[h] Error given as 95% CI: 177.5–205.0.

Determinations post-2004

Efron *et al.* (2007) used a 'stacking technique' to measure the *Dk* of five silicone hydrogel contact lenses on the market at the time of their experiment. All lenses were 1.00D in power to ensure they were approximately parallel-sided (Weissman and Fatt, 1989). The lenses were obtained through normal commercial channels without reference to the fact that they were to be used for *Dk* measurement.

In general terms, Efron *et al.* (2007) adhered to the procedures for measuring *Dk* as stipulated in ISO 9913-1.4 Prior to *Dk* measurement, lenses were removed from their blister packs, placed in glass vials containing phosphate buffered saline solution, and left overnight in a thermostatically controlled water bath at $35 \pm 0.5\,°C$. A single lens was placed on a polarographic oxygen sensor (Rehder Development Company, California, USA) comprising a pair of electrodes (gold cathode and silver anode) and a solid state temperature sensor. This assembly was housed in a chamber maintained at $35\,°C$ and was connected to an external polarographic amplifier. The electric current passing between the two electrodes was monitored on a digital display on the amplifier unit. The steady-state current was recorded once the current reading had stabilized, which was typically within 20 minutes of placing the lens on the polarographic oxygen sensor.

This process was repeated using separate stacks of 2, 3, 4, 5 and 6 lenses. Different lenses were used to create each stack, so 21 lenses were used for each lens type. This stacking technique has the advantage of allowing finished lenses to be used (rather than using specially manufactured lenses) without influencing measurement values (Weissman and Fatt, 1989). In each case, the thickness of the single lens and that of each of the stacks of 2, 3, 4, 5 and 6 lenses was measured using an electromechanical gauge (Rehder Development Company). The entire procedure was conducted twice.

Typically, to acquire a full dataset for each lens type using the procedure described above took about five working days. The order in which the lens types were measured was randomized and the investigator undertaking these procedures was masked with respect to the lens type under evaluation. Masking was achieved by removing the lenses from the blister packs in which they were supplied and placing them in coded glass vials containing 0.9% phosphate-buffered saline.

The *Dk/t* for each lens stack was calculated by multiplying the mean of the current in microamperes by 2.854×10^{-9}. This value is based on Faraday's constant, the partial pressure of oxygen in the atmosphere and the surface area of the electrode used in this work. A correction was made for the edge effect by using formulae given in the ISO standard. The values for the inverse of the calculated *Dk/t* (i.e. resistance) were plotted graphically against stack thickness; the inverse of the gradient of the line of best fit through the data points for this graph represents the Dk of the lens material. This process eliminates error due to the boundary effect.

Chhabra *et al.* (2007) described a novel polarographic apparatus that requires only a single soft contact lens to ascertain oxygen permeabilities of high-Dk lenses. Unlike the stacking technique, the apparatus they described requires only a single-lens thickness. This is accomplished by minimizing (or completely eliminating) edge effects, boundary-layer resistances and lens desiccation in the polarographic apparatus. By taking these effects into account, Chhabra *et al.* (2007) were able to obtain reliable Dk estimates of six silicone hydrogel lenses. These authors claimed that their single-lens device provides a reliable, efficient and economical method for measuring Dk of silicone hydrogel lenses.

The results of all of the studies described above, and the Dk values claimed by the manufacturers, are summarized in Table 11.2. Taking lotrafilcon A – the only lens measured by all authors – it can be seen that Dk estimates vary from 140 to 190.2 barrer. Five authors measured the Dk of balafilcon A, and results varied between 76 and 111 barrer. Given that (a) the stated error of measurement cited by all authors is considerably less than these ranges, and (b) the commercially supplied materials used by all authors were essentially identical, it would appear that the discrepancies in mean values between authors are largely a result of the different methodologies adopted. Indeed, various ingenious but different strategies were employed by the different authors so as to adapt their protocols to be suitable for measuring lenses of much higher Dk values than stipulated by ISO 9913-1.

The Dk values of three silicone hydrogel lenses were determined by both Efron *et al.* (2007) and Chhabra *et al.* (2007). Whereas these authors were in reasonable agreement for estimates of galyfilcon A (75 and 72 barrer, respectively) and senofilcon A (107 and 100 barrer, respectively), the values they reported for lotrafilcon B were discrepant (81 and 120 barrer, respectively).

Practitioners who fit contact lenses generally rely upon the specifications provided by the manufacturer, for the simple reason that such information is readily accessible. It seems that, with few exceptions, the values cited by the manufacturers are generally lower than those reported by independent studies. Putting these discrepancies aside, it is clear that silicone hydrogel lenses, with Dk values above 60 barrer, have a far superior oxygen performance than was previously available with conventional hydrogel lenses, which all had Dk values less than 35 barrer.

The relation between contact lens Dk and water content is shown in Fig. 11.4 for both conventional and silicone hydrogel lenses. Whereas Dk increases with increasing water content for conventional hydrogel lenses, the opposite is true for silicone hydrogel lenses.

The good fit of the data regression curve for conventional hydrogel lenses is attributed to hydrogels being considered as a single family of polymers. On the other hand, the different silicone hydrogel materials can be considered as being derived from different families of polymers, which is why the fit to the regression line is less accurate. Nevertheless, for silicone hydrogel materials, the principle is clear: since water is essentially a barrier to oxygen permeability, the less water present, the greater is the capacity for oxygen to flow through the material. The challenge for polymer chemists and clinicians is to find the right balance of material properties, whereby the silicone content is not so high as to compromise lens wettability and comfort, but not too low as to compromise oxygen performance.

11.3.3 Limitations of polarographic methodology

International standard ISO 9913-1 stipulates that Dk can be determined by measuring the current in a polarographic oxygen sensor when lens samples of various thickness are placed upon the sensor, as long as (a) the test samples have parallel or near-parallel anterior and posterior surfaces, (b) the thickest lens sample does not exceed 0.40 mm and (c) the resultant Dk is less than 100 barrer. As explained above, researchers have found it necessary to adapt the polarographic technique in different ways to measure the Dk of silicone hydrogel lenses, and in all cases ISO 9913-1 has been technically violated.

Compan $et\ al.$ (2002) and Young and Benjamin (2003) used powered lenses of non-uniform thickness. Morgan $et\ al.$ (2001) described four exceptions to the procedures described in ISO 9913-1 that they implemented when measuring Dk, and suggested that their modified technique could be used to measure soft lenses with Dk values up to 150 barrer. These authors criticized ISO 9913-1, stating that it '... did not contain sufficient, appropriate detail to unambiguously implement ... [the procedures described therein]'. Chhabra $et\ al.$ (2007) used an apparently effective but non-ISO-sanctioned method for eliminating edge and boundary effects.

Instead of using lens samples of different thickness as prescribed by ISO 9913-1, Efron $et\ al.$ (2007) used stacks of one to six parallel-sided lenses, all –1.00D, according to the methodology described by Weissman and Fatt (1989). Note 7 of ISO 9913-1 incorrectly states: 'The near parallel condition would correspond to dioptric powers within the range +0.50 to –0.50'; however, Weissman and Fatt (1989) have demonstrated that the best approximation to parallel-sided soft lenses is achieved by using lenses of –1.00D.

The thickest stack of six silicone hydrogel lenses measured by Efron $et\ al.$ (2007) reached 0.53 mm for lotrafilcon A. In addition, the resultant Dk values exceeded 100 barrer for two of the five silicone hydrogel lenses tested. Notwithstanding these technical violations of ISO 9913-1, Efron $et\ al.$ (2007) demonstrated that, using stacks of up to six lenses, when applying the polarographic methodology to the measurement of the Dk of silicone hydrogel contact lens materials, results in robust data acquisition. Indeed, when plotting resistance (t/Dk) versus stack thickness (t), an r^2 value of greater than 0.98 was obtained for all five silicone hydrogel lenses tested, and the 95% confidence limits of all Dk estimates were within 8% to 20% of the mean.

This stacking methodology has been previously validated by Weissman and Fatt (1989); however, a possible disadvantage of the stacking technique is the potential for additional fine layers of saline to form between the lenses in the stack, cumulatively adding to the resistance to oxygen flow as the stack become larger. This results in a potential underestimation of the true Dk value. Efron *et al.* (2007) demonstrated that, as more lenses are stacked on each other, the thickness of the stacks tends to be greater than that which would be expected based upon the individual lens thicknesses that comprise the stacks. This discrepancy, which occurred for all lens types assessed in their work, is probably due to non-perfect alignment of the lens surfaces, and gaps between stacked lenses filling with saline.

The results of these various authors indicate that polarographic methodology can be used for measuring the Dk of silicone hydrogel lenses, with suitable modifications to the procedures laid out in ISO 9913-1. There is a clear need for ISO 9913-1 to be updated so as to accommodate the measurement of contact lenses with Dk values in excess of 100 barrer, by adopting one or more of the novel modifications as outlined above.

11.4   Corneal oxygen availability with silicone hydrogel lenses

11.4.1 Oxygen flux

Clinicians are interested in the performance of contact lenses with respect to their impact on the physiology of the ocular surface. As such, they need to consider the amount of oxygen which reaches the ocular surface during lens wear, that is defined as the 'oxygen flux'. Oxygen flux indicates the volume of oxygen that reaches a unit area of the corneal surface in unit time. In a number of ways, therefore, this is a more important clinical parameter than Dk, which is a laboratory measure that takes no account of ocular conditions.

For the range of Dk values offered by conventional hydrogels, there is an approximately linear relationship between Dk and corneal oxygen flux. Figure 11.5 presents the relationship between oxygen flux and transmissibility for open-eye and closed-eye conditions, for lenses of various thickness, using a mathematical model proposed by Brennan (2001). It is evident that, for conventional hydrogel lenses, increases in Dk afford similar proportional

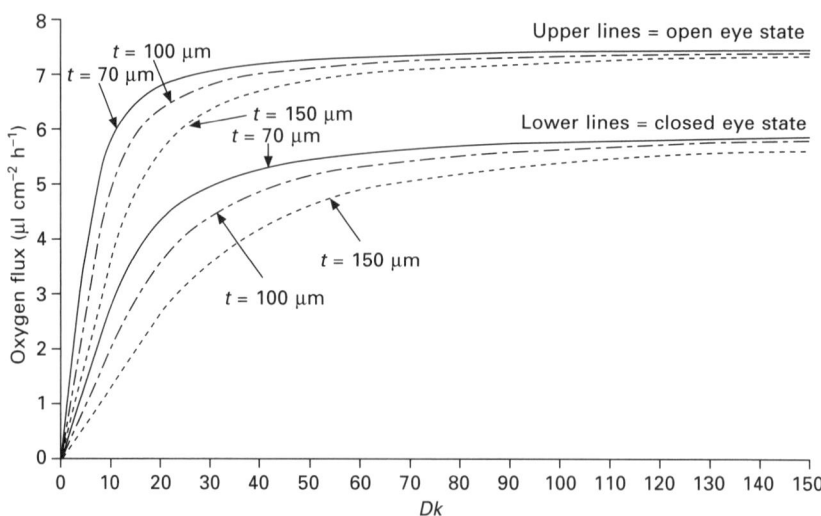

11.5 Relation between corneal oxygen flux versus *Dk* (barrers) for open- and closed-eye states during wear of contact lenses of 70 μm, 100 μm and 150 μm thickness.

changes in flux. As such, for conventional hydrogels, presenting values of *Dk* for contact lenses is reasonably informative in terms of understanding the amount of oxygen that reaches the ocular surface.

At higher levels of oxygen performance, however, it is clear that there is a system of 'diminishing returns'. That is, as measured contact lens *Dk* rises, the increase in the amount of oxygen that is delivered to the cornea reduces in magnitude. On this basis, it would seem that the use of *Dk* values in the era of silicone hydrogels is not appropriate. Corneal oxygen flux is a strong contender for replacing these parameters, although Brennan (2005), and more recently Chhabra *et al.* (2008) and Larrea and Büchler (2009), have argued for a more sophisticated and physiology-based approach which considers the amount of oxygen that is actually consumed by the cornea.

An important clinical ramification of flux theory as applied to contact lenses is that all silicone hydrogel lenses currently on the market are essentially equivalent in terms of corneal oxygen supply. This argument certainly applies to central corneal oxygenation. Alvord *et al.* (2007) have suggested that, for high minus-powered contact lenses, which are necessarily thicker in the lens periphery, oxygen flux can be significantly reduced in the peripheral cornea if silicone hydrogel lenses of lower *Dk* are fitted. This interpretation has been disputed by Brennan (2008), who argues that the minimum *Dk* required to fully oxygenate the peripheral cornea is only 30 barrer – not 125 barrer as suggested by the Alvord model.

11.4.2 Critical oxygen requirement

A vital question in understanding the issues relating to contact lens oxygen performance is the amount of oxygen that is required for normal corneal physiology. This has been addressed in many different ways historically. For open-eye (daily wear) conditions, the best known value is that of Holden and Mertz (1984), who suggested that a lens with Dk/t of 24.1 barrer/cm/would not induce corneal swelling during daily wear. At the time of the work, Dk values were not normally edge-corrected, and the edge-corrected equivalent Dk/t value is 21.8 barrers/cm (Table 11.3).

The situation for overnight wear is more complex. Holden and Mertz (1984) found that a lens with a transmissibility of 87 barrer/cm (73 barrer/cm if edge-corrected values are employed) would limit overnight corneal swelling to 4% – a value considered to be that of a non-lens wearer. Subsequent workers, using a variety of rationales, have reported thresholds up to 300 barrer/cm. Superficially, this seems to be a large range of values, which clearly must be in contradiction with each other. However, when these values are considered as flux measures, this difference is much reduced because of the relationship between oxygen flux and transmissibility.

Table 11.3 Estimates of critical oxygen transmissibility to avoid contact lens-induced corneal changes

Author	Year	Criterion	Dk/t (barrer/cm)
Holden and Mertz	1984	Zero day-wear oedema	24
Holden and Mertz	1984	Zero residual overnight oedema	34
Holden and Mertz	1984	Closed-eye oedema	87
O'Neal *et al.*	1984	Closed-eye oedema	75
Andrasko	1986	Closed-eye oedema	159
Ichijima *et al.*	1992	Epithelial cells	64
Tsubota and Laing	1992	PN/Fp ratio	59
Imayasu *et al.*	1993	LDH, MDH	64
Giasson and Bonanno	1994	Aqueous pH	18
Giasson and Bonanno	1994	Epithelial pH	300
Ichijima and Cavanagh	1994	LDH	84
Papas	1998	Open-eye limbal injection	125
Harvitt and Bonanno	1999	Oxygen profile modelling	125
Sweeney *et al.*	2004	Closed-eye oedema	125
Morgan *et al.*	2009a	Open-eye oedema – central cornea	20
Morgan *et al.*	2009a	Open-eye oedema – peripheral cornea	33

PN, pyridine nucleotides; Fp, Flavoproteins; LDH, lactate dehydrogenase; MDH, malate dehydrogenase.

11.5   Conclusions

The century-long battle to develop contact lenses that allow sufficient levels of oxygen to reach the anterior ocular surface during contact lens wear for normal corneal metabolism is over. Silicone hydrogel lenses have been measured by numerous authors to have very high Dk levels – in excess of 60 barrer for all contact lenses on the market today. Considerations of anterior eye corneal oxygen flux has lead to the conclusion that there is essentially no difference in oxygen performance between current-generation silicone hydrogel lenses.

However, the search for the perfect contact lens is not over. Although the issue of lens-induced hypoxia has largely been solved, other issues remain. For example, silicone hydrogel materials have a higher modulus (greater stiffness) than conventional hydrogels, which possibly confers a greater mechanical effect on the cornea. This can result in reduced lens comfort and mechanically induced effects such as disruption to the corneal and conjunctival epithelial surface (Alba-Bueno et al., 2009; Sorbara et al., 2009) and corneal infiltrative responses (Efron et al., 2005; Szczotka-Flynn and Diaz, 2007). Silicone hydrogel contact lenses are still associated with a risk of microbial keratitis, albeit low (Efron et al., 2005; Stapleton et al., 2008), and strategies need to be developed to reduce the risk of lens-associated infection even further. No doubt attention will now turn away from the question of oxygen and will begin to focus more acutely on some of these unresolved issues, in search of the 'perfect' contact lens.

11.6   References

Alba-Bueno F, Beltran-Masgoret A, Sanjuan C, Biarnés M and Marín J (2009), 'Corneal shape changes induced by first and second generation silicone hydrogel contact lenses in daily wear', *Cont Lens Anterior Eye*, **32**(2), 88–92.

Alvord L, Court J, Davis T, Morgan C F, Schindhelm K, Vogt J and Winterton L (1998), 'Oxygen permeability of a new high Dk soft contact lens material', *Optom Vis Sci*, **75**(1), 30–36.

Alvord L A, Hall W J, Keyes L D, Morgan C F and Winterton L C (2007), 'Corneal oxygen distribution with contact lens wear', *Cornea*, **26**(6), 654–664.

Andrasko G J (1986), 'Corneal deswelling response to hard and hydrogel extended wear lenses', *Invest Ophthalmol Vis Sci*, **27**(1), 20–23.

Brennan N A (2001), 'A model of oxygen flux through contact lenses', *Cornea*, **20**(1), 104–108.

Brennan N A (2005), 'Beyond flux: total corneal oxygen consumption as an index of corneal oxygenation during contact lens wear', *Optom Vis Sci*, **82**(6), 467–472.

Brennan N A (2008), 'Oxygen modeling of the peripheral cornea', *Cornea*, **27**(2), 258–259.

Brennan N A, Efron N, Holden B A and Fatt I (1987), 'A review of the theoretical concepts, measurement systems and application of contact lens oxygen permeability', *Ophthal Physiol Opt*, **7**(4), 485–490.

Chhabra M, Prausnitz J M and Radke C J (2007), 'A single-lens polarographic measurement of oxygen permeability (*Dk*) for hypertransmissible soft contact lenses', *Biomaterials*, **28**(30), 4331–4342.

Chhabra M, Prausnitz J M and Radke C J (2008), 'Diffusion and Monod kinetics to determine in vivo human corneal oxygen-consumption rate during soft contact-lens wear', *J Biomed Mater Res B Appl Biomater*, **90**(1), 202–209.

Compan V, Andrio A, Lopez-Alemany A, Riande E and Refojo M F (2002), 'Oxygen permeability of hydrogel contact lenses with organosilicon moieties', *Biomaterials*, **23**(13), 2767–2772.

Dumbleton K A (2003), 'Noninflammatory silicone hydrogel contact lens complications', *Eye Contact Lens*, **29**(1 Suppl), S186–S189.

Efron N (2004), *Contact Lens Complications*, Edinburgh, Butterworth-Heinemann.

Efron N and Ang J H B (1990), 'Corneal hypoxia and hypercapnia during contact lens wear', *Optom Vis Sci*, **67**(7), 512–521.

Efron N and Carney L G (1979), 'Oxygen levels beneath the closed eyelid', *Invest Ophthalmol Vis Sci*, **18**(1), 93–95.

Efron N, Morgan P B, Cameron I D, Brennan N A and Goodwin M (2007), 'Oxygen permeability and water content of silicone hydrogel contact lens materials', *Optom Vis Sci*, **84**(4), 328–337.

Efron N, Morgan P B, Hill E A, Raynor M K and Tullo A B (2005), 'Incidence and morbidity of hospital-presenting corneal infiltrative events associated with contact lens wear', *Clin Exp Optom*, **88**(4), 232–239.

Fleiszig SM (2006), 'The Glenn A. Fry award lecture 2005. The pathogenesis of contact lens-related keratitis', *Optom Vis Sci*, **83**(12), 866–873.

Giasson C and Bonanno J A (1994), 'Corneal epithelial and aqueous humor acidification during in vivo contact lens wear in rabbits', *Invest Ophthalmol Vis Sci*, **35**(3), 851–861.

Harvitt D M and Bonanno J A (1999), 'Re-evaluation of the oxygen diffusion model for predicting minimum contact lens oxygen transmissibility values needed to avoid corneal anoxia', *Optom Vis Sci*, **76**(10), 712–719.

Holden B A and Mertz G W (1984), 'Critical oxygen levels to avoid corneal edema for daily and extended wear contact lenses', *Invest Ophthalmol Vis Sci*, **25**(10), 1161–1167.

Ichijima H and Cavanagh H D (1994), 'Effects of rigid lens extended wear on lactate dehydrogenase activity and isozymes in rabbit tears', *Cornea*, **13**(5), 429–434.

Ichijima H, Petroll W M, Jester J V, Ohashi J and Cavanagh HD (1992), 'Effects of increasing Dk with rigid contact lens extended wear on rabbit corneal epithelium using confocal microscopy', *Cornea*, **11**(4), 282–287.

Imayasu M, Moriyama T, Ohashi J and Cavanagh HD (1993), 'Effects of rigid gas permeable contact lens extended wear on rabbit cornea assessed by LDH activity, MDH activity, and albumin levels in tear fluid', *CLAO J*, **19**(153), 153–157.

ISO (1996a), ISO International Standard 9913-1 'Optics and optical instrumentation – Contact lenses – Part 1: Determination of oxygen permeability and transmissibility by the Fatt method', Geneva, International Organization for Standardization.

ISO (1996b), ISO International Standard 9913-1 'Optics and optical instrumentation – Contact lenses – Part 2: Determination of oxygen permeability and transmissibility by coulometric method', Geneva, International Organization for Standardization.

Iwata J, Hoki T and Ikawa S (2005), 'Long wearable soft contact lens', Asahi Aime Co. Ltd, Tokyo, Napan.

Iwata J, Hoki T and, Ikawa S (2006), 'Silicone hydrogel contact lens', Asakikasei Aime Co. Ltd and CooperVision Inc., Tokyo, Napan.

Klyce S D (1981), 'Stromal lactate accumulation can account for corneal oedema osmotically following epithelial hypoxia in the rabbit', *J Physiol*, **321**, 49–64.

Künzler J and Ozark R (1994), 'Fluorosilicone hydrogels', US Patent 5321108.

Larrea X and Büchler P (2009), 'A transient diffusion model of the cornea for the assessment of oxygen diffusivity and consumption', *Invest Ophthalmol Vis Sci*, **50**(3), 1076–1080.

Loftstrom T and Kruse A (2005), 'A conjunctival response to silicone hydrogel lens wear', *Contact Lens Spectrum*, **20**(9), 42–44.

Maiden A C, Vanderlaan D G and Turner D C (2002), 'Hydrogel with internal wetting agent', Johnson & Johnson Vision Care Inc., Jacksonville, Florida, USA.

Maldonado-Codina C and Efron N (2005), 'Impact of manufacturing technology and material composition on the surface characteristics of hydrogel contact lenses', *Clin Exp Optom*, **88**(6), 396–404.

Maldonado-Codina C and Morgan P B (2007), 'In vitro water wettability of silicone hydrogel contact lenses determined using the sessile drop and captive bubble techniques', *J Biomed Mater Res A*, **83**(2), 496–502.

Maldonado-Codina C, Morgan P B, Efron N and Canry J-C (2004a), 'Characterization of the surface of conventional hydrogel and silicone hydrogel contact lenses by Time-of-Flight Secondary Ion Mass Spectroscopy', *Optom Vis Sci*, **81**(6), 455–460.

Maldonado-Codina C, Morgan P B, Schnider C M and Efron N (2004b), 'Short-term physiologic response in neophyte subjects fitted with hydrogel and silicone hydrogel contact lenses', *Optom Vis Sci*, **81**(12), 911–921.

Mandell R B (1988), 'Historical development', in Mandell R B (ed.), *Contact Lens Practice*, 4th edn, Springfield, Charles C. Thomas, p. 19.

McCabe K P, Molock F F and Hill G A (2004), 'Biomedical devices containing internal wetting agents', US Patent 6,822,016.

Mizutani Y, Iwashita H, Nozaki S and Tanahashi N (1992), 'The volumetric method of measuring the *Dk* of soft contact lens materials', *J Jpn Contact Lens Soc*, **34**, 283–288.

Morgan C F, Brennan N A and Alvord L (2001), 'Comparison of coulometric and polarographic measurement of a high-Dk hydrogel', *Optom Vis Sci*, **78**(1), 19–29.

Morgan P B and Efron N (1998), 'The oxygen performance of contemporary hydrogel contact lenses', *Cont Lens Anterior Eye*, **21**(1), 3–6.

Morgan P B, Maldonado-Codina C, Quhill W, Rashid K, Brennan NA and Efron N (2009a), 'Central and peripheral oxygen transmissibility thresholds for the avoidance of corneal swelling during open eye soft contact lens wear', *Biomaterials* (in press).

Morgan P B, Woods C A, Tranoudis I G, Efron N, Knajian R, Grupcheva C N, Jones D, Tan K O, Pesinova A, Ravn O, Santodomingo J, Vodnyanszky E, Montani G, Itoi M, Bendoriene J, van der Worp E, Helland M, Phillips G, González-Méijome J M, Radu S, Belousov V, Silih M S, Hsiao J C and Nichols J J (2009b), 'International contact lens prescribing in 2008', *Contact Lens Spectrum*, **24**(2), 28–32.

O'Neal M R, Polse K A and Sarver M D (1984), 'Corneal response to rigid and hydrogel lenses during eye closure', *Invest Ophthalmol Vis Sci*, **25**(7), 837–842.

Papas E (1998), 'On the relationship between soft contact lens oxygen transmissibility and induced limbal hyperaemia', *Exp Eye Res*, **67**(2), 125–131.

Pearson R M and Efron N (1989), 'Hundredth anniversary of August Müller's inaugural dissertation on contact lenses', *Surv Ophthalmol*, 34(2), 133–141.

Skotnitsky C, Sankaridurg P R, Sweeney D F and Holden B A (2002), 'General and local contact lens induced papillary conjunctivitis (CLPC)', *Clin Exp Optom*, **85**(3), 193–197.

Sorbara L, Jones L and Williams-Lyn D (2009), 'Contact lens induced papillary conjunctivitis with silicone hydrogel lenses', *Cont Lens Anterior Eye*, 32(2), 93–6.

Stapleton F, Keay L, Edwards K, Naduvilath T, Dart J K, Brian G and Holden B A (2008), 'The incidence of contact lens-related microbial keratitis in Australia', *Ophthalmology*, **115**(10), 1655–1662.

Sweeney D F, du Toit R, Keay L, Jalbert I, Sankaridurg P R, Stern J, Skotinsky C, Stephensen A, Covey M, Holden B A and Rao N (2004), 'Clinical performance of silicone hydrogel lenses', in Sweeney D F (ed.), *Silicone Hydrogels. Continuous Wear Contact Lenses*, Edinburgh, Butterworth-Heinemann, pp. 164–216.

Szczotka-Flynn L and Diaz M (2007), 'Risk of corneal inflammatory events with silicone hydrogel and low dk hydrogel extended contact lens wear: a meta-analysis', *Optom Vis Sci*, **84**(4), 247–256.

Tanaka K, Takahashi K and Kanada M (1979), 'Copolymer for soft contact lens, its preparation and soft contact lens made therefrom', US Patent 4139513.

Tighe B (2004), 'Silicone hydrogels: structure, properties and behaviour' in Sweeney D F (ed.), *Silicone Hydrogels. Continuous Wear Contact Lenses*, Edinburgh, Butterworth-Heinemann, pp. 1–27.

Tsubota K and Laing R A (1992), 'Metabolic changes in the corneal epithelium resulting from hard contact lens wear', *Cornea*, **11**(121), 121–126.

Weidemann K E and Lakkis C (2005), 'Clinical performance of microchannel contact lenses', *Optom Vis Sci*, **82**(6), 498–504.

Weissman B and Fatt I (1989), 'Stacking samples while measuring oxygen transmissibility of hydrogel contact lenses', *Optom Vis Sci*, **66**(4), 235–238.

Wichterle O (1978), 'The beginning of the soft lens' in Ruben M (ed.), *Soft Contact Lenses. Clinical and Applied Technology*, London, Baillière Tindall, pp. 3–5.

Wichterle O and Lim D (1960), 'Hydrophilic gels for biological use', *Nature*, **185**(4706), 117–118.

Young M D and Benjamin W J (2003), 'Oxygen permeability of the hypertransmissible contact lenses', *Eye Contact Lens*, **29**(1 Suppl), S17–21.

12
Extended wear contact lenses

B. J. TIGHE, Aston University, UK

Abstract: The chapter shows how the successful design of polymers for contact lens applications depends on the need to provide a balance of properties appropriate to the ocular environment. The principal relevant aspects of the anterior eye are tear film, eyelid and cornea, which govern the requirements for surface properties, modulus and oxygen permeability, respectively. In the case of extended (overnight) wear, oxygen permeability is the most critical because of the reduced availability of oxygen to the avascular cornea. The relationship between permeability requirements and the developing view of the needs of the cornea, in terms of oxygen consumption, are discussed and the particular roles of fluorine and silicon in the design of successful polymers described. The evolution of polymer design is taken as a background for the consideration of the current generation of silicone hydrogels, which have proved to be the most successful family of materials for this demanding application.

Key words: extended wear contact lenses, oxygen permeability, fluoropolymers, silicone hydrogels, ionic permeability.

12.1 Introduction

It is perhaps not immediately obvious that the use of polymers in contact lenses represents an excellent example of biomaterials design. The use of quite similar materials in joint replacement, heart valves, membrane oxygenators and haemodialysis membranes presents specific problems associated with, for example, their biocompatibility, strength and permeability that might seem to be absent in contact lenses. This is certainly not the case, however, and the general biomedical principle of designing the material to give a balance of properties appropriate to the particular environment is of prime importance. The situation is obviously less critical in the case of lenses intended for daily wear only, than for those intended for successive day and night periods, frequently referred to as extended wear. Nonetheless, properties very similar to those required for other biomedical applications are involved. Indeed, the research carried out into the use of hydrogels in contact lenses provides information on a range of materials that will assist future work on their use in other medical applications.

The properties that are relevant to the contact lens field are important in different ways and to different extents. Some are essential to the successful performance of the lens in the eye; others affect convenience of handling, while a third group govern the behaviour of the lens during manufacture. The relative importance of the various properties will further depend upon whether the lens is intended for daily wear or extended (overnight) wear. In addition, some properties such as refractive index and density vary by relatively small amounts within a given range of polymers, but will not greatly affect the potential usefulness of a material, whereas others have a critical and limiting effect on the ability of the lens to perform successfully.

In general terms, a lens for extended wear must be considered as an extension of the cornea. Thus, the lens must allow the cornea to respire normally, it must resist the deforming force of the eyelid and it must permit a continuous tear film to be maintained around the lens, while minimising the accumulation of deposits. These factors can be discussed in terms of oxygen permeability, rigidity modulus and surface properties. Some attempt must be made therefore to put quantitative limits on these very important properties, which are discussed in relation to hydrogel structure in Chapter 19. Once these fundamental requirements are met, there are properties controlling aspects of lens behaviour that relate to patient perception to consider. Perhaps the most important of these relates to long-term comfort and the maintenance of adequate lubrication of the lens throughout the day. This is the area of biotribology, reflected principally in the coefficient of friction between the lens and the eyelid, together with the changes in this property brought about by factors such as progressive lens dehydration and changes in the tear film. Since coefficient of friction is so affected by these environmental changes and is difficult to measure accurately and reproducibly, it has only recently been recognised as an important measurable parameter in assessing materials properties.

It is always instructive to consider the nature and properties of any biological environment that is to be interfaced with a synthetic biomaterial. Making a synthetic material equivalent to the cornea presents formidable difficulties, since corneal surface and bulk properties are separately governed by the epithelium and stroma, and their natures are quite different. Such information is valuable, however, in providing a basis for understanding the way in which contact lens materials behave in the eye, particularly in extended wear. Appropriate data are summarised in Table 12.1. These lead on naturally to a more detailed consideration of achievable properties of available materials in relation to their structure. Although this discussion is primarily concerned with the behaviour of hydrogel contact lenses in relation to the factors discussed in Chapter 19, it extends naturally to

Table 12.1 Typical properties of the cornea and its environment

Surface tension of tears	46 mN m^{-1}
Thickness of tear film	7–10 μm
Rigidity modulus of cornea	1 MPa
Critical surface tension of cornea	35 mN m^{-1}
Oxygen consumption of cornea	5×10^{-6} l cm^{-2} h^{-1}
Partial pressure of oxygen (open eye)	155 mm
Partial pressure of oxygen (closed eye)	55 mm

other materials that can satisfy, in whole or part, the very demanding requirements of successful extended wear of contact lenses.

There are three important couplings of aspects of the anterior eye and physicochemical properties of the lens material:

- cornea and transport properties;
- eyelid and mechanical properties;
- tears and surface properties.

The cornea is avascular when healthy and governs the oxygen permeability requirements of the material. The eyelid, which exerts a significant deforming force, governs the need for a balance between comfort and visual stability. The tear film, which maintains ocular lubrication and defence, governs the wettability and (together with the eyelid) frictional requirements. These links, and the properties shown in Chapter 19, Table 19.1, need to be considered in the context of the more detailed stuctural aspects of the anterior eye discussed elsewhere in this volume. The cornea is a complex composite structure with a high epithelial turnover rate. The tear film is 'structured' with a thin superficial lipid layer that 'breaks up' at time intervals (which are very patient dependent) of approximately 10 seconds. The aqueous component of the tear film has a volume of some 7–10 μl and is replenished at a rate of around 1 μl per minute. Lipid turnover is appreciably slower.

Set in this context, the various aspects of contact lens design seem to face very considerable problems, for the simple reason that the contact lens is some ten times thicker than the tear film. This means that the problems associated with lens wettability and tear film stability are more severe than those in the non-lens-wearing eye. A stable tear film needs to exist on both anterior and posterior surfaces of the lens and adequate post-lens tear flow needs to be maintained in order to remove cellular debris and metabolic waste products. The necessary lens movement means that the mechanical property requirements are not the same as those of the cornea itself. One important consequence of the fact that the lens is so much thicker than the tear film is that the tear film break-up time is markedly reduced and the lipid layer is progressively deposited on the anterior surface of the lens. If the lens material has an affinity for lipids, these are immobilised and exposed to oxygen and light for very much longer periods than is the case in the normal eye, where lipid turnover minimises such problems. As well as these problems, which are common to both daily wear and extended wear lenses, extended wear faces additional problems – one of which is central to the discussion in this chapter: this is the need to allow the cornea to respire in a substantially undisturbed fashion in an environment where the partial pressure of oxygen is reduced from around 155 mm to some 55 mm.

12.2   Oxygen: corneal requirements and the limitations of hydrogel permeability

The importance of oxygen to corneal metabolism and the physiological consequences of oxygen deprivation in this respect have long been recognised. A great deal of information has been published over the last 40 years as the quantitative aspects of the subject have been addressed with increasingly sophisticated techniques. Two questions have been addressed: how much oxygen is required to satisfy the requirements of the cornea, and how does that information convert to the required permeability of lens materials? The development of measurement techniques has been at the heart of the progress that has been made.

The oxygen requirement of the cornea has been expressed in various ways, including a direct figure for oxygen consumption (as shown in Table 12.1) and, alternatively, as the minimum partial pressure of oxygen required to maintain normal corneal metabolism. Such quantities are difficult to measure in such a manner that the techniques employed give unambiguous results and do not, in their use, influence corneal behaviour. Thus, the value accepted as the minimum partial pressure of oxygen required to prevent corneal oedema, which was 11–19 mmHg in 1970 had progressively risen to 23–37 mmHg by 1980. In the following decade, available techniques for measuring increases in corneal thickness increased in sensitivity. Experimental results show an approximately exponential decline in corneal thickness with increase in available oxygen, which makes it increasingly difficult to obtain an absolute correlation between the two values. In consequence, clinical assessments of the oxygen requirements at that time varied between 40 and 74 mmHg. A useful overview of these developments has been compiled by Efron and Brennan (1987). Although these considerations may seem somewhat obscure, they are central to the design of materials for extended wear contact lenses.

The translation of corneal oxygen requirement to the thickness and oxygen permeability (P) of a material can be approached in various ways. The minimal partial pressure of oxygen (sometimes called oxygen tension) required at the anterior surface of the epithelium is assumed to be the minimum oxygen tension required behind a contact lens during both- open and closed-eye conditions. This value can then be inserted into a simple relationship, which enables the oxygen flux (F) across the epithelial surface under a tight-fitting contact lens (i.e. assuming no leakage from the side) to be determined. As indicated above, in the 1970s a value of around 15 mmHg was considered to be appropriate, which produces a value for F of approximately $3.5 \times 10^{-6} \, 1 \, cm^{-2} \, h^{-1}$. This is taken as a minimum but sufficient oxygen flux to maintain corneal transparency. The resultant value can then be used in equation [12.1], which relates the oxygen flux (F) to the permeability (P) and thickness (t) of a polymer membrane, and the pressure gradient across the membrane (Δp). Δp will be the difference between the partial pressure of available oxygen (Table 12.1) and the minimum partial pressure required at the corneal surface.

$$F = P/t \times \Delta p \qquad [12.1]$$

It was on the basis of this, and similar, approaches that the figures for oxygen permeability requirements for daily wear and extended wear in the 1970s were widely accepted as 5–8 barrers and 25–30 barrers, respectively. From Chapter 19, it will be seen that this requirement is readily satisfied by hydrogels with equilibrium water contents (EWCs) of around 40% and around 70%, even with lenses of 0.1 mm centre thickness. At that period in contact lens history this was very much the accepted view. The relevant background including calculations, available data and relevant references are summarised elsewhere (Tighe, 1989).

As the 1980s progressed, the approach to extended wear and particularly the relationship between available oxygen and corneal health changed. Instrumentation for measurement of corneal oedema improved and clinical complications associated with chronic corneal hypoxia were reported. In addition, techniques for measurement of oxygen permeability were standardised, values quoted in manufacturer's literature became more conservative, and the widely accepted value for the partial pressure of oxygen in the closed eye was questioned. In 1984, Holden and Mertz published data to support their view that in order to prevent overnight hypoxia-induced oedema, extended wear contact lenses should have an oxygen transmissibility equivalent to a P/t of 87 (equation [12.1]). This corresponds to an oxygen permeability of 87 barrers for a lens of 0.1 mm centre thickness (Holden and Mertz, 1984). There has been an ongoing division of opinion about the merits of increasing this value, but it remains the most widely quoted baseline requirement for extended wear lenses.

12.3   The evolution of contact lens materials: the drive for increased permeability

In order to understand the permeability of polymers and the way in which the oxygen transport requirements for extended wear materials have been met, we have to look more closely at the nature of permeability. The coefficient, P, for a given species (the permeant) through a polymer is a product of two terms:

$$P = DS \qquad [12.2]$$

These two terms are the diffusion coefficient, D, and a solubility term, S. It has become conventional in the contact lens field to replace the term S by K, and to refer to the permeability coefficient as Dk. While the diffusion term is related to the mobility of the polymer chains and the ease with which the permeant (e.g. oxygen) molecule can meander through them, the solubility term is governed by the amount of oxygen that the material can dissolve at a given ambient partial pressure. Thus k is a partition coefficient. Values of Dk are conveniently quoted in barrers, where 1 barrer = 10^{-11} cm^{3}O$_2$ (STP) cm/s cm^2 mmHg.

Thus Dk (or P) is the permeability coefficient for a given material, and the transmissibility of a sample of a given thickness t (such as a contact lens) of that material becomes Dk/t. Since lenses are around 0.1 mm thick, the values of contact lens transmissibility are usually quoted with units of 10^{-9} (cm $\times$ mlO$_2$)/(s ml mmHg), which keeps them numerically similar to Dk values.

Chapter 19 shows that incorporation of water into a glassy polymer not only increases the ease of diffusion, but also provides a medium that dissolves oxygen. Not surprisingly, then, the more water that the polymer contains, the greater amount of oxygen that it will dissolve and the higher the resultant permeability. Additionally, the water acts as a plasticiser, as described in the same chapter, and progressively increases the ease of diffusion. There is, however, a limitation imposed by water as a transport medium. The product of diffusion and solubility (i.e. permeability or Dk) in a conventional hydrogel will always be significantly below the value for water itself, which at 34 °C is no more than 100 barrers. Given the fragility of high-EWC hydrogels, especially if lens thickness is reduced in order to increase Dk/t, there is no possibility of meeting the Holden and Mertz criterion with conventional hydrogel contact lenses. The story of contact lens material development has been driven by attempts to increase both D and k while maintaining levels of surface and mechanical properties appropriate to successful lens wear.

Several types of material have been used in contact lens production, some more successfully that others. The most significant, in approximate order of availability, are:

* glass;
* poly(methyl methacrylate) (PMMA);
* conventional hydrogels;
* silicone rubber;
* rigid gas permeable lenses (RGPs);
* silicone hydrogels.

Of these, all except glass and PMMA have been used in extended wear lenses. Currently, silicone hydrogels are growing dramatically in importance, RGPs have a very limited market appeal and silicone rubber has minimal use except in a medical setting. Each material has, however, contributed to the existence and current success of silicone hydrogels. In order to understand the emergence and unrivalled position of silicone hydrogels, it is necessary to examine some preliminary data.

The solubility of oxygen in water is relatively low – less than 5 ml oxygen/ ml water at 25 °C and atmospheric pressure. Workers in various fields have sought inert liquids of similar physical properties, for example, boiling point, in which to carry out oxygen-mediated processes more effectively. Typical silicone oils having molecular weights around 350 show oxygen solubilities of around 100 ml/100 ml silicone oil at 25 °C. Silicones are not the only organic compounds with high oxygen dissolution capabilities that have been harnessed in the contact lens field. Fluorocarbons show similar, although less marked, dissolution advantages over water; perfluoro-n-heptane, which also has a molecular weight of around 350 and a boiling point of 115 °C, shows an oxygen solubility of around 45 ml/100 ml fluorocarbon at 25 °C. Fluorine and silicon are complementary, rather than competitive elements in polymer design. Fluorine can replace hydrogen directly in many organic compounds but can not form chains. Silicon, on the other hand, can form chains with oxygen (the silicones) and can replace carbon in certain situations. Figure 12.1 illustrates this point and provides the basis for an interesting comparison of relative oxygen permeability values of structures incorporating fluorine and silicon. As Fig. 12.1 shows, poly(hexafluoroisopropyl methacrylate) has a Dk value around 100 times greater than that of PMMA. Poly(dimethyl siloxane), better known in the form of silicone rubber, has a Dk value at least 1000 times greater than that of PMMA. Not surprisingly, these properties have not gone unexploited in the contact lens field.

There is one unusual feature about the development of silicon-based (and to a much lesser extent, fluorine-based) polymers as biomaterials. There has been a growing tendency in recent years to exploit the principles of biomimesis in biomaterials development. This was certainly the case in both Wichterle's original work, and much of the subsequent innovation and development in the field of hydrogels. It is useful to put these organofluorine and organosilicon compounds into perspective and to speculate why the body has no need of structures with similarly high oxygen permeability.

The number of chemical elements exceeds 100 but the vast majority (over 95%) of living matter is made up of only 4 (carbon, nitrogen, oxygen and hydrogen). There is no biomimetic driving force to exploit silicon or fluorine, or even analogous structures on which the polymers contained in Fig. 12.1 might be loosely based. When it comes to the historic development of materials based on natural resources, the story is rather different. The four most abundant elements on Earth are oxygen, iron, silicon and magnesium – fluorine joins the list at 17th. Historically, materials science was driven by commonly available inorganic raw materials such as metals and ceramics. It is only since the field of biomaterials has developed that materials science has turned to the structure and function of the human body for inspiration. In this respect silicon is something of an anomaly. Its role in the formation of glass gave it an important position in civilisation because of the unique

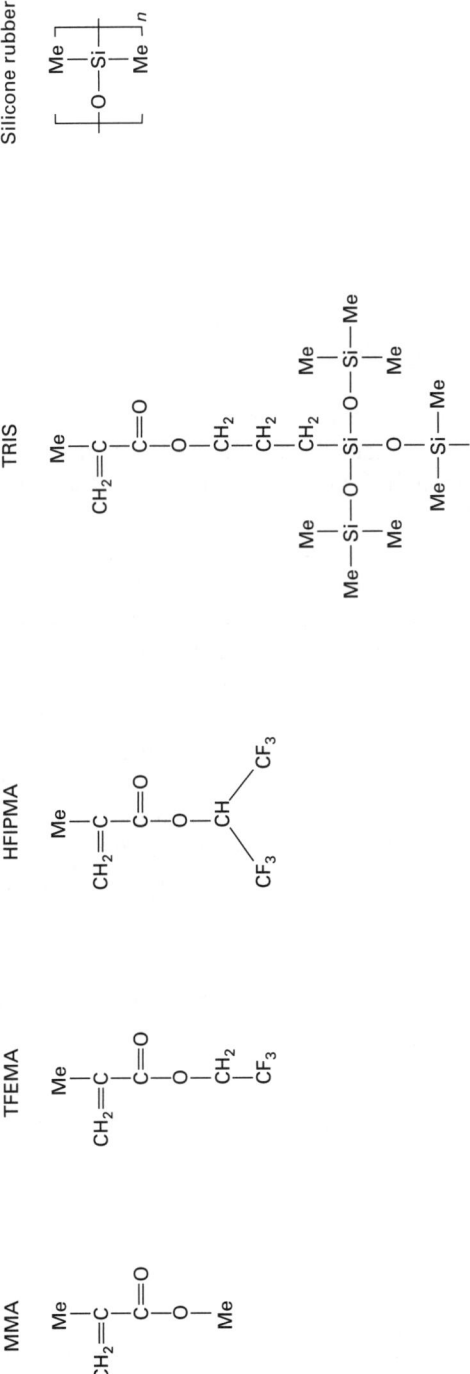

12.1 Fluorine-containing and silicon-containing polymers and their relative oxygen permeabilities. MMA, methyl methacrylate; TFEMA, trifluoroethyl methacrylate; HFIPMA, hexafluoroisopropyl methacrylate; TRIS, tris(trimethylsiloxy)-γ-methacryloxy-propylsilane; silicone rubber, poly(dimethyl siloxane). Oxygen permeability increases in the order: polyMMA < polyTFEMA < polyHFIPMA < polyTRIS < silicone rubber. Relative magnitude of increase c. 0.5, 25, 40, 300, 1000, respectively.

clarity and rigidity of this material. Because of these properties it was used in ancient cultures to represent living tissue – the eye – in statues of birds and animals. Much later glass was used to augment the function of the same organ, for example in tissue-contacting devices such as scleral contact lenses.

The fact that the element silicon is once more growing in importance in ophthalmic biomaterials is substantially unrelated to its place in materials history, however. Its new role is, on the face of it, unconnected to either its ability to form silicate glasses or its natural abundance. Nor is its use inspired by the way in which it performs in the human body – where it is largely absent. The very useful properties brought by silicon, and by fluorine, to the field of organic materials, and thence to polymer science, were discovered by experimentation rather than by design. The structures of the organic materials are quite different from those of their mineral precursors. Silicone groups contain the element silicon linked directly to both oxygen and to carbon atoms. Thus the terms siloxy and silicone refer to organic compounds of silicon, whereas silica and silicates are inorganic glasses containing oxygen but no organic carbon. Organofluorine compounds are also quite different from the naturally occurring fluorine minerals and certainly lack any biomimetic inspiration. The reason why a device such as the contact lens needs materials that are much more oxygen permeable than those present in the natural tissue seems fairly clear and relates to the fact that the contact lens is around ten times thicker than the tear film. Its thickness is not only a function of manufacturing constraints, but it is also a necessary consequence of the need for optical power and thus differential curvatures of anterior and posterior surface. It is in the blending of these curvatures to produce maximum comfort, reasonable lens movement and minimum possible disturbance to tear film stability that the skills of lens design are found.

12.4   Exploitation of silicon and fluorine: silicone rubber and rigid gas permeable lenses

The most useful characteristic that unites silicon and carbon is their ability to form polymers. One major difference between the siloxane (Si—O—Si) backbone and the carbon (C—C) backbone is in the ease of rotation resulting from differences in size, bond lengths and bond angles between the constituent atoms. These points are illustrated in Fig. 12.2. Their practical consequence in terms of permeability to oxygen is reflected in the fact that the Dk of silicone rubber is 40 times higher than that of the hydrocarbon analogue polyisobutylene. This widely known high gas permeability of silicone rubber led to its use in the medical field as a membrane oxygenator. The attractions of this material in the contact lens field were obvious. Silicone rubber lenses, surface treated to give acceptable wettability, were developed

Characteristic properties of C—C and Si—O bonds

	C—C	Si—O
Bond length (nm)	0.154	0.163
Bond angle (deg)	112	130
Rotational energy (kcal/mol)	3.6	30.2

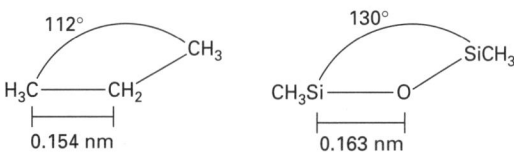

12.2 Characteristics of the Si—O—Si and C—C—C backbones.

in the mid 1960s and were found clinically to have little deleterious effect on corneal respiration. The problems of maintaining adequate surface properties, which were initially encountered in its routine clinical use, have never been fully overcome, despite a great deal of effort. The exceedingly hydrophobic nature of silicone elastomers resulted in poor lens wetting and rapid lipid deposition, which inevitably limited the use of these lenses. The uniquely high oxygen permeability, coupled with the resistance to tearing and general durability of the lens, led to its use in paediatric aphakia, where most of its applications still lie. Perhaps the best known silicone elastomer lens is Silsoft (Bausch & Lomb), which obtained US Food and Drug Administration (FDA) approval in 1984 as a 30-day extended wear lens for aphakia.

In retrospect, following many years of materials development and the study of the relationship between surface properties and mechanical properties, the behaviour of silicone rubber fits a clear pattern. Elastomers, such as silicone rubber, are in many ways intermediate between thermoplastics (such as PMMA) and hydrogels (such as polyhydroxyethyl methacrylate (PHEMA)). Thus, they possess to a degree the toughness associated with the former group of materials and the softness of the latter and in this sense they are ideal candidates for contact lens usage. Unfortunately, however, they all possess the same inherent disadvantage. The molecular features required for true elastic behaviour invariably produce polymers with hydrophobic surfaces. All polymers in this group, not only the silicone-based materials, require some form of surface modification to render them sufficiently hydrophilic for use as contact lenses, but because of the ease of chain rotation consequent upon their elastomeric characteristics, the surfaces slowly revert to their untreated state. This problem is made worse by the virtually instantaneous (dynamic) elastic recovery of the materials, which causes them to 'grab' the cornea after being deformed by the blink. This in turn displaces the posterior tear film and leads to lens binding. Despite the attempts to harness almost every available elastomeric material, as witnessed by the patent literature, no true elastomer has been successfully used as a commercial contact lens material. Current understanding of silicone hydrogel behaviour suggests a link between adherence to the ocular surface and inadequate fluid and ion transport. This indicates the fundamental difficulty in achieving reasonable lens movement with silicone elastomers, which coupled with the exceedingly hydrophobic nature which results in poor wetting and rapid lipid deposition, has led to very limited use of these lenses. The uniquely high oxygen permeability of the silicon–oxygen backbone has, however, been harnessed in two distinct types of contact lens material: the so-called rigid gas permeable (RGP) materials and the silicone hydrogels.

Once the need for a contact lens material with higher oxygen permeability than PMMA was established, a wide-ranging search began. A detailed account of the sequence of patents and products is given elsewhere (Tighe, 1989). If the principles of the separate contribution of diffusion and solubility to oxygen permeability are accepted, the logic of combining the ease of preparation of acrylics and the oxygen permeability of silicone rubber is inescapable. The siloxymethacrylates that form the basis of both current gas permeable and silicone hydrogel technology achieve this aim in a well-recognised, but nevertheless quite ingenious, way. The most widely used example is the siloxymethacrylate monomer tris(trimethylsiloxy)-γ-methacryloxy-propylsilane (Fig. 12.1), commonly referred to as TRIS. In essence, it consists of individual segments of silicone rubber structure assembled as pendant groups on to a modified methyl methacrylate molecule. This major advance was one aspect of the work of Norman Gaylord, which paved the way for the subsequent development of RGP contact lens materials. Another important aspect of Gaylord's work was the recognition of the value of incorporating fluoroalkyl methacrylates as comonomers, principally to enhance oxygen permeability (Gaylord, 1974, 1978).

The concept of a fluorine-containing contact lens was not entirely new, as the description of the advantages of contact lenses prepared from perfluoroalkylethyl methacrylates can be found in a series of DuPont patents (e.g. Cleaver, 1976). Whereas earlier descriptions of the advantages of fluorine incorporation went unexploited, however, Gaylord's patents led rapidly to commercial products. The underlying reason is that the fluoromethacrylates, on their own, do not produce a clinically significant balance of advantages over PMMA, whereas the gain in oxygen permeability of the siloxymethacrylates over conventional methacrylates is dramatic. The particular benefit of the fluorinated methacrylates comes when they are used to partially replace methyl methacrylate (as a comonomer) in copolymers with TRIS. The balance of the three components (fluoro methacrylate, methyl methacrylate and TRIS) is adjusted to optimise oxygen permeability, hardness (which influences processability) and wettability. Although Gaylord's patents marked the beginning of the inventive thread, several other workers made significant contributions to the development of lenses with advantages in clinical practice by identifying ways of optimising the balance of oxygen permeability, wettability and mechanical behaviour (Tighe, 1989). These led to the current commercially available high-*Dk* RGPs, which have *Dk* values above 100 barrers. They adequately meet the Holden and Mertz criterion and give excellent clinical outcomes with no significant adverse responses (Sweeney, 2004). There are, then, two distinct types of lens material that meet criteria for extended wear lenses, silicone rubber and RGPs. The properties of current commercial examples, together with those of PMMA for comparison, are summarised in Table 12.2.

Despite the fact that the Holden and Mertz criteria are exceeded by both these high-*Dk* material types, they have not given rise to successful high-volume cosmetic lenses. This is an illustration of the importance of addressing all the properties highlighted in Section 12.1 if successful lens performance is to be achieved. The materials in Table 12.2 have different shortcomings. Silicone elastomers suffer from poor wettability and high lipid deposition, which in turn cause problems with the lens adhering to the eye and subsequent adverse effects. The fact that lenses are not easy to manufacture in comfortable designs with good edge profiles adds to lens discomfort. RGP contact lens materials also have high *Dk* values, which undisputedly meet the corneal needs for oxygen. Although they have excellent tear flow behind the lens and produce no significant level of adverse responses, their popularity is poor with both practitioners and patients. Patients find them inherently uncomfortable and many practitioners experience difficulty in fitting the lenses, especially when compared with the current generation of single basecurve soft lenses.

12.5   The need for water: emergence of silicone hydrogels

The underlying concept that led to the development of the class of materials that have come to be called 'silicone hydrogels' follows logically from the description of the effect of water in conventional hydrogels. Since water

Table 12.2 Properties of silicone rubber and RGP contact lenses

Name (manufacturer/supplier)	Material type	*Dk* at 34°C (barrers)	Density	Refractive index
Equalens II (B&L/Polymer Tech)	Siloxy-fluoromethac copolymer (optifocon-A)	125	1.240	1.423
Fluoroperm 151 (Paragon Vision Sci)	Siloxy-fluoromethac copolymer (paflufocon-D)	151	1.10	1.442
Menicon SFP (Menicon Co.)	Siloxy-fluoromethac copolymer	102	1.120	N/A
Silicone rubber (Silsoft, B&L)	Silicone rubber	450	1.13	1.44
PMMA (for comparison)	Poly (methyl methacrylate)	0.5	1.195	1.49

B&L = Bausch & Lomb.

acts to dissolve oxygen and increase oxygen permeability of PMMA-like polymers, it follows that, if a substance showing greater solubility for oxygen than water could be incorporated in place of the conventional acrylic hydrogel backbone, a greater gain in oxygen permeability would follow. Additionally, and very importantly, the additional advantages of water described in Chapter 19 could be retained to some extent with potential advantage (at least over RGPs and silicone rubber) to both mechanical and surface properties.

The logical approach is to combine a typical hydrogel-forming monomer such as 2-hydroxyethyl methacrylate (HEMA) (Fig. 12.3) with the monomer that has been so successfully used in the preparation of RGP lens materials, commonly referred to as TRIS (Fig. 12.1). Although this is logical, there is one major difficulty. To combine hydrophobic TRIS with hydrophilic HEMA, and then hydrate the product, causes a degree of phase separation and does not readily yield an optically clear material. There are many ways around this problem, as witnessed by the growing number of commercial silicone hydrogel lenses based on subtly different chemistries and described in a range of patents (Tighe, 2000, 2004). The approaches described are not mutually exclusive and involve such strategies as:

- the synthesis of more hydrophilic variants of TRIS (Fig. 12.4);
- the synthesis of macromers (Fig. 12.5) consisting of short segments of

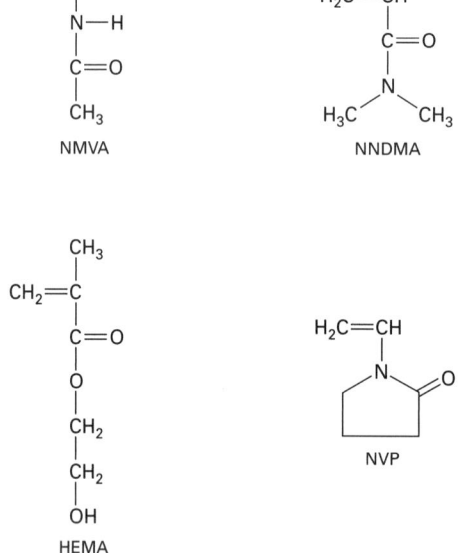

12.3 Hydrophilic monomers used in silicone hydrogel formation. HEMA, 2-hydroxyethyl methacrylate; NVP, *N*-vinyl pyrrolidone; NNDMA, *N,N*-dimethyl acrylamide; NMVA, *N*-methyl vinyl acetamide.

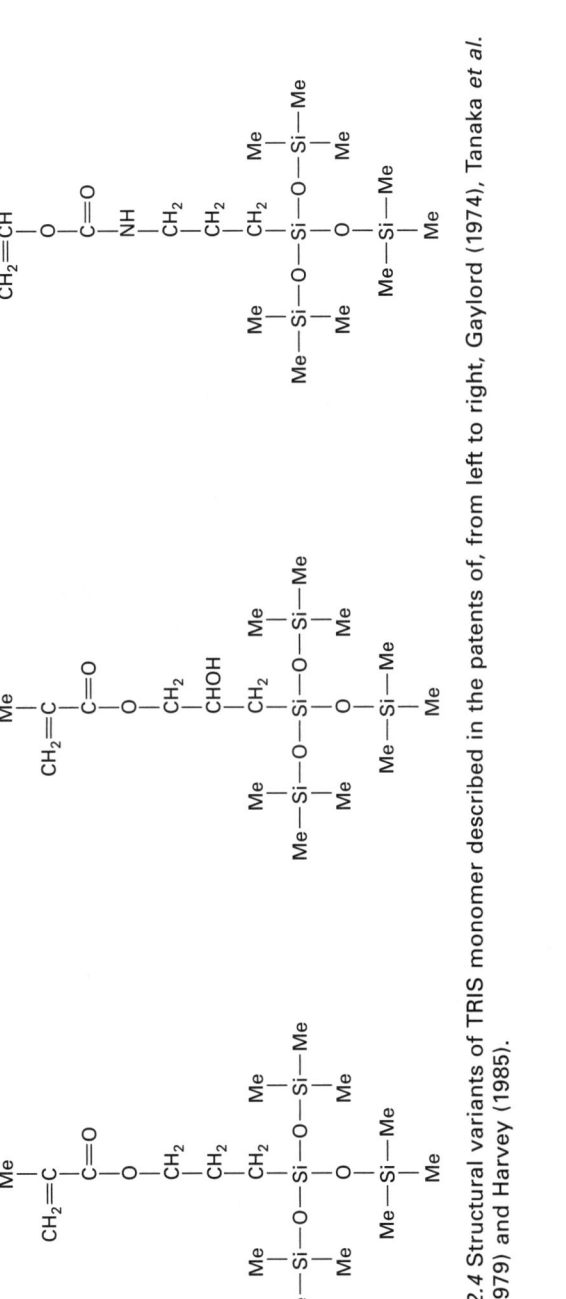

12.4 Structural variants of TRIS monomer described in the patents of, from left to right, Gaylord (1974), Tanaka *et al.* (1979) and Harvey (1985).

$$CH_2{=}\overset{\overset{\displaystyle CH_3}{|}}{C}{-}X{-}(OCH_2\,CH_2)_n{-}X{-}(O{-}\underset{\underset{\displaystyle CH_3}{|}}{\overset{\overset{\displaystyle CH_3}{|}}{Si}}{-})_n{-}X{-}(OCH_2\,CH_2)_n{-}X{-}\overset{\overset{\displaystyle CH_3}{|}}{C}{=}CH_2$$

(where n = 3–44, m = 25–40 and total molecular weight = 2000–10 000)

Siloxy-based polyether macromer

$$CH_2{=}\overset{\overset{\displaystyle CH_3}{|}}{C}{-}X{-}(O{-}\underset{\underset{\displaystyle CH_3}{|}}{\overset{\overset{\displaystyle CH_3}{|}}{Si}}{-})_n{-}X{-}(O\,CF_2\,CF_2)_m{-}X{-}(O{-}\underset{\underset{\displaystyle CH_3}{|}}{\overset{\overset{\displaystyle CH_3}{|}}{Si}}{-})_n{-}X{-}\overset{\overset{\displaystyle CH_3}{|}}{C}{=}CH_2$$

(where n = 5–100, but especially 14–28, and m = 10–30)

Siloxy-based polyfluoroether macromer

12.5 Examples of siloxy macromers (Nicholson *et al.*, 1996).

the siloxane chain alternating, for instance, with hydrophilic segments of poly(ethylene glycol);
- the use of monomers other than HEMA, for example, monomers that contain the $-N-CO-$ linkage (Fig. 12.3).

Two of these approaches have been at the heart of the development of successful silicone hydrogels over the last decade. The earliest patent to propose and exemplify a more hydrophilic version of TRIS was granted to the Toyo Contact Lens Company in 1979, with Kyoichi Tanaka as the principal inventor (Tanaka *et al.*, 1979). His solution to the problem involves inserting a hydroxyl group into the pendant propyl linkage – simple in concept but less simple to achieve in practice. The fact that another 20 years elapsed before the widespread launch of silicone hydrogel contact lenses illustrates the point that the problems are more complex than might have been initially assumed. This conclusion is further supported by the fact that additional approaches have been regularly described in the patent literature of the 1980s and 1990s, but it was not until the mid 1990s, however, that patents explicitly addressed the question of lens movement – which has proved to be a critical and contentious issue.

The second approach is the development of macromer technology. Macromers are large monomers formed by pre-assembly of structural units that are designed to bestow particular properties on the final polymer. This can be illustrated by a 1991 CIBA patent entitled 'Wettable, flexible, oxygen permeable contact lens containing block copolymer polysiloxane–polyoxyalkylene backbone units and use thereof', with Robertson, Su, Goldenberg and Mueller as the named inventors (Robertson *et al.*, 1991). The title describes very well the nature of the invention. The principle involved is the construction of a macromer that contains, typically, hydrophilic polyethylene oxide segments and oxygen permeable polysiloxane units. The patent formed the basis of CIBA's very significant 1996 patent, which has had such an influence on the field of silicone hydrogels, for reasons that will become apparent.

The property enhancement of silicone hydrogels by the incorporation of fluorine was a logical extension of previous knowledge and clearly offered potential benefits. A 1994 patent assigned to Bausch & Lomb and entitled 'Fluorosilicone hydrogels' is one of Jay Kunzler's many excellent contributions to the contact lens field (Kunzler and Ozark, 1994). It describes novel fluorosiloxane-containing monomers, which are claimed to be especially useful for the preparation of contact lenses. The monomers are designed to improve the compatibility of TRIS-like monomers in hydrophilic monomers thereby overcoming the compatibility problems outlined earlier. It was Kunzler who first illustrated the variation of oxygen permeability (Dk) with EWC of TRIS-based silicone hydrogels compared with the well-known Dk vs water content dependence of conventional hydrogels (Fig. 12.6).

The approaches described here, taken from patents over a 15-year period, highlight potentially successful synthetic approaches to the design of extended wear contact lens materials. Despite the length of time that the patents span and the range of companies – showing that synthetic expertise was widely spread – no successful commercial product emerged. The situation changed quite rapidly as the millennium approached. Until the mid 1990s, the three paradigm properties against which the potential success of new contact lens materials was judged were: wettability, mechanical behaviour and oxygen permeability. There were clearly other more or less obvious considerations such as optical clarity, cost, processibility, toxicity and deposit resistance

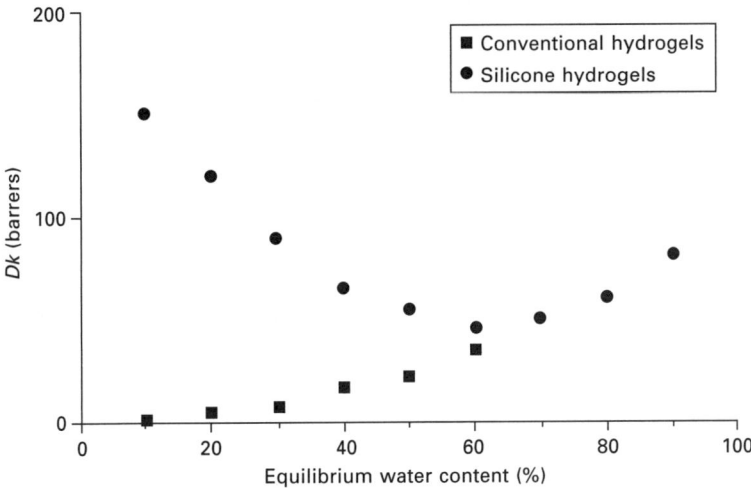

12.6 Variation of oxygen permeability (dk) with EWC of TRIS-based silicone hydrogels and conventional hydrogels.

but in terms of measurable physical properties that could be used (on the basis of acquired clinical experience) to predict minimum acceptable baseline performance of a material, reliance was inevitably placed upon measurement by appropriate methods of its wetting properties, oxygen permeability and mechanical properties. That situation lasted until the publication of an extensive CIBA patent (Nicholson *et al.*, 1996) that proposed a fourth type of property measurement, which is linked to lens movement on the eye – aqueous and ionic permeability.

12.6   CIBA patent WO 96/31792 (Nicholson *et al.*, 1996)

The CIBA patent WO96/31792(Nicholson *et al.*, 1996) entitled 'Extended wear ophthalmic lens', published on 10 October 1996, is so extensive and raises such important issues that have subsequently dominated the commercial arena that it must be considered here in some detail – although not specifically from the viewpoint of the patent lawyer. The patent encompasses a range of structures and methodologies (e.g. siloxy macromers with polyether and fluorine-modified polyether segments, biphasic structures, surface coating), which are central to the theme of the patent. The introductory sections of the patent are informative, highlighting the main issues and giving clues to the underlying philosophy of the invention. The background highlights what is perceived to be a shortcoming in the approach taken in previously described attempts to prepare successful silicone hydrogel extended wear materials and summarises the central object of the invention:

'... prior attempts at producing a true extended wear contact lens have been unsuccessful, either because of the effect of the extended-wear lens on corneal health or because the lens would not move on the eye. Thus, there remains a need for an ophthalmically compatible, transparent polymeric material, which is suited to extended periods of continuous contact with ocular tissue and tear fluid. An object of the invention is to provide a material having a balance of oxygen permeability, ion permeability, on-eye movement and tear exchange, all of which are sufficient for corneal health and wearer comfort during extended periods of continuous wear.'

One far-reaching feature of this patent is that the first (and arguably the most important) claim describes a principle or method upon the basis of which successful extended wear contact lenses may be designed. That is the combination of adequate oxygen permeability and adequate ionic or aqueous permeability. Much of the rest of the patent is concerned with a specific approach to the design of acceptable materials (the formation of biphasic structures) and with an appraisal of the link between ionic or aqueous permeability and lens movement on the eye.

12.6.1 Ionic permeability and biphasic structures

We now move to the principles involved in the improvements, which centre on the provision of both oxygen permeability and ion permeability in the lens together with a hydrophilic non-lipophilic coating. There are detailed descriptions of the ways in which an oxygen transmission pathway and an ion transmission pathway can be independently maintained. Their co-existence is made possible by the 'existence of a region of substantially uniform composition which is a distinct and physically separate portion of a heterogeneous polymeric material'. More particularly, with respect to the polymeric components of a lens, two different types of phase, an ionoperm phase and an oxyperm phase are described.

The picture that emerges is of a material that permits both oxygen and ions to permeate freely from front to back surface by means of two co-continuous phases. The water content range is subsequently defined as, desirably, 15–25% and the type of material involved is thus best described as a biphasic hydrogel with co-continuous ionopermeable and oxygen permeable phases. The term co-continuous highlights an important (in contact lens terms) and novel element of the invention since biphasic polymers frequently consist of one phase in isolated regions or droplets, within a second continuous phase; the major component normally forming the continuous phase. The oxyperm materials are described as monomers and macromers, which are siloxane-containing, fluorine-containing or carbon–carbon triple bond-containing. The ionoperm materials are simply hydrophilic monomers, which are known in hydrogel production, together with poly(ethylene glycol). These classes were already well known and have been described in the previous section.

There is nothing inherently novel in the broad description of the constituents of the invention as the novelty lies in the morphology, i.e. the existence of two co-continuous phases, coupled with optical clarity, and in the polymerisation methodology used in their formation. The achievement and maintenance of these two discrete co-continuous phases, which link the front and back surfaces of an optically clear lens, constitute the key inventive materials step of the patent. However, that is neither the only, nor arguably, the major feature of the patent. The patent is tied together with a clever knot. The co-continuous ionopermeable and oxygen permeable phases enable ion permeability and oxygen permeability to be independently modulated. This has enabled the first – and all-embracing – claim of the patent to be validated to the satisfaction of patent examiners. Thus, it established the basis upon which successful extended wear contact lenses may be designed: '…the combination of adequate oxygen permeability and adequate ionic or aqueous permeability'. The contribution of biphasic structures to the achievement of this requirement and the role of a 'hydrophilic non-lipophilic' coating to the success of an extended wear contact lens are important subsidiary aspects of the invention. The whole patent works together to define, with supporting evidence, the behavioural requirements for successful extended wear.

These four points – (a) the need for adequate oxygen permeability to satisfy corneal oxygen requirements; (b) the need for adequate ion permeability to promote lens movement; (c) the importance of biphasic structures in achieving ionic and oxygen permeability; and (d) the value of a coating in promoting compatibility with tear components – had not been previously identified collectively. The importance of oxygen and surface properties was well established, but the need for, and the use of, ion permeability as an indicator of successful extended wear had been nowhere referred to in previous work. The clever knot that links these points together does not require specific chemical structures to achieve this. Given the problems in achieving compatibility of inherently hydrophobic silicones and hydrophilic aqueous gels, it is probable that any silicone hydrogel will show some degree of segregation of hydrophilic and hydrophobic domains. Similarly, as water content increases, ion permeability will inevitably increase – independent of specific chemistry. When the range of commercial products is examined in a following section, it will be apparent that it is extremely difficult to develop a silicone hydrogel lens – even with novel chemistry – that does not fall within the scope of the concepts outlined above.

Although this patent contains a range of materials and different chemistries, the many compositions identified can be simplistically regarded as being formed from four components, a macromer (e.g. Fig. 12.5) plus TRIS monomer (Fig. 12.4), together with two 'solvents' (one of which is a hydrophilic monomer). The polymerisation involves an increase in molecular weight coupled with network formation together with a concurrent disappearance of one of the 'solvents' (usually *N,N*-dimethyl acrylamide (NNDMA); Fig. 12.3). The resultant network is left as a swollen gel in the 'permanent' solvent (e.g. ethanol). This polymerisation has all the features of a phase-inversion process, such as those used to form porous (sometimes asymmetric) membranes commonly used in separation processes. In the most common phase-inversion processes a mixture of solvents is evaporated from a polymer solution at differential rates. By control of the polymer precipitation and gelation process the microstructure of the resultant polymer is determined. In the process described here no evaporation occurs (if a closed mould is used) but the solvent properties change concurrently with the polymerisation by conversion of NNDMA monomer to matrix-bound copolymer. In conventional phase-inversion processes, the rate of solvent evaporation has a marked effect on the pore size and asymmetry of the product.

The consequence of successful polymerisation of this type is highlighted as the likely formation of porosity having dimensions in the region of 100 nm, reference also being made to the possible existence of an interphase region of distinct composition and structure. It is reasonable to comment that the patent has been, no doubt for commercial reasons, less explicit than it might have been in the exposition of the underlying principles of those features of the invention that underpin its success. It may be the intention to obscure a general principle that could be exploited by others with polymer structures that fall outside the scope of compositions claimed within the patent.

12.6.2 Ionic permeability: quantitative criteria for on-eye movement

In addition to describing optically clear phase-separated materials which allow ionic transport and oxygen transport to take place through separate phases, the CIBA patent establishes criteria for on-eye lens movement. These are essentially 'threshold values'; they can be best understood by examining the way in which sodium ion transport and aqueous transport relate to water content in conventional hydrogels. This is illustrated in Fig. 12.7. Conventional hydrogels behave in some ways as though they consist of dynamically fluctuating water-filled pores, the size of which diminishes as the water content decreases. Because water and oxygen molecules are similar in size, their permeability behaviour has many similarities. As a result, the way in which the oxygen curve in Fig. 12.7 varies with water content may be taken to represent the behaviour of water transport. This figure, for the remainder of the discussion, may be regarded as a representation of relative aqueous and sodium ion transport through all classes of non-phase-separated hydrogels. It is clear that sodium ion transport diminishes with water content more markedly than the transport of water itself and is totally impeded at

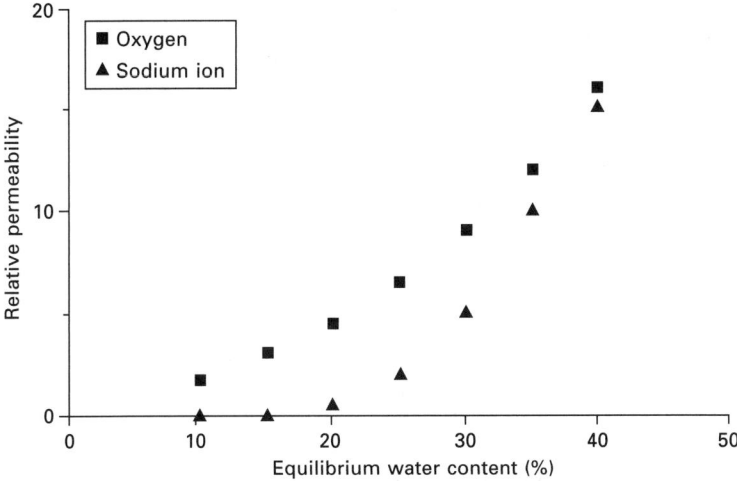

12.7 Comparative oxygen and sodium ion permeability as a function of water content.

water contents below 20%. The reason for this is the fact that sodium requires a shell of water molecules around it and is unable to diffuse through low water content membranes. This difference underpins the operating principle of desalination (reverse osmosis) membranes, which have a 'salt rejecting' polymer skin with a water content below 20%. This allows water to pass through under pressure, but 'rejects' sodium ions. It will be obvious from Fig. 12.7 that as the water content increases, the difference between ionic and aqueous permeability becomes unimportant, whereas as the water content falls, the ionic permeability becomes critical since the tear layer on both sides of the lens behaves as a dilute salt solution.

The extrapolation of these concepts to silicone hydrogels suggests that aqueous and ionic permeability will take place through the aqueous phase, whereas the transport of oxygen will take place predominantly through the silicone polymer phase. The patent goes on to describe and exemplify the limiting aqueous and ionic permeabilities that have been observed to be necessary for lens movement on eye. These have been overlaid on a graph of variation in sodium ion permeability with hydrogel water content in Fig. 12.8. The critical minimum sodium ion permeation value claimed in the patent to be necessary for lens movement $(0.2 \times 10^{-6} \text{ cm}^2\text{s}^{-1})$ is very similar to the reported literature value for PHEMA $(0.18 \times 10^{-6} \text{ cm}^2\text{s}^{-1})$. The patent claims that the same minimum value for aqueous permeability is required for lens movement $(0.2 \times 10^{-6} \text{ cm}^2\text{s}^{-1})$, which is consistent with the analysis suggested here. It also suggests that any hydrogel with a water content similar to that of PHEMA will have sufficient ion permeability to

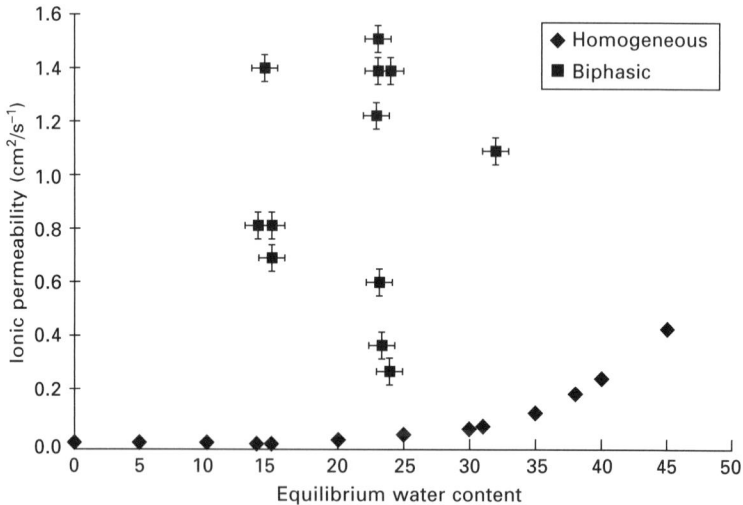

12.8 Variation in sodium ion permeability with hydrogel water content overlaid showing transition in lens movement (data from Nicholson *et al.*, 1996).

give adequate on-eye movement. The logical corollary is that only materials with water contents appreciably below this level (e.g. CIBA's Focus Night & Day contact lens material) will need the type of sophisticated bi-continuous biphasic described in this patent to achieve adequate on-eye movement. The effectiveness of the co-continuous biphasic structures in increasing the sodium ion permeability of such silicone hydrogels is illustrated in Fig. 12.9, with data taken from the patent.

12.7   Commercial products and further patents

The fact that the CIBA patent described above has proved to be so broad in the intellectual property net that it casts around the field of extended wear silicone hydrogel contact lenses has not inhibited further materials developments. It has rather had the effect of stimulating ingenuity as companies have sought to evade the all-inclusive intellectual property constraints. One aspect of this has been the development of ways of achieving sufficiently hydrophilic surfaces without the use of a separate surface coating or modification step. One approach is the incorporation of an internal wetting agent or hydrophilic interpenetrant polymer, either incorporated as such at the time of polymerisation or generated by *in situ* polymerisation. This fourth general strategy must be

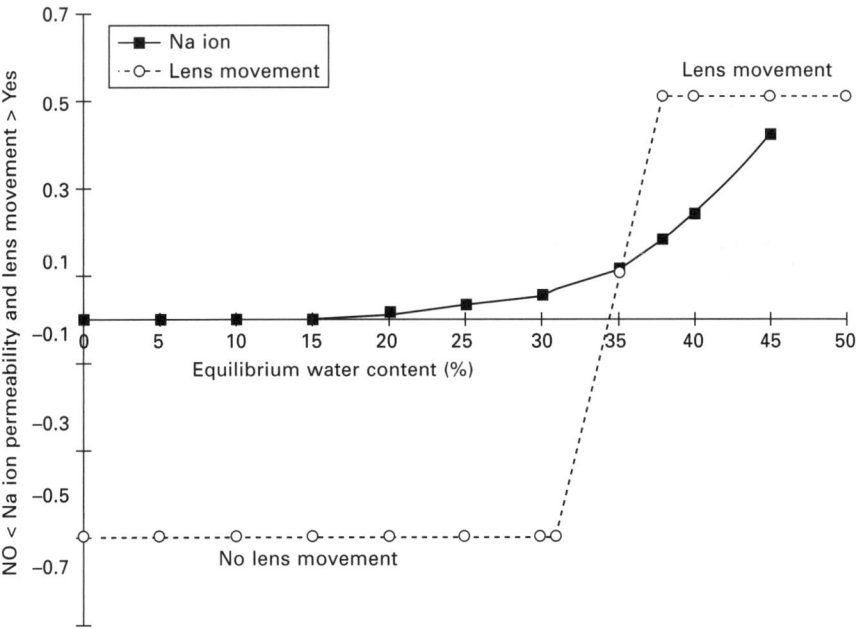

12.9 Variation in sodium ion permeability with hydrogel water content showing enhance permeabilities of biphasic structures (data from Nicholson *et al.*, 1996).

added to the three highlighted in Section 12.5 (hydrophilic TRIS variants, macromers and novel co-monomers). The first 10 years of silicone hydrogel extended wear lenses has seen a progressive change from (relatively) high modulus–low water content materials with surfaces modified by a separate discrete coating step, to lower modulus–higher water content materials with no coating. Even though these products are conceptually very different from the materials described in the CIBA patent of 1996, many of them fall within the broad behavioural criteria described in Section 12.6.2. As a result, there has been a steady stream of legal challenge, court case and royalty agreement reports in the press.

The most effective way of reviewing the technical developments is to follow the chronological appearance of commercial products (Table 12.3) commenting briefly on the underlying scientific features and advances described in their associated patents. Silicone hydrogel daily wear lenses whose oxygen transmissibilities do not meet the Holden and Mertz (1984) criteria are included since these sometimes serve to pave the way for the subsequent launch of an extended wear variant.

The first two commercial silicone hydrogels to be launched were the Bausch & Lomb PureVision (balafilcon A) lens and Focus Night & Day (lotrafilcon A) from CIBA Vision. Although they were launched within months of each other, patent issues have meant that sales of PureVision have been restricted to certain parts of the world. The PureVision material, balafilcon, is based on the approach of making more compatible versions of TRIS and employs the vinyl carbamate monomer illustrated in Fig. 12.4 (Bambury and Seelye, 1991, 1997). Unfortunately for Bausch & Lomb, CIBA Vision discovered a mid 1980s US patent (Harvey, 1985) that pre-disclosed the vinyl carbamate siloxy derivative. This surfaced among the intellectual property that came to them as part of the acquisition of Wessley-Jessen. The effect of this has been to prevent US sales of PureVision until the expiry of the Harvey patent. PureVision has a water content of 35% and a Dk of 110 barrers. It is said to have a water transport slightly (10%) in excess of that of PHEMA. This would put it above the critical minimum value of ionic and aqueous permeability for lens movement on the eye. This implies some degree of phase separation since the water transport value corresponds to a water content of 40% rather than 35%. Although Bausch & Lomb do not specifically claim that their material has biphasic characteristics, it has been shown to possess a degree of inhomogeneity (Lopez Alemany et al., 2002). In consequence, the material falls within the limits of the CIBA patent.

CIBA's approach, on the other hand, has been more focused on the macromers and polymerisation methodologies discussed in relation to the 1996 patent (Section 12.6). Two broad features underpin the Night & Day material. It is claimed to be a biphasic material with co-continuous channels enabling both high oxygen permeability and high ion (e.g. sodium) permeability to be

Table 12.3 Silicone hydrogel lens materials

				Proprietary name					
	PureVision	Focus Night & Day	Air Optix	Acuvue Advance	Acuvue Oasys	TruEye	Biofinity	Avaira	Clariti
United States adopted name	Balafilcon A	Lotrafilcon A	Lotrafilcon B	Galyfilcon A	Senofilcon A	Narafilcon A	Comfilcon A	Enfilcon A	N/A
Manufacturer	Bausch & Lomb	CIBA Vision	CIBA Vision	Vistakon	Vistakon	Vistakon	CooperVision	CooperVision	Sauflon
Water content (%)	36	24	33	47	38	54	48	46	58
Oxygen permeability (barrers)	99	140	110	60	103	100	128	100	60
Tensile modulus (psi)	148	238	190	65	92	96	105	80	80
Initial modulus (MPa)	1.1	1.4	1.2	0.4	0.6	0.66	0.8	0.5	0.5
Surface treatment	Plasma oxidation	Plasma coating	Plasma coating	Internal wetting agent (PVP)	Internal wetting agent (PVP)	Internal wetting agent (PVP)	None specified	None specified	None specified

achieved. In addition, it meets the defined minimum levels of ion or water permeation required to enable the lens to move adequately on the eye. The material (lotrafilcon A) is based on a fluoroether macromer of the general form shown in Fig. 12.5 copolymerised with TRIS monomer and NNDMA in the presence of a diluent. It is a fluoroether-based silicone hydrogel having a water content of 24% and a Dk of 140 barrers. With a water content as low as 24%, it is clear from Fig. 12.7 that neither sodium ion permeability nor aqueous permeability would approach that of PHEMA, if the structure were homogeneous. Because of the biphasic structure upon which the material is based, which allows oxygen and ionic permeability to be uncoupled (Fig. 12.9), the ionic permeability of the material exceeds that of PHEMA and consequently the lens is reported to have adequate on-eye movement.

One final difference between the PureVision and Focus Night & Day lenses lies in the surface treatment. Both are treated using gas plasma techniques but whereas Bausch & Lomb have opted for plasma oxidation, CIBA have chosen to apply a plasma coating. In the former case glassy islands are produced on the surface and on the latter a dense, 25 nm thick, high refractive index coating.

Much of the commercial realisation of this silicone hydrogel technology and especially the timing of product launches has been governed by patent ownership and litigation. Although Tanaka's monomer (3-methacryloxy-2-hydroxypropyloxy) propyl-bis(trimethylsiloxy)methylsilane (Fig. 12.4), was the first monomer of this type to be exemplified in the patent literature, it was not converted into a commercial silicone hydrogel in the lifetime of the patent. It formed the basis of not the first, but the third commercial silicone hydrogel lens. Tanaka's initial intent seems to have been to use it in RGP materials, primarily in an attempt to improve surface properties, although there is no evidence that it was successful in that role. Its use in silicone hydrogels did not come until the original 1979 patent had expired 25 years later. Despite the fact that the patent does contain details of silicone hydrogel lenses, these have proved very difficult to replicate using the synthetic methodologies described. In a well-thought out strategy, workers at Vistakon developed a much improved synthesis for the Tanaka monomer and were thus able to use it as a key component of Acuvue Advance (galyfilcon A), which was launched in 2004 upon the expiry of the original patent.

Galyfilcon A has a higher water content (47%), a lower Dk (60 barrers) and a much lower modulus than the two initial materials. Whereas both PureVision and Focus Night & Day are FDA approved for overnight use, Acuvue Advance is only approved for daily wear. The silicone hydrogel matrix is based on a combination of Tanaka's monomer, copolymerised with HEMA and NNDMA (Fig. 12.3), together with a simple siloxy macromer. The siloxy macromer is effectively a silicone rubber chain approximately 11 units long with a polymerisable methacrylate unit at the end of the chain.

The additional feature is the incorporation of poly(N-vinylpyrrolidone) (PVP) to enable an adequate degree of lens wettability to be achieved without subsequent surface treatment. The PVP is referred to as 'HydraClear™' technology and is sometimes described as functioning as an internal wetting agent (McCabe *et al.*, 2004).

Galyfilcon A was launched as a precursor to an extended wear version, senofilcon A, which has the name Acuvue Oasys. This material is based on the same chemistry, but has a water content of 38% and a *Dk* of 103 barrers. These second-generation silicone hydrogels are formulated quite differently from the first generation, as indicated by the much lower modulus of Acuvue Oasys in comparison to PureVision, which has a similar water content. The other marked difference is the absence of a coating, as PVP is serving to provide a wettable lubricious surface. In this general time frame, CIBA Vision launched a higher water content (33%) and lower *Dk* (110 barrers) version of Night & Day. This material (lotrafilcon B) was initially launched as O_2 Optix and subsequently renamed Air Optix. The marked difference in modulus of the CIBA Vision and Bausch & Lomb materials approach on the one hand and the Vistakon formulation on the other is clear from Table 12.3. The most recent development in the Vistakon portfolio is Acuvue TruEye (narafilcon A). Although this combines a water content of 54% with a *Dk* of 100 barrers (*Dk/t* = 117), it is currently sold as a daily disposable material suggesting that reformulation to achieve improvements in process technology have been the main driver. In 2008/2009 CibaVision introduced 'Aqua' versions of both Air Optix and Night & Day. These changes involve a surface modification step brought about by introducing an N-vinylpyrrolidone-co-N,N-dimethylaminoethyl methacrylate copolymer (commercially available as Copolymer 845, ISP Corporation) to the lens packing solution before the final autoclaving step. The intention is to increase initial comfort. Although no characterisation data are available as yet, it is interesting that this is effectively a means of producing a PVP surface.

The next silicone hydrogel lens to appear was the CooperVision Biofinity (comfilcon A). It combines a water content of 48% (marginally higher than Acuvue Advance) with an oxgen permeability of 128 barrers and a modulus intermediate between that of Air Optix and Acuvue Advance. A subsequent daily wear variant, Avaira (enfilcon A) has a similar water content (46%) coupled with a *Dk* of 100 barrers. The comfilcon material was immediately interesting for two reasons. The first was the absence of either surface treatment or an internal wetting agent. The second was the fact that the oxygen permeability is, on the basis of existing materials, unexpectedly high for its water content – as inspection of Table 12.1 shows. This is not, in principle, a completely unexpected development. The oxygen permeabilities of gas permeable materials vary over a wide range, indicating that the structure of the non-aqueous part of a silicone hydrogel will, equally, be capable of influencing the achievable oxygen permeability at a given water content. Similarly, the oxygen permeability of silicone rubber is appreciably higher than that of TRIS, indicating that replacing TRIS by more extensive linear sequences of siloxy material would lead to increased oxygen permeability. Examination of the relevant patent (Iwata *et al.*, 2006) indicates that this strategy has been used.

The technology underpinning the comfilcon material originates in a Japanese patent filed in December 2000 by the Asahikasei Aime Co., Ltd. Asahikasei Aime Company entered into an agreement with Ocular Sciences who subsequently became part of CooperVision leading to Iwata's 2006 patent. There are two interesting disclosures, which give a clue as to the reasons for the departure of comfilcon from the previous 'mould' in which silicone hydrogels had been developed. The first is the fact that the conventional 'TRIS' monomer and its derivatives are not used. Instead, the patent claims that two siloxy macromers of different sizes, one of which is only monofunctionalised (contains only one polymerisable double bond), when used together produce advantageously high oxygen permeabilities. The second is the use of vinyl amides as hydrophilic monomers. Whereas these monomers are well known (indeed NVP is a vinyl amide), the specific advantages of *N*-methyl-*N*-vinyl acetamide, which is a central component in the Iwata patent, have not been previously harnessed in silicone hydrogels. The patent contains other subtleties which, taken together, appear to have enhanced the compatibility of the silicone moieties with the hydrophilic domains and produced a very useful addition to the silicone hydrogel product portfolio.

The most recent silicone hydrogel to emerge is the only material produced by a UK company. The patent (Broad, 2008) has interesting features of novelty and ingenuity in this intensely competitive area. The essence of the patent is the production of a silicone hydrogel with a wettable surface without use of coating or added internal wetting agent. This aspect of the invention is achieved by incorporating sufficient NVP to ensure that the product contains a significant proportion of PVP homopolymer. This might be regarded as a sequential semi-interpenetrating network, which enables PVP to exert a similar surface influence to that encountered in patents that use preformed polymer in their formulation. The other element of novelty lies in the use of a siloxy monomer with a linear pendant polysiloxane chain – essentially a monofunctional macromer, which is used in conjunction with 3-methacryloxypropyl tris(trimethylsiloxy) silane. This, together with the use of hydrophilic monomer in addition to *N*-vinyl pyrrolidone enables an optically clear product to be obtained. The currently available lens (Clariti) based on this technology is a daily wear lens with a water content of 58%, a *Dk* of 60 barrers and a modulus equivalent to that of PHEMA.

12.8   Conclusions

12.8.1 Extended wear contact lenses: candidate materials

The criteria for successful extended wear, considered against the achievable properties of candidate materials, have led to the conclusion that, of the four families that have been examined for this type of contact lens, only three can meet current clinical requirements for oxygen transmissibility. Conventional hydrogels have many attractive features and from a theoretical standpoint it would be possible to meet the transmissibility requirements with ultra-thin (<50 μm), high water content (>75%) lenses. The practicalities of manufacturing an adequately durable lens to meet these constraints represents a considerable, but perhaps not insuperable, challenge. The combined approach of increasing water content and reducing lens thickness has received a considerable amount of attention in the past and has demonstrated that even if manufacturing and handling problems did not exist, there is a more major obstacle: lens dehydration. The proposed mechanisms and clinical consequences are beyond the scope of this discussion; suffice to say this has not proved to be a viable route to successful extended lens wear.

Each of the remaining candidate materials – silicone rubber, RGPs and silicone hydrogels – has attractions. Tables 12.2 and 12.3 summarise the oxygen transmissibilites of available examples of these materials and, in terms of oxygen transmissibilies alone, no single class would be excluded. The broad requirements discussed in Section 12.1, taken together with the clinical observations reported in Section 12.4, indicate that there is little or no prospect of success for a mass-market RGP or silicone rubber extended wear contact lens. Silicone hydrogels, in contrast, have developed into a wide-ranging family of materials as the information assembled in Table 12.3 shows.

12.8.2 Comparative properties of conventional and silicone-modified hydrogel materials

Until the mid 1990s the three paradigm properties against which the potential success of new contact lens materials was judged were wettability, mechanical behaviour and oxygen permeability. There were clearly other more or less obvious considerations – such as optical clarity, cost, processibility, toxicity and deposit resistance – but in terms of measurable physical properties that could be used (on the basis of acquired clinical experience) to predict minimum acceptable baseline performance of a material, reliance was inevitably placed upon measurement by appropriate methods of its wetting properties, oxygen permeability and mechanical properties. As a general observation, it can be said that the properties of silicone hydrogels are in many ways similar to those of conventional hydrogels. The earlier sections of this chapter have raised questions, however, as to the adequacy of the foregoing properties as criteria for the successful prediction of the clinical behaviour of silicone hydrogel lenses. Having brought information on a significant collection of these materials together, it is appropriate to assess wherein, and to what extent, their behaviour differs from the conventional hydrogels whose properties are discussed in Chapter 19.

Water content, permeability and mechanical properties

As a general rule of thumb, the most significant effect of increasing water content in silicone hydrogels is a decrease in both oxygen permeability and stiffness. The extensive CIBA 1996 patent (Section 12.6) proposed an additional type of permeability measurement, which is linked to lens movement on the eye – aqueous and ionic permeability. The patent, which underpins CIBA's Night & Day material, not only describes the preparation of biphasic materials with high oxygen permeability, it also defines minimum levels of ion or water permeation that are sufficient to enable silicone hydrogel lenses to move adequately on the eye. These levels of permeability correspond approximately to values independently measured for PHEMA. Because of this, the relevance of this property increases as water contents of silicone hydrogels fall markedly below that of PHEMA – especially since the elastomeric 'grab' of the materials also increases with decreasing water contents.

Although achievement of a threshold level of ion permeability was relevant in terms of the polymer design of Focus Night & Day and perhaps Air Optix, which have water contents significantly below that of PHEMA, the passage of time has made it less relevant to the development of new materials. The move to higher water contents and lower moduli, enabled by moves away from TRIS and its variants to longer siloxane sequences, has ensured that the materials produced have adequate ionic permeabilities as a consequence of their inherent water content. Nonetheless the teaching in the patent, and its translation to practice, has provided valuable information. The practical benefits of the biphasic approach appear to be primarily in the achievement of higher oxygen permeabilities while maintaining ion transport at the level achieved by conventional hydrogels. Now that there is such a wide range of available silicone hydrogels, the relative perceived importance of higher oxygen permeability, at a cost of compromise in other properties, will be demonstrated by practitioner and patient preference.

The relative oxygen permeabilities of the nine materials shown in Table 12.3 can be seen by inspection to show a general downward trend with increasing water content. Significantly, the permeabilities of the last four materials to be introduced all lie above the 'TRIS' line shown in Fig. 12.6. The primary advantage of materials with higher water contents is the consequent reduction in stiffness, and this is more important with silicone-containing than with conventional hydrogels. This is because the silicone content conveys elements of elastomeric behaviour, which becomes more apparent as silicone increases and water decreases. One aspect of this behaviour is that the stiffness changes as the rate of deformation increases – the faster the deformation, the stiffer the material appears to be. The deformational movement of the eyelid is rapid, whereas the deformation produced by handling a material is slow. There has been no need with conventional materials to employ sophisticated testing techniques but with silicone hydrogels the separate assessment of the viscous and elastic components gives important information. It does seem clear that the effect of these mechanical property characteristics, together with the contribution of silicone segments to the wetting behaviour – particularly the high hysteresis – was in significant part responsible for the clinical complications, such as SEALS (superior epithelial arcuate lesions), corneal erosions and CLPC (contact lens-induced papillary conjunctivitis), that were associated with the early years of silicone hydrogel use. The first generation of silicone hydrogels provided a clinical spearhead and brought a wealth of experimental data to the study of contact lens behaviour (Sweeney, 2004). The fact that the subsequent silicone hydrogels moved to higher water contents reflects two things. The first is that clinical research and opinion suggests that less stiff materials would be likely to produce better clinical outcomes. The second is that laboratory evaluation demonstrated that the aim of producing silicone hydrogels with mechanical properties more closely resembling those of conventional hydrogels entailed reduction of the high-frequency elastomeric behaviour described above. This, in turn, is much easier to eliminate as percentage water contents rise above the mid 30s.

Surface properties and spoilation

The most obvious measure of surface properties is wettability. There are several ways of measuring wettability, but perhaps the most generally valuable for contact lens materials is the dynamic contact angle technique in which a sample of material is repeatedly and cyclically immersed in, and removed from, a test solution (usually saline or water). The reason that this technique is so valuable is that it reflects the breaking and reformation of the tear film. Hydrogels undergo relatively rapid backbone rotation at an air interface with hydrophilic groups clustered into the gel and presenting hydrophobic groups externally. When covered by the tear film, the polar water-loving groups surround the hydrophobic polymer backbone. When the tear film breaks and leaves the surface of the hydrogel exposed to air or to a deposited lipid layer (both of which are relatively hydrophobic), the structure is more dominated by the relatively hydrophobic polymer backbone. The consequence of this change in the surface structure is that the intrinsic wettability of the polymer changes. This change is very effectively reflected in the change in contact angle as an aqueous layer advances over, and then recedes from, the surface. The advancing angle is designated as θ_A, the receding contact angle is designated as θ_R and the difference between them (the so-called contact angle hysteresis) is designated as θ_H.

There is a range of values of θ_A, θ_R and θ_H that have been found to correspond to minimum levels of clinical acceptability, and although values of around 70°, 20° and 50°, respectively, appear to be desirable for conventional hydrogels, materials showing lower wettabilities (i.e. higher values of θ_A and θ_R) perform reasonably well. It must be emphasised that wettability of unworn lenses as determined by dynamic contact angle is a necessary, but not sufficient, criterion for success. It is important that the material should retain its wettability (a) after spoilation by tear components, and (b) under load in friction studies.

For both conventional and silicone hydrogels, values of the receding contact angle generally lie between 25° and 45° with silicone hydrogels at the upper end of the range. The major difference between conventional and silicone hydrogels lies in the advancing contact angle, however. The advancing angle for silicone hydrogels is often around 100°, depending upon the time of exposure to air in the dipping cycle. A typical value for conventional hydrogels measured under the same conditions would be around 70°. All the currently available silicone hydrogels have wettabilities that are inferior to the best conventional hydrogels. This is not very marked until the materials are exposed to air – under these conditions that advancing contact angle rises sharply with time of exposure. The clinical consequence is that, as the front surface of the lens begins to dehydrate, it becomes very hydrophobic and consequently accumulates lipid deposits. This will be patient dependent and will be affected by a combination of tear break-up time and inter-blink period as well as tear lipid profile.

It is important to note that variations in individual tear chemistries frequently override differences between one material and another. There are, however, some useful generalisations to be made. The general tendency of hydrogels to undergo chain rotation, which is responsible for the differences in advancing contact angles of silicone hydrogels and conventional hydrogels, occurs much more readily in siloxane sequences than in carbon–carbon sequences. This has been discussed in Section 12.4. Additionally, silicones are hydrophobic, low surface energy materials. As a consequence, lipid accumulation is vastly greater on silicone hydrogel than on a conventional hydrogel surface. In contrast, protein accumulation on silicone hydrogels is very modest. For this reason, overall patterns of spoilation are quite different between the two classes of lens. Having commented that Focus Night & Day has the lowest water content and the highest modulus of the silicone hydrogels, it is important to indicate also that, because of the plasma coating on the lens, there is less opportunity for silicone group 'dynamics' at the surface. As a consequence, it has much more modest contact angle hysteresis and shows lower levels of surface lipid accumulation than the generality of silicone hydrogel lenses.

Biotribology and friction

Biotribology is concerned with lubrication, friction and wear at biological interfaces. The study of the biotribology of other body sites provides a sound basis for understanding the behaviour of the lens-wearing eye. The lubrication of the normal eye involves both aqueous and non-aqueous species (proteins, mucins, lipids, etc.) and mechanisms that are common to other body sites, such as articulating joints and lung alveoli. The contact lens influences these lubrication mechanisms, and when lubrication breaks down complications inevitably follow. In the *in vivo* situation, lid movement over the lens surface induces both movement of the lens on the cornea and transfer of shear forces to the ocular surface. Different contact lens materials show frictional differences, especially at start-up, but the presence and nature of the hydrodynamic lubricating layer are the single most important factors.

Because the retention of a liquid (hydrodynamic) layer is vital to the normal lens lubrication mechanism, it is clear that lens wettability is a necessary but not sufficient surface property criterion. Whereas measurement of advancing and receding contact angles provides information on the stability of the intrinsic wettability of the surface layer, measurement of the coefficient of friction under eyelid load gives an indication of the stability of the wetting layer during the blink. For conventional hydrogel lenses it has been demonstrated that, when this wetting layer (e.g. the tear film) is intact, the frictional behaviour of lenses is very similar. General observations about silicone hydrogels reflect the same behaviour but with differences of degree. The frictional coefficients of the silicone hydrogels with an intact lubrication layer are lower than those of most conventional hydrogels. This is a consequence of the techniques (internal wetting agent, etc.) that have been used to maintain the wettability of the lens. In contrast, changes of lubricating liquid and break-up of the lubricating layer cause appreciably greater increases in friction; a consequence of the inherent hydrophobicity and elastomeric character of the siloxy sequences.

It is clear that there is still some considerable margin for improvement in the surface properties of silicone hydrogel contact lenses. On the other hand, it must be emphasised that tremendous strides have already been made with this exciting group of materials. The properties of all the silicone hydrogel lenses described here are clinically acceptable and no one material is universally preferred. It is likely that perceived differences are driven as much by the patient as by the material. The problem of lipid deposition reflects this, because patient-to-patient variation in lipid levels is so marked and the propensity for lipid deposition is probably the single most undesirable feature of silicone hydrogels. Nonetheless, the development of silicone hydrogel extended wear lenses has been one of the major success stories in the history of the contact lens.

12.9   References

Bambury R E and Seelye D (1991), 'Vinyl carbonate and vinyl carbamate contact lens material monomers', US Patent 5070215.

Bambury R E and Seelye D (1997), 'Vinyl carbonate and vinyl carbamate contact lens material monomers', US Patent 5610252.

Broad R A (2008), to Sauflon CL Ltd, 'Contact Lens', WO/2008/061992.

Cleaver C S (1976), 'Contact lens having an optimum combination of properties', US Patent 3950315.

Efron N and Brennan N A (1987), 'In search of the oxygen requirement of the cornea', Contax, 1(6), 5–11.

Gaylord N G (1974), to Polycon Lab Inc., 'Oxygen-permeable contact lens composition methods and article of manufacture', US Patent 3, 808, 178.

Gaylord N G (1978), to Syntex USA Inc., 'Methods of correcting visual defects: compositions and articles of manufacture useful therein', US Patent 4, 120, 570.

Harvey T B (1985) Hydrophilic siloxane monomers and dimmers for contact lens materials and contact lenses fabricated therefrom US Patent 4,711,943.

Holden B and Mertz G (1984), 'Critical oxygen levels to avoid corneal edema for daily and extended wear contact lenses', Invest Ophthalmol Vis Sci, 25, 1161–1167.

Iwata J, Hoki T, Ikawa S and Back A (2006) Silicone hydrogel contact lens US Patent Application Number 11/213437.

Kunzler J and Ozark R (1994), 'Fluorosilicone hydrogels', US Patent 5321108.

Lopez-Alemany A, Compan V and Refojo M F (2002), 'Porous structure of Purevision versus Focus Night&Day and conventional hydrogel contact lenses', J Biomed Mater Res (Appl Biomat), 63, 319–325.

McCabe K, Molock F, Azaam A, Steffen R B, Vanderlaan D G and Young K A (2004), to Johnson & Johnson Vision Care Inc., 'Biomedical devices containing internal wetting agents', US Patent 6822016.

Nicholson P, Baron R, Chabrecek P et al. (1996), to CIBA Vision, 'Extended wear ophthalmic lens', WO 96/31792.

Robertson J R, Su K C, Goldenberg M S and Mueller K F (1991), 'Wettable, flexible, oxygen permeable contact lens containing block copolymer polysiloxane–polyoxyalkylene backbone units and use thereof', US Patent 5070169.

Sweeney D, Ed. (2004), Silicone Hydrogels (2nd Edition), Butterworth-Heineman, Oxford, UK.

Tanaka K, Takahashi K, Kanada M and Toshikawa T (1979), to Toyo Contact Lens Co. Ltd, Japan, 'Methyl di(trimethylsiloxy)silylpropyl glycerol methacrylate', US Patent 4 139 548.

Tighe B J (1989), 'Contact lens materials', Chapter 3 in Contact Lenses Practice (3rd Edition), Phillips A J and Stone J, Eds, Butterworths, London, pp. 72–124.

Tighe, B J (2000), Silicone hydrogel materials – how do they work? Chapter 1 in Silicone Hydrogels: the rebirth of continuous wear, Ed D Sweeney. Butterworth–Heineman, (pp 1-21).

Tighe, B J (2004), Silicone hydrogel materials – structure, properties and behaviour Chapter 1 in Silicone Hydrogels (2nd Edition), Ed D Sweeney. Butterworth–Heineman, (pp 1-27).

Part II

Applications in the posterior segment

13

Designing hydrogels as vitreous substitutes in ophthalmic surgery

K. E. SWINDLE-REILLY and N. RAVI, Washington
University in St Louis, USA

Abstract: In this chapter, the optimization of the design of vitreous
substitutes will be discussed. First, a review will explain the structure and
function of the vitreous humor and the need for a better vitreous substitute.
The approach taken in this work will be to develop a biomimetic vitreous
substitute. As a result, the next section will discuss the biomechanics of the
natural vitreous humor and the development of an animal model for the ideal
vitreous substitute. Mixture design is used to screen candidates rapidly for
use as *in situ*-forming polymeric hydrogel vitreous substitutes. Statistical
experimental design is used to determine the effects of the crosslinker
content, hydrophobic substitution, and polymer concentration in the hydrogel
on the optomechanical properties. In addition, the equilibrium swelling
properties are characterized and the osmotic pressure exerted by the hydrogel
is calculated to determine whether or not these hydrogels could tamponade
the retina via exertion of a slight osmotic pressure as vitreous substitutes.

Key words: vitreous substitutes, vitreous humor, *in situ*-forming hydrogel.

13.1   Introduction

For years, vitreous substitute research dealt primarily with looking for a
biocompatible fluid capable of approximating the retina to the posterior of the
eye. This has led to the development of several short-term vitreous substitutes.
However, they are not appropriate for long-term or permanent vitreous
substitution because of migration from the eye, toxic reactions, and other
unsuitable properties (Chirila *et al.*, 1998; Giordano and Refojo, 1998).

It would be more appropriate to design a vitreous substitute that mimics
the physical and mechanical properties of the natural vitreous humor.
Porcine, bovine, and human vitreous are natural hydrogels that have been
tested by rheological methods to determine their viscoelastic properties, and
the results have been recently summarized (Swindle and Ravi, 2007). It has
been determined that the vitreous behaves as a viscoelastic solid with higher
elasticity than viscosity.

Accordingly, the focus of recent vitreous substitute research has been on
polymeric hydrogels. Hydrogels are hydrophilic polymers that form a gel
network when crosslinked and are capable of absorbing several times their
weight in water. The result is typically a clear viscoelastic gel that strongly

339

resembles the natural vitreous humor. Hydrogels are more favorable vitreous substitutes because they are clear, tend to be biocompatible, and can act as a viscoelastic damper much like the natural vitreous (Chirila et al., 1998). Additionally, hydrogels exhibit controllable swelling in aqueous solution, which enables the substitute to push the retina into place by exerting osmotic pressure while swelling (Brannon-Peppas and Peppas, 1990).

The main problem with preformed polymeric hydrogels as vitreous substitutes is that they irreversibly shear upon injection into the eye during vitrectomy. This irreversible destruction of the network causes the hydrogels to lose some of their elasticity and become more fluid-like and viscous. Additionally, shearing of the hydrogels through injection breaks the crosslinks in the gels, potentially decreasing biocompatibility as a result of the uncrosslinked polymer chains infiltrating the posterior segment and causing irritation and variation in swelling pressure (Hong et al., 1996; Vijayasekaran et al., 1996; Chirila and Hong, 1998).

This problem has been addressed by our process of in situ regelation. Our group has achieved regelation in situ with disulfide chemical crosslinks, which are found in natural biopolymers such as proteins. These disulfide crosslinks form when the thiol-containing polymer comes into contact with oxygen. There are other methods of in situ gel formation such as thermally reversible gels and ionic gels (Suri and Banerjee, 2006). However, the formation of chemical crosslinks is preferable because it improves biocompatibility, increases retention in the eye, and mimics the natural vitreous.

The vitreous humor is an avascular network occupying the majority of the volume of the eye. The vitreous fills the space between the retina and the lens, allows for clear passage of light, holds the retina in place, and dampens eye movements. A schematic of the eye is shown in Fig. 13.1. It is known that the vitreous is a natural hydrogel composed of 99% water and a framework of collagen and hyaluronic acid. Even in a normal eye the vitreous undergoes syneresis or degradation. The collections of collagen fibers are frequently referred to as 'floaters', which may interfere with vision. Liquefaction of the gel structure can cause degeneration or detachment of the vitreous. Retinal detachment occurs when the neurosensory retinal segments separate from the retinal pigment epithelium. A number of vision-threatening phenomena, such as macular holes, retinal detachments, and vitreous hemorrhage, are associated with this transition (Los et al., 2003).

The vitreous humor undergoes liquefaction or transformation from a formed gel to a phase-separated fluid with advancing age, and in some cases it causes retinal detachments that can lead to blindness. The vitreous is removed during some surgical procedures and replaced with a vitreous substitute. No permanent vitreous substitutes are currently available, and the use of silicone oil as a vitreous substitute accelerates the formation of cataracts (Federman and Schubert, 1998).

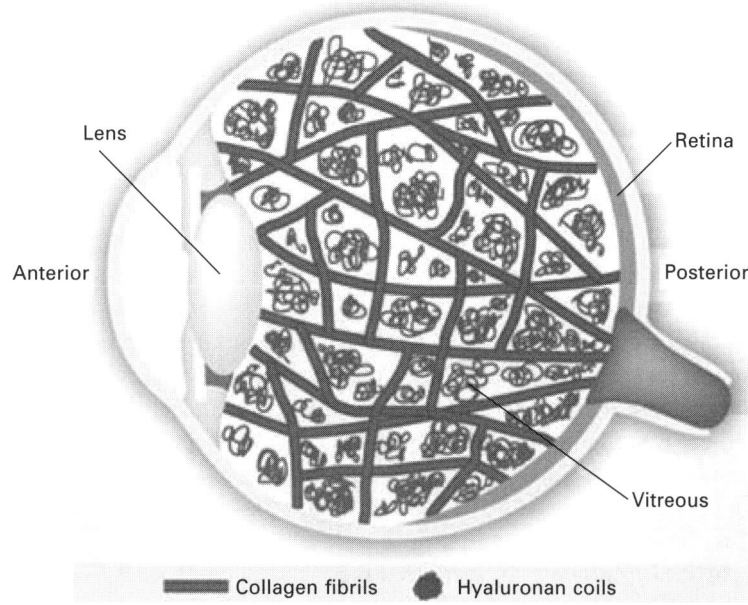

13.1 Ocular anatomy (Swindle and Ravi, 2007).

In recent years, research into vitreous substitutes has focused on polymeric hydrogels, and these have been reviewed extensively (Chan *et al.*, 1984; Chirila *et al.*, 1998; Soman and Banerjee, 2003 Swindle and Ravi, 2007). However, these preformed equilibrium-swollen hydrogels disintegrate when injected and sheared through a small gauge needle (Chirila and Hong, 1998). We have previously designed, synthesized, and characterized water-soluble thiol-containing copolymers that gel in the presence of oxygen (Foster *et al.*, 2006). Thus, prior to injection, they exist in polymeric form. The use of a reversible disulfide crosslinker in the initial formation of the hydrogel enables chemical reduction to a substantially pure thiol-containing copolymer that can undergo subsequent exhaustive purification and can regel under physiological conditions in the eye. In this work, the young porcine vitreous was characterized and used as an animal model for the development of the specification for vitreous substitutes. Then, potential vitreous substitutes that are *in vivo*-forming hydrogels were developed and characterized to meet the criteria established via testing of the natural vitreous humor.

13.2   Biomechanics of the vitreous humor

13.2.1 Background

The vitreous humor is a viscoelastic gel, which means that it exhibits both solid- and liquid-like behavior. The vitreous has a higher storage modulus

(G') than loss modulus (G''), which indicates its viscoelastic solid behavior. G' represents the elastic or recoverable component, whereas G'' represents the viscous component or dissipated energy. Its viscosity is highest in the posterior and decreases toward the anterior segment (Lee *et al.*, 1992).

The mechanical properties of the vitreous humor have been studied by several groups. Beginning in 1976, Bettelheim and Wang tested the viscoelastic properties of bovine eyes by inserting compression chucks in the vitreous cavity. A dynamic viscoelastometer applied compressional sinusoidal strain via electromagnetic transducers. In bovine vitreous, the storage and loss moduli were found to be 4.2–4.7 Pa and 1.9–3.7 Pa, respectively. They hypothesized that hyaluronic acid contributed to the viscosity and collagen contributed to the elasticity. Their results showed that the elastic and viscous components were of the same magnitude, but the elasticity was slightly higher (Bettelheim and Wang, 1976). The two biopolymers in the vitreous interact to form a stable hydrogel without syneresis or mechanical collapse when subjected to conditions that would normally destroy collagen networks (Chirila *et al.*, 1998).

In 1980, Zimmerman measured the viscoelasticity of the human vitreous *in vivo* by light scattering. He reported an elastic shear modulus of 0.05 Pa (Zimmerman, 1980). Tokita *et al.* used a torsional pendulum to measure the complex shear modulus of bovine vitreous at low frequencies, giving a shear modulus value of 0.5 Pa (Tokita *et al.*, 1984).

In the early 1990s, a magnetic microrheometer was developed by Lee *et al.* because typical rotational rheometers may destroy the vitreous structure. The fluid was stressed by moving a microscopic iron sphere in a horizontal direction under the influence of magnetic force magnets. They then used an empirical four-parameter viscoelastic model to calculate the creep compliance of human, bovine, and porcine vitreous. The model is mathematically equivalent to an ideal Burgers model, but the parameters are valid for their data from the microrheometric creep test. The Maxwell viscosity represents the unrecoverable viscosity, while the Kelvin viscosity represents the internal viscosity (Lee *et al.*, 1994). Several conclusions could be drawn from their work. The human vitreous has lower retardation times than the bovine or porcine vitreous, indicating faster recovery in the human eye. The vitreous humor is most viscous at the posterior in order to protect the retina and is less viscous at the anterior in order to allow rapid accommodation. The mechanical properties of the human vitreous are more similar to the porcine than to the bovine vitreous, and the human vitreous most closely resembles that of the central region of the porcine vitreous. Their results indicate that the porcine vitreous would serve as a suitable animal model for the human vitreous humor (Lee *et al.*, 1994).

A novel cleat geometry was recently developed to overcome wall slip in shear rheometry (Nickerson *et al.*, 2005). Initial G' and G'' values were 30

Pa and 16 Pa for bovine vitreous, and 9.5 Pa and 3.6 Pa for porcine vitreous, respectively. The final steady-state values were 6.5 Pa and 2.0 Pa for bovine vitreous, and 2.6 Pa and 0.65 Pa for porcine vitreous, respectively. Nickerson *et al.* reported storage moduli higher than all other sources, and postulated that the moduli are even higher *in vivo* owing to the noticeable decrease in modulus with time outside the eye. The hyaluronan trapped in the vitreous *in vivo* increases the modulus by placing the collagen network under internal tension as it swells to its equilibrium state. The release of tension would provide a driving force for modulus reduction and fluid expulsion when the vitreous was removed from the eye and hyaluronan was no longer trapped (Nickerson *et al.*, 2005).

As shown in Fig. 13.2 the human vitreous humor acts as a viscoelastic polymeric hydrogel. The high molecular weight elements, such as collagen and hyaluronic acid, provide a system that absorbs stress and protects eye tissues during eye movement and activity (Balazs, 1987). The combination of collagen and hyaluronic acid creates a mesh with primary stress supported by collagen fibrils and hyaluronic acid coils protecting the network from

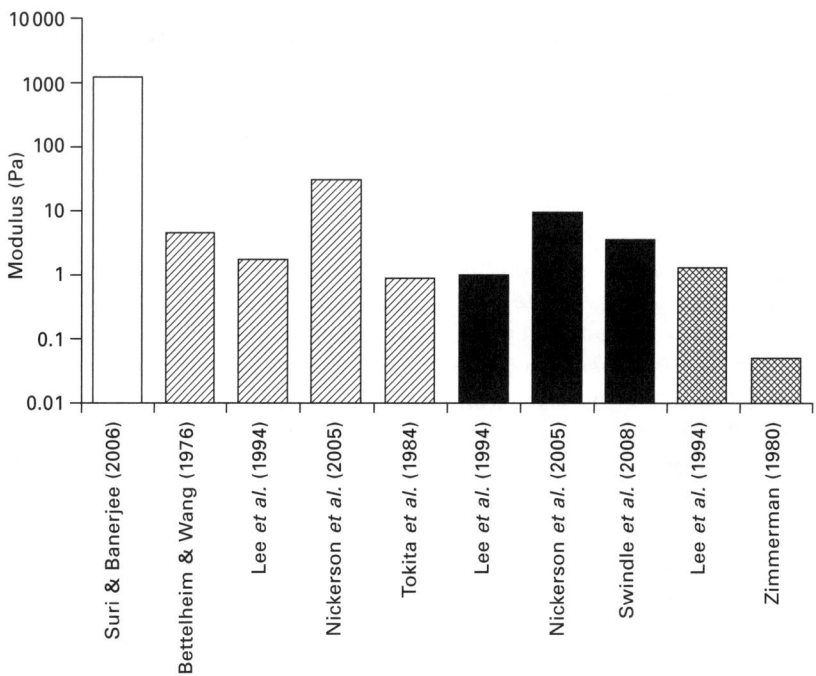

13.2 Literature values for modulus of vitreous humor. G', storage modulus; G_k, internal elastic modulus; g elastic shear modulus. Reproduced from *Expert Rev Ophthalmol*, **2**(2), 255–265 (2007) with permission from Expert Reviews Ltd (Swindle and Ravi, 2007).

collapse (Balazs, 1973). It is evident that a vitreous substitute should mimic the natural vitreous by being viscoelastic and transparent.

13.2.2 Experimental methods

Porcine eyes ($N = 90$) were used for analysis of the physical and mechanical properties of the natural vitreous humor. The eyes were obtained from 6-month-old pigs from a local abattoir (Weyhaupt Brothers Packing Company, Belleville, IL, USA). All eyes were tested within 12 hours of death to ensure retention of vitreous structure. Rheological analysis of the porcine vitreous is challenging because of the nature of the vitreous humor. The natural vitreous is a heterogeneous gel with solid gel components and liquid components that flow easily.

The sclera was cut around the exterior of the cornea and lens. The anterior segment of the eye was removed with tweezers, while the vitreous body remained attached to the lens. Finally, the vitreous was placed in a Petri dish and the lens was gently removed from the vitreous sample. When initially removed from the eye, the vitreous is a viscoelastic solid, but with time the structure degrades and the gel becomes fluidic and slowly starts to creep.

Viscoelastic properties were determined using the Vilastic-3 oscillatory capillary rheometer (Vilastic, Austin, TX, USA). The capillary rheometer was used for rheological evaluation because it enables testing of small samples and the central section of the porcine vitreous rather than the encapsulated vitreous body, which showed slippage effects on a parallel plate rheometer (Nickerson *et al.*, 2005). The capillary tube had an inner diameter of 0.149 cm. The anterior segment was removed from fresh porcine eyes, the vitreous was removed from the vitreous cavity, and approximately 0.5 cm^3 of the intact vitreous was aspirated for testing.

Samples were tested at 25 °C rather than at physiological temperature because Tokita *et al.* showed that the mechanical properties of the vitreous were temperature invariant from approximately 10 to 40 °C (Tokita *et al.*, 1984). The porcine vitreous was analyzed by frequency scans from 0.05 to 20 Hz at 0.05 strain, increasing shear rate from 0.05 to 30 s^{-1} at 2 Hz, or for 30 minutes at 2 Hz constant frequency and 0.5 s^{-1} shear rate. A frequency of 2 Hz was chosen for the constant frequency experiments because it was found to be the region most sensitive to changes in moduli (Buchsbaum *et al.*, 1984), and it was the frequency used by other groups that analyzed the vitreous humor (Nickerson *et al.*, 2005).

13.2.3 Results and disscussion

Porcine eyes ($N = 50$) were analyzed at a constant frequency of 2 Hz with shear rate increasing from 0.05 to 30 s^{-1} to simulate the degradation of a preformed hydrogel that may occur during the injection process. The data from nine eyes were considered statistical outliers. This could be due to the handling of the eyes before dissection, which sometimes resulted in samples with phase separation or retinal detachments. Figure 13.3 shows the average storage and loss moduli for porcine vitreous humor ($N = 41$) with increasing shear rate at an oscillation frequency of 2 Hz.

The storage modulus is slightly higher than the loss modulus, which indicates that the vitreous humor behaves as a viscoelastic solid. In addition, both the storage modulus and the loss modulus decrease with increasing shear rate. This indicates irreversible destruction of the fragile vitreous structure, which precludes the use of natural vitreous humor as a vitreous substitute.

A frequency scan was run on the porcine vitreous ($N = 34$) from 0.05 to 20 Hz at a constant strain of 5%. The data from eight eyes were determined to be outliers. The storage moduli and loss moduli of the porcine vitreous ($N = 26$) versus frequency are shown in Fig. 13.4. The frequency scan also shows a higher storage modulus than loss modulus for all frequencies tested. The modulus increased with increasing frequency, indicating that the sample was not allowed to relax between sample times at high frequencies.

As shown previously by other groups, the porcine vitreous humor is the best animal model for the human vitreous (Lee *et al.*, 1994). The porcine vitreous humor had never before been analyzed by capillary rheometry. Ninety eyes were evaluated, so a thorough depiction of the mechanical properties of the vitreous humor was achieved. The values obtained for storage and loss

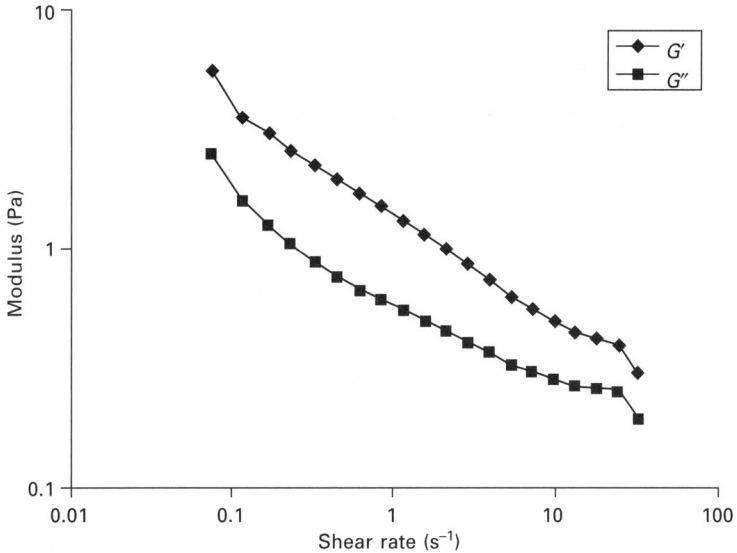

13.3 Porcine vitreous storage and loss moduli at 2 Hz.

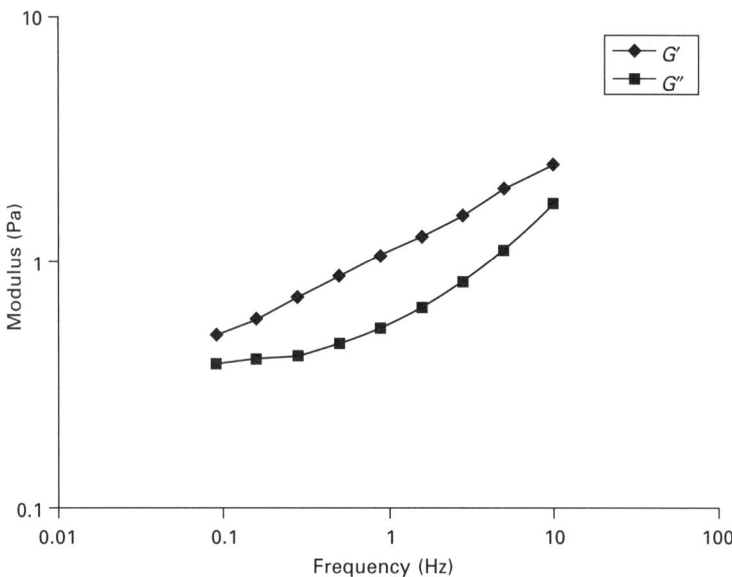

13.4 Porcine vitreous storage and loss moduli versus frequency.

moduli compare well with those obtained by other groups that analyzed the porcine vitreous humor by other methods. The viscoelastic properties obtained were used as the animal model for targeting the ideal vitreous substitute.

13.3   Vitreous substitutes

13.3.1 Background

A vitrectomy is a surgical procedure where the vitreous is cut and aspirated, and this is normally followed by replacement with an artificial substitute. A vitrectomy is usually performed for relief of traction and removal of blood from the ocular cavity. Currently, gases (air, sulfur hexafluoride, or perfluoropropane), perfluorocarbon liquids, fluorosilicone oil, or silicone oil (polydimethylsiloxane) are used as temporary vitreous substitutes to tamponade the detached retina against the posterior of the eye. These substitutes are not satisfactory for several reasons. For example, depending on the location of the retinal tear, these substitutes may require the patients to position themselves face down for days (Colthurst *et al.*, 2000). Silicone oil can be difficult to remove, has shown toxicity to intraocular structures, is capable of emulsification, and has been associated with glaucoma and corneal decompensation, both of which can lead to blindness (Leaver and Billington, 1989; Giordano and Refojo, 1998; Jonas *et al.*, 2001). Silicone oil is only 70% effective in retinal reattachment (Jonas *et al.*, 2001), and often the patient has to undergo subsequent cataract surgery after use of silicone oil as a tamponade (Leaver and Billington, 1989). Most importantly, none of these clinically available substitutes can be left in the eye safely for more than a few months (Giordano and Refojo, 1998). While silicone oil has been successful in retinal reattachment in some severe cases, it is evident that a better long-term vitreous substitute is needed. Silicone oils, perfluorocarbon liquids, and gases as vitreous substitutes have been extensively reviewed (Leaver and Billington, 1989; Sparrow *et al.*, 1990; Giordano and Refojo, 1998; Colthurst *et al.*, 2000; Jonas *et al.*, 2001; Versura *et al.*, 2001; Wolf *et al.*, 2003).

Initial research on vitreous substitutes focused on replacing the vitreous humor with vitreous from animals. However, because of the degradation of the vitreous outside the eye, these failed as vitreous substitutes (Deutschmann, 1906; Cutler, 1947). Next, researchers focused on developing vitreous substitutes from the natural components. However, the failure of collagen (Pruett *et al.*, 1972; Pruett *et al.*, 1974) Nakagawa *et al.*, 1997; Nayak, 1999; Liang *et al.*, 1998 and hyaluronic acid (Pruett *et al.*, 1979; Nakagawa *et al.*, 1997) to mimic the natural vitreous led to research into synthetic polymers. These synthetic polymeric vitreous substitutes, uncrosslinked and crosslinked hydrogels, are discussed below. Work with synthetic polymers began in the 1950s after poly(methyl methacrylate) was used in lens and cornea prostheses (Refojo, 1971).

In recent years, research of vitreous substitutes has focused on polymeric hydrogels, and these have been reviewed extensively (Chan *et al.*, 1984; Chirila *et al.*, 1998; Soman and Banerjee, 2003; Swindle and Ravi, 2007). However, these preformed equilibrium-swollen hydrogels disintegrate when injected and sheared through a small-gauge needle (Chirila and Hong, 1998). We have developed reversible hydrogels from acrylamide and N, N'-*bis*(acryloyl) cystamine (BAC), a disulfide crosslinker. The disulfide bonds were reduced to thiol groups, enabling purification and removal of all unreacted toxic monomer and low molecular weight polymers (Aliyar *et al.*, 2004). Gel elasticity was maintained after injection in human cadaver eyes (Foster *et al.*, 2006) and porcine eyes (Swindle *et al.*, 2006) *ex vivo*. The patient would not have to remain face-down for extended periods of time as is required for vitrectomy with traditional materials (Aliyar *et al.*, 2004). This work confirmed that these gels may be formed in the eye and that it is possible for a hydrogel to produce osmotic pressure in the vitreous cavity (Foster *et al.*, 2006). The addition of a hydrophobic monomer, N-phenylacrylamide (NPA), to the acrylamide and BAC greatly improved biocompatibility. Toxicity tests on Chinese Hamster Ovary (CHO) cells showed a viability of approximately 100% after 5 days at a concentration of 15 mg/mL. Additionally, rheological testing showed that the storage and loss moduli of this hydrogel formulation matched those of the natural porcine vitreous (Swindle *et al.*, 2008).

The future of vitreous substitutes is to find a formulation that can be left in the eye in the long term. Additionally, it would be preferable to mimic the mechanical properties, water content, and light transmittance of the natural vitreous humor. Silicone oil, currently the most commonly employed vitreous substitute, accomplishes none of these things. Polymeric hydrogel vitreous substitutes developed and tested experimentally have proven capable of matching these properties. Rheological testing can help match the mechanical properties of the polymeric substitutes to those of the natural vitreous. Furthermore, the process of *in situ* gelation is the key to viable vitreous substitutes because polymers that are injected as gels rather than as liquids fragment due to shear, lose their elasticity, and can cause inflammatory reactions in ocular tissues. In the future, there will be further research conducted on *in situ* gelling polymeric vitreous substitutes. Polymers can be tailored to alter their mechanical properties to match those of the natural vitreous humor. The goal is to match those properties, have a transparent hydrogel that is 99% water, and to find a substitute that will not cause cytotoxic reactions and will be retained in the eye.

13.3.2 Experimental methods

Statistical experimental design

Statistical experimental design is a useful tool for rapid screening of candidates and for determining important factors. Scheffe simplex-lattice designs were developed specifically to analyze mixture designs. Mixture design of experiments is used to determine the optimum concentration of chemical constituents that elicit a particular response while minimizing the number of experiments to be run. In a mixture experiment, the independent factors are proportions of different components of a blend and must sum to 100%. The purpose of the mixture design is to be able to predict empirically the response of a mixture for any combination of ingredients, or measure the influence of each component singly and in combination with others on the response (Anderson and Whitcomb, 2000). A range of polymeric hydrogel formulations may be analyzed using a mixture design with the monomer components along the backbone treated as mixture variables and the polymer concentration in the final hydrogel as a process factor.

StatEase Design-Expert 7.1 software (Minneapolis, MN, USA) enabled rapid selection of experimental parameters and analysis of data. The fundamentals are rooted in statistical experimental design, in which the test formulations chosen have monomer feed ratios and polymer concentrations within the ranges specified, as well as midpoints to determine non-linearity and error. The assumptions used in factorial design apply to mixture design. After the experimental data were obtained, analysis of variance (ANOVA) was used to determine which factors were statistically significant in contributing to specified properties, which in our case were viscoelasticity and refractive index. Those factors were the individual factors, such as the monomer feed ratios, and the interactions between those parameters. The factors that were deemed significant are utilized in the model, and the model was then used to predict the optimal formulation for the polymeric hydrogel.

It was shown that these hydrogels are capable of exerting small osmotic pressures at the low concentrations being evaluated. The osmotic pressure modeling for poly(acrylic acid) (PAA) was promising because of its higher sweling affinity compared with polyacrylamide. Therefore, the method of statistical experimental design was extended to a new polymer system to be evaluated as *in vivo*-forming vitreous substitutes. PAA was analyzed by mixtures design in an attempt to rapidly identify a candidate that could act as a biomimetic vitreous substitute.

Synthesis of copolymers

Acrylic acid (AA), BAC, NPA, *N,N,N',N'*-tetramethylethylenediamine (TEMED), dithiothreitol (DTT), 5,5'-dithio-*bis*(2-nitrobenzoic acid) (DTNB) (all from Sigma, Saint Louis, MO, USA), ammonium persulfate (APS), methanol, diethyl ether, acetone, and sodium diphosphate buffer (all from Aldrich, Milwaukee, WI, USA) were purchased and used without further purification, with the exception of AA which was purified by vacuum distillation at 80 °C to remove the inhibitor. All other reagents used were analytical grade. The chemical structures of AA, NPA, and BAC crosslinker are shown in Fig. 13.5.

The PAA hydrogels were synthesized in 25% ethanol in water (w/w) at an initial monomer concentration of 7.5% by weight. Owing to the low pH of the AA monomer and the inactivation of the disulfide bonds in the BAC

13.5 Chemical structures of acrylic acid (AA), *N*-phenylacrylamide (NPA), and *N,N'-bis*(acryloyl)cystamine (BAC).

crosslinker under acidic conditions, the pH of AA had to be raised to 7.0–7.5 before the BAC was added to the reaction mixture. This was accomplished by adding at 0.5 M sodium diphosphate buffer 10% of the volume of the total volume of the mixture, and with the addition of sodium hydroxide. The hydrogels were formed by free-radical polymerization with 10% APS and TEMED.

StatEase Design Expert was used to analyze the effects of the concentration of hydrophobic monomer (NPA), crosslinker (BAC), and polymer in the hydrogel on refractive index and viscoelastic properties. A crossed model was used that treated the monomer components as mixture components while incorporating the polymer concentration in the hydrogel as a numeric process factor. The compositions tested are shown in Table 13.1.

Reductive liquefaction and purification

After exhaustive washing with double distilled water, hydrogel formulations were reduced from the S—S crosslinks to linear polymers with S—H groups with DTT. In order to improve the biocompatibility and decrease polydispersity, the reduced polymer solutions were dialyzed with Spectra/Por tubing with a 25 kDa molecular mass cut-off, in nitrogen-bubbled water at pH 4 to prevent oxidation. The dialysis washing solution was changed three times over 72 hours. After dialysis, the polymers were precipitated in either acetone or a 25:75 mixture of methanol and diethyl ether. Precipitation in acetone was advantageous when large batches were produced because the solvent was more readily available than the diethyl ether. However, precipitation in diethyl ether produced a white powder that did not aggregate as it had a tendency to do in acetone. The precipitate was freeze-dried in a lyophilizer and was stored under vacuum to prevent oxidation.

Regelation

The reduced polymers were regelled by air oxidation at physiological pH of 7.4 in Dulbecco's phosphate buffered saline (DPBS). Figure 13.6 shows the complete reaction scheme of the AA copolymer, and the reaction mechanism for oxidative regelation of the polymers with air is shown in Fig. 13.7.

Table 13.1 Poly(acrylic acid) hydrogel compositions tested

Variable	Lower limit	Upper limit
AA (%)	90	94
BAC (%)	3	5
NPA (%)	3	5
Gel (%)	1	3

13.6 Acrylic acid copolymer regelation procedure: A, initial polymerization and crosslinking; B, reduction, C, regelation *in situ*.

$$AB-SH + {}^-OH \rightleftharpoons AB-S^- + H_2O$$

$$AB-S^- + O_2 \longrightarrow AB-S^\bullet + O_2^-$$

$$2\,AB-S^\bullet \longrightarrow AB-SS-AB$$

13.7 Free radical regelation procedure. AB, acrylamide or acrylic acid; B, BAC crosslinker; SS, crosslinked disulfide bond; SH, thiol group when not cross linked.

Hydrogel analysis

An Abbe refractometer was used to measure the refractive index of each tested sample (ATAGO Abbe Refractometer NAR-1T, Kirkland, WA, USA). The testing was done at a visible light wavelength of 552 nm at 37 °C. Storage and loss moduli of the hydrogels were determined using the Vilastic-3 oscillatory capillary rheometer. All samples were evaluated at 37 °C at 2 Hz, with the shear rate increasing from 0.1 to 100 s^{-1}. Additionally, the samples were analyzed at increasing frequency at a constant shear rate. Several samples were too stiff to be analyzed on the capillary rheometer, so they were analyzed on the cone and plate rheometer by frequency scan at 5% strain or strain scan at 2 Hz frequency.

Toxicity testing was carried out following the tetrazolium-based colorimetric (MTT) assay described by Bruining *et al.* (2000), in which 3-(4,5-dimethylthiol-2-yl)-2,5-diphenyl tetrazolium bromide (thiazolyl blue) is converted to formazan, an insoluble precipitate, by an enzymatic reaction performed only by living cells. Human retinal pigment epithelial (RPE) cells (ARPE-19, American Type Culture Collection (ATCC), Manassas, VA, USA) were used for cytotoxicity evaluation because they are the cells that would actually come into contact with the vitreous substitute *in vivo*.

RPE cells were plated at a density of 15 000 cells per 16-mm well in 1 mL of 10% calf serum (CS) minimum essential medium (MEM) with antibiotics. Media were aspirated after 24 hours and replaced with fresh media containing polymeric materials. Cells were incubated 72 hours. Media containing polymer were replaced by 0.5 mL 10% CS M199 medium without phenol red with 0.65 mg/mL thiazolyl blue. After 4 hours, the media were aspirated and formazan precipitate was dissolved in 200 μL dimethylsulfoxide. Absorbance was measured at 540 nm in a microtiter plate. All samples were tested in quadruplicate. To test for toxicity, polymer solutions of varying concentrations were added to acidified (pH 6) MEM media, dissolved, and gelled by air oxidation at pH 7.4 at final concentration of 15 mg/mL in 10% CS MEM. The viability was calculated as a percentage of absorbance of the test sample with respect to the control sample (Bruining *et al.*, 2000).

13.3.3 Results and discussion

The adhesive property of the polymer was one of the reasons why PAA was selected as a potential vitreous substitute (Park and Robinson, 1987). The natural vitreous humor attaches to the retina at several points, and it would be desirable to replace the vitreous with a hydrogel that could adhere to the retina and could mimic those attachment points.

Table 13.2 summarizes the PAA formulations tested, and the results for storage modulus, loss modulus, and refractive index. More midpoints, axial points, and replicates were chosen for the PAA in an attempt to gather information about the non-linear factors that may contribute to the modulus of the hydrogel vitreous substitutes.

Figure 13.8 plots the refractive indices of the hydrogel formulations and compares them to the natural vitreous humor. The noticeable trend is that the refractive index is dependent primarily upon polymer concentration in the hydrogel, as expected. It is also important to note that hydrogel formulations near 1% polymer concentration match the refractive index of the vitreous humor. By comparison, the refractive index of silicone oil is 1.4.

Figures 13.9 and 13.10 show storage modulus and loss modulus, respectively, versus frequency at 5% strain for all PAA hydrogels analyzed. Even at 1% polymer concentration, these hydrogels were stronger than the natural vitreous humor. All formulations have a higher storage modulus than loss modulus and act as viscoelastic solids, like the natural vitreous humor.

For analysis of the storage and loss moduli, the data underwent a log transformation. The retractive index results required no data transformation. A quadratic Scheffe model was used to correlate the data. The models for storage modulus, loss modulus, and retractive index were all significant, with p values of 0.0001 for storage modulus and retractive index, and 0.0004 for loss modulus. The p, R^2, and F values are summarized in Table 13.3.

The resultant equations produced to predict the values of storage modulus, loss modulus, and refractive index are shown below. In the equations below,

Table 13.2 Poly(acrylic acid) data summary

BAC (%)	NPA (%)	AA (%)	Gel (%)	G′ (Pa)	G″ (Pa)	RI
3	3	94	1.0	17.0	2.8	1.3348
3	3	94	1.0	17.9	4.3	1.3352
3	3	94	2.0	31.4	5.7	1.3359
3	3	94	3.0	130.1	54.0	1.3382
3	3	94	3.0	140.4	6.8	1.3382
3	5	92	1.0	24.8	3.9	1.3341
3	5	92	1.0	22.9	4.0	1.3343
3	5	92	2.0	91.7	8.4	1.3360
3	5	92	3.0	164.3	18.9	1.3376
3	5	92	3.0	195.5	29.5	1.3363
4	3	93	1.5	74.4	3.7	1.3343
4	4	92	1.0	18.0	4.6	1.3348
4	4	92	1.5	36.8	7.0	1.3359
4	4	92	2.0	46.4	8.2	1.3365
4	4	92	3.0	64.5	7.6	1.3376
4	5	91	1.5	37.2	6.3	1.3356
4	5	91	2.5	88.5	9.2	1.3373
5	3	92	1.0	38.7	17.2	1.3350
5	3	92	2.0	274.4	17.6	1.3366
5	3	92	3.0	363.8	27.8	1.3380
5	3	92	3.0	388.9	188.3	1.3378
5	4	91	1.0	15.2	12.4	1.3348
5	4	91	3.0	156.5	39.8	1.3386
5	5	90	1.0	40.8	13.1	1.3347
5	5	90	2.0	89.8	14.1	1.3366
5	5	90	3.0	151.6	42.3	1.3381

AA, BAC, NPA, and Gel refer to the percentage concentrations. For example, 1% AAB5N5 would have the input values of 1 for Gel, 90 for AA, 5 for BAC, and 5 for NPA.

$$\log(G') = 0.618 \times BAC + 0.514 \times NPA - 0.016 \times AA - 0.128$$
$$\times BAC \times NPA - 0.002 \times BAC \times Gel - 0.025$$
$$\times NPA \times Gel + 0.006 \times AA \times Gel \qquad [13.1]$$

$$\log(G'') = 0.289 \times BAC + 0.058 \times NPA - 0.010$$
$$\times AA - 0.031 \times BAC \times Gel - 0.035 \times NPA$$
$$\times Gel + 0.006 \times AA \times Gel \qquad [13.2]$$

$$RI = 1.3331 + 0.0016 \times Gel \qquad [13.3]$$

Statistical analysis of the results using the targeted values for the refractive index and moduli shown in Table 13.4 produced an optimal hydrogel formulation of 1.20% AAB3N4, or a hydrogel containing 1.20% polymer by weight with 3% crosslinker and 4% NPA along the backbone. The predicted

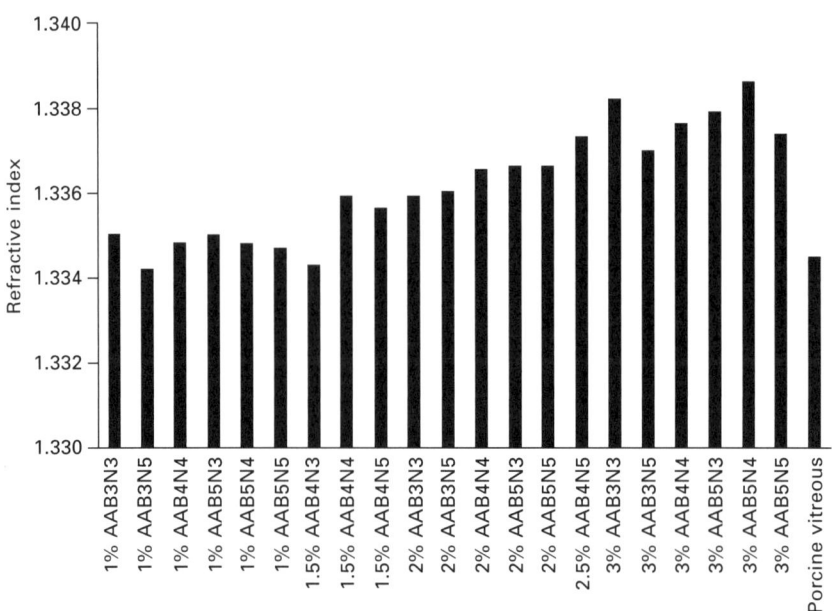

13.8 Refractive indices of poly(acrylic acid) formulations.

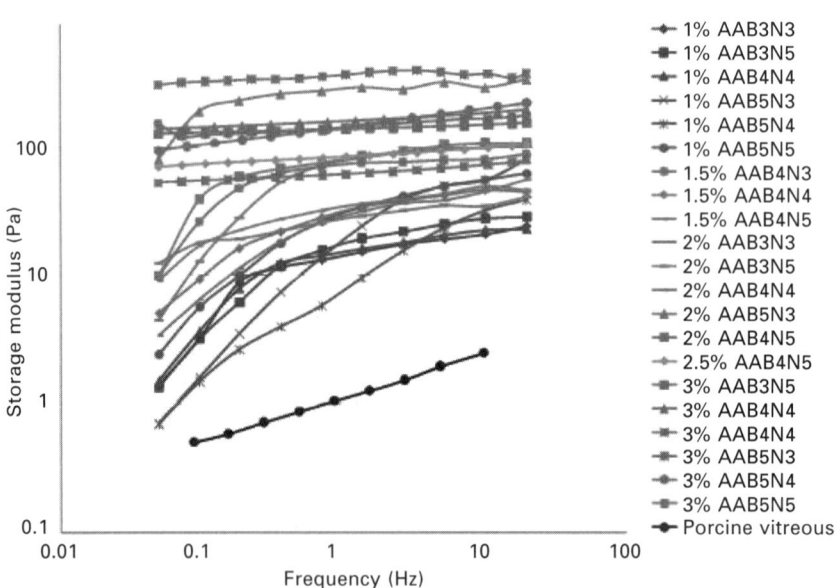

13.9 Poly(acrylic acid) storage modulus versus frequency at 5% strain.

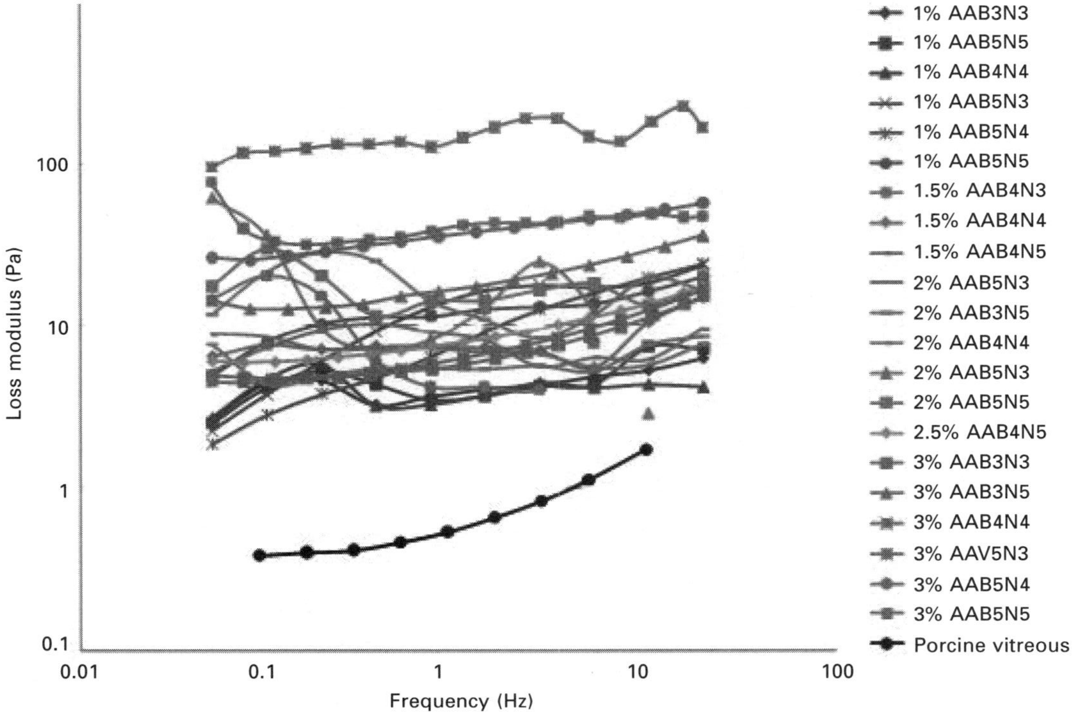
Loss modulus (Pa)
100
10
1
0.1
0.01
0.1
1
10
100
Frequency (Hz)
1% AAB3N3
1% AAB5N5
1% AAB4N4
1% AAB5N3
1% AAB5N4
1% AAB5N5
1.5% AAB4N3
1.5% AAB4N4
1.5% AAB4N5
2% AAB5N3
2% AAB3N5
2% AAB4N4
2% AAB5N3
2% AAB5N5
2.5% AAB4N5
3% AAB3N3
3% AAB3N5
3% AAB4N4
3% AAV5N3
3% AAB5N4
3% AAB5N5
Porcine vitreous

13.10 Poly(acrylic acid) loss modulus versus frequency at 5% strain.

Table 13.3 Statistical analysis of poly(acrylic acid)
model results

Model	p	R^2	F
G'	0.0001	0.85	17.25
G''	0.0004	0.66	7.62
RI	0.0001	0.87	167.72

Table 13.4 Experimental design targets for
vitreous substitutes

Target	Lower Limit	Upper Limit
G' (Pa)	5.0	15.0
G'' (Pa)	0.5	5.0
RI	1.3340	1.3360

Table 13.5 Predicted and measured properties of
optimized poly(acrylic acid) formulation

Property	Predicted	Actual
G' (Pa)	11.8	3.2
G'' (Pa)	3.6	2.7
RI	1.335	1.334

and experimental values for this formulation are shown in Table 13.5. The storage and loss moduli of 1.2% AAB3N4 are plotted against frequency in Fig. 13.11.

The statistical model results are represented graphically in several plots. The darker shaded portions of the figures illustrate the regions that have storage modulus values between 5 and 15 Pa, loss modulus values between 0.5 and 5 Pa, and refractive index values between 1.334 and 1.336. Figures 13.12 to 13.14 show the targeted areas for 0.75%, 1.00%, and 1.25% hydrogels, respectively. A 1% hydrogel is a desirable formulation to owing due to its similar water content to the natural vitreous humor and lower viscosity than formulations containing higher polymer content.

The following plots represent graphically the full range of possibilities for PAA formulations that could behave as biomimetic vitreous substitutes. Figures 13.15 to 13.17 show storage modulus, loss modulus, and refractive index, respectively. Finally, the darker shaded region of Fig. 13.18 shows all possible PAA formulations that fall within the targeted values of the optomechanical properties of the ideal vitreous substitute.

Microindentation of several formulations of PAA hydrogels at 7.5% polymer concentration revealed a trend in elastic modulus. The results are summarized in Table 13.6. As expected, an increase in crosslinker

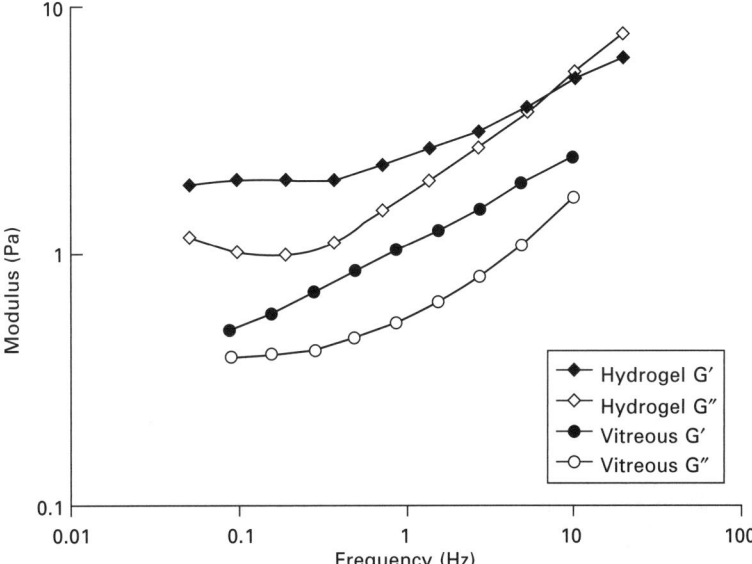

13.11 Moduli of 1.2% AAB3N4 poly(acrylic acid) formulation versus frequency.

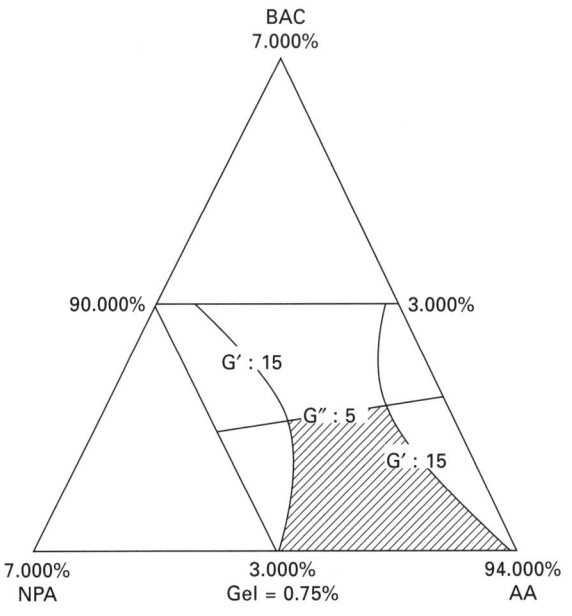

13.12 Mode 1 predictions for the 0.75% poly(acrylic acid) hydrogel.

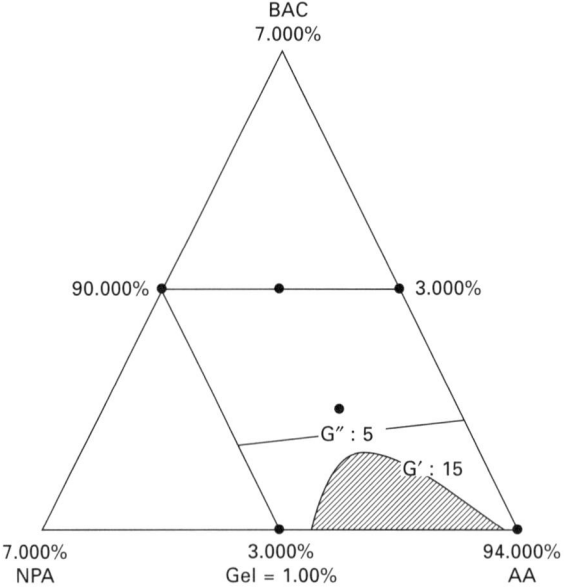

13.13 Model predictions for the 1.00% poly(acrylic acid) hydrogel.

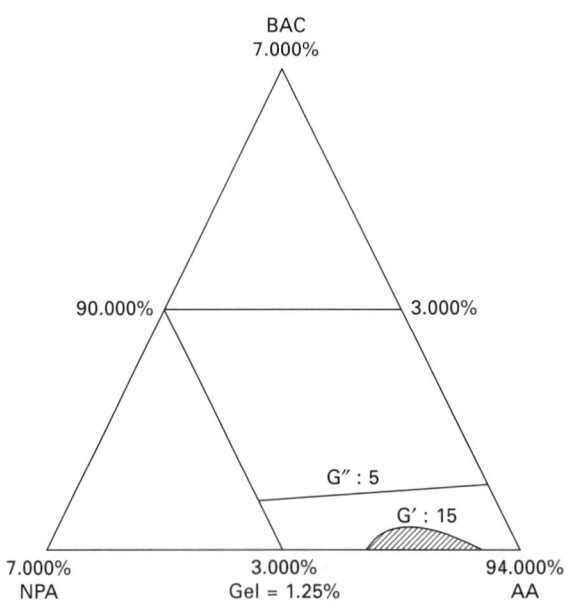

13.14 Model predictions for the 1.25% poly(acrylic acid) hydrogel.

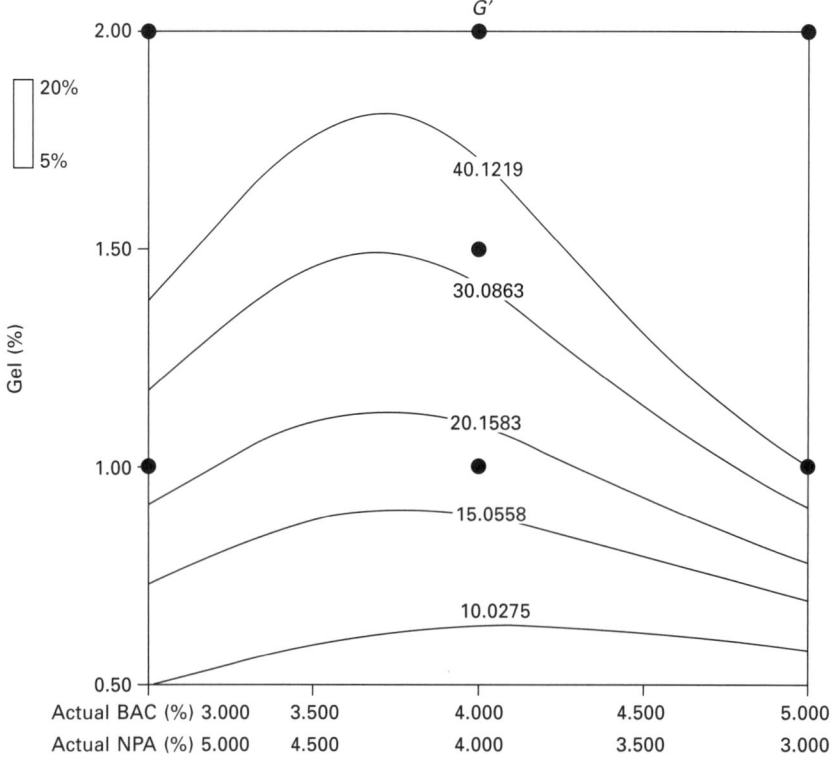

13.15 Model predictions for poly(acrylic acid) storage modulus.

concentration increased the modulus of the hydrogel. However, it is also noticeable that an increase in the NPA content decreased the modulus. This is due to ineffective crosslinking in the hydrogels containing more NPA. These hydrogels often form more intramolecular crosslinks because of the clustering of the hydrophobic groups along the polymer backbone.

In addition to the determination of the refractive index, storage modulus, and loss modulus, the *in vitro* toxicity of PAA was determined using RPE cells. The results of four formulations are shown in Fig. 13.19. Upon first glance, the PAA hydrogel vitreous substitutes appear to be more toxic than the polyacrylamide vitreous substitutes (Swindle *et al.*, 2008). There are a few confounding factors. The polyacrylamide formulations were tested using CHO cells, which are less sensitive than RPE cells. In addition, the PAA formulations are far more viscous and adhere to the cells, so some error resulted when the cells stuck to the polymer samples and therefore did not remain in the culture dish, resulting in an artificially diminished number due to aspiration rather than cell death. These results are not discouraging because the toxicity shown corresponds to the linear polymer chains and

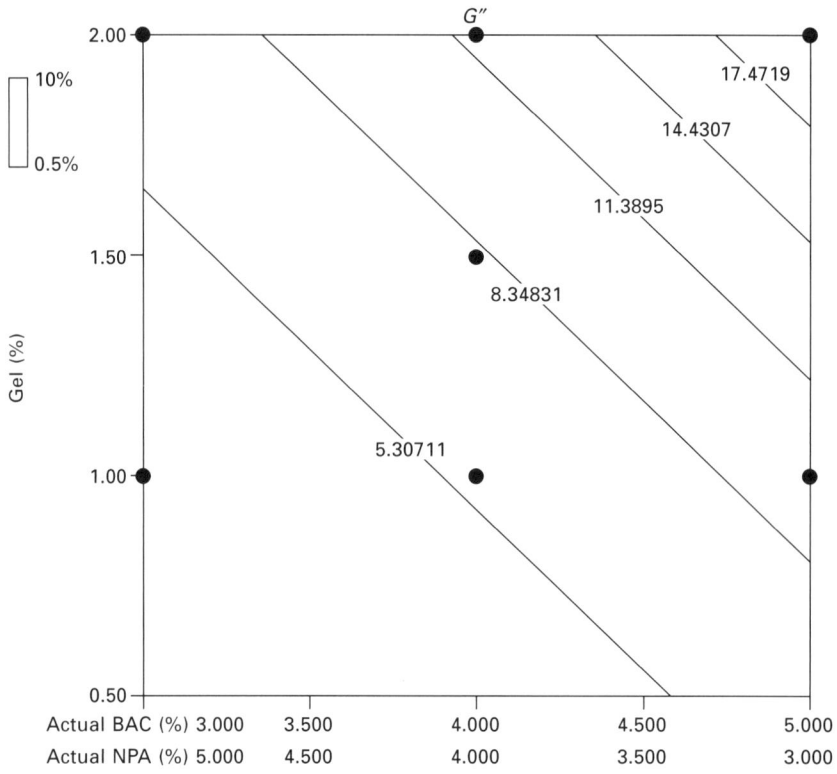

13.16 Model predictions for poly(acrylic acid) loss modulus.

not the less toxic crosslinked hydrogels. An important trend to note is that the higher the concentration of NPA along the backbone, the higher the *in vitro* biocompatibility. This was also noted in preliminary toxicity studies with CHO cells and polyacrylamide hydrogels.

The refractive index and viscoelasticity of the natural vitreous humor can be mimicked by a number of different formulations of PAA copolymeric hydrogels. The optimal formulation determined by the statistical design models had refractive index, storage modulus, and loss modulus values very close to ose of the natural vitreous humor.

13.4   Osmotic pressure

13.4.1 Background

A hydrogel is a crosslinked hydrophilic polymer that can absorb several times its weight in water without dissolving. It absorbs water as a result of hydrophilic functional groups along the polymeric backbone and resists

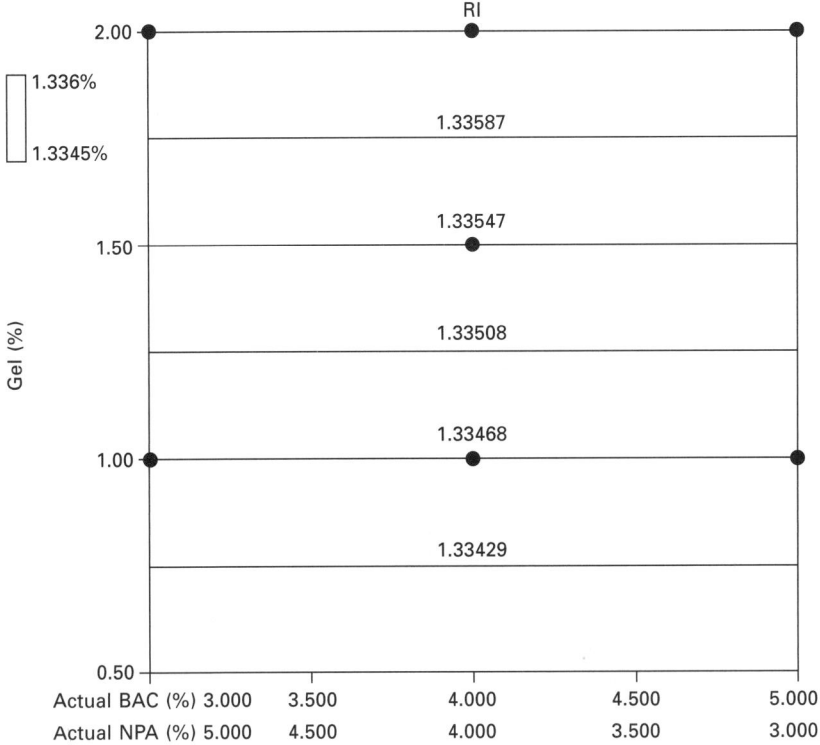

13.17 Model predictions for poly(acrylic acid) refractive index.

dissolution as a result of crosslinks. Ionic hydrogels respond to changes in pH, ionic strength, and temperature. Their interactions are changed by use of good or poor solvents. Hydrogels have strong orientation-dependent interactions (hydrogen bonds), which influence swelling equilibrium. Inhomogeneities in hydrogels can arise from crosslinking inefficiency. Imperfections are caused by pre-existing order, network defects, or phase separation.

Flory equilibrium swelling theory states that the polymer absorbs solvent until chemical potentials in the gel phase and in the free solution are equal. Gels swell when solvent penetrates the polymer mesh. Swelling equilibrium occurs when the net osmotic pressure equals zero and when cohesive energy density and solubility of solvent equal those of the polymer. Polymer chains are stretched when the gel is swollen. Swelling properties depend upon polymer functionality, crosslink density, ionic content, and solvent characteristics (Flory and Rehner, 1943). Peppas and Lucht modified the Flory–Rehner equation to describe swelling behavior for non-Gaussian networks crosslinked in solution (Peppas and Lucht, 1984).

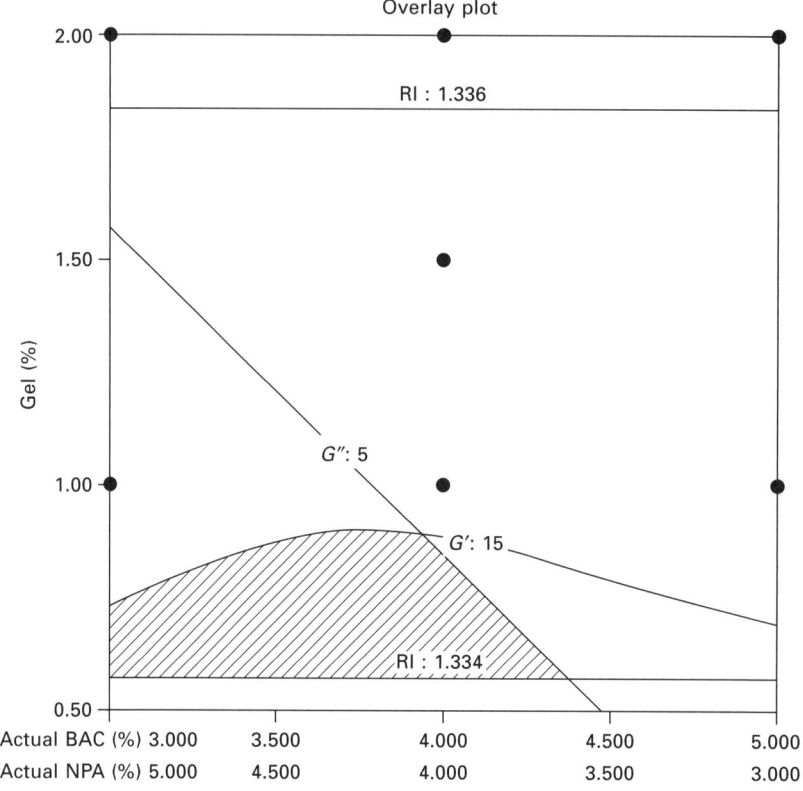

13.18 Model predictions for poly(acrylic acid) target values.

Table 13.6 Microindentation of 7.5%
poly(acrylic acid) hydrogels

Hydrogel	Modulus (Pa)
AAB3N4	950 ± 60
AAB3N5	1930 ± 90
AAB5N3	4640 ± 140
AAB5N4	2770 ± 260

$$\frac{1}{M_c} = \frac{2}{M_n} - \frac{(v/V_1)[\ln(1-v_{2s})+v_{2s}+\chi_1 v_{2s}^2][1-(1/N)(v_{2s}/v_{2r})^{2/3}]^3}{v_{2r}[(v_{2s}/v_{2r})^{1/3}-0.5(v_{2s}/v_{2r})][1+(1/N)(v_{2s}/v_{2r})^{1/3}]^2}$$

[13.4]

In Equation 13.4, v is the specific volume of the polymer, V_1 is the molar
volume of the solvent, v_{2s} is the polymer fraction in the swollen state, v_{2r} is
the polymer fraction in the relaxed state, N is the number of chain linkages,

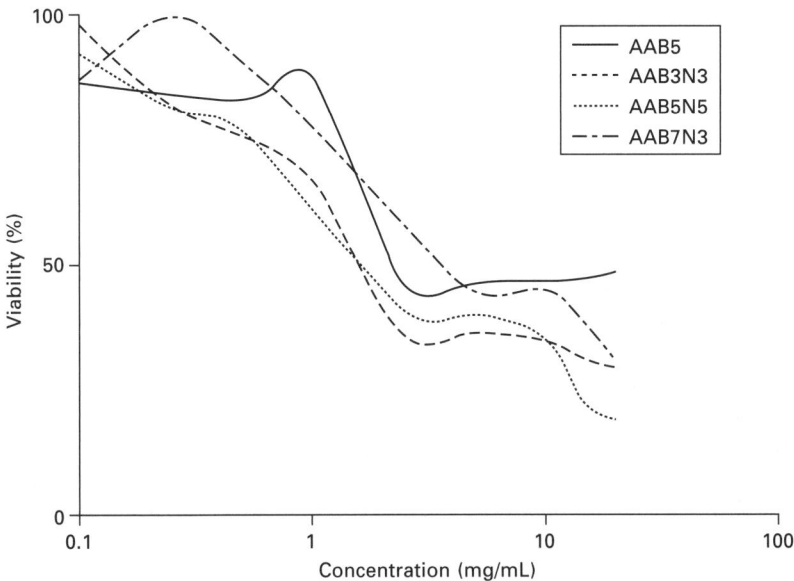

13.19 Poly(acrylic acid) toxicity in RPE cells.

M_c is the molecular weight between crosslinks, M_n is the number-averaged molecular weight, and ξ_1 is the Flory–Huggins polymer–solvent interaction parameter. The relaxed state of the polymer is the condition immediately after initial polymerization. The gel contains some water in the relaxed state because it was polymerized in solution.

According to Peppas and Brannon-Peppas (1990), N can be calculated as follows:

$$N = \frac{2M_c}{M_r} \qquad [13.5]$$

where M_r is the molecular weight of the polymer repeating unit. The copolymers synthesized in this project are tetrafunctional and follow the phantom network model. They are highly swollen gels and not all the chains may interact with each other. The polymers were treated as highly crosslinked non-Gaussian networks, so the Peppas-Lucht equation was utilized.

The degree of swelling decreases with initial monomer concentration because of the decreased likelihood of cyclization during reaction, increased entanglements, and decreased mesh size. Swelling increases as a result of higher molecular weights between crosslinks, porosity, conversion, and fewer defects. The degree of swelling decreases with hydrophobicity because of hydrophobic physical interactions and the change in the χ_1 parameter. As a result, the gel density increases and the modulus increases. The modulus is higher in a collapsed state than in a swollen state due to physical crosslinks (Bajpai *et al.*, 2004).

Copolymerization with hydrophilic monomers increases water sorption and swelling. Addition of hydrophobic copolymeric groups will decrease the degree of swelling. Ions repel each other, which leads to swelling. Hydrophilicity decreases interfacial tension which also leads to swelling. Swelling decreases with increased crosslink density. This also causes increased homogeneity and decreased solvent diffusivity. The effective crosslink density can be increased by entanglements. At high crosslink densities, some gels can have two phases: an unswollen core and an outer swollen shell (Bajpai *et al.*, 2004).

As previously mentioned, equilibrium swelling occurs when the net osmotic pressure is zero. The equilibrium swelling ratio, Q, is the swollen volume, V_s, divided by the dry volume of the polymer, V_d.

$$Q = \frac{V_s}{V_d} \qquad [13.6]$$

The volumes V can be calculated by dividing the mass W by the density ρ.

$$V = \frac{W}{\rho} \qquad [13.7]$$

In the present study, the crosslink density is the reciprocal of the thiol content. It can be compared to the theoretical value of the crosslink density, which is calculated as

$$M_c = \frac{\text{mol\%}_{\text{monomer}}}{\text{mol\%}_{\text{crosslinker}}} M_r \qquad [13.8]$$

Hydrogels swell rather than dissolve in solution. A good solvent ($\xi_1 < 0.5$) is one in which repulsion between polymer chains occurs, resulting in swelling. A poor solvent ($\chi_1 > 0.5$) results in interchain attractive forces and shrinking behavior. The energy of swelling behavior is described by Flory–Rehner (Flory and Rehner, 1943) equations below based on Gibbs free energy (ΔG) of mixtures. At equilibrium swelling, ΔG is minimized and the osmotic pressure (Π) terms sum to zero. This is represented mathematically by the equations below, in which $\Delta\mu_1$ is chemical potential and n_1 is moles.

$$\Delta G = \Delta G_{\text{mixture}} + \Delta G_{\text{elastic}} + \Delta G_{\text{ionic}} + \Delta G_{\text{electrolyte}} \qquad [13.9]$$

$$\Delta\mu_1 = \frac{d\Delta G_{\text{mixture}}}{dn_1} + \frac{\Delta G_{\text{elastic}}}{dn_1} + \frac{d\Delta G_{\text{ionic}}}{dn_1} + \frac{\Delta G_{\text{elec}}}{dn_1} \qquad [13.10]$$

$$\Pi_{\text{swell}} = \Pi_{\text{mix}} + \Pi_{\text{elastic}} + \Pi_{\text{ion}} + \Pi_{\text{elec}} \qquad [13.11]$$

Equations [13.9] to [13.11] show that the swelling osmotic pressure is a result of the contribution of four terms: the mixing effects between the polymer and solvent, the elastic component due to the contraction of polymer chains, the effects of ions, and the electrolytic effects. The PAA synthesized in this project was synthesized at neutral pH in the sodium salt form, and no electric potential was applied, so the electrolyte term can be discarded. The mixture and elastic potentials are given by Equations [13.12] and [13.13], respectively.

$$\Pi_{mix} = -\frac{RT}{V_1}[\ln(1-\phi) + \phi + \chi_1\phi^2]$$

[13.12]

$$\Pi_{elastic} = -RT \frac{(v/V_1)[\ln(1-v_{2s}) + v_{2s} + \chi_1 v_{2s}^2]}{v_{2r}[v_{2s}/v_{2r})^{1/3} - 0.5(v_{2s}/v_{2r})]} \frac{[1 - (1/N)(v_{2s}/v_{2r})^{2/3}]^3}{[1 + (1/N)(v_{2s}/v_{2r})^{1/3}]^2}$$

[13.13]

In Equations [13.12] and [13.13], R is the gas constant, T is the temperature, ϕ is the polymer functionality, and the other terms are as defined previously.

For swelling in physiological salt solutions, an additional osmotic pressure term must be added. Following the Donnan ion exclusion theory, the ionic effects can be calculated as:

$$\Pi_{ion} = -RT \left(\frac{1}{4I}\right)\left(\frac{fv_{2s}}{v}\right)^2\left(\frac{K_a}{(10^{-pH} + K_a)}\right)^2$$

[13.14]

where I is the salt concentration in DPBS, f is the fraction of ionized polymer, K_a is the acid dissociation constant of the polymer, and pH is that of the solvent. For PAA swollen in DPBS, the parameters are $I = 0.101$ mol/L, $f = 1$, $K_a = 5.5 \times 10^{-5}$, and $pH = 7.4$ (Jabbari et al., 2007). To determine the osmotic pressure exerted by the hydrogel, the elastic, mixing, and ionic osmotic terms in Equations [13.12] to [13.14] are summed, resulting in Equation 13.15.

$$\Pi_{swell} = -\frac{RT}{V_1}[\ln(1-\phi) + \phi + \chi_{12}\phi^2] - RT\left(\frac{1}{4I}\right)\left(\frac{fv_{2s}}{v}\right)^2\left(\frac{K_a}{(10^{-pH} + K_a)}\right)$$
$$- RT \frac{(v/V_1)[\ln(1-v_{2s}) + v_{2s} + \chi_1 v_{2s}^2][1 - (1/N)(v_{2s}/v_{2r})^{2/3}]^3}{v_{2r}[v_{2s}/v_{2r})^{1/3} - 0.5(v_{2s}/v_{2r})][1 + (1/N)(v_{2s}/v_{2r})^{1/3}]^2}$$

[13.15]

The Flory–Huggins interaction parameter used in the swelling equations was calculated using known swelling parameters, and Equation [13.15] was used to determine the osmotic pressure exerted by a hydrogel in physiological saline (Horkay *et al.*, 2000).

13.4.2 Experimental methods

Synthesis of copolymers

The PAA hydrogels were synthesized in 25% ethanol in water (w/w) at an initial monomer concentration of 7.5% by weight. Owing to the low pH of the AA monomer and the inactivation of the disulfide bonds in the BAC crosslinker under acidic conditions, the pH of the AA had to be raised to 7.0–7.5 before the BAC was added to the reaction mixture. This was accomplished by adding 0.5 M sodium diphosphate buffer at 10% of the volume of the total volume of the mixture, and with the addition of sodium hydroxide. The hydrogels were formed by free-radical polymerization with 10% APS and TEMED. The initial composition tested for equilibrium swelling was AAB4N3, or a copolymer containing 93% AA, 4% BAC crosslinker, and 3% NPA.

Equilibrium swelling

The hydrogels formed at 7.5% initial monomer concentration were swollen in DPBS, pH 7 water, or pH 4 water. The swelling solution was changed every 24 hours for 1 week. By 7 days, the hydrogels had reached equilibrium, as determined by constant mass between consecutive weighings.

13.4.3 Results and discussion

AAB4N3 hydrogels synthesized at 7.5% concentration were swollen in DPBS, pH 7 water, or pH 4 water. The equilibrium swelling ratios and final weight concentrations were calculated and are shown in Table 13.7. In Table 13.7, the equilibrium swelling ratio is the ratio of the hydrogel in its swollen state with respect to its relaxed state, or the state at which the hydrogel was synthesized in solution. For reference, the equilibrium swelling ratios from the dry polymer state are also included.

The swelling ratio of the 7.5% AAB4N3 hydrogel in water was 12.7. For PAA, all the parameters in the swelling equations were known except

Table 13.7 Equilibrium swelling results for AAB4N3

Swelling media	Swelling ratio	Final concentration	Swelling ratio dry
DPBS	5.9 ± 0.1	1.28%	170 ± 3
Distilled H_2O, pH 4	10.4 ± 0.2	0.72%	300 ± 7
Distilled H_2O, pH 7	12.7 ± 0.6	0.59%	340 ± 18

for the polymer–solvent interaction parameter. At equilibrium swelling, the osmotic pressure is zero. Therefore, by using data from equilibrium swelling studies on the hydrogels, the polymer–solvent interaction parameter was determined. The parameter was calculated to be 0.44, which corresponds to the value reported in literature of 0.45 (Jabbari *et al.*, 2007). Using the known parameters, the osmotic pressure was calculated for formulations with variations in crosslinker content and polymer concentration in the hydrogel. The results are summarized in Figs. 13.20 and 13.21.

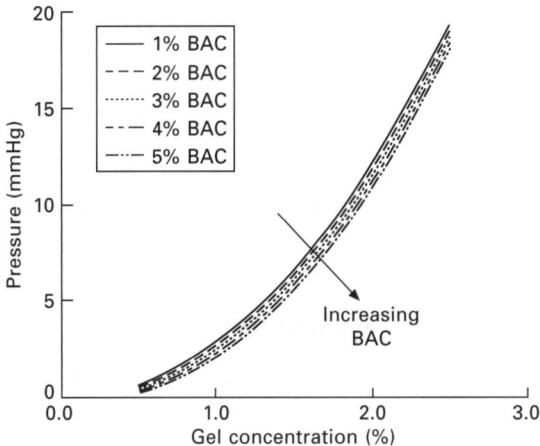

13.20 Poly(acrylic acid) osmotic pressure exerted in DPBS versus gel concentration.

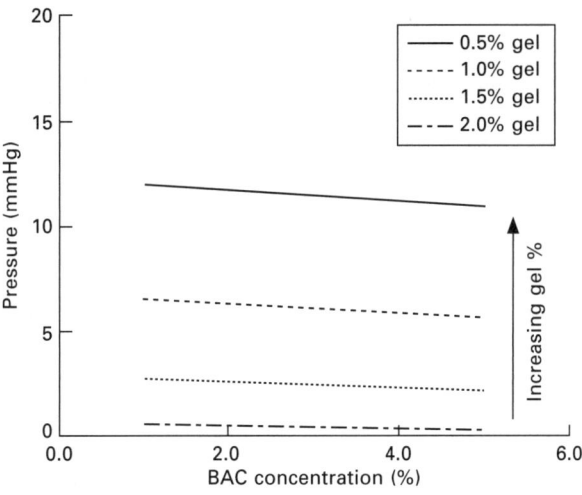

13.21 Poly(acrylic acid) osmotic pressure exerted in DPBS versus crosslinker content.

As expected, the osmotic pressure exerted by the hydrogel increased with polymer concentration in the hydrogel and with decreasing crosslinker concentration. There is a non-linear increase in osmotic pressure with polymer concentration and a linear decrease with the crosslinker concentration. The polymer concentration has the most significant impact on osmotic pressure.

For all formulations analyzed with polymer concentration between 0.5 and 2.0% and crosslinker content between 1 and 5%, the gels will swell slightly and exert a small osmotic pressure. The osmotic pressure is plotted in mmHg because the intraocular pressure is routinely expressed in this unit. Therefore, none of these hydrogel formulations exceed the normal intraocular pressure of 15 mmHg and should not cause glaucoma (Tasman and Jaeger, 2006). However, the swelling pressure may be sufficiently high that it may maintain healthy ocular function and tamponade the retina. This confirms that PAA is a good candidate for vitreous substitution because of its ability to exert a slight osmotic pressure even at low polymer concentrations in the hydrogel.

13.5   Conclusions and recommendations

Knowledge of the mechanical behavior of the vitreous humor was acquired to develop *in situ*-forming hydrogels as permanent vitreous substitutes. One of the objectives of this research was to examine and understand fully the viscoelastic behavior of the vitreous humor and its application to its function in the eye. Its mechanical properties have been objectively tested using rheometry. A large number of porcine vitreous samples were analyzed using capillary rheometry, and the storage and loss moduli match those found by other groups who used different methods. The data showed that the vitreous humor had a higher storage modulus than loss modulus, indicating viscoelastic solid behavior similar to that of a polymeric hydrogel.

Additionally, it has been definitively shown that the composition of the vitreous humor is a mesh of collagen with hyaluronic acid coils interspersed in a gel of 99% water (Foulds, 1987). This research made it possible to develop a better, permanent vitreous substitute by mimicking the natural vitreous in form and function. Additionally, this knowledge could lead to a better understanding of the mechanism of retinal detachment and vitreous syneresis, improving the knowledge base for practicing ophthalmologists in diagnostics. The disciplines of chemical engineering, polymer chemistry, ophthalmology, and biology were applied to examine the vitreous humor from a multifaceted perspective. The results show that the vitreous body could be tested intact, which had not been done before, by employing capillary rheometry.

The review of the literature shows that there is obviously a need for a better vitreous substitute. Hence, the second objective of this work focused on the design of a biomimetic prosthetic. It has been shown that the refractive index and viscoelastic properties of the natural vitreous can be mimicked by a copolymeric hydrogel network composed of PAA. The incorporation of a hydrophobic moiety along the polymer backbone enables hydrogel formation at lower polymer concentrations, which minimizes both the refractive index and the modulus.

The concept that sets these vitreous substitutes apart from the others is the process of *in situ* gelation. It has been shown that *in situ* gelation greatly improves the biocompatibility and efficacy of the vitreous substitute. The reversible disulfide crosslinker enables the synthesized copolymers to be liquefied and extensively purified. By the time the copolymers come into contact with ocular tissues, all monomers and low molecular weight components were removed, greatly improving biocompatibility (Swindle *et al.*, 2008). The method of gelation *in vivo* also has practical benefits. Implantation of a preformed hydrogel into the ocular cavity is not feasible, and injection of a preformed hydrogel is difficult and leads to some loss of elasticity and cohesiveness.

It was also shown through modeling that the osmotic pressures exerted by these *in situ*-forming vitreous substitutes were low enough to avoid surgical and post-surgical complications, while high enough to tamponade the retina. The osmotic pressure that will be exerted by the vitreous substitute can be tailored by modifying the polymer concentration, crosslinker content, or the hydrophobic content.

A mixture design was used to optimize the formulation of *in situ*-forming hydrogel vitreous substitutes. This method of hydrogel design optimization enabled rapid screening of candidate formulations that matched the optical and mechanical properties of the natural vitreous humor. This statistical experimental design method was applied to novel polymer formulations in order to rapidly screen for an *in situ*-forming hydrogel vitreous substitute to be used eventually in a long-term animal study and possibly clinical trials.

By acquiring the properties of the vitreous humor, better vitreous substitutes were developed that are capable of forming *in situ* due to the incorporation of the disulfide crosslinker. In conclusion, the viscoelastic properties of the vitreous humor were determined, the method of *in situ* regelation was proven, the mechanism of retinal attachment via exertion of osmotic pressure was proven through modeling, and biomimetic hydrogel vitreous substitutes were rapidly screened using a mixture design.

13.6   Future trends

The future of vitreous substitutes lies in developing a biomimetic replacement. The animal model for the ideal vitreous substitute has been thoroughly characterized, and can serve as the target values for refractive index and modulus for a biomimetic vitreous substitute. Polymeric hydrogels formed at low concentrations should be able to match both the refractive index and viscoelastic properties of the natural vitreous humor.

The concept of an *in situ*-forming hydrogel vitreous substitute has been proven *in vitro* and *in vivo* using model polymeric systems. The process of injecting a liquid into the eye and having it form a gel in the shape of the ocular cavity is preferable. Additionally, the use of an *in situ*-forming hydrogel as a vitreous substitute would require no change in the current vitrectomy technique, allowing for easier adoption by the surgical community. Other novel polymer systems with improved biocompatibility can be applied as vitreous substitutes with the incorporation of a disulfide crosslinker along the backbone, or by using other *in situ* crosslinking methods. A mixture design should be used to rapidly screen these new polymeric candidates and to target the formulation that will yield a biomimetic vitreous substitute.

It is possible that an *in vivo*-forming hydrogel vitreous substitute could be used in clinical trials shortly. Several of the fundamental questions have been answered through the completion of osmotic pressure modeling and optimization of the design of the vitreous substitutes. These methods can be applied to other polymeric systems to rapidly screen for vitreous substitute candidates for future animal studies and possibly clinical trials.

13.7   Sources of further information and advice

Refojo explored polymers as ophthalmic prostheses and reviewed vitreous substitutes (Refojo, 1971; Chan *et al.*, 1984; Giordano and Refojo, 1998). Chirila's group pioneered the modern research by evaluating synthetic polymeric hydrogels as vitreous substitutes. They were also the first to evaluate the viscoelastic properties of vitreous substitutes (Chirila *et al.*, 1998; Chirila and Hong, 1998). Experimental vitreous substitutes have also been reviewed extensively by several groups (Chan *et al.*, 1984; Chirila *et al.*, 1998; Soman and Banerjee, 2003; Swindle and Ravi, 2007). The development of *in situ*-forming hydrogel vitreous substitutes has been explored by a couple of groups recently (Foster *et al.*, 2006; Suri and Banerjee, 2006; Swindle *et al.*, 2008).

13.8   References

Aliyar HA, Foster WJ, Hamilton PD and Ravi N (2004), 'Towards the development of an artificial human vitreous', *Polym Prepr*, **45**, 469–470.

Anderson MJ, Whitcomb PJ (2000), *DOE Simplified: Practical Tools for Effective Experimentation*, New York, Productivity Press.

Bajpai AK, Bajpai J, Shukla S and Kulkarni RA (2004), 'Modulation in sorption dynamics of a pH-sensitive interpenetrating polymer network (IPN)', *J Macromol Sci*, **A41**(2), 211–230.

Balazs EA (1973), 'Fine structure and function of ocular tissues. The vitreous', *Int Ophthalmol Clin*, 13, 169–187.

Balazs EA (1987), 'Functional anatomy of the vitreous', in *Biomedical Foundations of Ophthalmology*, Duane TA, Jaeger EA, eds, Philadelphia, J.B. Lippincott Company, pp. 1–16.

Bettelheim FA and Wang TJY (1976), 'Dynamic viscoelastic properties of bovine vitreous', *Exp Eye Res*, **23**, 435–441.

Brannon-Peppas L and Peppas NA (1990), 'The equilibrium swelling behavior of porous and non-porous hydrogels', *Absorbent Polym Technol*, **4**, 67–102.

Bruining MJ, Blaauwgeerss HGT, Kuijer R, Pels E, Nuijts RMMA and Koole LH (2000), 'Biodegradable three-dimensional networks of poly(dimethylamino ethyl methacrylate). Synthesis, characterization and in vitro studies of structural degradation and cytotoxicity', *Biomaterials*, **21**, 595–604.

Buchsbaum G, Sternklar M, Litt M, Grunwald JE and Riva CE (1984), 'Dynamics of an oscillating viscoelastic sphere: a model of thge vitreous humor of the eye', *Biorbeology*, **21**, 285–296.

Chan IM, Tolentino FI, Refojo MF, Fournier G and Albert DM (1984). 'Vitreous substitute: experimental studies and review', *Retina*, **4**, 51–59.

Chirila TV and Hong Y (1998), 'Poly(1-vinyl-2-pyrrolidinone) hydrogels as vitreous substitutes: a rheological study', *Polym Int*, **46**, 183–195.

Chirila T V, Hong Y, Dalton P D, Constable I J and Refojo M F (1998), 'The use of hydrophilic polymers as artificial vitreous', *Prog Polym Sci*, **23**, 475–508.

Colthurst MJ, Williams RL, Hiscott PS and Grierson I (2000), 'Biomaterials used in the posterior segment of the eye', *Biomaterials*, **21**, 649–665.

Cutler NL (1947) 'Vitreous transplantation', *Trans Am Acad Ophthalmol Otolaryngol*, **52**, 253–259.

Deutschmann R (1906), 'Zur operativen Behandlung der Netzhautablosung', *Klin Monastbl Augenheilkd*, **44**, 364–370.

Federman JL and Schubert HD (1988), 'Complications associated with the use of silicone oil in 150 eyes after retina-vitreous surgery', *Ophthalmology*, **95**, 870–876.

Flory PJ and Rehner J, Jr (1943), 'Statistical mechanics of cross-linked polymer networks. I. Rubberlike elasticity', *J Chem Phys*, **11**(11), 513–526.

Foster WJ, Aliyar HA, Hamilton P and Ravi N (2006). 'Internal osmotic pressure as a mechanism of retinal attachment in a vitreous substitute', *J Bioact Compat Polym*, **21**, 221–235.

Foulds WS (1987), 'Is your vitreous really necessary?', *Eye*, **1**, 641–664.

Giordano GG and Refojo MF (1998), 'Silicone oils as vitreous substitutes', *Prog Polym Sci*, **23**, 509–532.

Hong Y, Chirila TV, Vijayasekaran S, Dalton PD, Tahija SG, Cuypers MJH and Constable IJ (1996), 'Crosslinked poly (1-vinyl-2-pyrrolidinone) as a vitreous substitute', *J Biomed Mater Res A*, **30**(4), 441–448.

Horkay F, Tasaki I and Basser PJ (2000), 'Osmotic swelling of polyacrylate hydrogels in physiological salt solutions', Biomacromolecules, **1**, 84–90.

Jabbari E, Tavakoli J and Sarvestani AS (2007), 'Swelling characteristics of acrylic acid polyelectrolye hydrogel in a dc electric field', *Smart Mater Struct*, **16**, 1614–1620.

Jonas JB, Knorr HLJ, Rank RM and Budde WM (2001), 'Retinal redetachment after removal of intraocular silicone oil tamponade', *Br J Ophthalmol*, **85**, 1203–1207.

Leaver PK and Billington BM (1989), 'Vitrectomy and fluid/silicone-oil exchange for giant retinal tears: 5 years follow-up', *Graefe's Arch Clin Exp Ophthalmol*, **227**, 323–327.

Lee B, Litt M and Buchsbaum G (1992), 'Rheology of the vitreous body. Part I: viscoelasticity of human vitreous', *Biorheology*, **29**, 521–533.

Lee B, Litt M and Buchsbaum G (1994), 'Rheology of the vitreous body. Part 2. Viscoelasticity of bovine and porcine vitreous', *Biorheology*, **31**, 327–338.

Liang C, Peyman GA, Serracarbassa P, Calixto N, Chow AA, and Rao P (1998), 'An evaluation of methylated collagen as a substitute for vitreous and aqueous humor', *Int Ophthalmol*, **22**, 13–18.

Los LI, van der Worp RJ, van Luyn MJA and Hooymans JMM (2003), 'Age-related liquefaction of the human vitreous body: LM and TEM evaluation of the role of proteoglycans and collagen', *Invest Ophthalmol Vis Sci*, **44**, 2828–2833.

Nakagawa M, Tanaka M and Miyata T (1997), 'Evaluation of collagen gel and hyaluronic acid as vitreous substitutes' *Ophthalmic Res*, **29**, 409–420.

Nayak PL (1999), 'Biodegradable polymers: opportunities and challenges', *JMS-Rev Macromol Chem Phys*, **C39**, 481–505.

Nickerson CS, Karageozian HL, Park J and Kornfield JA (2005), 'Internal tension: A novel hypothesis concerning the mechanical properties of the vitreous humor', *Macromol Symp*, **227**, 183–189.

Park H and Robinson JR (1987), 'Mechanisms of mucoadhesion of poly(acrylic acid) hydrogels', *Pharm Res*, **4**(6), 457–464.

Peppas NA and Brannon-Peppas L (1990), 'Hydrogels at critical conditions. Part 1. Thermodynamics and swelling behavior', *J Memb Sci*, **45**, 281–290.

Peppas NA and Lucht LM (1984), 'Macromolecular structure of coals. I. The organic phase of bituminous coals as a macromolecular network', *Chem Eng Commun*, **30**, 291–310.

Pruett RC, Calabria GA and Schepens CL (1972), 'Collagen vitreous substitute: I. Experimental study', *Arch Ophthalmol*, **88**, 540–543.

Pruett RC, Schepens CL and Freeman HM (1974), 'Collagen vitreous substitute: II. Preliminary clinical trials', *Arch Ophthalmol*, **91**, 29–32.

Pruett RC, Schepens CL and Swann DA (1979), 'Hyaluronic acid vitreous substitute: a six-year clinical evaluation', *Arch Ophthalmol*, **97**, 2325–2330.

Refojo MF (1971), 'Polymers in ophthalmic surgery', *J Biomed Mater Res*, **5**, 113–119.

Soman N and Banerjee R (2003), 'Artificial vitreous replacements', *Biomed Mater Eng*, **13**, 59–74.

Sparrow JR, Ortiz R, MacLeish PR and Chang S (1990), 'Fibroblast behavior at aqueous interfaces with perfluorocarbon, silicone, and fluorosilicone liquids', *Invest Ophthalmol Vis Sci*, **31**, 638–646.

Suri S and Banerjee R (2006), 'In vitro evaluation of in situ gels as short term vitreous substitutes', *J Biomed Mater Res*, **79A**, 650–664.

Swindle KE, Hamilton PD and Ravi N (2006), 'Advancements in the development of artificial vitreous humor utilizing polyacrylamide copolymers with disulfide crosslinkers', *Polym Prepr*, **47**, 59–60.

Swindle KE, Hamilton PD and Ravi N (2008), 'In situ formation of hydrogels as vitreous substitutes: viscoelastic comparison to porcine vitreous', *J Biomed Mater Res A*, **87**(3), 656–665.

Swindle KE and Ravi N (2007), 'Recent advances in polymeric vitreous substitutes' *Expert Review Ophthalmol*, **2**(2), 255–265.

Tasman W and Jaeger EA (2006), *Duane's Ophthalmology*, Philadelphia, Lippincott Williams & Wilkins.

Tokita M, Fujiya Y and Hikichi K (1984), 'Dynamic viscoelasticity of bovine vitreous body', *Biorheology*, **21**, 751–756.

Versura P, Cellini M, Torreggiani A, Bernabini B, Rossi A, Moretti M, Caramzza R (2001), 'The biocompatibility of silicone, fluorosilicone and perfluorocarbon liquids as vitreous tamponades: an ultrastructural and immunohistochemical study', *Ophthalmologica*, **215**, 276–283.

Vijayasekaran S, Chirila TV, Hong Y, Tahija SG, Dalton PD, Constable IJ and McAllister IL (1996), 'Poly(1-vinyl-2-pyrrolidinone) hydrogels as vitreous substitutes: histopathological evaluation in the animal eye', *J Biomater Sci Polym Ed*, **7**(8), 685–696.

Wolf S, Schon V, Meier P and Wiedemann P (2003), 'Silicone oil–RMN3 mixture ("heavy silicone oil") as internal tamponade for complicated retinal detachment', *Retina*, **23**, 335–342.

Zimmerman RL (1980), 'In vivo measurements of the viscoelasticity of the human vitreous humor', *Biophys J*, **29**, 539–544.

14
Retinal repair and regeneration

G. A. LIMB and J. S. ELLIS, UCL Institute of
Ophthalmology, UK

Abstract: Regeneration of neural retina to restore visual function constitutes
a major challenge in the ophthalmic field. Various sources of stem/progenitor
cells capable of developing into retinal neurons have been identified in the
human retina and much research into the feasibility of developing cell-based
therapies using autologous or syngeneic stem cells has been undertaken in
recent years. Several approaches have been used to deliver these cells, but
very little success has been achieved so far. In order to develop retinal cell-
based therapies, it is important to understand the pathways that lead to the
differentiation and maturation of this specialized neural tissue, the structure
and neural interaction in the normal adult retina and the pathological features
that develop as a result of retinal disease. New scientific developments have
resulted in the introduction of biomaterials for tissue regeneration, and the
retina is an amenable organ in which such technologies may potentially be
applied. This chapter addresses various aspects of retinal development and
degeneration and the potential contributions that biomaterials may provide to
the development of cell-based therapies to regenerate neural retina.

Key words: retina, regeneration, retinal progenitor cells, Müller stem cells,
biomaterials.

14.1 Introduction

The retina is a unique sensory organ with a network of specialized neurons
responsible for light perception and construction of visual images in the
brain. Widespread damage of retinal neurons leads to irreversible blindness,
for which new advances in stem cell research provide a hope for restoration
of visual function in patients affected by retinal degenerative conditions.
Major retinal degenerative diseases that may potentially benefit from stem
cell therapies include: age-related macular degeneration (AMD), which
affects between 20 and 25 million people worldwide (Chopdar *et al.*, 2003);
proliferative diabetic retinopathy (PDR), which affects more than 35% of
individuals after 20 years of diabetes (Kohner *et al.*, 1998); other common
retinal disorders such as end-stage glaucoma, retinitis pigmentosa (RP),
proliferative vitreoretinopathy and inherited retinal diseases, which affect
a large number of individuals during their productive life (Rosenberg and
Sperazza, 2008).

Recent studies in the adult human eye have uncovered various sources of
neural retinal progenitors, which under appropriate regenerative conditions

may potentially be used to promote retinal regeneration. Although the retina harbours these cells in adulthood, they appear to remain quiescent and there is no evidence that they re-enter the cell cycle or undergo neural differentiation following retinal injury. This brings us to speculate that the developed retina may provide an inhibitory environment for these cells to proliferate or differentiate *in situ*. However, unravelling the mechanisms that promote their quiescence in adulthood may help to identify factors to promote the growth and differentiation of these cells without the need for transplantation. Alternatively, retinal stem cells may potentially be expanded *in vitro* for autologous or syngeneic grafting, and this approach may require demanding and specialized resources. Understanding developmental pathways, cell requirements for *in vivo* expansion and survival, and the microenvironment in which progenitor cells are to be transplanted are essential for the development of successful cell-based therapies. To date, several methods have been used experimentally to deliver stem cells with limited success, but research in the field is rapidly expanding. Cell transplantation into the retina may require structural support, and new advances in the biomaterials field may lead to the development of appropriate scaffolds for cell delivery, which may promote the survival of transplanted cells and therefore facilitate the establishment of such treatments.

14.2 Retinogenesis and stem cells in the adult human eye

The eye develops from three different types of embryonic tissue: the cornea and sclera develop from the mesoderm, the lens develops from the surface ectoderm and the retina and retinal pigmented epithelium (RPE) from the neural ectoderm (Graw, 1996). Although most of the studies in retinal neurogenesis have been performed in small species such as fish, amphibians, avians and rodents, there is a general consensus that similar developmental pathways occur in the human eye. Neural cell differentiation in the embryonic retina first occurs in the central optic cup, near the optic nerve head (Prada *et al.*, 1991). This is followed by the migration of differentiating cells along the proximo-distal axis, i.e., in the direction of the central retina to the iris (Galli-Resta *et al.*, 1997; Reese *et al.*, 1995). During late retinogenesis, an increase in the proportion of postmitotic cells is observed and new cells are generated in a proliferative zone, the neuroblast layer, from where differentiating neurons migrate into laminating cell layers. Retinal ganglion cells are the first differentiated retinal neurons that emerge, followed in overlapping phases by horizontal cells, cone photoreceptors, amacrine cells, rode photoreceptors, bipolar cells and finally Müller glia (Cepko *et al.*, 1996; Young, 1985).

Stem cells located at the margin of the neural retina immediately adjacent to the ciliary epithelium were first identified in fish and amphibians. This region, known as the ciliary marginal zone (CMZ), is known to harbour retinal progenitors responsible for the regeneration of neural retina in these species throughout life (Hollyfield, 1968; Raymond and Hitchcock, 1997). The presence of a region similar to the fish CMZ has also been shown in avians and small mammals during early postnatal life (Fischer and Reh, 2001; Ooto *et al.*, 2004), and a similar anatomical region has now been described in the human eye (Bhatia *et al.*, 2009). Another population of neural retinal progenitor cells has also been identified within the ciliary epithelium of the postnatal mammalian eye (Gu *et al.*, 2007; Tropepe *et al.*, 2000). However, much confusion has occurred with the understanding of the origin of these cells as a result of various reports giving different descriptions of the anatomical region from which ciliary epithelial cells with progenitor characteristics have been isolated from the mammalian eye. While reporting the presence of neural progenitors in the adult mammalian eye, various groups have failed to identify the anatomical provenance of these cells accurately. The first report that identified these cells in the mouse eye described them as 'pigmented ciliary margin cells' (Tropepe *et al.*, 2000), while in the human eye they were reported to 'derive from the pars plicata and pars plana of the ciliary margin' (Coles *et al.*, 2004). A more recent report described a 'comparison of retinal progenitor cells isolated from the pars plana with a population of progenitors isolated from the ciliary body' (MacNeil *et al.*, 2007). It is therefore important to clarify that both the pars plana and the pars plicata are adjacent areas of the ciliary body (Bron *et al.*, 1997), that the ciliary body is formed by two epithelial cell layers – one pigmented and the other non-pigmented (Bron *et al.*, 1997) – and that the term 'ciliary margin' has traditionally been given to the marginal region of the neural retina, which is adjacent, yet different, to the ciliary body and which has been shown to harbour populations of neural progenitors in some species (Perron and Harris, 2000) (Fig. 14.1). Clarifying the fact that the ciliary body is not part of the neural retina may help us to understand the different nature of the various progenitor populations so far identified in the human eye. Interestingly, at the time of publication of this book, it has become clear that not only the anatomical origin of these so-called 'ciliary margin' cells has been incorrectly cited by many authors, but also the 'stem cell nature' of these cells in the adult eye has become incorrectly a dogma. Extensive evidence has now been presented that ciliary epithelial cells are not retinal stem cells (Cicero *et al.*, 2009) but only ciliary epithelium that express pan-neuronal markers and does not form *bona fide* retinal neurons or glia *in vivo* or *in vitro* (Cicero *et al.*, 2009). In this context, it might be important to clarify whether these properties of the ciliary epithelium vary within species and during different developmental stages.

During development, Müller glia and retinal neurons share a common progenitor that is multipotent at all stages of retinal histogenesis (Raymond

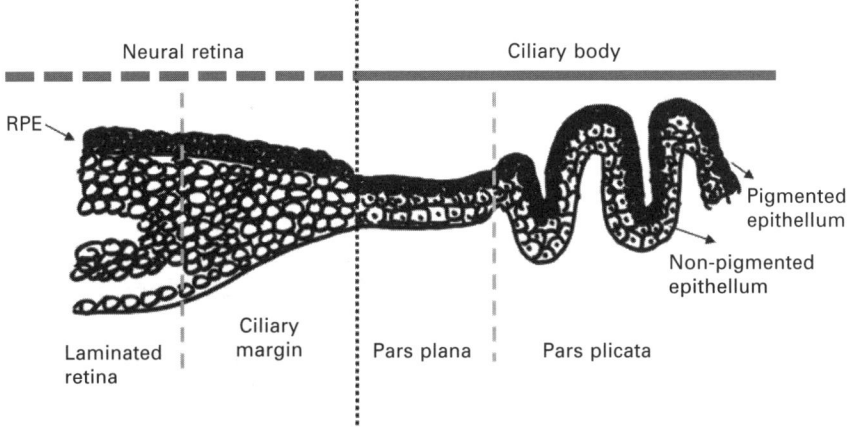

14.1 Diagram showing the anatomical localization of the ciliary body and the neural retina in the mammalian eye. The non-laminated ciliary marginal zone is present in fish and amphibians throughout life (Raymond and Hitchcock, 1997) and has also been observed in early postnatal life of avians and mammals (Fischer and Reh, 2001; Ooto *et al.*, 2004).

and Hitchcock, 1997). This evidence derives from examination of the progeny of a single mouse retinal progenitor cell transfected with a retrovirus, which generated clones containing up to three types of neurons, while others contained a combination of neurons and Müller glia, Müller glia alone or a single type of neuron (Raymond and Hitchcock, 1997). Müller glia have been identified as a source of progenitor cells and retinal regeneration in the postnatal chick (Fischer and Reh, 2001). They have also been shown to proliferate and to produce some neuronal cell types (bipolar and rod photoreceptors) after neurotoxic injury to the adult rat retina (Ooto *et al.*, 2004). Subsequent studies have unequivocally demonstrated that Müller glia exhibit neurogenic characteristics in the adult zebra fish (Raymond *et al.*, 2006), and that these cells form the retinal stem cell niche, which is able to generate neurons after retinal injury in this species (Raymond *et al.*, 2006). More recent investigations have shown that a population of Müller glial cells with stem cell characteristics is also found in the adult human retina (Bhatia *et al.*, 2009; Lawrence *et al.*, 2007) (Fig. 14.2), suggesting that humans may have some potential for neural retinal regeneration.

Retinal progenitor/stem cells can be isolated and induced to proliferate *in vitro* from the foetal and adult neural retina of the human eye using enzymatic dissociation methods (Kelley *et al.*, 1995; Klassen *et al.*, 2004; Lawrence *et al.*, 2007). To promote their proliferation, retinal stem cells can be cultured in the presence of growth and differentiation factors such as fibroblast growth factor (FGF) and epidermal growth factor (EGF) (Kelley

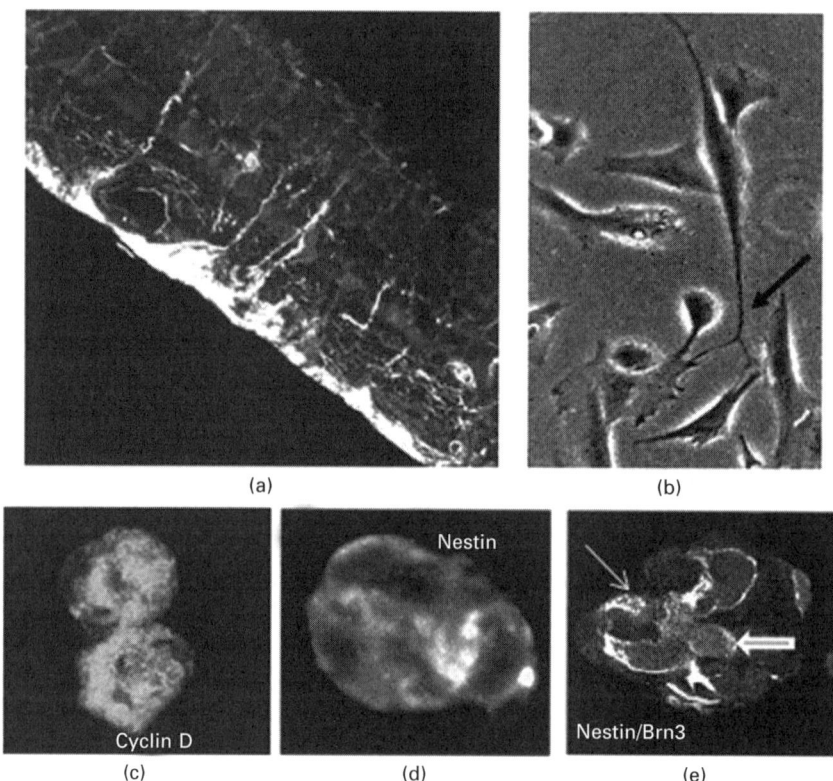

14.2 A population of Müller glia from the adult human retina exhibit neural stem cell characteristics. (a) A small proportion of Müller glia cells that expand across the width of the retina express markers of neural progenitors such as nestin (fluorescent label shown in white). (b), These cells can be isolated from the human neural retina and become spontaneously immortalized. In culture they show long processes that resemble Müller glia *in situ* (black arrow). (c), Müller stem cells cultured at low density in the presence of fibroblast growth factor 2 (FGF2) form neurospheres and express cyclin D, a marker of proliferating cells. (d) and (e) Neurospheres stain for nestin and cells contained within them express markers of differentiated retinal neurons such as rhodopsin (a photoreceptor marker, thin arrow) and Brn3 (a ganglion cell marker, open arrow showing nuclear staining). scale bars, 50 μm.

et al., 1995; Lawrence *et al.*, 2007). Retinal stem/progenitor cells can be identified by the expression of markers of neural progenitors, such as nestin and βIII tubulin (Fischer and Reh, 2003; Kelley *et al.*, 1995; Lawrence *et al.*, 2007), as well as various transcription factors and proteins expressed by retinal stem cells during development. Some of the factors used to identify stem cells from the neural retina include: (a) Pax6, a regulatory factor that promotes multipotency of retinal progenitor cells (Marquardt and Gruss, 2002); (b) sonic hedgehog protein (Shh), which promotes proliferation and differentiation of progenitor cells into ganglion cells (Moshiri and Reh, 2004); (c) Chx10, one of the earliest markers of the developing retina, which is required for retinal cell proliferation and formation of bipolar cells (Chen and Cepko, 2000); (d) basic helix–loop–helix (bHLH) transcription factors, such as Math 5 and NeuroD, which drive progenitor cells towards the ganglion cell and amacrine lineages, respectively (Ahmad et al., 1995); and (e) Sox2, a transcription factor found in early neurogenesis, which is downregulated as cells differentiate and migrate to the different retinal cell layers (Taranova et al., 2006). Expression of Sox2 has also been found to be an important marker of Müller stem cells in the adult human retina (Bhatia et al., 2009; Lawrence et al., 2007). Retinal stem cells that proliferate under the influence of growth factors may also be induced to differentiate into cells expressing markers of retinal neurons by modifications in culture conditions, such as the presence of extracellular matrix proteins and the addition of differentiation factors such as FGF, retinoic acid, insulin and the thyroid hormone T_3 (Kelley et al., 1995; Klassen et al., 2004; Lawrence et al., 2007).

14.3   Regeneration of neural retina

The first studies investigating the possibility of regenerating retina involved the transplantation of whole eyes to genetically eyeless salamanders (Harris, 1982). Implantation of peripheral nerves into adult rat retina (So and Aguayo, 1985), and grafting of embryonic rat retina into damaged adult rat retina have also been performed (Turner et al., 1986), but without success. Several investigations using various models of retinal degeneration have been developed; with various sources of stem cells used for retinal transplantation. These have included brain-derived stem cells (Young et al., 2000), embryonic retinal progenitor cells, ciliary epithelium and stem cells from the postnatal eye (Chacko et al., 2003), human embryonic stem cells (Banin et al., 2006), umbilical cord tissue cells and mesenchymal stem cells (Lund et al., 2007), bone marrow stem cells (Otani et al., 2004) and Müller stem cells (Lawrence et al., 2007). However, despite intensive research in the field, there is no evidence for widespread stem cell integration into the retina, long-term graft survival or complete restoration of visual function.

Neural progenitors obtained from the hippocampus have been shown to survive for very short periods of time after transplantation into the retina, and have failed to express markers of terminally differentiated retinal neurons, such as rhodopsin (Young et al., 2000). Lack of retinal marker expression has also been seen when other brain-derived precursor cell lines have been used for grafting into degenerating retina (Warfvinge et al., 2001). In contrast, progenitor cells obtained from the foetal retina have shown, in addition to good survival, expression of photoreceptor-specific markers after retinal transplantation. However, they have not integrated as well as hippocampal-derived progenitor cells (Chacko *et al.*, 2000). Damaged, dystrophic or degenerating retinae have been shown to promote the migration and integration of grafted retinal progenitors (Chacko *et al.*, 2003; Mellough *et al.*, 2004). These observations suggest that factors that regulate neuronal differentiation and synaptic connectivity during development might be reactivated by retinal degenerative processes (Sheen and Macklis, 1995).

Restoration of retinal function by transplanted stem cells requires the functional restoration of neural synapses, and the potential success of such therapies would depend on the ability of grafted cells to undergo neural differentiation and restoration of synaptic pathways within the host retina. On this basis it is more likely that retinal-specific stem cells from the adult eye that have undergone the developmental stages to become retinal neurons, may constitute more suitable candidates for cell-based therapies to restore retinal function than stem cells derived from embryos or other adult tissues.

At present, it is not known which conditions are needed to achieve optimal integration and long-term survival of transplanted stem cells. Whether better integration, neural differentiation and long-term graft survival may be obtained by transplantation of cell suspensions or cells supported by biomaterial scaffolds, or whether previously differentiated stem cells *in vitro* may functionally integrate better than non-differentiated cells, is not known. Experimental studies in a mouse model of retinal degeneration have suggested that efficient integration and differentiation of retinal progenitors into functional photoreceptor cells may be observed when specific neural precursors are transplanted (MacLaren *et al.*, 2006). On this basis, *in vitro* differentiation of retinal stem cells may be necessary before transplantation and this may require intensive and careful laboratory procedures to protect their biological integrity and to avoid carcinogenesis. In addition to the type of stem cells potentially considered for cell-based therapies, the environment in which the cells are to be transplanted may need to be well thought-out, as abnormal deposition of extracellular matrix and the presence of pro-inflammatory cells that characterize retinal gliosis, may prevent the migration, differentiation and long-term survival of the grafts. Moreover, growth factors known to induce differentiation of neural stem cells during *in vivo* development could potentially be used as adjuvant therapies to induce neural differentiation and proliferation of adult retinal stem cells *in situ*. Following this line of research, recent evidence has shown that Shh, a protein that plays an important role in regulating neurogenesis during retinal development, and wingless-type protein-a (Wnt3a), a transcription factor important for neurogenesis, are able to induce *in situ* proliferation of Müller stem cells and generation of photoreceptors derived from these cells following neurotoxic damage or degeneration of mammalian retina (Osakada *et al.*, 2007; Wan *et al.*, 2007).

14.4   Natural barriers for stem cell transplantation to regenerate neural retina

Retinal remodelling after injury, similar to the remodelling seen in other parts of the central nervous system (CNS), is triggered by photoreceptor degeneration and often results in the formation of a glial scar (Fawcett and Asher, 1999). In order to deliver therapeutic progenitor cells, this glial scar itself must be broken down. Inhibitory axon guidance molecules – such as the chondroitin sulphate proteoglycans (CSPGs) aggrecan, versican and neurocan – have been identified in the human retina. These molecules are produced during the normal development of the retina and optic nerve (Popp et al., 2004) and their developmental time course in the retina parallels that seen in other areas of the CNS. Expression of CSPGs has been shown to be associated with reduction of neurite outgrowth in an experimental model of glial scarring following CNS injury (McKeon et al., 1999), suggesting that such molecules may be involved in limiting the growth of regenerating axons following injury. There is evidence that microcrush injury in the rat optic nerve induces formation of a glial scar rich in CSPGs, which is thought to contribute to the failure of retinal garglion cell regeneration (Selles-Navarro et al., 2001).

Degradation of CSPGs using chondroitinase ABC in rat spinal cords enhances the neurite-promoting potential of spinal cord tissue (Zuo et al., 1998). In addition, regeneration of CNS axons in the lesioned rat nigrostriatal tract (Moon and Fawcett, 2001) and dorsal columns (Bradbury et al., 2002) is enhanced following treatment of the CSPG-rich scar with chondroitinase ABC. This treatment has also demonstrated restoration of postsynaptic activity below the lesion and functional recovery (Bradbury et al., 2002). The retina, being part of the CNS, would be amenable to similar treatments to facilitate the migration and integration of transplanted stem cells. CSPGs (such as neurocan) act as barriers in the developing CNS and are associated with the guiding of axonal pathways (Margolis and Margolis, 1997). They are expressed in the normal rodent retina, although the expression decreases with age (Popp et al., 2004). However, increased production and accumulation of CSPGs have been described in the dystrophic RCS rat retina (Chu et al., 1992; Zhang et al., 2003). These observations have shed sufficient evidence that degenerated adult retina does not provide a permissive environment for the integration or neural differentiation of transplanted stem cells, and abnormal extracellular matrix deposition and microglia accumulation undoubtedly constitute a major barrier for retinal transplantation. The fact that CSPGs deposited in the degenerating retina play an important role in the inhibition of migration and integration of transplanted stem cells to regenerate retina is illustrated by recent observations that degradation of CSPGs by chondroitinase ABC promoted the migration and integration of transplanted Müller stem cells into the degenerating retina of the RCS (Royal college of Surgeons) rat (Singhal *et al.*, 2008).

In addition to changes in the extracellular matrix, resident microglial cells become activated by injury or disease. Experimental evidence indicates that microglia activation occurs with retinal degenerative diseases (Thanos *et al.*, 1993). These cells, which are normally present in the inner retinal layers, migrate to the outer layers when photoreceptors are damaged. Upon recruitment, they proliferate, secrete cytokines, chemokines and neurotoxins, and potentially amplify retinal degeneration (Langmann, 2007). Macrophages also have the ability to produce CSPGs (Lindholm *et al.*, 2005), and recent studies have shown that microglia release these extracellular matrix proteins at the site of retinal damage (Singhal *et al.*, 2008), therefore contributing to the inhibition of migration of the transplanted cells. This has been demonstrated by observations that CSPGs co-localize with microglia at the sites of photoreceptor damage in the RCS rat retina, and that targeted anti-inflammatory therapy that prevents microglia accumulation, in conjunction with administration of chondroitinase ABC, markedly facilitates the migration of transplanted stem cells into the degenerating retina of the RCS rat (Singhal *et al.*, 2008).

14.5   Biomaterials in retinal repair and regeneration

Biomaterials are being extensively investigated for their use in the retinal field, not only for their use in tissue engineering, but also for drug delivery. Biomaterials may potentially be used to provide scaffolds for neural cell differentiation and to facilitate their alignment into structures resembling the retina. Biomaterials may also be used to deliver proteins (Wyatt and Saltzman, 1997), DNA or RNA (Kumar *et al.*, 2004), drugs (Molpeceres *et al.*, 1997) and encapsulated cells (Beck *et al.*, 2007) to target the retina. Polymeric microparticles or nanoparticles made of poly(lactide-co-glycolide) (PLGA) and poly(lactic acid) (PLLA), have been shown to diffuse rapidly through the neural retina and remain in the RPE for up to 4 months following intravitreal injection (Bourges *et al.*, 2003). These particles have been shown to provide a vehicle for the delivery of neurotrophins into the retina (Jiang *et al.*, 2007), enabling the delivery of these molecules over an extended period of time. Another type of biomaterial used for delivery of neuroprotective factors into the retina are hydrogels. A hydrogel is a network of cross-linked polymers which absorb a large quantity of water and therefore swell in its presence (Lin and Metters, 2006). While maintaining water, the cross-linked polymers remain insoluble, providing great flexibility to the solid material (Lin and Matters, 2006). An example of a polymer that can be used in the preparation of hydrogels is poly(ethylene glycol) (PEG), a water-soluble polymer, which is highly hydrophilic. This hydrophilicity decreases the adsorption of proteins and therefore can be used to modify interactions between materials, tissues and cells (Ifkovits *et al.*, 2008). Photopolymerizable PEG hydrogels have been used for encapsulation of porcine islets of Langerhans for transplantation into experimental models of insulin-dependent diabetes mellitus (Cruise *et al.*, 1999), as well as for chondrocyte encapsulation for cartilage tissue engineering (Bryant *et al.*, 2008). Experimental evidence has demonstrated the potential use of hydrogels for human mesenchymal stem cell differentiation and function, for application to bone regeneration (Benoit *et al.*, 2006). In addition, thermo-responsive hydrogel scaffolds have been shown to promote neurite outgrowth from primary neurons and neural stem cells and to provide a useful tool for the repair of spinal cord injury (Nisbet *et al.*, 2009). Studies have also been undertaken to develop various hydrogels to promote differentiation of neural stem cells (Hynes *et al.*, 2008). However, much research still needs to be done in the field in order to provide conclusive evidence for the use of these materials as carriers for stem cell transplantation to regenerate retina.

In contrast to other biomaterials, natural extracellular matrix proteins have an ordered nanoscale structure that can modulate cell behaviour and promote directional migration of grafted stem cells (Alsberg *et al.*, 2006). Extracellular matrix proteins used as biomaterials for tissue engineering include collagen, fibrin, fibrinogen, elastin, hyaluronic acid, chondroitin sulphate and gelatin (Venugopal *et al.*, 2008). Compared with nanoscaffolds made of synthetic polymers, nanoscaffolds made of these biomaterials appear to provide better mechanical and physical properties for the growth and delivery of stem cells (Venugopal *et al.*, 2008). It has been shown that biocompatible scaffolds made of fibrin nanofibrils support adhesion and spreading of human microvascular endothelial cells (Alsberg *et al.*, 2006), while agarose covalently coupled to laminin has been shown to enhanced neurite extensions of embryonic chick dorsal ganglia significantly in a three-dimensional cell culture system (Yu *et al.*, 1999). Laminin coupled to PLLA nanofibres has also been shown to enhance PC12 cell viability and neurite outgrowth (Koh *et al.*, 2008), and nanofibres of collagens type I and II have been shown to act as scaffolds that support growth of human dermal fibroblasts for skin regeneration (Venugopal *et al.*, 2006).

The extracellular matrix present in stem cell niches is thought to play an important role in the programming of these cells to differentiate. Studies have shown that individual components of the extracellular matrix, such as laminin or collagen, do not influence the growth of embryonic stem cells (Philp *et al.*, 2005). In contrast, complex preparations containing multiple extracellular matrices induce embryonic stem cells to differentiate into structures that are similar to the tissue from which the matrix is derived (Philp *et al.*, 2005). Other studies support the importance of the extracellular matrix for stem cell differentiation, as shown by observations that differentiation of adult retinal stem cells into cells expressing markers of retinal neurons is influenced by the type of extracellular matrix proteins in which these cells are cultured *in vitro* (Lawrence *et al.*, 2007). In this context, use of nanofibres made of matrix proteins found in the normal retina may be advantageous compared with the use of synthetic polymers to build cellular scaffolds for retinal transplantation, and this merits extensive investigations.

Scaffolds made of biomaterials have been used with the aim of promoting survival of transplanted cells and promoting the differentiation of retinal progenitor cells (Lavik *et al.*, 2005). Retinal progenitor cells delivered on PLLA/PLGA substrates to the mouse subretinal space have been shown to survive much longer than cells transplanted as a conventional bolus injection, as well as promoting the expression of markers of differentiated neurons *in vivo*. This has been shown by observations that cells that migrated into the retinal laminae adjacent to the graft, expressed typical markers of mature cells including GFAP (glial fibrillary acidic protein – glial marker), recoverin and rhodopsin (Tomita *et al.*, 2005). Polymer composites have also been shown to promote *in vitro* differentiation of mouse retinal progenitors into cells expressing mature retinal markers, and to provide grafts with laminar organization and structural guidance channels (Lavik *et al.*, 2005).

Other polymers, such as poly(methyl methacrylate) (PMMA) (Tao *et al.*, 2007) and poly(glycerol sebacate) (PGS), have been used to manufacture scaffolds for retinal transplantation (Neeley *et al.*, 2008). Investigations on the growth of retinal progenitors on PMMA built with either smooth or porous laminin-coated surfaces showed that cells can be cultured with similar results on either surface. However, transplantation of cells with non-porous scaffolds showed limited progenitor retention, while porous scaffolds demonstrated enhanced cell adherence during transplantation. This was shown to facilitate cell migration into the retina (Tao *et al.*, 2007).

Although advances in the biomaterial field have been made, at present there are several problems with the use of biomaterials as scaffolds for retinal regeneration. This is due to the nature of these materials, such as their slow biodegradability and lack of flexibility, which makes some scaffolds difficult to manipulate for insertion into the retina (Tao *et al.*, 2007; Tomita *et al.*, 2005). In addition, we cannot disregard the potential inflammatory responses that biopolymers may trigger in the retinal microenvironment, as illustrated by observations that these polymers are able to elicit severe microglial activation (Wong *et al.*, 2007).

14.6   Conclusions

Although advances in the retinal stem cell field have been made, development of methods for retinal regeneration still constitutes a major challenge in ophthalmology. Different types of stem cells can potentially be used for regeneration of the diseased human retina, but it may be more appropriate to use adult cells that have already undergone crucial developmental stages that commit them to become retinal neurons. Alternatively, development of methods to induce proliferation and differentiation of resident stem cells *in situ* may constitute a practical and safer therapeutic substitute for cell transplantation. It is also necessary to identify and control natural barriers caused by retinal degenerative processes, which have shown to limit the ability of transplanted cells to integrate, differentiate and survive. Recent advances in the biomaterial field provide an interesting area of research that can be explored in order to deliver retinal stem cell therapies safely while promoting restoration of visual function.

14.7   References

Ahmad I, Zaqouras P, Artavanis-Tsakonas S (1995) Involvement of Notch-1 in mammalian retinal neurogenesis: association of Notch-1 activity with both immature and terminally differentiated cells. *Mech Dev* **53**: 73–85.

Alsberg E, Feinstein E, Joy MP, Prentiss M, Ingber DE (2006) Magnetically guided self-assembly of fibrin matrices with ordered nano-scale structure for tissue engineering. *Tissue Eng* **12**: 3247–3256.

Banin E, Obolensky A, Idelson M, Hemo I, Reinhardtz E, Pikarsky E, Ben-Hur T, Reubinoff B (2006) Retinal incorporation and differentiation of neural precursors derived from human embryonic stem cells. *Stem Cells* **24**: 246–257.

Beck J, Angus R, Madsen B, Britt D, Vernon B, Nguyen KT (2007) Islet encapsulation: strategies to enhance islet cell functions. *Tissue Eng* **13**: 589–599.

Benoit DS, Nuttelman CR, Collins SD, Anseth KS (2006) Synthesis and characterization of a fluvastatin-releasing hydrogel delivery system to modulate hMSC differentiation and function for bone regeneration. *Biomaterials* **27**: 6102–6110.

Bhatia B, Singhal S, Lawrence JM, Khaw PT, Limb GA (2009). Distribution of Müller stem cells within the neural retina: evidence for the existence of a ciliary margin-like zone in the adult human eye. *Exp Eye Res.* **89**: 373–382.

Bourges JL, Gautier SE, Delie F, Bejjani RA, Jeanny JC, Gurny R, BenEzra D, Behar-Cohen FF (2003) Ocular drug delivery targeting the retina and retinal pigment epithelium using polylactide nanoparticles. *Invest Ophthalmol Vis Sci* **44**: 3562–3569.

Bradbury EJ, Moon LD, Popat RJ, King VR, Bennett GS, Patel PN, Fawcett JW, McMahon SB (2002) Chondroitinase ABC promotes functional recovery after spinal cord injury. *Nature* **416**: 636–640.

Bron AJ, Tripathi RC, Tripathi BJ (Eds) (1997) The posterior chamber and ciliary body. In *Wolff's Anatomy of the Eye and Orbit* Chapman & Hall, London), pp. 336–341.

Bryant SJ, Nicodemus GD, Villanueva I (2008) Designing 3D photopolymer hydrogels to regulate biomechanical cues and tissue growth for cartilage tissue engineering. *Pharm Res* **25**: 2379–2386.

Cepko CL, Austin CP, Yang X, Alexiades M, Ezzeddine D (1996) Cell fate determination in the vertebrate retina. *Proc Natl Acad Sci USA* **93**: 589–595.

Chacko DM, Das AV, Zhao X, James J, Bhattacharya S, Ahmad I (2003) Transplantation of ocular stem cells: the role of injury in incorporation and differentiation of grafted cells in the retina. *Vision Res* **43**: 937–946.

Chacko DM, Rogers JA, Turner JE, Ahmad I (2000) Survival and differentiation of cultured retinal progenitors transplanted in the subretinal space of the rat. *Biochem Biophys Res Commun* **268**: 842–846.

Chen CM, Cepko CL (2000) Expression of Chx10 and Chx10-1 in the developing chicken retina. *Mech Dev* **90**: 293–297.

Chopdar A, Chakravarthy U, Verma D (2003) Age related macular degeneration. *BMJ* **326**: 485–488.

Chu Y, Walker LN, Vijayasekaran SL, Cooper RL, Porrello KV, Constable IJ (1992) Developmental study of chondroitin-6-sulphate in normal and dystrophic rat retina. *Graefes Arch Clin Exp Ophthalmol* **230**: 476–482.

Cicero SA, Johnson D, Reyntjens S, Frase S, Connell S, Chow LML, Baker SJ, Sorrentino BP, Dyer MA (2009) Cells previously identified as retinal stem cells are pigmented ciliary epithelial cells. *Proc Nat Acad Sci U S A* **106**: 6685–6690.

Coles BL, Angenieux B, Inoue T, Del Rio-Tsonis K, Spence JR, McInnes RR, Arsenijevic Y, van der KD (2004) Facile isolation and the characterization of human retinal stem cells. *Proc Natl Acad Sci U S A* **101**: 15772–15777.

Cruise GM, Hegre OD, Lamberti FV, Hager SR, Hill R, Scharp DS, Hubbell JA (1999) *In vitro* and *in vivo* performance of porcine islets encapsulated in interfacially photopolymerized poly(ethylene glycol) diacrylate membranes. *Cell Transplant* **8**: 293–306.

Fawcett JW, Asher RA (1999) The glial scar and central nervous system repair. *Brain Res Bull* **49**: 377–391.

Fischer AJ, Reh TA (2001) Muller glia are a potential source of neural regeneration in the postnatal chicken retina. *Nat Neurosci* **4**: 247–252.

Fischer AJ, Reh TA (2003) Potential of Muller glia to become neurogenic retinal progenitor cells. *Glia* **43**: 70–76.

Galli-Resta L, Resta G, Tan SS, Reese BE (1997) Mosaics of islet-1-expressing amacrine cells assembled by short-range cellular interactions. *J Neurosci* **17**: 7831–7838.

Graw J (1996) Genetic aspects of embryonic eye development in vertebrates. *Dev Genet* **18**: 181–197.

Gu P, Harwood LJ, Zhang X, Wylie M, Curry WJ, Cogliati T (2007) Isolation of retinal progenitor and stem cells from the porcine eye. *Mol Vis* **13**: 1045–1057.

Harris WA (1982) The transplantation of eyes to genetically eyeless salamanders: visual projections and somatosensory interactions. *J Neurosci* **2**: 339–353.

Hollyfield JG (1968) Differential addition of cells to the retina in *Rana pipiens* tadpoles. *Dev Biol* **18**: 163–179.

Hynes SR, Rauch MF, Bertram JP, Lavik EB (2008) A library of tunable poly(ethylene glycol)/poly(L-lysine) hydrogels to investigate the material cues that influence neural stem cell differentiation. *J Biomed Mater Res A*. **89**: 499–509.

Ifkovits JL, Padera RF, Burdick JA (2008) Biodegradable and radically polymerized elastomers with enhanced processing capabilities. *Biomed Mater* **3**: 34104.

Jiang C, Moore MJ, Zhang X, Klassen H, Langer R, Young M (2007) Intravitreal injections of GDNF-loaded biodegradable microspheres are neuroprotective in a rat model of glaucoma. *Mol Vis* **13**: 1783–1792.

Kelley MW, Turner JK, Reh TA (1995) Regulation of proliferation and photoreceptor differentiation in fetal human retinal cell cultures. *Invest Ophthalmol Vis Sci* **36**: 1280–1289.

Klassen H, Ziaeian B, Kirov II, Young MJ, Schwartz PH (2004) Isolation of retinal progenitor cells from post-mortem human tissue and comparison with autologous brain progenitors. *J Neurosci Res* **77**: 334–343.

Koh HS, Yong T, Chan CK, Ramakrishna S (2008) Enhancement of neurite outgrowth using nano-structured scaffolds coupled with laminin. *Biomaterials* **29**: 3574–3582.

Kohner EM, Aldington SJ, Stratton IM, Manley SE, Holman RR, Matthews DR, Turner RC (1998) United Kingdom Prospective Diabetes Study, 30: diabetic retinopathy at diagnosis of non-insulin-dependent diabetes mellitus and associated risk factors. *Arch Ophthalmol* **116**: 297–303.

Kumar MN, Mohapatra SS, Kong X, Jena PK, Bakowsky U, Lehr CM (2004) Cationic poly(lactide-co-glycolide) nanoparticles as efficient in vivo gene transfection agents. *J Nanosci Nanotechnol* **4**: 990–994.

Langmann T (2007) Microglia activation in retinal degeneration. *J Leukoc Biol* **81**: 1345–1351.

Lavik EB, Klassen H, Warfvinge K, Langer R, Young MJ (2005) Fabrication of degradable polymer scaffolds to direct the integration and differentiation of retinal progenitors. *Biomaterials* **26**: 3187–3196.

Lawrence JM, Singhal S, Bhatia B, Keegan DJ, Reh TA, Luthert PJ, Khaw PT, Limb GA (2007) MIO-M1 cells and similar Muller glial cell lines derived from adult human retina exhibit neural stem cell characteristics. *Stem Cells* **25**: 2033–2043.

Lin C-C, Metters AT (2006) Hydrogels in controlled release formulations: Network design and mathematical modeling. *Adv Drug Del Rev* **58**: 1379–1408.

Lindholm MW, Nilsson J, Moses J (2005) Low density lipoprotein stimulation of human macrophage proteoglycan secretion. *Biochem Biophys Res Commun* **328**: 455–460.

Lund RD, Wang S, Lu B, Girman S, Holmes T, Sauve Y, Messina DJ, Harris IR, Kihm AJ, Harmon AM, Chin FY, Gosiewska A, Mistry SK (2007) Cells isolated from umbilical cord tissue rescue photoreceptors and visual functions in a rodent model of retinal disease. *Stem Cells* **25**: 602–611.

MacLaren RE, Pearson RA, MacNeil A, Douglas RH, Salt TE, Akimoto M, Swaroop A, Sowden JC, Ali RR (2006) Retinal repair by transplantation of photoreceptor precursors. *Nature* **444**: 203–207.

MacNeil A, Pearson RA, MacLaren RE, Smith AJ, Sowden JC, Ali RR (2007) Comparative analysis of progenitor cells isolated from the iris, pars plana, and ciliary body of the adult porcine eye. *Stem Cells* **25**: 2430–2438.

Margolis RU, Margolis RK (1997) Chondroitin sulfate proteoglycans as mediators of axon growth and pathfinding. *Cell Tissue Res* **290**: 343–348.

Marquardt T, Gruss P (2002) Generating neuronal diversity in the retina: one for nearly all. *Trends Neurosci* **25**: 32–38.

McKeon RJ, Jurynec MJ, Buck CR (1999) The chondroitin sulfate proteoglycans neurocan and phosphacan are expressed by reactive astrocytes in the chronic CNS glial scar. *J Neurosci* **19**: 10778–10788.

Mellough CB, Cui Q, Spalding KL, Symons NA, Pollett MA, Snyder EY, Macklis JD, Harvey AR (2004) Fate of multipotent neural precursor cells transplanted into mouse retina selectively depleted of retinal ganglion cells. *Exp Neurol* **186**: 6–19.

Molpeceres J, Aberturas MR, Chacon M, Berges L, Guzman M (1997) Stability of cyclosporine-loaded poly-sigma-caprolactone nanoparticles. *J Microencapsul* **14**: 777–787.

Moon LD, Fawcett JW (2001) Reduction in CNS scar formation without concomitant increase in axon regeneration following treatment of adult rat brain with a combination of antibodies to TGFbeta1 and beta2. *Eur J Neurosci* **14**: 1667–1677.

Moshiri A, Reh TA (2004) Persistent progenitors at the retinal margin of ptc+/- mice. *J Neurosci* **24**: 229–237.

Neeley WL, Redenti S, Klassen H, Tao S, Desai T, Young MJ, Langer R (2008) A microfabricated scaffold for retinal progenitor cell grafting. *Biomaterials* **29**: 418–426.

Nisbet DR, Moses D, Gengenbach TR, Forsythe JS, Finkelstein DI, Horne MK (2009) Enhancing neurite outgrowth from primary neurones and neural stem cells using thermoresponsive hydrogel scaffolds for the repair of spinal cord injury. *J Biomed Mater Res A* **89**: 24–35.

Ooto S, Akagi T, Kageyama R, Akita J, Mandai M, Honda Y, Takahashi M (2004) Potential for neural regeneration after neurotoxic injury in the adult mammalian retina. *Proc Natl Acad Sci U S A* **101**: 13654–13659.

Osakada F, Ooto S, Akagi T, Mandai M, Akaike A, Takahashi M (2007) Wnt signaling promotes regeneration in the retina of adult mammals. *J Neurosci* **27**: 4210–4219.

Otani A, Dorrell MI, Kinder K, Moreno SK, Nusinowitz S, Banin E, Heckenlively J, Friedlander M (2004) Rescue of retinal degeneration by intravitreally injected adult bone marrow-derived lineage-negative hematopoietic stem cells. *J Clin Invest* **114**: 765–774.

Perron M, Harris WA (2000) Retinal stem cells in vertebrates. *Bioessays* **22**: 685–688.

Philp D, Chen SS, Fitzgerald W, Orenstein J, Margolis L, Kleinman HK (2005) Complex extracellular matrices promote tissue-specific stem cell differentiation. *Stem Cells* **23**: 288–296.

Popp S, Maurel P, Andersen JS, Margolis RU (2004) Developmental changes of aggrecan, versican and neurocan in the retina and optic nerve. *Exp Eye Res* **79**: 351–356.

Prada C, Puga J, Perez-Mendez L, Lopez AR, Ramirez G (1991) Spatial and temporal patterns of neurogenesis in the chick retina. *Eur J Neurosci* **3**: 559–569.

Raymond PA, Barthel LK, Bernardos RL, Perkowski JJ (2006) Molecular characterization of retinal stem cells and their niches in adult zebrafish. *BMC Dev Biol* **6**: 36.

Raymond PA, Hitchcock PF (1997) Retinal regeneration: common principles but a diversity of mechanisms. *Adv Neurol* **72**: 171–184.

Reese BE, Harvey AR, Tan SS (1995) Radial and tangential dispersion patterns in the mouse retina are cell-class specific. *Proc Natl Acad Sci USA* **92**: 2494–2498.

Rosenberg EA, Sperazza LC (2008) The visually impaired patient. *Am Fam Physician* **77**: 1431–1436.

Selles-Navarro I, Ellezam B, Fajardo R, Latour M, McKerracher L (2001) Retinal ganglion cell and nonneuronal cell responses to a microcrush lesion of adult rat optic nerve. *Exp Neurol* **167**: 282–289.

Sheen VL, Macklis JD (1995) Targeted neocortical cell death in adult mice guides migration and differentiation of transplanted embryonic neurons. *J Neurosci* **15**: 8378–8392.

Singhal S, Lawrence JM, Bhatia B, Ellis JS, Kwan AS, MacNeil A, Luthert PJ, Fawcett JW, Perez MT, Khaw PT, Limb GA (2008) Chondroitin sulfate proteoglycans and microglia prevent migration and integration of grafted Muller stem cells into degenerating retina. *Stem Cells* **26**: 1074–1082.

So KF, Aguayo AJ (1985) Lengthy regrowth of cut axons from ganglion cells after peripheral nerve transplantation into the retina of adult rats. *Brain Res* **328**: 349–354.

Tao S, Young C, Redenti S, Zhang Y, Klassen H, Desai T, Young MJ (2007) Survival, migration and differentiation of retinal progenitor cells transplanted on micro-machined poly(methyl methacrylate) scaffolds to the subretinal space. *Lab Chip* **7**: 695–701.

Taranova OV, Magness ST, Fagan BM, Wu Y, Surzenko N, Hutton SR, Pevny LH (2006) SOX2 is a dose-dependent regulator of retinal neural progenitor competence. *Genes Dev* **20**: 1187–1202.

Thanos S, Mey J, Wild M (1993) Treatment of the adult retina with microglia-suppressing factors retards axotomy-induced neuronal degradation and enhances axonal regeneration *in vivo* and *in vitro*. *J Neurosci* **13**: 455–466.

Tomita M, Lavik E, Klassen H, Zahir T, Langer R, Young MJ (2005) Biodegradable polymer composite grafts promote the survival and differentiation of retinal progenitor cells. *Stem Cells* **23**: 1579–1588.

Tropepe V, Coles BL, Chiasson BJ, Horsford DJ, Elia AJ, McInnes RR, van der KD (2000) Retinal stem cells in the adult mammalian eye. *Science* **287**: 2032–2036.

Turner JE, Blair JR, Chappell ET (1986) Peripheral nerve implantation into a penetrating lesion of the eye: stimulation of the damaged retina. *Brain Res* **376**: 246–254.

Venugopal J, Low S, Choon AT, Ramakrishna S (2008) Interaction of cells and nanofiber scaffolds in tissue engineering. *J Biomed Mater Res B Appl Biomater* **84**: 34–48.

Venugopal JR, Zhang Y, Ramakrishna S (2006) In vitro culture of human dermal fibroblasts on electrospun polycaprolactone collagen nanofibrous membrane. *Artif Organs* **30**: 440–446.

Wan J, Zheng H, Xiao HL, She ZJ, Zhou GM (2007) Sonic hedgehog promotes stem-cell potential of Muller glia in the mammalian retina. *Biochem Biophys Res Commun* **363**: 347–354.

Warfvinge K, Kamme C, Englund U, Wictorin K (2001) Retinal integration of grafts of brain-derived precursor cell lines implanted subretinally into adult, normal rats. *Exp Neurol* **169**: 1–12.

Wong DY, Hollister SJ, Krebsbach PH, Nosrat C (2007) Poly(epsilon-caprolactone) and poly (L-lactic-co-glycolic acid) degradable polymer sponges attenuate astrocyte response and lesion growth in acute traumatic brain injury. *Tissue Eng* **13**: 2515–2523.

Wyatt TL, Saltzman WM (1997) Protein delivery from nondegradable polymer matrices. *Pharm Biotechnol* **10**: 119–137.

Young MJ, Ray J, Whiteley SJ, Klassen H, Gage FH (2000) Neuronal differentiation and morphological integration of hippocampal progenitor cells transplanted to the retina of immature and mature dystrophic rats. *Mol Cell Neurosci* **16**: 197–205.

Young RW (1985) Cell differentiation in the retina of the mouse. *Anat Rec* **212**: 199–205.

Yu X, Dillon GP, Bellamkonda RB (1999) A laminin and nerve growth factor-laden three-dimensional scaffold for enhanced neurite extension. *Tissue Eng* **5**: 291–304.

Zhang Y, Rauch U, Perez MT (2003) Accumulation of neurocan, a brain chondroitin sulfate proteoglycan, in association with the retinal vasculature in RCS rats. *Invest Ophthalmol Vis Sci* **44**: 1252–1261.

Zuo J, Neubauer D, Dyess K, Ferguson TA, Muir D (1998) Degradation of chondroitin sulfate proteoglycan enhances the neurite-promoting potential of spinal cord tissue. *Exp Neurol* **154**: 654–662.

15

Development of tissue-engineered membranes for the culture and transplantation of retinal pigment epithelial cells

A. S. L. KWAN, T. V. CHIRILA and S. CHENG,
Queensland Eye Institute, Australia

Abstract: The idea of retinal cell transplantation as a potential treatment for age-related retinal degeneration, a leading cause of blindness in the Western world, has been around for a number of years. To date, however, it has not been entirely successful; one of the main reasons for this is the lack of an ideal substratum for the retinal cells, specifically for the growth of retinal pigment epithelial cells prior to transplantation. This chapter reviews the reasoning behind this potential treatment, the development of animal transplantation models for human trials, the prerequisites of an ideal substratum, the past and current research on substratum materials, and the potential for future developments in this area.

Key words: macular degeneration, biomaterials, Bruch's membrane, retinal pigment epithelium, retinal transplantation, substratum.

15.1   Introduction

Retinal degeneration and especially age-related macular degeneration is a leading cause of blindness in the Western world. Patients suffer from extensive visual loss due to degenerative change in the retina and its adjacent layers, loss of functioning cells, abnormal vascular ingrowth, and subsequent scar formation at the macula. Cell transplantation has been explored, without success, as a potential treatment and one of the reasons for this lack of success is the lack of a suitable tissue as support for cell transplantation. The acronyms ARM, ARMD, and AMD are often used interchangeably in the literature. Early disease is sometimes referred to as age-related maculopathy (ARM), and late disease in the form of geographic atrophy (GA) or exudative choroidal neovascular membrane (CNVM) is referred to as age-related macular degeneration (AMD or ARMD). The use of these terminologies is not universal. For simplicity, AMD is used here to refer to the spectrum of disease. This chapter looks at the potential of using an artificial layer as a supportive layer for cell culture and cell transplantation in AMD.

15.2   The scale of the problem of age-related macular degeneration

AMD is one of the leading causes of blindness in the Western world. In the United States, its prevalence is 0.05% before the age of 50 years and that rises to 11.8% after 80 years of age (Friedman *et al.*, 2004). In Australia, the most common cause of blindness (presenting visual acuity of less than 6/60) was AMD (48%), and the predicted number of Australians who will have low vision or blindness will almost double over the years 2000 to 2024 (Taylor *et al.*, 2005). This estimation was mirrored in the American study with the prevalence of AMD expected to double in the coming decades because of the projected increase in ageing populations (Friedman *et al.*, 2004). The direct health cost for macular degeneration was estimated to be A$19.4 million in 2004 and this did not include the special allocated funding for photodynamic therapy, the best available treatment at the time, which was estimated to be between A$30 and 40 million per annum (Taylor *et al.*, 2006). This estimate will undoubtedly be significantly higher as a number of governments worldwide have approved funding for one of the pharmacological treatments for AMD – intravitreal injection of anti-vascular endothelial growth factor (anti-VEGF) ranibizumab (Lucentis). There is clearly an urgent and important need for further research on the management of macular degeneration.

15.3   Retinal pigment epitheliun–Bruch's membrane complex and the effect of ageing

15.3.1   Normal retinal pigment epitheliun

Retinal pigment epithelium (RPE) is a monolayer of pigmented cells derived from the neuroectodermal layer of the optic cup and constitutes the outermost layer of retina. RPE is known to secrete various factors promoting retinal photoreceptor survival and differentiation. The RPE cell exhibits an apical–basal polarity characteristic for a transporting epithelium. The subretinal space which is the extracellular space at the apical RPE surface is filled with inter-photoreceptor matrix. RPE projects specialized microvilli into the subretinal space serving to maintain the retinal adhesion. The infolded basal RPE surface rests on Bruch's membrane and forms the outer part of the blood–retinal barrier by the tight junctions between RPE cells. The barrier isolates the subretinal space from the porous choriocapillaris, allowing selective transport of nutrients and metabolic end products between the subretinal space and choriocapillaris (Strauss, 2005). There is a geographical difference in the differentiated RPE cells. In the macula, for example, RPE cells are more tightly packed together (14 μm × 12 μm), and contain higher amounts of melanin. Higher degradation enzyme activities found in this region allow for the maintenance of greater numbers of macular photoreceptors compared with the peripheral RPE cells, which are larger in size (60 µm) and variable in height (Harman *et al.*, 1997; Panda-Jonas *et al.*, 1996; Strauss, 2005).

RPE helps to absorb light energy focused by the lens on to the retina. The heat generated is dissipated by choriocapillaris perfusion. RPE melanins in the melanosome and lipofuscin which are initially beneficial but later accumulate to toxic levels, help absorb the damaging blue light. RPE plays a critical role in the visual cycle where all-trans-retinol from photoreceptors is isomerized to 11-*cis*-retinal within the RPE cells and re-delivered back to photoreceptors to bind with opsin and initiates the photo-transduction cascade. RPE is also responsible for photoreceptor outer segment renewal in a circadian-controlled fashion. The shed outer segment is phagocytosed by RPE via specific binding of apical RPE membrane receptors, such as CD36, MerTK (receptor tyrosine kinase c-mer) and integrin receptors responsible for regulating the internalization process (Harman *et al.*, 1997; Panda-Jonas *et al.*, 1996; Strauss, 2005).

Growth factor, trophic and paracrine secretory functions of RPE are essential for retinal homeostasis and normal function. The health of RPE is therefore critically important in maintaining the normal retinal function and subretinal homeostasis. Any disturbance to the physiological levels of growth factors may lead to an altered homeostasis of the retinal micro-environment, and such changes in RPE secretory activity are found to be associated with retinal proliferative diseases (Binder *et al.*, 2007).

15.3.2 Ageing retinal pigment epithelium

RPE cells undergo significant age-related changes with observed increase in β-galactosidase staining, telomere loss, mitochondrial deoxyribonucleic acid (DNA) damage, nuclear DNA damage, protein crosslinking and lipid hydroperoxidation, many of which are non-reversible in such post-mitotic cells (de Jong, 2006; Handa, 2007; Zarbin, 2004). RPE in early AMD was observed to contain more melano-lipofuscin and melano-lysosomes than pure melanin and the number of lipofuscin granules increased. Melanosomes contained within the RPE are exposed to a variety of environmental and metabolic insults. There are suggestions that aged human melanosomes are highly phototoxic and can result in RPE dysfunction, while young melanosomes appear to confer photoprotection (Rozanowski *et al.*, 2008). Age-related changes in melanosomes, possibly the result of oxidative damage, include disorientation within the RPE, decline in number after the age of 40 years, increase in melanosome complexes with lysosomes and/or lipofuscin, loss of melanin resulting in fading of eye colour with age, and increases in shorter wavelength blue spectrum absorption.

Preferential accumulation of lipofuscin in ageing RPE within the macula is a heterogeneous mixture of non-degradable lipid peroxidation products. These products originate from conjugates formed by visual cycle retinoid in photoreceptor cells that accumulate in RPE cells due to the inability of the RPE cells to convert all all-*trans*-retinol into 11-*cis*-retinal. RPE lipofuscin is a potent generator of reactive oxygen species. It is hypothesized that such species, including reactive fragments from lipids and retinoids, contribute to the mechanisms of RPE lipofuscin pathogenesis (Ng *et al.*, 2008).

Lipofuscin autofluoresces a yellowish orange colour due to its composition being a heterogeneous mixture of cytotoxic fluorophore *N*-retinylidene-*N*-retinylethanolamine (A2E) and its photo-isomers A2E epoxides. There are suggestions of a possible link between A2E's role in interfering with normal lipid metabolism and a resultant delay in lipid degradation and accumulation, leading to increased RPE sensitivity to blue light. The above degenerative RPE changes ultimately lead to the formation of basal deposits, drusen, RPE cell apoptosis, followed by secondary damage to choriocapillaris and neurosensory retina, and resulting in (de Jong, 2006; Handa, 2007; Zarbin, 2004).

15.3.3 Bruch's membrane and ageing changes

The anatomy of human Bruch's membrane displays a penta-laminar structure (1–4 μm thick) composed of a 50 nm, thin acellular RPE basal lamina, an inner collagen layer (ICL), an elastin layer (EL), an outer collagen layer (OCL), and the choriocapillaris basal lamina (Strauss, 2005).

Most dysfunction within AMD starts in the ICL, with drusen-like material accumulating either side of the RPE basal lamina and invasion of the ICL tissue plane by CNVM in advanced AMD. Drusen is the clinical hallmark of AMD. The punctate hard drusen of size <63 μm in diameter is not associated with AMD. However, large (>63 μm) drusen size and, to a lesser extent, the number of indistinct soft drusen are found to correlate positively with progression to advanced AMD. The EL underneath is also found to become pathologically fragmented. Apart from age-related collagen crosslinking change in the OCL, extracellular deposits (drusen, lipid deposits) appear to spare this layer and accumulate mainly within the ICL.

It is thought that, once the EL and ICL are filled with debris, lipoprotein deposits continue to accumulate near the RPE. This possibly explains why no further accumulation was found in the OCL (Huang *et al.*, 2008). Interestingly, CNVM only penetrates through, but does not invade the OCL. Perhaps this is due to the age-related decrease in endostatin levels in these structures, which may be permissive for CNVM formation (Bhutto *et al.*, 2004). In addition, unlike the RPE basal lamina, there is no evidence of deposit formation on either side of the choriocapillaris basal lamina as a function of advancing age.

15.3.4 Relationship between the retinal pigment epithelium and Bruch's membrane

The intricate relationship between the photoreceptor, RPE, and Bruch's membrane is fundamental to normal retinal function. Age-related alterations in the molecular composition and ultrastructures of human Bruch's membrane make it an unfavourable substratum for the attachment and survival of grafted RPE cells (Tezel et al., 1999; Tezel and Del Priore, 1999). Attempts have been made, by way of in vitro re-engineering, to 'clean' the Bruch's membrane (especially the inner collagen layer) with a non-ionic detergent and refurbish it with extracellular matrix (ECM) proteins (laminin, vitronectin, fibronectin) (Tezel et al., 2004). This may be why these attempts to repopulate the RPE defects with native or transplant RPE cells alone have not met with great success. The presence of disease within the host's Bruch's membrane, iatrogenic removal of the inner layers of Bruch's membrane, and immune rejection of the transplant have all been blamed for limiting visual recovery after RPE cell transplantation studies (Del Priore et al., 2006).

15.4 Summary of the aetiology and management of age-related macular degeneration

The aetiology of AMD is multi-factorial – including physiological ageing, genetic, inflammatory, and environmental factors – but the end result is a complex series of events that lead to a significant change in the RPE–Bruch's membrane–choroidal complex, also known as Ruysch's complex (de Jong, 2006). This is accompanied by loss of RPE and photoreceptors, and eventually fibrovascular membrane and scar formation. Different potential therapies have been tried including: dietary/vitamin supplement; laser treatment with or without photosensitizing dye; submacular membranectomy with or without RPE transplantation or translocation; macular translocation surgery; radiotherapy; gene therapy; and pharmacological treatment (e.g. angiostatic steroid and anti-VEGF therapy). Despite these treatments, many patients lose their vision from chorioretinal fibrovascular scaring following the formation of CNVM, therefore alternative treatments are still being explored (Binder et al., 2007).

Ninety per cent of severe visual loss from AMD is due to the 'wet' type of macular degeneration – i.e. CNVM formation (Smith et al., 2001). Unfortunately, simple excision of the CNVM in AMD results in RPE defects because the original RPE is removed along with the neovascular complex; this is because the CNVM found in AMD is situated beneath the ageing native RPE layer (Grossniklaus et al., 1994). The loss of RPE following this surgery leads to progressive loss of the underlying choriocapillaris and the overlying photoreceptors (Del Priore et al., 2006). The end result is similar to a subtype of dry macular degeneration – geographic atrophy, with equally devastating effects.

15.5   Retinal pigment epithelium transplantation from animals to human

In order to address the problem of RPE loss, studies on RPE transplantation in animal models of retinal degeneration were carried out. It has been proven in principle that RPE transplantation can lead to photoreceptor rescue and functional improvement in the Royal College of Surgeons (RCS) rat (Lund *et al.*, 2001), which has retinal degeneration with a mutation in its Mertk gene (D'Cruz *et al.*, 2000). Other cell types have been tried, including stem cells (Schraermeyer *et al.*, 2001) and Schwann cells (Lawrence *et al.*, 2000), but RPE cell transplantation remains the benchmark as most of the other cell types have so far failed to achieve the same degree of rescue and the ethical issues, associated with obtaining these cells, remain a problem. Armed with the success in the laboratory, Peyman and coworkers performed one of the first RPE transplantations in humans, whereby submacular scar excisions were followed by translocation of an autologous RPE pedicle flap or transplantation of an allogenic RPE–Bruch's membrane explant in two patients (Peyman *et al.*, 1991). This was followed by trials of transplantation of foetal human RPE patches following subretinal membrane removal. These patients were able to fixate over the area of the RPE graft initially but cystoid macula oedema ensued and eventually the grafts were encapsulated by fibrotic scars; these might be a result of immune rejection as none of the patients were immunologically suppressed. Because of the rejection, autologous iris pigment epithelial (IPE) cells have been used to replace the lost or damaged RPE cells in the macular area (Thumann *et al.*, 2000). However, transplantation of suspensions of autologous IPE cells has also not resulted in a prolonged improvement of vision in AMD patients. One of the reasons for this failure was probably because the transplanted IPE cells did not fully differentiate into cells that had the morphological and physiological properties of RPE cells *in situ*. Binder and coworkers transplanted suspensions of autologous RPE cells into eyes with wet type AMD after removal of CNVM membranes (Binder *et al.*, 2002). They reported that these eyes had significantly better reading acuity than controls with CNVM removal only. However, obtaining sufficient numbers of RPE cells was sometimes difficult, and in some patients the aspirated RPE cells were not transplanted because of insufficient numbers or haemorrhage. In most of these studies, suspensions of isolated cells were injected into the subretinal space, one problem with IPE/RPE cells in the suspension is that photoreceptor cells survived well when a monolayer of pigment epithelial cells was transplanted, but the photoreceptors did not survive when the transplanted cells clustered into a mound-like shape (Crafoord *et al.*, 2002). Moreover, RPE cells in suspension may not settle in the subretinal space but instead find their way into the vitreal cavity where they de-differentiate, become fibroblastic in nature, and eventually migrate and contract in the form of epiretinal membrane or proliferative vitreoretinopathy. These may result in macular pucker and retinal detachment, which will have a detrimental effect on the visual outcome. Despite these early problems, recently, three surgical techniques (macular translocation and combining surgical removal of CNVM and RPE–choroid transplantation) have been used to restore foveal photoreceptor contact to an area of relative healthy RPE, albeit ageing RPE; the techniques met with some success and serve as a proof of the principle that some foveal (photoreceptor) function can be restored in AMD (Chen *et al.*, 2009; MacLaren *et al.*, 2007; Toth *et al.*, 2004).

These studies have therefore provided a compelling argument for RPE transplantation as a treatment option for atrophic AMD and exudative AMD. It represents a plausible cell-based therapeutic strategy with the aim of rescuing the remaining viable photoreceptors and preventing postoperative subfoveal choriocapillaris atrophy by replacing the diseased RPE/iatrogenic RPE loss secondary to membranectomy of the CNVM. Furthermore, early transplant intervention can prevent the onset of inner retinal changes secondary to remodelling processes (Wang *et al.*, 2005). Visual acuity appears to have the plasticity to maximize any visual signals it receives.

With the cell-based RPE transplantation, it is possible to modify many different biochemical pathways simultaneously and reduce the chance of 'escape' associated with currently available pharmacological monotherapy. In addition, it may offer benefits that complement those of pathway-based pharmacological therapy and/or gene therapy (Binder *et al.*, 2007).

15.6   Biomaterials for retinal pigment epithelium cell culture and transplantation

15.6.1 Search for an ideal substratum

In vitro, RPE has been grown on a number of potential substrata with different degrees of success. In addition to the biopolymers and synthetic polymers that will be described in the next section, substrata have been developed from microspheres with crosslinked fibrinogen (Oganesian *et al.*, 1999), amniotic membrane (Capeans *et al.*, 2003), anterior lens capsule (Hartmann *et al.*, 1999), Descemet's membrane (Thumann *et al.*, 1997), cryoprecipitated extracellular matrix membranes (Farrokh-Siar *et al.*, 1999), and cadaver Bruch's membrane (Castellarin *et al.*, 1998). Despite a general consensus that most of these materials are able to promote the formation of RPE cell layers with the retention of some of their phenotype characteristics, and therefore might be useful as temporary substrata for subretinal transplantation, few of the materials have been tested *in vivo* in animal models, and none of the materials has managed to encompass all the qualities for an ideal substratum. In order to mimic the native RPE layer on Bruch's membrane and to maximize the chance of normal function and survival, the ideal RPE layer for transplantation will need to have a number of properties: (a) it should be a monolayer of RPE cells with good adhesion to a substratum; (b) it should have the correct orientation/polarity, normal morphology, and expression of differentiated RPE cell features; (c) the substratum should be thin, suitably porous to allow the transport of both nutrients and waste from the underlying tissues to the transplanted RPE monolayer, strong and yet manipulable for ease of introduction to the subretinal space; (d) it should display biostability and biocompatibility, and be immunologically inert so that it does not cause inflammation and rejection. The material may or may not be biodegradable as long as no adverse effects are observed.

15.6.2 Biomaterials as substrata for retinal pigment epithelium cell culture and transplantation

The importance for the growth of RPE cells of substrata made of naturally derived and/or synthetic biomaterials was revealed indirectly some time ago. For instance, the effect of the ECM on the proliferation of RPE cells was investigated by using a synthetic polymer substratum (tissue culture polystyrene) coated with collagen, Matrigel™ (a commercially available synthetic basement membrane derived from a mouse sarcoma tumour cell line), poly(D-lysine), or undefined matrices deposited by either RPE cells or retinal glial cells (Williams and Burke, 1990). A crucial study demonstrating that the RPE cells cannot survive and undergo apoptosis when separated from their natural ECM if they do not have the opportunity to reattach to a substratum was also based on the use of tissue culture polystyrene used on its own or coated with ECM components, and of untreated polystyrene used on its own or coated with agents preventing cell adhesion (Tezel and Del Priore, 1997). However, a relatively small range of biomaterials have been proposed and investigated as substrata for transplantable RPE constructs.

In this section we will discuss both the processed biopolymers and the synthetic polymers that have been investigated to date as potential substrata for the growth of RPE cells. Collagen type I was used as a substratum for human foetal RPE cells to create sheet-like constructs, which were then transplanted *in vivo* into the subretinal space of non-pigmented rabbit eyes (Bhatt *et al.*, 1994). Two different collagen substrata were used, uncrosslinked and crosslinked (by ultraviolet (UV) irradiation). The crosslinked collagen transplants were unsuccessful as a result of the detachment of the RPE cells, which was explained by increased stiffness of the substratum. In the eyes containing the uncrosslinked collagen transplants, a layer of pigmented RPE was visible and the retina remained normal until the end of experiments (for 6 weeks). In spite of such promising results, there has been no record of using collagen substrata again until very recently. In this study (Thumann *et al.*, 2006), porcine primary RPE and IPE cells were grown to confluence on a 10 μm thick collagen type I membrane available commercially as ResoFoil® (from RESORBA Wundversorgung GmbH & Co. KG, Nuremberg, Germany). Both RPE and IPE cells readily attached to, and proliferated and formed monolayers on, the collagen substratum, and acquired differentiated properties. These constructs were then transplanted into the subretinal space of enucleated porcine eyes, and further assays showed that the cells maintained viability following this manipulation. In a more recent study (Lu *et al.*, 2007), the attention was focused towards fabricating collagen layers with the same thickness and properties as the natural Bruch's membrane. Membranes were produced from a collagen available commercially as Vitrogen 100® (Angiotech BioMaterials Corp., Palo Alto, CA, USA) to a thickness around 2.4 μm and having physical properties similar to Bruch's membrane. Cells from an immortalized human RPE cell line (ARPE-19) were successfully grown on these membranes; they showed normal morphology and intercellular tight junctions, and were able to phagocytize *in vitro* the photoreceptor outer segments. In spite of such promising results, there is no reported use of collagen substrata in human patients.

Gelatin was the substratum of choice in other studies, and it has to be accoladed as the only material used so far in human clinical trials. In one approach (Ho *et al.*, 1996), ECM was prepared from a layer of RPE cells, coated with a layer of gelatin, and then cooled to 4 °C when the gelatin solidified. Patches of ECM–gelatin were transferred to another tissue culture dish and RPE cells were seeded on to them. In another approach (Ho *et al.*, 1997), RPE were first cultured to confluence on tissue culture dishes, then covered with liquid gelatin and cooled to 4 °C. The RPE–gelatin blocks were easily cut and transferred to another tissue culture dish. Upon incubation at 37 °C, the gelatin melted and encased the cells, so providing a vehicle for the transplantation of the RPE constructs. Based on these developments, RPE cellular constructs encased in gelatin were transplanted into a human elderly patient affected by AMD (Del Priore *et al.*, 2001). The cells were harvested from a human donor. While the retina remained attached, the patient's vision did not improve over the follow-up period. As this patient died from unrelated causes about 4 months after operation, a complete histopathological examination of the eye was possible, revealing the presence at the transplant site of clusters of pigmented cells that failed to form a uniform layer. Recently, the transplantation of allogeneic RPE cell sheets encased in gelatin was reported in 12 patients affected by exudative AMD (Tezel *et al.*, 2007). The patients were followed for 1 year. Rejection of implants was prevented by administration of immunosuppressants, but other postoperative complications were observed, and there was no improvement in visual function.

The best-known and most accessible synthetic biodegradable polymers, the poly(α-hydroxyesters), represented mainly by polylactides and polyglycolides, have attracted much interest as potential substratum materials, to the extent that a review has been possible on this particular topic (Lu *et al.*, 2001b). Biodegradability is an attractive feature of the potential substrata, as it assures that the foreign material will be resorbed and will dissipate in time. Significant work has been carried out by Mikos' group (Giordano *et al.*, 1997; Lu *et al.*, 1998; Lu *et al.*, 2001a; Lu *et al.*, 2001b; Thomson *et al.*, 1996). They have developed substrata from poly(L-lactic acid) (PLLA) and poly(lactic-co-glycolic acid) (PLGA), with a thickness of at least 10 µm, and have demonstrated that foetal or adult RPE cells were able to attach to the polymer surface and to proliferate. At confluence, the cells expressed ZO-1 protein confirming the existence of normal tight junctions between cells. However, the cells appear more elongated prior to reaching confluence. Based on their own previous investigations regarding the effect of surface micropatterning on RPE cell growth on to glass (Lu *et al.*, 1999), the group demonstrated in a subsequent study that a topography can be created on the PLGA surface that promotes the characteristic cuboidal morphology of the RPE cells (Lu *et al.*, 2001a). This was achieved by using a microcontact printing technique enabling the creation of defined arrays of PLGA (which promotes cell adhesion but not an ideal cell morphology) separated by regions of a block copolymer, poly(DL-lactic acid)/poly(ethylene glycol) (PLA/PEG). The latter is a polymer substratum that inhibits cell adhesion. The resulting pattern promoted a cuboidal morphology of the cultured RPE cells. Other investigators have also focused their attention on these polymers. Porcine and human RPE cell cultures were established from post-mortem sources and grown on PLA or PLGA films, 10–30 µm in thickness, with the aim of evaluating them as substrata for RPE cells (Hadlock *et al.*, 1999). The cells proliferated readily on the films and retained their phenotype and functional characteristics. In another study, commercial poly(DL-lactide-*co*-glycolide) was used to prepare films of 35–50 µm thickness (Rezai *et al.*, 1999). Sheets of human foetal RPE cells dissected from foetal eyes were attached to these films and incubated in growth media. Within days, the attached cells generated spheroids, which were then dissociated and further characterized. This study was actually designed to investigate the formation of spheroids and to evaluate their long-term behaviour *in vitro*. The particular use of biodegradable polymers does not really appear to be any more justified than the use of any polymer able to promote cell adhesion. More recently, natural biodegradable polymers have been proposed as an alternative to the synthetic polymers. Poly(3-hydroxybutyrate-*co*-3-hydroxyvalerate), a copolymer produced by certain microorganisms, was assessed as a substratum for the RPE cell line D407 (Tezcaner *et al.*, 2003). In order to enhance cell adhesion, the polymer surface was treated in an oxygen plasma reactor. Cell counts showed that this treatment led to an increased number of attached cells. The authors' suggestion that this is a result of enhanced hydrophilicity of the polymer surface is, however, at odds with the well-known interrelation between cell adhesion and substratum hydrophilicity.

Although rather extensively assessed as substrata for RPE cells, PLA and PLGA were assessed *in vivo* as substratum materials only in experiments involving different cells – the retinal progenitor cells (RPCs) (Lavik *et al.*, 2005). Murine RPCs were cultured on porous PLA or PLGA scaffolds. Seeded scaffolds were then either co-cultured with degenerating mouse retinal explants or inserted into the subretinal space of rats. The results suggested that the scaffold may assist in the differentiation to photoreceptor phenotype. However, the same group subsequently used ultra-thin layers of laminin-coated poly(methyl methacrylate) (PMMA) as a substratum for RPCs with similar results (Tao *et al.*, 2007). Apparently, the investigators were not concerned by the non-biodegradability of PMMA.

Thermoresponsive polymers constitute another class of polymers, which have been evaluated over the last decade as substrata for the RPE cells. These polymers display a so-called 'lower critical solution temperature (LCST)'. In principle, at temperatures above the LCST, the polymer is hydrophobic and consequently supports the attachment of cells, which can be grown to confluent sheets. Water is partially displaced from the macromolecular coil, the hydrogen bonds involving water are weakened, and the hydrophobic interactions between polymer segments become dominant, resulting in the polymer chains having a compact conformation that prevents the penetration of water. Below the LCST, the polymer surface turns hydrophilic, as the hydrogen bonding between the hydrophilic segments and water molecules becomes dominant and leads to chains with an extended conformation. As soon as the surface turns hydrophilic, the cells detach (because of a lower tendency of cells to attach to hydrated surfaces) and they can be harvested as single uninterrupted sheets. This technique, coined 'cell sheet engineering', has so far been applied in ocular surface reconstruction, myocardial tissue engineering, and other therapies (Yang *et al.*, 2006). It has the advantage that it allows separation of cells without using enzymes.

The polymers based on *N*-isopropylacrylamide (NIPAAm) include some of the most studied synthetic thermoresponsive materials. The routine cell incubation temperature (37°C) is well above their LCST, which assures normal growth of cells on these surfaces when they are in a hydrophobic state. A copolymer of NIPAAm and aminostyrene, modified with cinnamoyl functions, was studied as a substratum for the growth and fabrication of RPE cell sheets (von Recum *et al.*, 1998a; von Recum *et al.*, 1998b; von Recum *et al.*, 1999a; von Recum *et al.*, 1999b). RPE cells from various sources (chicken, post-mortem human, or D407 line) were able to attach and grow on this substratum, and stable cell sheets could be detached and manipulated. Importantly, the RPE cells maintained a normal retinoid metabolism, a function usually lost during cell culture. Owing to the chemistry of the surface of the copolymer, growth factors could be easily immobilized on to the surface, a treatment that improved the proliferation of RPE cells. Other types of RPE cells (rat, ARPE-19) showed similar behaviour when the substratum was the structurally simpler homopolymer, poly(NIPAAm) (Abe *et al.*, 2006; Kubota *et al.*, 2006).

Although both biodegradable and thermoresponsive polymers have been the synthetic materials most studied as substrata for RPE cells, there is no record of any *in vivo* or clinical application so far.

There have also been episodic reports of individual polymers evaluated as potential substrata for RPE cell constructs. For instance, membranes made from a proprietary synthetic hydrogel based on methacrylamide (Organogel Canada, Quebec), coated with poly(D-lysine) and fibronectin, were used as substrata for human RPE cells *in vitro* (Singh *et al.*, 2001). Although the growth and behaviour of cells was deemed as successful as that seen on lens capsule substrata, we are not aware of any further developments involving this hydrogel. A group at the University of Liverpool (UK) reported the *in vitro* evaluation of a series of commercial polyurethanes (Williams *et al.*, 2005) and of a commercial silicone elastomer (Krishna *et al.*, 2007), which were plasma-treated for the enhancement of cell adhesion. Although the RPE cells readily proliferated and the assays showed the maintenance of the main cellular functions, it is to be noted that these polymers are not biodegradable and consequently they would be retained indefinitely after transplantation. Nevertheless, the authors perceived this as an advantage over the biodegradable substrata because of the potential release of toxic breakdown products from the latter.

Some advanced materials based on the allotropic forms of carbon have been contemplated as substrata for RPE cell growth. Such a material was 'bucky paper' (sometimes worded as 'buckypaper'). Bucky paper is a member of the fullerenes, which are molecular structures composed entirely of carbon and include spherical, cylindrical, and planar molecules – known, respectively, as buckyballs, carbon nanotubes (CNTs), and graphenes. Bucky paper is an entangled aggregate of CNTs held together as a planar film. Conventionally, the thickness of bucky paper is between 50 and 500 μm. This material can be generated by a variety of methods based on the dispersion of CNTs (using surfactants, acid oxidation, etc.) followed by filtration. Recently, a method ('frit filtration') has been established (Whitby *et al.*, 2008) that avoids some of the disadvantages associated with the previous methods. Although there are contradictory reports on the biocompatibility of CNTs (Zanello *et al.*,

2006), bucky paper has attracted attention as a potential substratum for cell growth because of its inertness, adjustable thickness and porosity, and mechanical properties. Collaborative work at Stanford University and NASA Ames Research Center proved that bucky paper can function as a substratum for RPE cells (Leng *et al.*, 2003; Loftus *et al.*, 2006). Both human RPE cells (ARPE-19) and IPE cells (harvested from rabbit eyes) were cultured successfully on sheets of bucky paper (50–100 µm in thickness) in serum-supplemented media, although the IPE cells did not from a uniform layer. The *in vivo* biocompatibility of bucky paper was investigated by implantation of sheets into the subretinal space of rabbits and was followed-up for 1 month. The bucky paper sheet was easy to handle and the material was well tolerated in the subretinal space. The issue of the non-biodegradability of bucky paper was not mentioned by these investigators. We are not aware of any continuation of this work.

15.6.3 Preliminary evaluation of silk fibroin as a substratum for retinal pigment epithelium cells

We have recently proposed and evaluated a protein isolated from natural silk as a substratum material for the growth of RPE cells (Kwan *et al.*, 2007). Silk proteins belong to the group of fibrous proteins, which also includes collagens, elastins, and myosins. There is an enormous range of silks, which are produced predominantly by the larvae of insects from the order Lepidoptera (i.e. moths and butterflies) and by spiders (Araneae). We have focused our attention on the silk produced by the domesticated silkworm (*Bombyx mori*), which is basically constituted from fibroin and sericin. There is much interest in using the silkworm silk as a biomaterial (Altman *et al.*, 2003; Hakimi *et al.*, 2007; Wang *et al.*, 2006). In fact, this silk has a long record of use as surgical sutures, in spite of frequent inflammatory response in the eye (Moore and Aronson, 1969; Salthouse *et al.*, 1977; Soong and Kenyon, 1984), which was attributed to the allergenic activity of sericin. By removing the sericin, this problem can be avoided (Altman *et al.*, 2003), although reportedly fibroin itself may trigger delayed hypersensitivity (Kurosaki *et al.*, 1999).

In our project, we evaluated a membrane based on a silkworm silk fibroin (*Bombyx mori* silk fibroin, henceforth BMSF), and assessed the feasibility of using such a tissue as a scaffold for growing a monolayer of RPE cells. We believe that one of the features that makes silk fibroin attractive as a substratum for the tissue-engineered RPE constructs is its ability to degrade in the presence of enzymes at a rate that suits the ideal duration for such an application. In addition, silk membrane is a flexible and pliable material, and is mechanically strong even as a very thin film. This physical consistency makes it a potential material for carrying RPE cells into the subretinal space.

In a pilot study, we evaluated BMSF as a substratum for RPE culture both alone or coated with a selection of ECM proteins, and with or without serum. The ARPE-19 cell line was seeded on to tissue culture plastic (TCP), BMSF membrane alone, or BMSF membrane coated with laminin, vitronectin, fibronectin, a laminin–vitronectin–fibronectin combination (LVF), or collagen type IV. Samples were cultured in media containing foetal bovine serum (FBS) for 72 hours, then fixed and stained with nuclear stain Hoechst, and the cells attached were counted. Experiments were repeated with serum-starved ARPE-19 cells, which were seeded on to the different substrata, and cultured under serum-free conditions for 24 hours. The results showed that ARPE-19 cell growth on the BMSF membrane demonstrated no statistical difference ($P > 0.05$) when compared with TCP in FBS-containing culture conditions. The ARPE-19 cell count on the BMSF membrane alone in serum-free culture conditions was 50% of that on standard TCP in FBS ($P = 0.01$). However, the cell counts on BMSF membranes coated with ECM proteins surpassed unmodified BMSF membrane alone (vitronectin > collagen IV > fibronectin > LVF > laminin). Furthermore, cell attachment on BMSF membranes coated with vitronectin or collagen IV in serum-free conditions was found to be comparable with that seen in medium containing FBS on TCP (Kwan *et al.*, 2007). We are looking further into the characteristics of RPE cells growing on BMSF and different conditions that may enhance their cellular expression and survival.

15.7   Conclusions and future trends

In conclusion, there is a need to identify the ideal substratum for RPE cell growth and potential RPE transplant as current clinical therapies are inadequate for curing the different presentations of AMD. Although there have been some advances in the development of potential substrata for RPE cell growth and maintenance, it remains unclear as to what represents the best substratum (e.g. material), the most suitable vascular components (e.g. underlying vascular scaffold), the best microenvironment (e.g. combination of growth factors), the ideal cell type (e.g. RPCs vs genetically modified cells), and the most appropriate timing of the surgery. All these factors pose a great challenge to both scientists and clinicians in finding a cure for AMD, but if this enigma could be solved it would make a tremendous impact on the lives of AMD sufferers in the future.

15.8   Acknowledgements

We would like to thank Drs Damien Harkin, Zeke Barnard, and Zainuddin for providing their expertise in cell culture and production of silk fibroin membranes. We are also grateful for support from the Prevent Blindness

Foundation through Viertels' Vision, Queensland, Australia. Funding for the project through an ORIA/Vision Australia research grant is also acknowledged.

15.9   References

Abe T, Hojo M, Saigo Y, Yamato M, Okano T, Wakusawa R, and Tamai M (2006), 'Retinal pigment epithelial cells from thermally responsive polymer-grafted surface reduce apoptosis', *Adv Exp Med Biol*, **572**, 363–366.

Altman G H, Diaz F, Jakuba C, Calabro T, Horan R L, Chen J, Lu H, Richmond J, and Kaplan D L (2003), 'Silk-based biomaterials', *Biomaterials*, **24**, 401–416.

Bhatt N S, Newsome D A, Fenech T, Hessburg T P, Diamond J G, Miceli M V, Kratz K E, and Oliver P D (1994), 'Experimental transplantation of human retinal pigment epithelial cells on collagen substrates', *Am J Ophthalmol*, **117**, 214–221.

Bhutto I A, Kim S Y, McLeod D S, Merges C, Fukai N, Olsen B R, and Lutty G A (2004), 'Localization of collagen XVIII and the endostatin portion of collagen XVIII in aged human control eyes and eyes with age-related macular degeneration', *Invest Ophthalmol Vis Sci*, **45**, 1544–1552.

Binder S, Stanzel B V, Krebs I, and Glittenberg C (2007), 'Transplantation of the RPE in AMD', *Prog Retin Eye Res*, **26**, 516–554.

Binder S, Stolba U, Krebs I, Kellner L, Jahn C, Feichtinger H, Povelka M, Frohner U, Kruger A, Hilgers R D, and Krugluger W (2002), 'Transplantation of autologous retinal pigment epithelium in eyes with foveal neovascularization resulting from age-related macular degeneration: a pilot study', *Am J Ophthalmol*, **133**, 215–225.

Capeans C, Pineiro A, Pardo M, Sueiro-Lopez C, Blanco M J, Dominguez F, and Sanchez-Salorio M (2003), 'Amniotic membrane as support for human retinal pigment epithelium (RPE) cell growth', *Acta Ophthalmol Scand*, **81**, 271–277.

Castellarin A A, Sugino I K, Vargas J A, Parolini B, Lui G M, and Zarbin M A (1998), 'In vitro transplantation of fetal human retinal pigment epithelial cells onto human cadaver Bruch's membrane', *Exp Eye Res*, **66**, 49–67.

Chen F K, Patel P J, Uppal G S, Rubin G S, Coffey P J, Aylward G W, and Da Cruz L (2009), 'A comparison of macular translocation with patch graft in neovascular age-related macular degeneration', *Invest Ophthalmol Vis Sci*, **50**, 1848–1855.

Crafoord S, Geng L, Seregard S, and Algvere P V (2002), 'Photoreceptor survival in transplantation of autologous iris pigment epithelial cells to the subretinal space', *Acta Ophthalmol Scand*, **80**, 387–394.

D'Cruz P M, Yasumura D, Weir J, Matthes M T, Abderrahim H, LaVail M M, and Vollrath D (2000), 'Mutation of the receptor tyrosine kinase gene Mertk in the retinal dystrophic RCS rat', *Hum Mol Genet*, **9**, 645–651.

de Jong P T (2006), 'Age-related macular degeneration', *N Engl J Med*, **355**, 1474–1485.

Del Priore L V, Kaplan H J, Tezel T H, Hayashi N, Berger A S, and Green W R (2001), 'Retinal pigment epithelial cell transplantation after subfoveal membranectomy in age-related macular degeneration: clinicopathologic correlation', *Am J Ophthalmol*, **131**, 472–480.

Del Priore L V, Tezel T H, and Kaplan H J (2006), 'Maculoplasty for age-related macular degeneration: reengineering Bruch's membrane and the human macula', *Prog Retin Eye Res*, **25**, 539–562.

Farrokh-Siar L, Rezai K A, Patel S C, and Ernest J T (1999), 'Cryoprecipitate: An autologous substrate for human fetal retinal pigment epithelium', *Curr Eye Res*, **19**, 89–94.

Friedman D S, O'Colmain B J, Munoz B, Tomany S C, McCarty C, de Jong P T, Nemesure B, Mitchell P, and Kempen J (2004), 'Prevalence of age-related macular degeneration in the United States', *Arch Ophthalmol*, **122**, 564–572.

Giordano G G, Thomson R C, Ishaug S L, Mikos A G, Cumber S, Garcia C A, and Lahiri-Munir D (1997), 'Retinal pigment epithelium cells cultured on synthetic biodegradable polymers', *J Biomed Mater Res*, **34**, 87–93.

Grossniklaus H E, Hutchinson A K, Capone A, Jr, Woolfson J, and Lambert H M (1994), 'Clinicopathologic features of surgically excised choroidal neovascular membranes', *Ophthalmology*, **101**, 1099–1111.

Hadlock T, Singh S, Vacanti J P, and McLaughlin B J (1999), 'Ocular cell monolayers cultured on biodegradable substrates', *Tissue Eng*, **5**, 187–196.

Hakimi O, Knight D P, Vacanti J P, and McLaughlin B J (2007), 'Spider and mulberry silkworm silks as compatible biomaterials', *Composites B*, **38**, 324–337.

Handa J T (2007), 'New molecular histopathologic insights into the pathogenesis of age-related macular degeneration', *Int Ophthalmol Clin*, **47**, 15–50.

Harman A M, Fleming P A, Hoskins R V, and Moore S R (1997), 'Development and aging of cell topography in the human retinal pigment epithelium', *Invest Ophthalmol Vis Sci*, **38**, 2016–2026.

Hartmann U, Sistani F, and Steinhorst U H (1999), 'Human and porcine anterior lens capsule as support for growing and grafting retinal pigment epithelium and iris pigment epithelium', *Graefes Arch Clin Exp Ophthalmol*, **237**, 940–945.

Ho T C, Del Priore L V, and Kaplan H J (1996), 'En bloc transfer of extracellular matrix in vitro', *Curr Eye Res*, **15**, 991–997.

Ho T C, Del Priore L V, and Kaplan H J (1997), 'Tissue culture of retinal pigment epithelium following isolation with a gelatin matrix technique', *Exp Eye Res*, **64**, 133–139.

Huang J D, Curcio C A, and Johnson M (2008), 'Morphometric analysis of lipoprotein-like particle accumulation in aging human macular Bruch's membrane', *Invest Ophthalmol Vis Sci*, **49**, 2721–2727.

Krishna Y, Sheridan C M, Kent D L, Grierson I, and Williams R L (2007), 'Polydimethylsiloxane as a substrate for retinal pigment epithelial cell growth', *J Biomed Mater Res A*, **80**, 669–678.

Kubota A, Nishida K, Yamato M, Yang J, Kikuchi A, Okano T, and Tano Y (2006), 'Transplantable retinal pigment epithelial cell sheets for tissue engineering', *Biomaterials*, **27**, 3639–3644.

Kurosaki S, Otsuka H, Kunitomo M, Koyama M, Pawankar R, and Matumoto K (1999), 'Fibroin allergy. IgE mediated hypersensitivity to silk suture materials', *Nippon Ika Daigaku Zasshi (J Nippon Med Sch)*, **66**, 41–44.

Kwan A, Cheng S, Barnard Z, Zainuddin, Harkin D, and Chirila T (2007), 'Development of retinal pigment epithelial cell culture on *Bombyx mori* silk fibroin (BMSF) membrane for retinal transplantation', *Clin Exp Ophthalmol*, **35** (suppl 1), A40.

Lavik E B, Klassen H, Warfvinge K, Langer R, and Young M J (2005), 'Fabrication of degradable polymer scaffolds to direct the integration and differentiation of retinal progenitors', *Biomaterials*, **26**, 3187–3196.

Lawrence J M, Sauve Y, Keegan D J, Coffey P J, Hetherington L, Girman S, Whiteley S J, Kwan A S, Pheby T, and Lund R D (2000), 'Schwann cell grafting into the retina of the dystrophic RCS rat limits functional deterioration. Royal College of Surgeons', *Invest Ophthalmol Vis Sci*, **41**, 518–528.

Leng T, Huie P, Bilbao K, Blumenkranz M S, Loftus D J, and Fishman H A (2003), 'Carbon nanotube bucky paper as an artificial support membrane and Bruch's membrane patch in subretinal RPE and IPE transplantation', *Invest Ophthalmol Vis Sci*, **44** (suppl), E-Abstract 481.

Loftus D J, Leng T, Huie P, and Fishman H A (2006), 'Bucky paper as a support membrane in retinal cell transplantation', US Patent 7,135,172.

Lu J T, Lee C J, Bent S F, Fishman H A, and Sabelman E E (2007), 'Thin collagen film scaffolds for retinal epithelial cell culture', *Biomaterials*, **28**, 1486–1494.

Lu L, Garcia C A, and Mikos A G (1998), 'Retinal pigment epithelium cell culture on thin biodegradable poly(DL-lactic-co-glycolic acid) films', *J Biomater Sci Polym Ed*, **9**, 1187–1205.

Lu L, Kam L, Hasenbein M, Nyalakonda K, Bizios R, Gopferich A, Young J F, and Mikos A G (1999), 'Retinal pigment epithelial cell function on substrates with chemically micropatterned surfaces', *Biomaterials*, **20**, 2351–2361.

Lu L, Nyalakonda K, Kam L, Bizios R, Gopferich A, and Mikos A G (2001a), 'Retinal pigment epithelial cell adhesion on novel micropatterned surfaces fabricated from synthetic biodegradable polymers', *Biomaterials*, **22**, 291–297.

Lu L, Yaszemski M J, and Mikos A G (2001b), 'Retinal pigment epithelium engineering using synthetic biodegradable polymers', *Biomaterials*, **22**, 3345–3355.

Lund R D, Kwan A S, Keegan D J, Sauve Y, Coffey P J, and Lawrence J M (2001), 'Cell transplantation as a treatment for retinal disease', *Prog Retin Eye Res*, **20**, 415–449.

MacLaren R E, Uppal G S, Balaggan K S, Tufail A, Munro P M, Milliken A B, Ali R R, Rubin G S, Aylward G W, and da Cruz L (2007), 'Autologous transplantation of the retinal pigment epithelium and choroid in the treatment of neovascular age-related macular degeneration', *Ophthalmology*, **114**, 561–570.

Moore T E, Jr and Aronson S B (1969), 'Suture reaction in the human cornea', *Arch Ophthalmol*, **82**, 575–579.

Ng K P, Gugiu B G, Renganathan K, Davies M W, Gu X, Crabb J S, Kim S R, Rozanowska M B, Bonilha V L, Rayborn M E, Salomon R G, Sparrow J R, Boulton M E, Hollyfield J G, and Crabb J W (2008), 'Retinal pigment epithelium lipofuscin proteomics', *Mol Cell Proteomics*, **7**, 1397–1405.

Oganesian A, Gabrielian K, Ernest J T, and Patel S C (1999), 'A new model of retinal pigment epithelium transplantation with microspheres', *Arch Ophthalmol*, **117**, 1192–1200.

Panda-Jonas S, Jonas J B, and Jakobczyk-Zmija M (1996), 'Retinal pigment epithelial cell count, distribution, and correlations in normal human eyes', *Am J Ophthalmol*, **121**, 181–189.

Peyman G A, Blinder K J, Paris C L, Alturki W, Nelson N C, Jr, and Desai U (1991), 'A technique for retinal pigment epithelium transplantation for age-related macular degeneration secondary to extensive subfoveal scarring', *Ophthalmic Surg*, **22**, 102–108.

Rezai K A, Farrokh-Siar L, Botz M L, Godowski K C, Swanbom D D, Patel S C, and Ernest J T (1999), 'Biodegradable polymer film as a source for formation of human fetal retinal pigment epithelium spheroids', *Invest Ophthalmol Vis Sci*, **40**, 1223–1228.

Rozanowski B, Cuenco J, Davies S, Shamsi F A, Zadlo A, Dayhaw-Barker P, Rozanowska M, Sarna T, and Boulton M E (2008), 'The phototoxicity of aged human retinal melanosomes', *Photochem Photobiol*, **84**, 650–657.

Salthouse T N, Matlaga B F, and Wykoff M H (1977), 'Comparative tissue response to six suture materials in rabbit cornea, sclera, and ocular muscle', *Am J Ophthalmol*, **84**, 224–233.

Schraermeyer U, Thumann G, Luther T, Kociok N, Armhold S, Kruttwig K, Andressen C, Addicks K, and Bartz-Schmidt K U (2001), 'Subretinally transplanted embryonic stem cells rescue photoreceptor cells from degeneration in the RCS rats', *Cell Transplant*, **10**, 673–680.

Singh S, Woerly S, and McLaughlin B J (2001), 'Natural and artificial substrates for retinal pigment epithelial monolayer transplantation', *Biomaterials*, **22**, 3337–3343.

Smith W, Assink J, Klein R, Mitchell P, Klaver C C, Klein B E, Hofman A, Jensen S, Wang J J, and de Jong P T (2001), 'Risk factors for age-related macular degeneration: Pooled findings from three continents', *Ophthalmology*, **108**, 697–704.

Soong H K and Kenyon K R (1984), 'Adverse reactions to virgin silk sutures in cataract surgery', *Ophthalmology*, **91**, 479–483.

Strauss O (2005), 'The retinal pigment epithelium in visual function', *Physiol Rev*, **85**, 845–881.

Tao S, Young C, Redenti S, Zhang Y, Klassen H, Desai T, and Young M J (2007), 'Survival, migration and differentiation of retinal progenitor cells transplanted on micro-machined poly(methyl methacrylate) scaffolds to the subretinal space', *Lab Chip*, **7**, 695–701.

Taylor H R, Keeffe J E, Vu H T, Wang J J, Rochtchina E, Pezzullo M L, and Mitchell P (2005), 'Vision loss in Australia', *Med J Aust*, **182**, 565–568.

Taylor H R, Pezzullo M L, and Keeffe J E (2006), 'The economic impact and cost of visual impairment in Australia', *Br J Ophthalmol*, **90**, 272–275.

Tezcaner A, Bugra K, and Hasirci V (2003), 'Retinal pigment epithelium cell culture on surface modified poly(hydroxybutyrate-co-hydroxyvalerate) thin films', *Biomaterials*, **24**, 4573–4583.

Tezel T H and Del Priore L V (1997), 'Reattachment to a substrate prevents apoptosis of human retinal pigment epithelium', *Graefes Arch Clin Exp Ophthalmol*, **235**, 41–47.

Tezel T H and Del Priore L V (1999), 'Repopulation of different layers of host human Bruch's membrane by retinal pigment epithelial cell grafts', *Invest Ophthalmol Vis Sci*, **40**, 767–774.

Tezel T H, Del Priore L V, Berger A S, and Kaplan H J (2007), 'Adult retinal pigment epithelial transplantation in exudative age-related macular degeneration', *Am J Ophthalmol*, **143**, 584–595.

Tezel T H, Del Priore L V, and Kaplan H J (2004), 'Reengineering of aged Bruch's membrane to enhance retinal pigment epithelium repopulation', *Invest Ophthalmol Vis Sci*, **45**, 3337–3348.

Tezel T H, Kaplan H J, and Del Priore L V (1999), 'Fate of human retinal pigment epithelial cells seeded onto layers of human Bruch's membrane', *Invest Ophthalmol Vis Sci*, **40**, 467–476.

Thomson R C, Giordano G G, Collier J H, Ishaug S L, Mikos A G, Lahiri-Munir D, and Garcia C A (1996), 'Manufacture and characterization of poly(alpha-hydroxy ester) thin films as temporary substrates for retinal pigment epithelium cells', *Biomaterials*, **17**, 321–327.

Thumann G, Aisenbrey S, Schraermeyer U, Lafaut B, Esser P, Walter P, and Bartz-Schmidt K U (2000), 'Transplantation of autologous iris pigment epithelium after removal of choroidal neovascular membranes', *Arch Ophthalmol*, **118**, 1350–1355.

Thumann G, Hueber A, Dinslage S, Schaefer F, Yasukawa T, Kirchhof B, Yafai Y,

Eichler W, Bringmann A, and Wiedemann P (2006), 'Characteristics of iris and retinal pigment epithelial cells cultured on collagen type I membranes', *Curr Eye Res*, **31**, 241–249.

Thumann G, Schraermeyer U, Bartz-Schmidt K U, and Heimann K (1997), 'Descemet's membrane as membranous support in RPE/IPE transplantation', *Curr Eye Res*, **16**, 1236–1238.

Toth C A, Lapolice D J, Banks A D, and Stinnett S S (2004), 'Improvement in near visual function after macular translocation surgery with 360–degree peripheral retinectomy', *Graefes Arch Clin Exp Ophthalmol*, **242**, 541–548.

von Recum H, Kikuchi A, Okuhara M, Sakurai Y, Okano T, and Kim S W (1998a), 'Retinal pigmented epithelium cultures on thermally responsive polymer porous substrates', *J Biomater Sci Polym Ed*, **9**, 1241–1253.

von Recum H, Kikuchi A, Yamato M, Sakurai Y, Okano T, and Kim S W (1999a), 'Growth factor and matrix molecules preserve cell function on thermally responsive culture surfaces', *Tissue Eng*, **5**, 251–265.

von Recum H A, Kim S W, Kikuchi A, Okuhara M, Sakurai Y, and Okano T (1998b), 'Novel thermally reversible hydrogel as detachable cell culture substrate', *J Biomed Mater Res*, **40**, 631–639.

von Recum H A, Okano T, Kim S W, and Bernstein P S (1999b), 'Maintenance of retinoid metabolism in human retinal pigment epithelium cell culture', *Exp Eye Res*, **69**, 97–107.

Wang S, Lu B, and Lund R D (2005), 'Morphological changes in the Royal College of Surgeons rat retina during photoreceptor degeneration and after cell-based therapy', *J Comp Neurol*, **491**, 400–417.

Wang Y, Kim H J, Vunjak-Novakovic G, and Kaplan D L (2006), 'Stem cell-based tissue engineering with silk biomaterials', *Biomaterials*, **27**, 6064–6082.

Whitby R L, Fukuda T, Maekawa T, James S L, and Mikhalovsky S V (2008), 'Geometric control and tuneable pore size distribution of buckypaper and buckydiscs', *Carbon*, **46**, 949–956.

Williams D F and Burke J M (1990), 'Modulation of growth in retina-derived cells by extracellular matrices', *Invest Ophthalmol Vis Sci*, **31**, 1717–1723.

Williams R L, Krishna Y, Dixon S, Haridas A, Grierson I, and Sheridan C (2005), 'Polyurethanes as potential substrates for sub-retinal retinal pigment epithelial cell transplantation', *J Mater Sci Mater Med*, **16**, 1087–1092.

Yang J, Yamato M, Nishida K, Ohki T, Kanzaki M, Sekine H, Shimizu T, and Okano T (2006), 'Cell delivery in regenerative medicine: the cell sheet engineering approach', *J Control Release*, **116**, 193–203.

Zanello L P, Zhao B, Hu H, and Haddon R C (2006), 'Bone cell proliferation on carbon nanotubes', *Nano Lett*, **6**, 562–567.

Zarbin M A (2004), 'Current concepts in the pathogenesis of age–related macular degeneration', *Arch Ophthalmol*, **122**, 598–614.

Part III

Other applications

16

Hydrogel sealants for wound repair in ophthalmic surgery

M. WATHIER and M. W. GRINSTAFF, Boston
University, USA

Abstract: Each year, 15 million individuals worldwide seek treatment
for the repair of ocular wounds. New hydrogel sealants – crosslinked
polymer matrices that possess a large fraction of water by weight – have
been successfully used to repair a variety of different types of trauma and
surgically induced ocular wounds. This chapter recounts the recent advances
in the development of hydrogel materials and the ongoing work to design the
ideal ophthalmic sealant.

Key words: hydrogel, ocular wounds, ophthalmic sealant, biomaterials,
dendrimers.

16.1   Introduction

Today, the use of sutures is the most common method to repair ocular wounds;
however, this technique has many drawbacks due to its application and
properties. Indeed, among the drawbacks, this technique induces new trauma
and new sites for infection, inflammation, and vascularization, while often
leading to uneven healing. Furthermore, it is a time-consuming procedure
and requires technical skill. Within the last 8 years, there has been significant
research into the development of new alternatives, with some notable successes.
The expansion of material engineering and macromolecular sciences has
enabled the development of new hydrogel sealants – crosslinked polymer
matrices that possess a large fraction of water by weight – that have been
successfully used to repair a variety of different types of trauma and surgically
induced ocular wounds. Herein, we recount these recent accomplishments
in the development of hydrogel materials and the ongoing work to design
the ideal ophthalmic sealant.

16.2   Background and clinical needs

Each year more than 15 million individuals worldwide seek treatment for
the repair of ocular wounds. Of these ocular wounds, there are numerous
ophthalmic conditions and procedures that result in corneal wounds,
including corneal ulcers, lacerations, perforations, transplants (0.1 million),
incisions for cataract removal and intraocular lens (IOL) implantation (11

million), and laser-assisted *in situ* keratomileusis (LASIK) (3 million). Today, the standard procedure for repairing ocular injuries involves using nylon sutures. Unfortunately, the use of these sutures constitutes an invasive surgical procedure and gives rise to a host of other complications. In addition to the potential for further trauma to corneal tissue (to include corneal inflammation and vascularization), the site itself is often more prone to infection. Instances of uneven healing and even astigmatism have also been reported. These drawbacks in and of themselves are problematic, and when one also considers that sutures may loosen or break postoperatively, or that they require removal after surgery, the need to find viable alternatives becomes all the more pressing.

Therefore, the need for alternative methods to repair ocular wounds is of current basic and clinical interest. Of the methods being explored, the use of polymeric adhesives or sealants has attracted significant attention. Polymers that adhere to tissue are of clinical value for applications where surgical procedures using sutures are not effective. It is for this reason that tissue sealants are an attractive alternative to sutures. It is hypothesized that the negative effects largely associated with sutures can be minimized by the use of tissue sealants. The goal of tissue sealant therapy is to provide immediate restoration of structural integrity and to prevent further tissue thinning. In fact, there is a precedent for the use of glues in ophthalmology, particularly in the management of corneal perforations. Previous ophthalmic sealants based on synthetic and/or natural polymers – such as cyanoacrylates, fibrin, and modified chondroitin sulfate–aldehyde systems – are not ideal for a number of reasons (including lack of biocompatibility, degradation, expensive cost, limitations in sealing only small ocular wounds, and/or complex methods of application). A new trend in ophthalmic sealant development is the use of hydrogels for repairing corneal perforations, and thus these hydrogel sealants must meet a number of requirements. Ideally, they should: (a) be biocompatible; (b) adhere to the moist corneal surface; (c) have a suitable polymerization time to set the polymer on the wound; (d) restore quickly the intraocular pressure (IOP); (e) possess a degradation time that matches the normal healing process; (f) be more elastic than corneal tissue, so as to disfavor formation of an astigmatism during healing; (g) be transparent and soft, making them the ideal adhesive sealant; and (h) be easily delivered to the tissue site.

The following sections describe the major uses of natural and synthetic hydrogel-based adhesives (see Fig. 16.1 for examples) in ophthalmology with an analysis of their uses in amniotic membrane transplants, scleral lacerations, corneal wounds, corneal transplants, and retinal detachments.

16.1 Example of chemical structures used to make hydrogels. (a) G1 poly(glycerol-succinic acid)-poly(ethylene glycol) hybrid dendrimer ([G1] PGLSA-MA-PEG) (Carnahan et al., 2002; Velazquez et al., 2004; Berdahl et al., 2009). (b) bovine serum albumin (BSA) bearing chlorine e6 (BSA-ce6) (Khadem et al., 2004). Cysteine-based dendron (C1) and PEG dialdehyde (C2) (Wathier et al., 2004; Wathier et al., 2006a). (d) Modified hylauronic acid (HA) with methacrylate groups (Miki et al., 2002). PEG N-hydroxy-succinimidyl (e1) and PEG-NH₂ (E2) (Margalit et al., 2000). Figure adapted from: Carnahan et al. (2002), Velazquez et al. (2004), Berdahl et al. (2009), Khadem et al. (2004), Wathier et al. (2004), Wathier et al. (2006a), and Margalit et al. (2000).

(c) (2)

(c) (1)

(d)

(e1)

(e2)

16.1 Continued

16.3   Hydrogel sealants

16.3.1 Amniotic membrane transplantation (AMT)

One of the exciting uses for a hydrogel sealant is to secure an amniotic membrane (AM) after its placement on the ocular surface. Amniotic membranes are used in ophthalmic surgeries/procedures when conventional treatments fail to restore the integrity of the tissue (i.e. epithelium or sclera). Specifically, the AM is used as a scaffold or temporary graft on which the tissue can re-grow. It is the innermost layer of the fetal membrane, which consists of an endodermal layer of epithelia cells. This membrane is an avascular stromal matrix which: (a) inhibits blood vessel growth in bordering tissues (Koizumi *et al.*, 2000); (b) promotes epithelialization (Tseng *et al.*, 1997); (c) exhibits anti-inflammatory properties (Kim *et al.*, 2000; Solomon *et al.*, 2001); and (d) assists in cellular migration to the treated areas (Tseng *et al.*, 1997); therefore, this technique minimizes scar tissue, making it very appealing for ophthalmic applications. Unfortunately, to secure this graft, the surgeon usually uses 10-0 nylon sutures, which inflict new trauma and unwanted scarring (Azuara-Blanco *et al.*, 1999). In order to overcome this problem, Takaoka and coworkers evaluated a sutureless AMT using either fibrin glue (Sekiyama *et al.*, 2007) or, even more recently, a Schiff base hydrogel sealant (Takaoka *et al.*, 2008). Fibrin glues are a two-component adhesive made from fibrinogen and thrombin delivered by a two-barrel syringe bearing a 'needle' mixing chamber. The thrombin converts the fibrinogen to fibrin by enzymatic reaction which can be controlled by the amount of thrombin added. Fibrin glues have been used for more than 20 years in Europe and have been approved since 1998 in the United States for cardiac surgeries but not for ophthalmic use, so these applications are considered off-label use. Even though good results were achieved using fibrin glue to seal the transplant, this technique has three main drawbacks. First, the preparation of the fibrin glue is difficult and time consuming. Second, since the fibrin glue has two main components, fibrinogen and thrombin directly extracted from blood plasma, some viruses, such as parvovirus B19 (HPV B19) which is particularly difficult to remove or inactivate, can lead to infection (Hino *et al.*, 2000; Kawamura *et al.*, 2002). Third, fibrin glue contains fibrinogen, which is well known to have a fundamental role in the process of inflammation that slows down the healing process (Tang, 1998; Forsyth *et al.*, 2001; Hu *et al.*, 2001; Rubel *et al.*, 2001). In order to overcome these drawbacks, the same group also studied a Schiff base hydrogel made from ε-poly(L-lysine) and aldehyde-derivatized polysaccharide to seal the AMT to sclera tissue as shown in Fig. 16.2 (Takaoka *et al.*, 2008). For ease of application, they used a double-barrel syringe with a mixing chamber needle for this study. One barrel contained a 14 wt% solution of aldehyde Dextran (0.43 aldehyde per sugar unit, molecular weight (MW) 75 kDa) and the other barrel contained

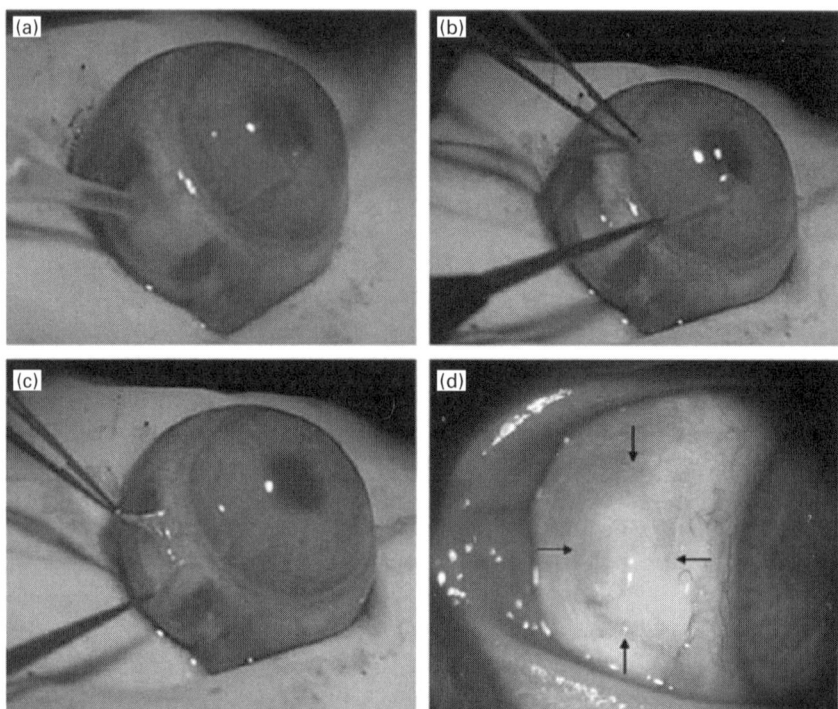

16.2 Representative photographs of the sutureless AMT. A drop of the bioadhesive was put on to the bare sclera from the tip of the syringe (a), and then the squarely trimmed AM was transferred into place with the epithelial basement membrane side up (b) and (c). Excess fluid that extruded from the interface was rubbed off with the sponge and approximately 3 min elapsed before the AM was fixed. Immediately after placement, the AM was firmly secured on the bare sclera (d). Pictures extracted from Takaoka *et al.* (2008) and displayed with the publisher's authorization.

a 7wt% solution of ε-poly(L-lysine) (containing 2.1 wt% acetic acid). The composition of these two solutions was set to give a hydrogel in approximately 30 seconds and one that would biodegrade in 4 days.

Even though histology has not shown any obvious *in vivo* cytotoxicity, it is likely that this material may pose some toxicity problems given the high half-maximal inhibitory concentration values (IC_{50}) of the two components. This is the concentration at which 50% of the cells are dead. The authors reported an IC_{50} 1000 times lower than formaldehyde and glutaraldehyde (6 and 10 mg/ml vs 1.7 and 3.9 mg/mL, respectively) but the observed cytotoxicity with this concentration is still much higher (20 and 7 times, respectively) than the concentration of the material used in the sealant (140 mg/mL (14 wt%)) and 70 mg/mL (7 wt%), respectively), and could produce a potential cytotoxic hydrogel in the case of poor mixing or incompleted reaction between both components.

16.3.2 Scleral lacerations (conjunctival wound, pterygium, vitrectomy)

Scleral lacerations are usually the result of surgical procedures such as pterygium surgery, sclerotomy, or vitrectomy. Even though many of the drawbacks inherent to sutures are not relevant for this type of surgery (e.g. astigmatism), the development of new hydrogel sealants will benefit both the patient and the surgeon by decreasing the risk of infection, inflammations, and procedure time. Very few studies have been completed using adhesives instead of sutures. In 2004, Krzizok used commercial fibrin glue to treat (Fig. 16.3), in a clinical setting, more than 100 patients (Krzizok, 2004). From this study, he found that fibrin glue was as effective as sutures in the healing process of the conjunctiva but with the added advantages of no infections or inflammations. Another advantage was the reduced procedural time (1–2 min vs 4–8 min for suturing).

Unfortunately, he discovered that this method was not applicable to children showing extended Tenon's fascia. In addition, it is well known that, since fibrin glues are directly extracted from human plasma, virus transmission, in particular prion diseases, is a possible risk (Hennis *et al.*, 1992). In order to overcome this viral transmission risk with human derived products, a synthetic hydrogel was designed and evaluated by Wathier and coworkers on enucleated porcine eyes (Wathier *et al.*, 2006b). A two-component formulation, a polyethylene glycol (PEG) succinimidyl ester (MW 3400)

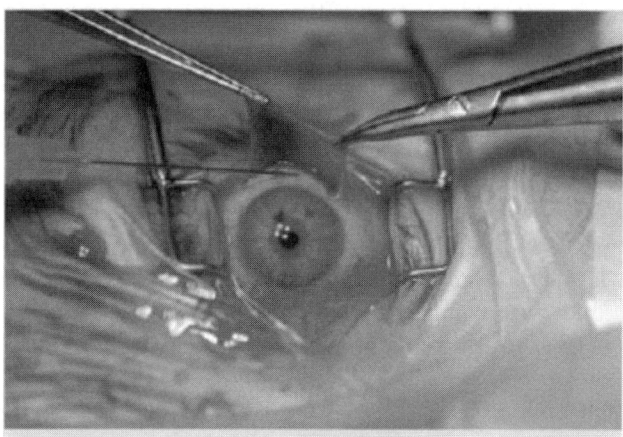

16.3 Sealing of the sclera wound with fibrin glue. Pictures extracted from Krzizok (2004) and displayed with the publisher's authorization.

and generation 1 and 2 of PEG- and lysine-based dendrimers, was used. By screening these different formulations of dendrimers, they found the lysine first-generation (G1) dendrimer to be the best candidate in terms of rheological and swelling properties to seal a sclera incision. This hydrogel sealant was transparent, easy and quick to set up; furthermore, it was strong and elastic, and had only moderate swelling. Using 5–10 µL of this formulation, they were able to seal a 1.4 mm full-thickness sclerotomy wound to an IOP of up to 250 mmHg, while the control groups – those left untreated and those using sutures – were only able to hold to 6 and 140 mmHg, respectively. This research also demonstrated the ability of the synthetic hydrogel sealant to be tuned in order to match the clinical requirement for a scleral sealant.

16.3.3 Corneal wounds

Corneal laceration

In the United States, approximately 50 000 eye laceration surgeries are performed each year. If the corneal wound is left untreated, it could result in permanent damage of the visual acuity over time caused by a decrease of the IOP that changes the curvature of the lens. Current repair strategies are insufficient for inducing normal tissue regeneration and complete visual recovery. The current clinical standard of care is suture fixation, which can cause trauma to the wound site, astigmatism, and infection. Cyanoacrylate glues have also been used off-label, but they are opaque and cytotoxic, as well as abrasive. In order to overcome these drawbacks, the use of a hydrogel adhesive is very appealing, since it can be made to be soft, non-toxic, transparent, and elastic enough to prevent astigmatism. The first report of a hydrogel sealant for cornea wound repair was published by the Grinstaff group (Miki *et al.*, 2002). Specifically, the authors developed and evaluated a new hydrogel formed from modified hyaluronic acid (HA). Their idea was to use this biological macromolecule present in the eye, as it may likely afford a biocompatible hydrogel material. They modified HA with methacrylate groups that can be photopolymerized by exposure to the radiation emitted by an argon laser (514 nm, 200 mW) to afford a crosslinked HA hydrogel. The new hydrogel sealant was tested *in vivo* on a rabbit model by performing either a 3 mm linear laceration or a 3 mm stellate laceration at the center of the cornea, and the results were compared with those treated with standard sutures. In a follow-up examination of the rabbit at 28 days, the authors used a slit-lamp (Fig. 16.4) to detect inflammation or infection, a Seidel test to check for wound leakage, and a Schiotz tonometer to measure the IOP at different time intervals (6 hours, and 1, 4, 7, 14, 21, and 28 days). At day 28, they euthanized the animal and performed histology on the corneas to check for inflammation and the quality of epithelial, stromal, and endothelial healing.

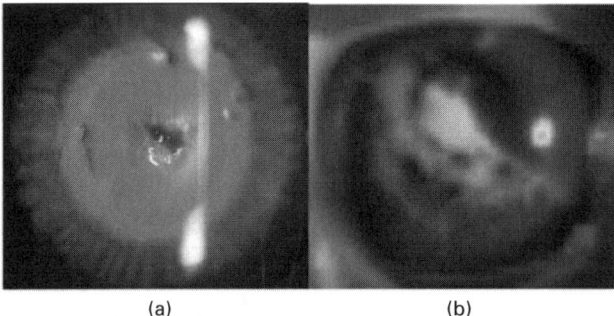

(a)   (b)

16.4 Clinical appearance over time of a stellate laceration with epithelial removal in the eye of a representative rabbit that was treated with the laser-activated HA– methyl acrylate (MA) polymer. (a) Slit-lamp photograph with retroillumination 1 day after the experimental laceration was sealed. The anterior chamber had reformed and the sealant filled the laceration which was still a gaping wound. (b) Seidel test showing that the sealant was still present, the laceration was closed, and no leakage was detected. Pictures extracted from Miki *et al.* (2002) and displayed with the publisher's authorization.

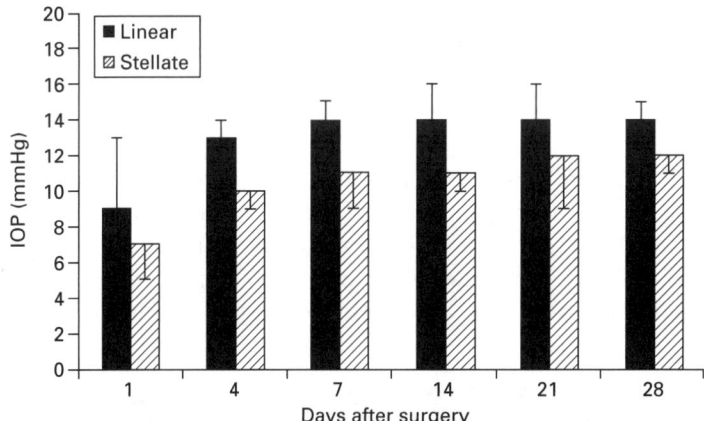

16.5 IOP from day 1 to day 28 following application and photopolymerization of HA–MA on experimental linear and stellate corneal lacerations in rabbit eyes. Linear lacerations, N = 8, black bar. Stellate lacerations, N = 14, white bar. Data for eyes with and without epithelial removal were combined since the results were not significantly different. Data extracted from Miki *et al.* (2002) and displayed with the publisher's authorization.

Almost all (37/38) of the rabbits had their IOP restored by day 7 (Fig. 16.5) and 97% (37/38) of the rabbit corneas healed with no signs of inflammation or infection. Additionally, the integrity of the cornea was re-established by stroma cell proliferation, which created new connective tissue.

In 2002, the Grinstaff group also published a report of another argon laser photocurable hydrogel using synthetic polymers, in particular, dendritic macromolecules composed of glycerol, succinic acid, and PEG (Carnahan *et al.*, 2002; Velazquez *et al.*, 2004). The advantage of using dendritic structures is that their physicochemical and rheological properties can be tuned to match the design requirements for treating corneal wounds. By screening the generations of their dendrimers on enucleated human eyes, they found that generation 1 (G1) was the most efficient for sealing 4.1 mm linear and 3 × 4 mm stellate central corneal lacerations. Indeed, using a methacrylate modified G1 poly(glycerol-succinic acid)–poly(ethylene glycol) hybrid dendrimer ([G1] PGLSA-MA-PEG), they were able to contain the leakage of the eye to 100 mmHg for the 4.1 mm laceration and to 78 mmHg for the stellate laceration. Compared with the control groups (either three interrupted 10-0 sutures for the 4.1 mm laceration or four interrupted 10-0 sutures for the stellate laceration which held only 78 and 57 mmHg, respectively), these results show the potential of these new hydrogels – which are soft, elastic, and non-toxic – to be effective cornea sealants.

Very recently, the Grinstaff group completed a comprehensive *in vivo* study with a chicken model (Berdahl *et al.*, 2009). Specifically, they evaluated the photocrosslinkable dendrimer-based hydrogel sealants used to repair full-thickness 4.1 mm central cornea lacerations. They used their successful hydrogel sealant ([G1] PGLSA-MA-PEG) developed in early 2002. Using slit-lamp photographs, Seidel test, and histology they compared the adhesive group (30 chickens) with a suture group (30 chickens treated with 3 interrupted 10-0 nylon sutures) at 28 days after treatment. The results were positive and very encouraging. The sealant sealed all the wounds at day 1 (Seidel negative) and was even better than sutures with respect to scarring and surface regularity starting at day 5 (Fig. 16.6). In addition, the hydrogel sealant was five times faster to apply than the sutures (1 min vs

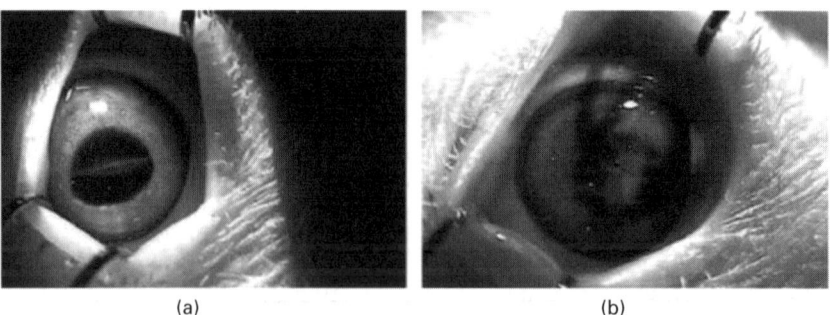

(a)   (b)

16.6 Postoperative day 5 corneas. (a) Adhesive; (b) sutured. Pictures extracted from Berdahl *et al.* (2009) and displayed with the publisher's authorization.

5 min). Finally, since it is elastic, the sealant should lead to a reduced risk of astigmatism.

Fibrin glue in conjunction with an AMT procedure has been used to treat three patients with a 2 mm central corneal laceration resulting from an ulcer (Duchesne *et al.*, 2001). The lacerations were secured with the fibrin glue and an AMT was placed on top of them to prevent failure that might result from the mechanical rubbing on the plug owing to the movements of the eyelids. Using this combination of treatment, they were able to seal these lacerations successfully but unfortunately they had to use a bandage contact lens for 3 weeks after surgery, which is not the ideal outcome for hydrogel sealant.

In 2003, Kalayci and coworkers reported the use of a modified, commercially available hydrogel (Confluent Surgical Inc.) to seal corneal wounds in an *ex vivo* rabbit model (Kalayci *et al.*, 2003). Central corneal lacerations from 1 to 5 mm wide were used. This hydrogel was made from two different PEG solutions, one containing a PEG bearing succinimidyl ester groups and the other amine functions. The hydrogel was applied to the wound using a spray system with only relative success, since the reproducibility of the coating was very difficult to control. Too much spraying led to a thick and bumpy layer, whereas too little spraying led to a thin coating unable to hold high IOPs. In spite of the difficulty of spraying the hydrogel, they were still able to get better results on all laceration sizes than those of the control group, which used one 10-0 nylon suture. This result was very promising, for they were able to secure (well above normal IOP) lacerations as wide as 5 mm with a non-toxic, soft, transparent, and elastic adhesive sealant that auto-set quickly without heat generation.

A BSA-based adhesive hydrogel was recently reported (Khadem *et al.*, 2004), which can be activated using the radiation emitted by a diode laser (665 nm, 300 mW, 2 min) instead of that from an argon ion laser. Two different photochemical initiators, chlorine e6 and Janus Green, were used to covalently bond the collagen surfaces together. The first was a BSA bearing chlorine e6 (BSA-ce6) and the second was a BSA bearing Janus Green (BSA-JG). Both hydrogel sealants were tested (2 wt%) *in vivo* on a 6 mm linear central corneal laceration in rats. The animals were assessed up to 14 days, and before they were killed the IOP was measured and samples were sent for histology. The hydrogel was completely gone at day 14 (and was only occasionally present at day 7), and satisfactory healing results (from the histology) with only minimal inflammation and hyperemia were obtained. The sealed lacerations were able to withstand IOP well above normal. The advantageous properties of hydrogel sealants combined with the promising *ex vivo* and *in vivo* results in corneal wound repair will lead to the development of a hydrogel sealant for ophthalmic application in the clinic.

Laser-assisted in situ keratomileusis

Laser-assisted *in situ* keratomileusis, or more commonly LASIK, is a procedure where the stromal layer is reshaped to correct improper corneal geometry. Before reshaping the stroma, the surgeon has to create a flap using a microkeratome to reveal the stroma. At the end of the surgery, this flap is carefully repositioned over the treated area. In the conventional LASIK procedure this flap remains in position by natural adhesion and no sutures or adhesives are used to hold it in place during the duration of the natural healing process. Leaving this flap unsealed requires the patients not to displace it (by rubbing their eyes, for example), so as to prevent an infection. Moreover, this unsealed wound is susceptible to epithelial ingrowth and other postoperative complications.

Three separate studies of fibrin hydrogel glues used to treat postoperative epithelial ingrowth resulting from a LASIK have been published (Anderson and Hardten, 2003; Julio *et al.*, 2006; Yeh *et al.*, 2006). Two of the three clinical cases used fibrin to secure LASIK flaps in patients that returned to the clinic at least 1 year after their initial surgery to be treated for recurring epithelial ingrowth which had been treated unsuccessfully by enhancement procedure (Anderson and Hardten, 2003; Julio *et al.*, 2006). The third clinical case involved the use of fibrin glue to treat a flap dislocation (Fig. 16.7) that occurred in an injury 21 months after LASIK surgery (Yeh *et al.*, 2006). Even though these three studies show success, it is difficult to use them as objective data, since no control group was used and only successful patient data were reported.

In order to keep the flap in place after surgery and to avoid postoperative infections, Kang and coworkers evaluated two different dendron-based

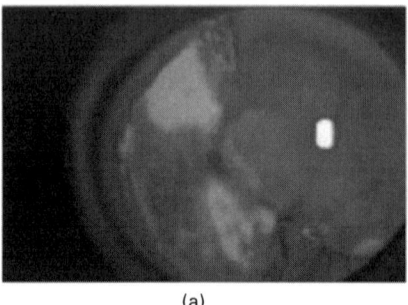 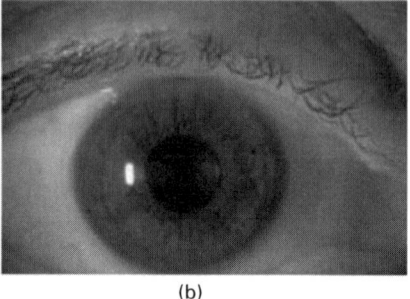

(a)   (b)

16.7 Appearance of patient's right eye after repositioning of a traumatic LASIK flap dislocation by a blackberry bush (a). Slit-lamp photograph demonstrating successful wound apposition (b). Two weeks later, the glue has dissolved, the flap is well positioned, and there is no evidence of epithelial ingrowth recurrence. Pictures extracted from Yeh *et al.* (2006) and displayed with publisher's authorization.

synthetic hydrogels in an *in vitro* set-up using human cadaver eyes (Kang *et al.*, 2005). These two dendron-based hydrogels differ in the polymerization technique that has been used; one used an argon laser and the other used self-gelling chemistry. The laser-activated hydrogel sealant was made from a first-generation PGLSA (poly(glycerol-succinic acid)) dendrimer that has methacrylate groups on its outer surface. After applying 60 μL of a 5 wt% adhesive solution by using the bottom side of a keratome blade on the flap edge, low intensity pulses of argon laser (Coherent SE 2000 argon ion laser, λ_{max}= 488 and 514 nm, 200 mW, 100 1-second exposures) were used to induce the polymerization of the solution into a clear, soft, flexible hydrogel, which secured the flap even when excessive force was applied with the Merocel sponge. To reduce the laser exposure to the patient and to obtain faster adhesive curing time (5 min in total with the laser-activated hydrogel), a self-gelling adhesive was tested. This two-component self-gelling adhesive cures via a chemical reaction, and it was prepared by mixing aqueous solutions of a cysteine-based dendron (33 wt% in phosphate buffer, 7.4 pH) and PEG di-aldehyde (55 wt% in phosphate buffer, 7.4 pH). After mixing these two solutions for 5 seconds, the bottom side of a keratome blade was used to apply the hydrogel on the flap edge. The hydrogel cured within 30 seconds, resulting again in a clear, soft, flexible hydrogel that was able to secure the flap even when excessive force was applied with the Merocel sponge. Fluorescein was also injected under the flap to verify if this adhesive could, in addition to securing the flap, potentially prevent ocular surface fluid from entering the sealed flap. None of the six eyes used in this study showed fluorescein leakage after application of the hydrogel, demonstrating that this sealant could be an effective protective barrier for the wound site.

Corneal transplants (penetrating keratoplasty and posterior lamellar keratoplasty)

Even though corneal transplants are the most successful human tissue transplants, they still represent a significant surgical challenge for ophthalmic surgeons. The conventional method (use of sutures) requires high surgical skill in order to prevent the occurrence of astigmatisms or infections. Currently, the graft is secured to the recipient's eye using either multiple sutures (typically 16) or uninterrupted running sutures. Sutures induce additional trauma and lead to corneal distortion, which may, in turn, cause astigmatism. In order to reduce distortion, surgeons usually use one or two uninterrupted running sutures, but these techniques require more technical skills and may still lead to infection through the corneal gap. Hydrogel sealants, therefore, have been envisioned to improve clinical outcomes by preventing astigmatism, reducing or eliminating altogether additional suture trauma, securing graft–host tissue gaps, and acting as a barrier against infections. In 2006, Pirouzmanesh and coworkers published promising results on the sutureless treatment of a 300 mm thick posterior lamellar keratoplasty (PLK) using a chondroitin-sulfate-aldehyde-based hydrogel sealant on human cadaver eyes (Pirouzmanesh *et al.*, 2006). The use of partial flap keratectomy in conjunction with a sutureless procedure using this hydrogel sealant led to a significant decrease in astigmatism (Fig. 16.8). Diopters decreased from 3.08 or the sutures group (five interrupted sutures) to 1.13 for the hydrogel-treated group. Unfortunately, the authors detected a great variability of graft stability (leaking pressure) in both groups ranging from around 55 to 110 mmHg. This lack of stability could be highly problematic since it may lead to infections and delayed healing times. Furthermore, since the graft is not secure (only the flap), possible slippage could occur which would lead to astigmatism.

Another study assessed laser-activated dendrimer hydrogels for sealing corneal transplants. In this study (Degoricija *et al.*, 2007), PEG-core, first-generation acrylated dendrimers were used to seal penetrating keratoplasty (PKP). Several dendrimer concentrations and PEG-core molecular weights were screened to find the best sealant for this application. According to the previous results obtained from a 4.1 mm central laceration study, the Grinstaff group evaluated the [G1] PGLSA-MA)$_2$-PEG dendrimers possessing PEG cores with MWs of 3400, 10 000, and 20 000, to secure enucleated porcine eyes. In this study, the authors used either 16 or 8 interrupted 10-0 nylon sutures and the dendrimer-based hydrogel adhesive; 100 μL of the adhesive solutions were applied to the PKP, so as to coat the sutures and wound interface. The solutions were then cured with a pulsed argon-ion laser to

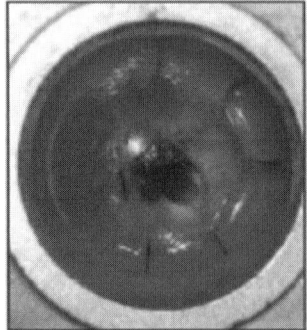

16.8 Postoperative view, suture group. The flap keratectomy is held in place by five interrupted 10-0 nylon sutures. The disk with posterior stroma and endothelium is secured underneath the flap without sutures. Pictures extracted from Pirouzmanesh *et al.* (2006) and displayed with publisher's authorization.

form the hydrogel adhesive. Using a 20% (w/v) of [G1] PGLSA-MA-PEG, containing either 3400, 10000, or 20000 PEG cores and 16 sutures, the leaking pressures were measured to be 103 ± 13, 114 ± 7, and 98 ± 14 mmHg, respectively, significantly greater than an autograft sealed with 16 sutures alone that held to 45 ± 10 mmHg. Next, they determined the leaking pressures of corneal autografts, initially secured with only 8 sutures, followed by the application and photocrosslinking of these three hydrogel adhesives at 20% (w/v). These studies were initiated to determine if, by using a sealant, a reduced number of sutures could be used to seal a PKP in order potentially to reduce the likelihood of astigmatism, to decrease overall surgery time, and to reduce tissue damage during the surgery. Using hydrogel sealants of 20% (w/v) of ([G1]-PGLSA-MA)$_2$-PEG$_{10000}$, and ([G1]-PGLSA-MA)2-PEG$_{20000}$ gave leaking pressures of 85 ± 22, and 81 ± 30 mmHg, respectively. For reference, the autografts sealed with 8 sutures had a leaking pressure of less than 5 mmHg. The capability of these adhesives to prevent bacterial infection was also assessed using an India ink method described elsewhere (Mcdonnell *et al.*, 2003). Even after several cycles of increasing and lowering the IOP, no India ink was detected, neither in the wound tissue interface nor inside the ocular cavity. These positive results show the potential benefits (namely, reductions in bacterial infection, astigmatism, and surgical time) of using a hydrogel sealant as a new alternative to secure corneal transplants with the standard number or a reduced number of sutures.

Next, Wathier and coworkers evaluated the ability of a self-crosslinking dendrimer-based hydrogel to seal PKP on human enucleated eyes (Wathier *et al.*, 2006a). For this study, a self-gelling hydrogel made from two components was used. The first component was a solution of modified PEG (MW 3400) bearing ester–aldehyde moieties at each end. The second component was a solution of lysine-based dendrimer bearing cysteine moieties on its periphery. Using this new ester–aldehyde system, the authors were able to use a new hydrogel crosslinking reaction (an intramolecular *O,N*–acyl rearrangement) that resulted in a hydrogel adhesive more stable (month vs days) than their previously reported self-crosslinking hydrogel (Wathier *et al.*, 2004), and therefore more effective for this type of surgery which involves a longer healing time. In this study, either 16 or 8 sutures were used in addition to the hydrogel sealant to secure the PKP. As a case in point, using 60 µL of a 50 wt% hydrogel mixture and 8 sutures, the PKP held to a leaking pressure of 77 mmHg compared with 5 mmHg for the 8 sutures-treated group). The India ink method mentioned above (Mcdonnell *et al.*, 2003) was again used to assess the ability of these hydrogels to act as a barrier to the flow of surface ocular fluid as a model for prevention of microbial infections. The hydrogel sealant secures the wound site preventing fluid from entering or exiting the wound. These new materials were also evaluated for their ability to decrease the duration of the surgical procedure and to reduce the number of sutures to prevent astigmatism. They concluded that the new hydrogels were easy to use and to apply, also they were transparent, soft enough to avoid eye irritation, elastic enough to prevent astigmatisms stable enough to keep the wound sealed during the healing process, strong enough to hold the IOP, and sealed enough to prevent microbial infections. Even though these parameters are all requirements for an ideal ocular hydrogel sealant, no *in vivo* data have yet been reported on these materials.

Clear corneal laceration cataract

Since Fine introduced the sutureless self-sealing cataract incision (Fine 1994), several papers have reported a correlated increase in endophthalmitis following surgery. The cause of the infections is the lack of a sealed wound and the resulting flow of ocular surface fluid (carrying the bacteria) into the chamber. This ocular surface fluid movement is the result of dynamic changes of the gap geometry, especially at low pressure and IOP fluctuations (Mcdonnell *et al.*, 2003; Taban *et al.*, 2005; Thoms *et al.*, 2007) or the use of topical anesthesia, which does not prevent long-term extraocular muscle akinesia (Ellis, 2003; Faulkner, 2007). In all cases, endophthalmitis might be prevented if the wound could be secured with a hydrogel adhesive. Thus, to evaluate a hydrogel adhesive for sealing a cataract incision, Grinstaff, in collaboration with Kim at Duke University (North Carolina, USA), used dendritic hydrogels to secure a cataract incision (Wathier *et al.*, 2004; Johnson *et al.*, 2009). A two-component adhesive was used in these studies, one part being a lysine-based dendrimer bearing cysteine moieties on its periphery, and the other part being a PEG di-aldehyde (MW 3400). Even though the early study showed promising results, the system was further improved by using a slightly different PEG and, additionally, using the India ink method (Mcdonnell *et al.*, 2003) it was confirmed that these hydrogel sealants could act as a barrier for microbial infections. In this study the wound was sealed up to 140 mmHg (± 22 mmHg), whereas an untreated wound leaked at 77 mmHg (± 14 mmHg). It was also noteworthy that even at low or high IOP the wound did not leak, confirming the effectiveness of hydrogel sealants in securing and the tissue preventing surface ocular fluid from penetrating the eye with IOP fluctuations.

Given the high number of cataract procedures performed each year and the significant clinical interest in preventing endophthalmitis, Reyes and coworkers also explored the use of a chondroitin sulfate (CS)-based hydrogel adhesive to secure a 3 mm clear corneal laceration (Reyes *et al.*, 2005). Their self-gelling hydrogel was made from CS-aldehyde with poly(vinyl alcohol-*co*-vinyl amine) (PVA-A) as a bridging reagent. This gel set in less than 30 seconds after mixing the two components as a consequence of a Schiff base reaction. The authors tested the leaking pressure of their hydrogel by increasing the IOP of the eye using a saline solution on enucleated rabbit eyes and compared their results with two control groups: one using only one 10-0 nylon suture (group 1) and the other using three 10-0 nylon sutures (group 2). Using this hydrogel, they were unable to detect a leak up to 100 mmHg (upper limit of their laboratory set-up), whereas suture groups 1 and 2 leaked at 26 and 44 mmHg, respectively. Once again these results support the use of a hydrogel adhesive to secure corneal wounds. As before, sealants that can effectively seal the tissue and prevent surface ocular fluid from entering the eye will likely reduce the risk of endophthalmitis.

16.3.4 Retinal applications

Retinal detachment may lead to vision loss and blindness if not treated rapidly. The peeling of the retina is mainly a result of either injury or inflammation; this inflammation is initially more localized before spreading to the whole ocular globe if not treated. The use of a hydrogel sealant for repairing a retinal detachment is more challenging than in the cases of corneal or scleral wounds, since the sealant has to be applied under wet conditions. Margalit and coworkers used a variety of different adhesives to treat retinal detachment, among them four hydrogel adhesives, one fibrin and three PEG-based hydrogels (Margalit *et al.*, 2000). After preliminary *in vitro* studies, they found the fibrin glue to be inadequate to treat this kind of wound since the hydrogel made from it, in wet conditions, is too weak. Thus, they focused their study on the three PEG-based hydrogels. The three different hydrogel mixtures were: SS-PEG (succinic succinimidyl ester) plus PEG-NH$_2$, SPA-PEG (propionic succinimidyl ester) plus PEG-NH$_2$, and ST-PEG (thiol) plus PEG-NHS (succinimidyl ester). First, they checked the strength of the hydrogel adhesive on retinal tissue using a laboratory strain gauge set-up. They found the three formulations to be strong enough to hold the retina in place. The next step was to check the *in vivo* cytotoxicity of these materials in rabbits by injecting 0.1 mL of the hydrogel into the ocular globe. The SPA-PEG/PEG-NH$_2$ formulations showed severe inflammation responses, which hampers their potential clinical use. The other two formulations caused only a mild inflammatory response that disappeared after the first week of treatment. Unfortunately, the histology of the ST-PEG/PEG-NHS formulation showed moderate damage to the photoreceptor layer of the retina, which also removed it from the list of potential retinal adhesives. Despite a short lasting time (72 hours), the SS-PEG/PEG-NH$_2$ formulation could be used as new hydrogel sealant in the treatment of those wounds that only require a short healing time.

In 2007, Sueda and coworkers re-examined the use of PEG-NHS in conjunction with an amine (a tripeptide of lysine) as a hydrogel sealant to fix retinal breaks (Sueda *et al.*, 2007). In their study, the authors used a modified formulation of a commercially available product, DuraSeal (Confluent Surgical Inc., Massachusetts, USA), which was designed to seal the dura. Unfortunately, even though this new hydrogel did not show signs of inflammation or abnormality by histology after 90 days in rabbit, its use in the *in vivo* study led to a 67% failure rate (re-detachment of the retina). This high failure rate was explained by poor mixing of the components and by the difficulty of application of this hydrogel under wet conditions. The authors noted that additional studies are under way to fix these drawbacks and to allow this hydrogel to be used for retinal surgery.

Another study evaluated a new gelatin-based adhesive that formed a hydrogel in the presence of an enzyme, microbial transglutaminase (mTG), to repair a retinal detachment (Chen *et al.*, 2006). Using a lap-shear test and scleral tissue flaps, the authors showed that this hydrogel can glue both flaps together up to 15–45 kPa, even under wet conditions. Furthermore, to evaluate the cytotoxicity of this hydrogel, they injected it into the vitreous cavity of rats. After 2 weeks, the animals were killed and histological sections of the eyes were obtained. No signs of necrosis, severe tissue damage, or inflammation were noted in the treated group.

16.4   Short commentary on future trends

The future is extremely positive and bright for the use of hydrogel sealants in ophthalmology. Given the successes with both natural and synthetic hydrogel sealants when used to repair corneal wounds, fix retinal detachments, secure amniotic membrane transplants, and seal scleral lacerations, a clear definition of the design requirements has emerged. These requirements, in addition to the obvious one of biocompatibility, include: restoration of the tissue function; adhesion to moist corneal, scleral, or retinal tissue; set-up time to facilitate application to the wound and subsequent sealing; degradation time of sealant to match the healing process; mechanical properties to favor tissue function while preventing further complications (e.g. astigmatism); transparency for clinical observation after treatment; and easy delivery to the tissue site by the clinician.

The next steps for hydrogel sealants are threefold. First, there must be continued research and development of sealants for applications in the back of the eye. Much of the work completed has focused solely on the front of the eye. Second, the use of these hydrogels for drug delivery applications should continue to be explored. Drug delivery in the eye is still a major challenge and the lessons learned in these studies should be applicable to advancing this area. Third, the work in the laboratory must lead to the transition of hydrogel sealant technology for repairing wounds to the clinic and must result in development of a product. There has been significant progress on this front. The team at HyperBranch Medical Technology (HBMT) has developed and commercialized the first ophthalmic bandage (OcuSeal^{TM}). After extensive *in vitro* and *in vivo* studies, as well as successful completion of the required pre-clinical safety studies, HBMT conducted a clinical trial for use of OcuSeal^{TM} to seal cataract incisions. In the fall of 2007, they obtained a CE Mark to sell the product in Europe. Today, thousands of cataract incisions have been sealed with OcuSeal^{TM}. In addition to providing a closed wound, the hydrogel bandage is delivered in a unique device that enables the clinician to 'paint' the sealant on the wound.

Continued research, development, and commercial activities with hydrogel sealants will advance our scientific and engineering knowledge of these materials and, perhaps more importantly, help patients through improved ways to treat ocular wounds. What else may be possible in the future? The possibilities are many and, by working together as a multidisciplinary team consisting of chemists, engineers, and clinicians, we will continue to solve current challenges as well as propose innovative solutions for our unmet clinical needs. In the ophthalmic sealant area, we see: (a) task-specific hydrogel sealants designed for a particular wound type, and (b) hydrogel sealants designed for an individual based on his/her own genetics and wound-healing capabilities, i.e. personalized medical sealants.

16.5   Sources of further information and advice

Articles have been found using either (a) key words (e.g. hydrogel, ocular sealant or glue, gel, adhesive, etc.) on the following search engines: SciFinder, Google scholar, and Web of Science or (b) publication citations. The articles have been downloaded online directly from the publisher or Science Direct when available, or they have been ordered through the library exchange system. More information about the OcuSeal™ ophthalmic bandage can be found at http://www.hyperbranch.com/. Other resources may be found at the American Academy of Ophthalmology (http://www.aao.org/) or at the Association for Research in Vision and Ophthalmology (ARVO) http://www.arvo.org.

16.6   Acknowledgements

Our research has been supported in part by the National Institutes of Health (NIH), the Pew Foundation, and Boston University. We would like to thank our collaborator, Dr Terry Kim (Duke University Eye Center), and his fellows and students who worked on these projects. We would also like to thank the following past and current graduate students and postdoctoral fellows from the Grinstaff Laboratory for their hard work and dedication to ophthalmic adhesive research: Jason Berlin, Michael Carnahan, Lovorka

Degoricija, Nathanael Luman, Meredith Morgan, Abigail Oelker, Kimberly Smeds, and Serge Söntjens.

Conflict of interest: M.W.G. is a co-founder of HBMT.

16.7   References

Anderson N J and Hardten D R (2003), 'Fibrin glue for the prevention of epithelial ingrowth after laser in situ keratomileusis', *J Cataract Refract Surg*, **29**, 1425–1429.

Azuara-Blanco A, Pillai C T and Dua H S (1999), 'Amniotic membrane transplantation for ocular surface reconstruction', *Br J Ophthalmol*, **83**, 399–402.

Berdahl J P, Johnson C S, Proia A D, Grinstaff M W and Kim T (2009), 'Comparison of sutures and new dendritic polymer adhesives for corneal laceration repair in an in vivo chicken model.' *Arch Ophthalmol*, **127**(4), 442–447.

Carnahan M A, Middleton C, Kim J, Kim T and Grinstaff M W (2002), 'Hybrid dendritic–linear polyester–ethers for in situ photopolymerization', *J Am Chem Soc*, **124**, 5291–5293.

Chen T H, Janjua R, Mcdermott M K, Bernstein S L, Steidl S M and Payne G F (2006), 'Gelatin-based biomimetic tissue adhesive. Potential for retinal reattachment', *J Biomed Mater Res Part B-Appl – Biomater*, **77B**, 416–422.

Degoricija L, Johnson C S, Wathier M, Kim T and Grinstaff M W (2007), 'Photo cross-linkable biodendrimers as ophthalmic adhesives for central lacerations and penetrating keratoplasties', *Invest Ophthalmol Vis Sci*, **48**, 2037–2042.

Duchesne B, Tahi H and Galand A (2001), 'Use of human fibrin glue and amniotic membrane transplant in corneal perforation', *Cornea*, **20**, 230–232.

Ellis M F (2003), 'Topical anaesthesia: a risk factor for post-cataract-extraction endophthalmitis?' *Clin Exp Ophthalmol*, **31**, 125–128.

Faulkner H W (2007), 'Association between clear corneal cataract incisions and postoperative endophthalmitis', *J Cataract Refract Surg*, **33**, 562–562.

Fine I H (1994), 'Clear corneal incisions', *Int Ophthalmol Clin*, **34**, 59–72.

Forsyth C B, Solovjov D A, Ugarova T P and Plow E F (2001), 'Integrin alpha(M) beta(2)-mediated cell migration to fibrinogen and its recognition peptides', *J Exp Med*, **193**, 1123–1133.

Hennis H L, Stewart W C and Jeter E K (1992), 'Infectious disease risks of fibrin glue', *Ophthalmic Surg*, **23**, 640–640.

Hino M, Ishiko O, Honda K I, Yamane T, Ohta K, Takubo T and Tatsumi N (2000), 'Transmission of symptomatic parvovirus B19 infection by fibrin sealant used during surgery', *Br J Haematol*, **108**, 194–195.

Hu W J, Eaton J W and Tang L P (2001), 'Molecular basis of biomaterial-mediated foreign body reactions', *Blood*, **98**, 1231–1238.

Johnson C S, Wathier M, Kim T and Grinstaff M W (2009), 'In vitro sealing of clear corneal cataract incisions with a novel biodendrimer adhesive', *Arch Ophthalmol*, **127**, 430–434.

Julio N, Arun C and Kenneth C (2006), 'Treatment of epithelial ingrowth after LASIK enhancement with a combined technique of mechanical debridement, flap suturing, and fibrin glue application', ' *Cornea*, **25**, 1115–1117.

Kalayci D, Fukuchi T, Edelman P G, Sawhney A S, Mehta M C and Hirose T (2003), 'Hydrogel tissue adhesive for sealing corneal incisions', *Ophthalmic Res*, **35**, 173–176.

Kang P C, Carnahan M A, Wathier M, Grinstaff M W and Kim T (2005), 'Novel tissue adhesives to secure laser in situ keratomileusis flaps', *J Cataract Refract Surg*, **31**, 1208–1212.

Kawamura M, Sawafuji M, Watanabe M, Horinouchi H and Kobayashi K (2002), 'Frequency of transmission of human parvovirus B19 infection by fibrin sealant used during thoracic surgery', *Ann Thorac Surg*, **73**, 1098–1100.

Khadem J, Martino M, Anatelli F, Dana M R and Hamblin M R (2004), 'Healing of perforating rat corneal incisions closed with photodynamic laser-activated tissue glue', *Lasers Surg Med*, **35**, 304–311.

Kim J S, Kim J C, Na B K, Jeong J M and Song C Y (2000), 'Amniotic membrane patching promotes healing and inhibits proteinase activity on wound healing following acute corneal alkali burn', *Exp Eye Res*, **70**, 329–337.

Koizumi N, Inatomi T, Sotozono C, Fullwood N J, Quantock A J and Kinoshita S (2000), 'Growth factor mRNA and protein in preserved human amniotic membrane', *Curr Eye Res*, **20**, 173–177.

Krzizok T (2004), 'Fibrin glue for closing conjunctival wounds in ophthalmic surgery', *Ophthalmologie*, **101**, 1006–1010.

Margalit E, Fujii G Y, Lai J C, Gupta P, Chen S J, Shyu J S, Piyathaisere D V, Weiland J D, De Juan E and Humayun M S (2000), 'Bioadhesives for intraocular use', *Retina*, **20**, 469–477.

Mcdonnell P J, Taban M, Sarayba M, Rao B, Zhang J, Schiffman R and Chen Z P (2003), 'Dynamic morphology of clear corneal cataract incisions', *Ophthalmology*, **110**, 2342–2348.

Miki D, Dastgheib K, Kim T, Pfister-Serres A, Smeds K A, Inoue M, Hatchell D L and Grinstaff M W (2002), 'A photopolymerized sealant for corneal lacerations', *Cornea*, **21**, 393–399.

Pirouzmanesh A, Herretes S, Reyes J M G, Suwan-Apichon O, Chuck R S, Wang D A, Elisseeff J H, Stark W J and Behrens A (2006), 'Modified microkeratome-assisted posterior lamellar keratoplasty using a tissue adhesive', *Arch Ophthalmol*, **124**, 210–214.

Reyes J M G, Herretes S, Pirouzmanesh A, Wang D A, Elisseeff J H, Jun A, Mcdonnell P J, Chuck R S and Behrens A (2005), 'A modified chondroitin sulfate aldehyde adhesive for sealing corneal incisions', *Invest Ophthalmol Vis Sci*, **46**, 1247–1250.

Rubel C, Fernandez G C, Dran G, Bompadre M B, Isturiz M A and Palermo M S (2001), 'Fibrinogen promotes neutrophil activation and delays apoptosis', *J Immunol*, **166**, 2002–2010.

Sekiyama E, Nakamura T, Kurihara E, Cooper L J, Fullwood N J, Takaoka M, Hamuro J and Kinoshita S (2007), 'Novel sutureless transplantation freeze-dried amniotic membrane surface reconstruction', *Invest Ophthalmol Vis Sci*, **48**, 1528–1534.

Solomon A, Rosenblatt M, Monroy D, Ji Z H, Pflugfelder S C and Tseng S C G (2001), 'Suppression of interleukin 1 alpha and interleukin 1 beta in human limbal epithelial cells cultured on the amniotic membrane stromal matrix', *Br J Ophthalmol*, **85**, 444–449.

Sueda J, Fukuchi T, Usumoto N, Okuno T, Arai M and Hirose T (2007), 'Intraocular use of hydrogel tissue adhesive in rabbit eyes', *Jpn J Ophthalmol*, **51**, 89–95.

Taban M, Behrens A, Newcomb R L, Nobe M Y, Saedi G, Sweet P M and Mcdonnell P J (2005), 'Acute endophthalmitis following cataract surgery – A systematic review of the literature', *Arch Ophthalmol*, **123**, 613–620.

Takaoka M, Nakamura T, Sugai H, Bentley A J, Nakajima N, Fullwood N J, Yokoi N,

Hyon S H and Kinoshita S (2008), 'Sutureless amniotic membrane transplantation for ocular surface reconstruction with a chemically defined bioadhesive', *Biomaterials*, **29**, 2923–2931.

Tang L P (1998), 'Mechanisms of fibrinogen domains: biomaterial interactions', *J Biomater Sci Polymer Ed*, 9, 1257–1266.

Thoms S S, Musch D C and Soong H K (2007), 'Postoperative endophthalmitis associated with sutured versus unsutured clear corneal cataract incisions', *Br J Ophthalmol*, **91**, 728–730.

Tseng S C G, Prabhasawat P and Lee S H (1997), 'Amniotic membrane transplantation for conjunctival surface reconstruction', *Am J Ophthalmol*, **124**, 765–774.

Velazquez A J, Carnahan M A, Kristinsson J, Stinnett S, Grinstaff M W and Kim T (2004), 'New dendritic adhesives for sutureless ophthalmic surgical procedures – *In vitro* studies of corneal laceration repair', *Arch Ophthalmol*, **122**, 867–870.

Wathier M, Johnson C S, Kim T and Grinstaff M W (2006a), 'Hydrogels formed by multiple peptide ligation reactions to fasten corneal transplants', *Bioconjugate Chem*, **17**, 873–876.

Wathier M, Johnson M S, Carnahan M A, Baer C, Mccuen B W, Kim T and Grinstaff M W (2006b), 'In situ polymerized hydrogels for repairing scleral incisions used in pars plana vitrectomy procedures', *ChemMedchem*, **1**, 821–825.

Wathier M, Jung P J, Camahan M A, Kim T and Grinstaff M W (2004), 'Dendritic macromers as in situ polymerizing biomaterials for securing cataract incisions', *J Am Chem Soc*, **126**, 12744–12745.

Yeh D L, Bushley D M and Kim T (2006), 'Treatment of traumatic LASIK flap dislocation and epithelial ingrowth with fibrin glue', *Am J Ophthalmol*, **141**, 960–962.

17
Orbital enucleation implants: biomaterials and design

D. A. SAMI, Children's Hospital of Orange County, USA;
S. R. YOUNG, California Pacific Medical Center, USA

Abstract: New biomaterials and design evolutions have improved rehabilitation, and reduced complication rates after enucleation. This evolution of thought and practice is the subject of this chapter. Topics covered include: orbital anatomy and physiology after enucleation, the current state of knowledge on implant motility, developments in the use of porous implants, and considerations for pediatric enucleation. A comprehensive review of implant types, in relation to implant motility and biocompatibility, is included.

Key words: enucleation, orbital enucleation implants, socket implants, orbital implant motility, orbital biomaterials.

17.1   Introduction

New biomaterials and design evolutions have improved rehabilitation and reduced complication rates after enucleation. The evolution of thought and practice, in relation to orbital enucleation implants is the subject of this chapter. A brief summary of the important themes and conclusions of the chapter are outlined here.

Animal studies and modern imaging techniques have changed our understanding of the physiology and anatomy of the post-enucleation orbit. Previous opinions (Soll 1982; Soll 1986) about the contribution of fat atrophy to orbital volume loss after enucleation have been challenged (Manson *et al.* 1986; Kronish *et al.* 1990a; Kronish *et al.* 1990b; Smit *et al.* 1990b). Following enucleation, there is a redistribution of intraorbital fat downward and forward in the anophthalmic orbit, with associated inferior displacement of the superior rectus-levator complex. (Soll 1986; Smit *et al.* 1990b). Placement of a spherical implant within Tenon's capsule counteracts this change. This is true even when an implant is placed late after enucleation. (Smit *et al.* 1991b).

Since their introduction in the late 1980s, porous implant have become widely adopted by surgeons who perform enucleations in North America (Hornblass *et al.* 1995; Su & Yen 2004). Are the porous implants truly superior to non-porous implants? In general, it appears that the incidence of implant extrusion and socket infection is lower with porous implants. (Chuah *et al.*

433

2004). When muscles are imbricated over the surface of a sphere, implant migration occurs substantially more frequently with non-porous implants. (Allen 1983; Trichopoulos & Augsburger 2005). This supports theoretical considerations that vascular ingrowth helps to anchor the implant and permits immune surveillance. The rough surface of unwrapped hydroxyapatite implants appears to be associated with a higher exposure rate when compared with buried non-porous implants. Overall, donor sclera-covered hydroxyapatite implants appear to have higher late exposure rates than sclera-covered silicone implants. (Nunery *et al.* 1993b; Custer *et al.* 2003). Exposure rates for porous polyethylene implants wrapped in absorbable material appear to be similar to those for unwrapped porous polyethylene. (Li *et al.* 2001; Blaydon *et al.* 2003). Excellent outcomes have been reported by suturing the rectus muscles independently to a 20 mm spherical silicone implant reinforced with autogenous fascia or preserved sclera, with no cases of implant migration (an extrusion rate of 0.84% (1 of 119) over a 10-year study period) (Nunery *et al.* 1993a).

The basic science of the major factors that determine implant and ocular prosthesis motility is poorly understood. To date, no objective difference has been documented for implant or prosthetic motility with respect to porous and spherical alloplastic implants (Custer *et al.* 2003). Placement of a peg may improve horizontal excursions (Guillinta *et al.* 2003) but is associated with a significant rate of complications (chronic discharge, pyogenic granuloma formation and peg extrusion) (Jordan *et al.* 1999b). When enucleation is performed in infancy, implant exchange may be necessary to stimulate adequate orbital growth. As such, porous implants in young children (less than 2–3 years of age) are controversial, in that implant exchange is difficult after a porous implant has vascularized. Although there are only a handful of studies in children, scleral wrapped porous implants appear to have a reduced exposure rate compared with unwrapped implants (De Potter *et al.* 1994; Karcioglu *et al.* 1998; Christmas *et al.* 2000; Lee *et al.* 2000; Nolan *et al.* 2003).

17.2   Historical perspective on enucleation

In the process of mummification, the ancient Egyptians would remove the eyes, fill the orbit with wax, and use precious stones to simulate the iris. However, there are no recorded techniques of enucleation or evisceration in the living until the late sixteenth century in Europe (Kelley 1970; Luce 1970). This early technique was known as extirpation, which was, essentially, subtotal exenteration without anesthesia.

The first written record of the operation is credited to George Bartisch, published in his '*Augendienst*' in Dresden, 1583 (Luce 1970). The operation was so painful and dangerous that it was rarely used. In preparation, the patient was tied down and bled to a state of delirium for pain control. A thick suture was passed through the globe to permit forward traction, and a curved knife was used to sever attachments (Fig. 17.1). In the process, the globe, along with conjunctiva, orbital fascia, and portions of eye muscles were removed. Profuse bleeding was controlled with ice water (Snyder 1965). The cavity left behind would eventually granulate-in, and was not suitable for fitting an ocular prosthesis. Extirpation remained virtually unchanged for over 250 years (Snyder 1965; Soll 1986).

Enucleation involves making a circumcorneal conjuncival incision which is extended peripherally to separate Tenon's capsule from the sclera. The muscle insertions are cut and the optic nerve is severed close to the globe. The procedure was described by Cleoburey in 1826 and again, independently, by O'Ferral (Dublin) and Bonnet (Paris) in 1841. O'Ferral reported a new tissue, the tunica vaginalis oculi, which was in fact the same fascia discovered by Jacques Rene Tenon in 1806, now known as Tenon's capsule (Guyton 1948; Snyder1965; Luce 1970; Vistnes 1987). In separating this fascia from the sclera, and severing the muscles at their insertion to the globe, surgeons found that the globe could be removed with little blood loss (Guyton 1948; Soll 1986).

In 1885, P. H. Mules placed a spherical hollow glass implant into an eviscerated globe (Mules 1885). Subsequently Frost (1887) placed a similar implant in Tenon's capsule after enucleation, while Lang (1887) carried

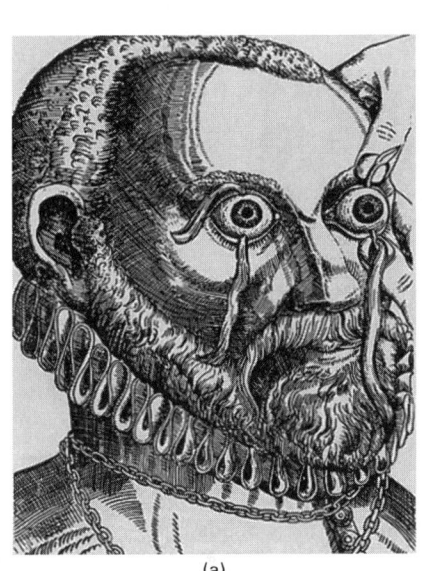 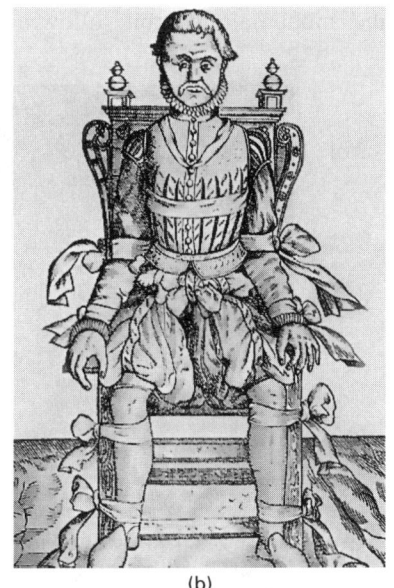

(a)   (b)

17.1 Preparation for extirpation of the eye. Reproduced from '*Augendienst*' 1583 by George Bartisch.

out a similar procedure using a celluloid sphere (Lang 1887). This was an important advance, expanding the definition of enucleation into simple enucleation (enucleation without implant) and enucleation with implant. Insertion of an implant at the time of enucleation has become the standard of care for the great majority of enucleations (Hornblass *et al.* 1995; Custer *et al.* 2003). Over the past two centuries, an extensive variety of materials have been used to fabricate orbital implants – some with disastrous results (Fig. 17.2). Table 17.1 outlines this experience.

17.3   Orbital anatomy and physiology after enucleation

Culler (in 1951) devised an orbital model to describe anatomic changes after enucleation (Culler 1952). Some of his theoretical predictions have been validated by human radiographic studies (Smit *et al.* 1990b). In theory, contraction of the extraocular muscles following enucleation results in retraction and collapse of Tenon's capsule (Culler 1952). In practice, surgeons have recognized that orbital tissue contraction produces a disfiguring entropion of the eyelids, particularly the upper eyelid (Allen 1970; Tyers & Collin 1982). These changes, while minimal in young children, manifest themselves quickly in older individuals (days to weeks) when enucleation without implantation is performed.

There is a redistribution of intraorbital fat downward and forward in the anophthalmic orbit following enucleation, which has been validated

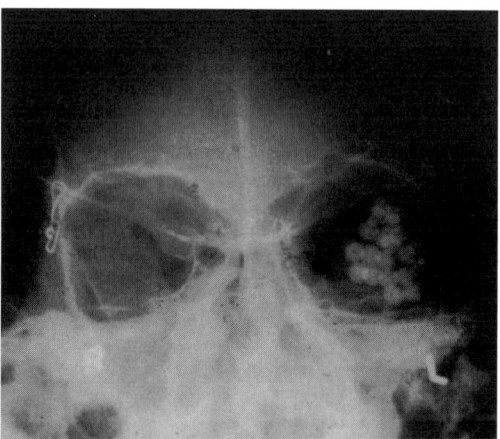

17.2 Skull X-ray showing placement of glass beads in an enucleated left orbit. Although glass is considered to be inert as an orbital biomaterial, glass beads were quickly abandoned as there were complications with migration of the beads into the sinuses, even the brain.

Table 17.1 Materials used for enucleation implants

Agar
Aluminum
Asbestos
Bone
Cartilage
Cat gut
Cellulose
Charred bone
Coral (hydroxyapatite)*
Cork
Fascia lata
Fat*
Glass (single hollow ball or beads)
Gold
Ivory
Paraffin
Peat
Plastic
Platinum
Poly(methyl-methacrylate) (PMMA)*
Polyvinyl sponge
Rubber
Silicone (solid or inflatable)*
Silk
Silver
Stainless steel
Tantalum
Vaseline
Vitallium
Wool

---

*Biomaterials that are still in common use.

by human radiographic studies (Smit *et al.* 1990b). The associated inferior displacement of the superior rectus–levator complex produces a hollow and sunken appearance of the superior lid sulcus (superior sulcus deformity) (Culler 1952).

The net effect of volume loss from enucleation (inferior displacement of the superior rectus–levator complex, downward and forward distribution of intraorbital fat) is a rotation of intraorbital contents. (Smit *et al.* 1990b) (Fig. 17.3). The large ocular prosthesis necessary to replace volume has a characteristic shape: thin on the inferior edge, becoming thicker superiorly and temporally. Despite its compensatory shape, the ocular prosthesis is often tilted: depressed superiorly and pushing against the lower eyelid inferiorly (Fig. 17.3). Superiorly, the ocular prosthesis does not adequately support the SR–levator complex. This translates into variable amounts of ptosis and deepening of the superior sulcus. These features are responsible for the

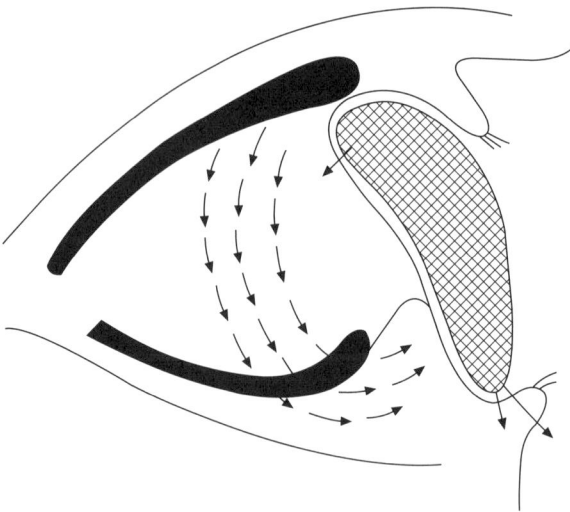

17.3 Volume loss from enucleation produces a downward and forward distribution of intraorbital fat (arrows). The large prosthesis necessary to replace volume is typically depressed superiorly and pushes against the lower eyelid inferiorly.

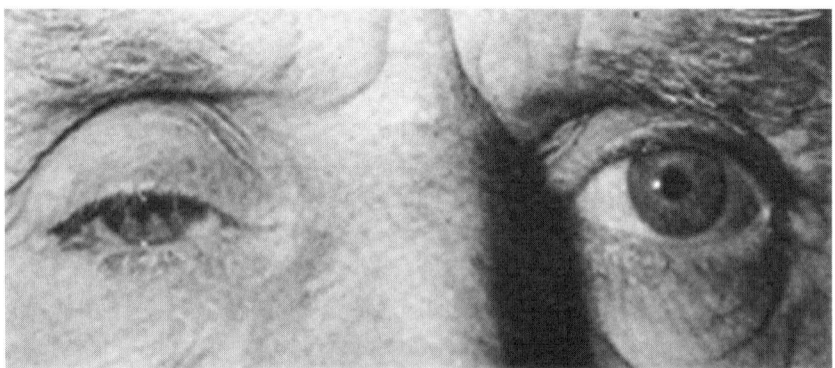

17.4 Photograph illustrating right-sided enopthalmos, deepening of the superior lid sulcus and ptosis – as part of the post-enucleation socket syndrome.

post-enucleation socket syndrome (Fig. 17.4): (a) deepening of the upper lid sulcus; (b) variable amounts of upper lid dysfunction – from lagophthalmos to severe ptosis; and (c) stretching of the lower lid with inadequate eyelid closure (Tyers & Collin 1982; Tyers & Collin 1985). Over time, the lower lid/inferior fornix becomes progressively stretched from ocular prosthesis tilt and the gravitational effect of the heavy ocular prosthesis. An ectropion often develops, which further compromises the fornix available to support the ocular prosthesis. This sets up a vicious cycle. As the lower lid and sulcus stretch inferiorly, the ocular prosthesis begins to sink, requiring a larger ocular prosthesis to re-establish normal appearance, which in turn places more weight on the lower eyelid.

Fat atrophy has previously been cited as a contributor to volume loss in the anophthalmic orbit (Soll 1982). This was based on thermogram studies showing a colder post-enucleation orbit (compared with the contralateral normal orbit), suggesting a presumed decrease in orbital metabolism, leading to fat atrophy (Soll 1982; Soll 1986). Alternatively, the change in the orbital thermal image may simply reflect removal of the eye, which has a rich uveal circulation. (Kronish et al. 1990a). More recent evidence based on animal and radiographic (human) studies suggest that accelerated fat atrophy is not a sequel of enucleation. (Manson et al. 1986; Kronish et al. 1990a; Kronish et al. 1990b; Smit et al. 1990b). Still, deepening of the superior sulcus over time, which is out of proportion to the contralateral normal eye, is well known. It may be that with age the normal atrophy of fat associated with both orbits becomes more apparent in an already volume-deficient socket.

Volume loss appears to be the major determinant of post-enucleation anatomic changes (Smit et al. 1990a; Smit et al. 1990b; Smit et al. 1991b). Human radiographic studies have confirmed that placement of a spherical implant within Tenon's capsule counteracts the post-enucleation rotation of intraorbital contents (and associated back-tilt of the ocular prosthesis). This is true even when the implant is placed late after enucleation (Smit et al. 1991b). Partial volume replacement permits a thinner ocular prosthesis, thus relieving weight on the lower eyelid and minimizing associated ectropion formation.

Traditionally, enucleation is thought to produce about a 7.0 ml loss of orbital volume, based on an average ocular axial length of 24 mm (Table 17.2). Recent studies suggest the average volume loss is higher: about 7.5–8.0 ml (Custer & Trinkaus 1999), emphasizing that there is substantial variability (5.5–9.0 ml) (Thaller 1997). A 20 mm spherical implant has a volume of 4.2 ml (Table 17.2). The remaining volume (about 3–4 ml) must be replaced by the ocular prosthesis. However, the physical dimensions of the palpebral fissure and conjunctival cul-de-sac, as well as problems associated with lower lid laxity produced by a heavy ocular prosthesis, limit the practical maximum size and volume of the ocular prosthesis. The average ocular prosthesis volume is 2.0–2.5 ml. A recent study suggested that the upper limit of prosthetic volume is about 4.2 ml (in the presence of a small implant). Interestingly, among patients with implant sizes of 14–22 mm and optimal prosthetic fit as judged by an ocularist, the average ocular prosthesis volumes were remarkably similar: 2.2–2.3 ml (Kaltreider 2000).

Table 17.2 Relationship between implant diameter and volume

Sphere diameter (mm)	Volume (mm³)
12	0.9
13	1.1
14	1.4
15	1.8
16	2.1
17	2.6
18	3.1
19	3.6
20	4.2
21	4.9
22	5.6
23	6.4
24	7.2

Thus when a small implant is used, the overall volume deficit may be even greater.

Volume deficit = [orbital volume loss from enucleation – (implant + prosthetic volume)]

Placing an implant with diameter >22 mm carries a higher risk of exposure in the early post-operative period – as Tenon's capsule must be closed with greater tension (Kim *et al.* 1994). At the extreme end, a large implant (usually >24 mm) will prevent the ocularist from fitting an artificial eye with enough antero-posterior depth (4 mm) to create a realistic anterior chamber depth (Neuhaus & Shorr 1982; Tyers & Collin 1985; Thaller 1997; Custer *et al.* 1999). In addition, crowding of the conjunctival fornices could restrict ocular prosthesis movement. In 1967, Soll devised an inflatable silicone implant filled with silicone gel (Soll 1969). Using a 30 gauge needle, saline or antibiotic solution could be injected centrally through a self-sealing area. The implant was designed to preferentially expand superiorly, to address superior sulcus deficit (Soll 1969; Gougelmann 1970).

The smaller overall diameter of the implant as compared with the natural globe, alters the functional length and pivot point of the levator complex (Tyers & Collin 1982; Gale *et al.* 1985) with possible associated decreased levator function and ptosis (Vistnes 1976; Vistnes 1987). Clinically, the situation may be improved by adding to the superior margin of the ocular prosthesis, to restore functional length and create a more anatomic pivot point for the levator muscle (Allen & Webster 1969; Vistnes 1987) (Fig. 17.5).

17.4   Motility implants

The earliest implants were simple spheres placed within Tenon's capsule (Mules 1885). The extraocular muscles were disinserted from the globe

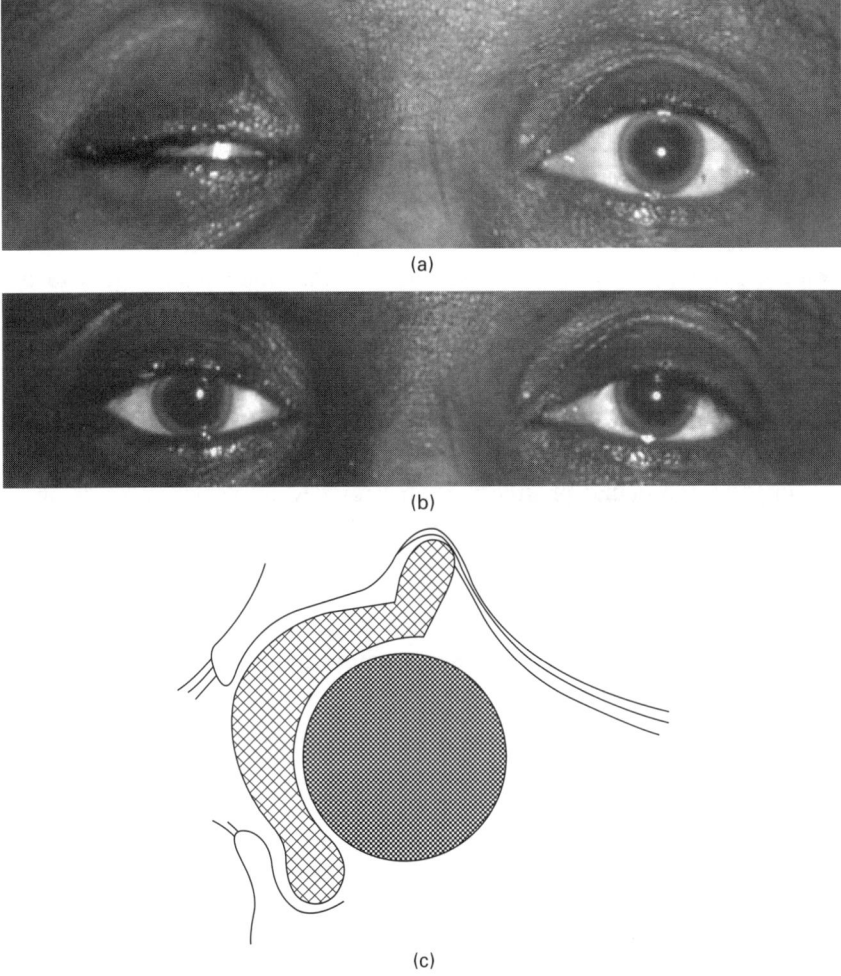

17.5 The smaller overall diameter of the implant as compared with the natural globe, may affect the functional length and pivot point of the levator muscle, with resultant decreased levator function and associated ptosis (a). The situation may be significantly improved by adding to the superior margin of the prosthesis (as illustrated), to restore functional length and create a more anatomic pivot point for the levator muscle. (b) and (c)).

and left to contract within the socket. The best outcome was an artificial eye with limited movement (Allen 1970) and inadequate rehabilitation. The next logical step was to attach muscles to the implant to anchor the implant, reducing extrusion rates, and to allow conjugate movement with the contralateral normal eye.

Attachment of the extraocular muscles to the implant has since become a source of some confusion in terminology, particularly over the meaning of 'integration'. This question was brought to the 2002 scientific panel of the ASO and AAO (American Society of Ocularists and American Academy of Ophthalmology): 'The definition of integrated implants does not appear to be consistent. Some refer to integration as the attachment of the extraocular muscles to the implant. Others define integration by the nature of physical contact between the implant and ocular prosthesis. What is the correct nomenclature?' The panel's consensus was that integration refers to the nature of fit between the ocular prosthesis and implant. Attachment of the extraocular muscles to the implant *does not* imply integration.

Based on the above consensus statement, implants are best categorized (Gougelmann 1970) as follows:

1. *Buried* – uninterrupted conjunctival lining. Smooth apposition between implant and ocular prosthesis. Some refer to implantation of a sphere without muscle attachment, as 'simple buried'.
2. *Exposed integrated* – interrupted conjunctival lining allowing direct coupling of implant to ocular prosthesis.
3. *Buried integrated* – no interruption of conjunctival lining. Irregular anterior surface of implant to improve translation of implant movement to ocular prosthesis.

In efforts to address the problem of implant exposure and extrusion, surgeons began to tie together the rectus muscles over smooth spherical plastic implants (i.e. imbrication of muscles – see Fig. 17.6). In addition to providing an extra layer of tissue for anterior closure, the tension of the imbricated muscles held the implant back, decreasing pressure/tension on the wound. This seemed like a logical approach, especially since it provided some motility to the implant as well. However, it proved to be problematic: a smooth implant with the rectus muscles imbricated over its anterior surface can slip between the imbricated muscles (Bosniak *et al.* 1989). Typically, the sphere migrates supero-temporally into the space between the superior and lateral rectus. (Allen 1983) (Fig. 17.6). Lee Allen attributed this propensity of migration to the presence of Lockwood's ligament inferiorly and the retracted obliques nasally – i.e. the implant migrates in the path of least resistance. In order to minimize this problem, later implants (Allen, Iowa and Universal implants) incorporated various types of grooves to receive the rectus muscles.

The first true motility implants were introduced in the early 1940s (Gougelmann 1970; Danz 1990). Their evolution mirrored rapid advances in the fabrication of ocular prosthetics. The battle casualties of the Second World War created a large demand for artificial glass eyes, which were mainly produced in Germany. The war-time shortage of glass eyes imported

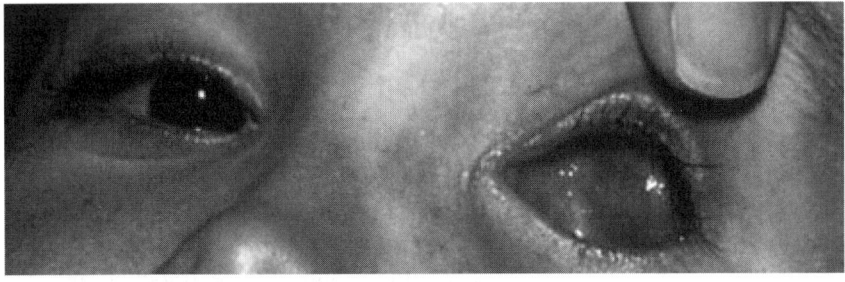

(a)

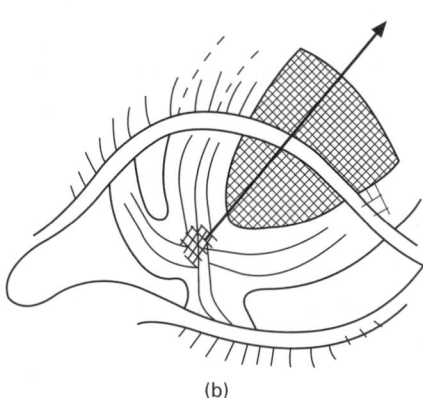

(b)

17.6 A smooth non-porous implant with the rectus muscles imbricated over its anterior surface can slip between the muscles. In this photograph of a child (a), the implant has migrated supero-temporally (between the lateral and superior rectus). The corresponding diagram (b) shows the imbricated muscles, the direction of migration (arrow) and part of the spherical implant (cross-hatched area).

from Germany led to development of the acrylic poly(methyl-methacrylate) (PMMA) ocular prosthesis (Murphey *et al.* 1945). Pink acrylic for dentures had already been used to make post-operative conformers (Kelley 1970). The acrylic ocular prosthesis permitted custom fitting of the prosthetic to the implant and was critical to development of the motility implants. Evolution of the exposed and buried integrated implants was concurrent.

17.4.1 Exposed integrated implants

Ruedemann's PMMA implant (1945) was a combined motility implant and ocular prosthesis. The posterior portion of the implant was covered with tantalum mesh to allow attachment of the rectus muscles, Tenon's capsule and conjunctiva (Ruedemann 1945). The inability to remove the ocular prosthesis for cleaning, the need for custom prefabrication prior to implantation and problems with positional deviations led to its abandonment (Durham 1949).

In 1947, Cutler described a PMMA 'ball and ring' implant. The exposed face had a square female receptacle, into which a 14 kt gold square male peg of the ocular prosthesis would fit. The rectus muscles were looped around and sutured to the ring (Cutler 1947), Other similar pegtype implants were produced. The Hughes enucleation implant was similar to Cutler's in shape, but was made of vitalium (an inert lightweight alloy of cobalt, chromium and molybdenum) (Hughes 1948). Whitney coupled the extraocular muscles to an implant by incorporating tantalum gauze around an acrylic sphere. Stone designed implants with metallic prongs on to which the rectus muscles were impaled. The Rolf implant incorporated a ring for muscle attachment and tantalum mesh anteriorly for conjunctival attachment (Gougelmann 1970).

Direct coupling of the ocular prosthesis to the implant significantly improved motility, apparently by eliminating slippage between the implant and ocular prosthesis. The supporting peg also helped to create a fuller upper lid sulcus and reduced the weight placed on the lower eyelid. Unfortunately, excessive secretions, recurrent granulations and chronic infection were common complications of exposed integrated implants (Drucker 1951; Perry 1991). In a review of the outcomes of 91 exposed integrated implants (74 hollow tantalum, 17 gold ring and cylinder), 50% of the hollow tantalum implants survived at 2 years while 60% of the gold ring implants survived after 3 years. Infection was the reason for extrusion/removal in 80% of cases (Choyce 1952). In retrospect this was the expected outcome of a chronically disrupted epithelial lining. This unifying failure led to the adoption of buried integrated implants.

17.4.2 Buried integrated implants

In theory a buried integrated implant combines the advantages of the smooth buried and exposed integrated implants in providing: (a) an uninterrupted conjunctival lining to minimize discharge and infection related to exposures, and (b) an irregular surface to translate implant movement to ocular prosthesis movement and to partially support the weight of the ocular prosthesis – reducing pressure on the lower lid and permitting a fuller upper lid sulcus.

In 1942, Dimitry described and patented the creation of an elevated stump on the implant surface, meant to fit into a ocular prosthesis with a posterior concavity – but he did not report any actual results (Guyton 1948). Cutler introduced a basket implant in 1945. This implant had four openings through which the rectus muscles were pulled and sutured together with conjunctiva closed over it. The ocular prosthesis had a knob on its posterior surface that fitted into the concavity of the implant (Cutler 1946). As with the exposed integrated implants, others developed similar types of implants. The King implant consisted of a pear-shaped tantalum mesh. The rectus muscles were attached to the base of the mesh and conjunctiva closed over it (Gougelmann 1970).

Among the better known of the buried integrated implants is the Allen implant. The story of this implant nicely captures the progression of orbital implant design/philosophy from the mid 1940s to the mid 1980s. What eventually became known as the Allen implant initially began life in 1946 as an exposed integrated implant (Allen 1950). In contrast to the Cutler design (Cutler 1947) (female implant), the Allen design incorporated the peg into the implant (male). Each rectus muscle was passed through a peripheral tunnel, split lengthwise to straddle the gold peg and sutured to its antagonist. Most such implants were retained only a few months before they extruded or were removed because of secondary infection. Consequently, the peg was removed and muscles were sutured together (i.e. imbricated) through a central 6 mm opening. Tenon's capsule and conjunctiva were completely closed over the flat surface of the implant. This design also turned out to be problematic: repeated exposures over the flat anterior plastic surface. It was thought that the exposures were related to an inadequate subconjunctival tissue bed. Thus the central anterior opening was enlarged from 6 to 15 mm. Imbrication of muscles within the ring created a broad, flat surface, permitting excellent translation of movement (since flat surfaces do not slip past each other as easily as curved surfaces) (Allen 1950).

Translation of movements was perhaps too good, as prosthetic edge show on extreme gaze and torsional end-point movements were particular problems of the Allen implant (Jordan et al. 1987). A possible explanation is that the flat apposition between the implant and the ocular prosthesis prevents the implant from slipping underneath the ocular prosthesis when the ocular prosthesis is restricted by the conjunctival fornices on side gaze. Any imbalance between the superior and inferior forces acting on the ocular prosthesis will create a rotational movement. Adding more to the peripheral edges to decrease edge show was impractical as it often created discomfort with opposite gaze. Late exposures over the outer ring were long-term complications (Fan & Robertson 1995) (Fig. 17.7). Since the flat surface did not support the weight of the ocular prosthesis well against gravity, lower lid droop and exaggeration of the upper lid sulcus were noticeable in some patients. In 1979, Jahrling reported a 19% incidence of extrusion among 168 Allen implants (40% in 43 Allen implants placed after severe trauma) (Jahrling 1979). Other investigators, however, have found much lower extrusion rates (2/186 = 1%) (Fan & Robertson 1995).

The successor to the Allen enucleation implant was the Iowa enucleation implant (Spivey 1970). The Iowa I implant was first reported in 1959. The

Iowa II implant was similar in shape but nearly one-third larger in volume (Allen *et al*. 1969). Like the Allen implant this was a buried integrated implant, originally reported as a 'quasi-integrated' implant (Allen *et al*. 1960). The Iowa implant was made of methyl-methacrylate resin and had four peripheral mounds (of 5 mm height) on its anterior surface designed to integrate with four depressions on the back of the ocular prosthesis. The rectus muscles were brought together through the valleys between the mounds, overlapped (5.0–5.5 mm) and tied together at a central anterior depression. Holes were made through parts of the implant in the hope of permitting fibrovascular tissue growth into the implant. This implant addressed many of the problems with the Allen implant. The four surface mounds supported the ocular prosthesis and reduced the gravitational effect on the lower lid (Jordan *et al*. 1987). Gaze-dependent ocular prosthesis edge show and torsional movements were also corrected (Allen *et al*. 1969; Spivey *et al*. 1969; Spivey 1970). When Iowa implants exposed, it was often over the surface of mounds (Spivey *et al*. 1969). This was likely due to localized pressure necrosis. As a result the Universal implant was introduced in 1987, with lower and more rounded mounds (Fig 17.7). (Jordan *et al*. 1987; Jordan 2000) Experience with the Universal implant was limited by the introduction of a new generation of porous implants.

17.4.3 Magnetic implants

Magnetic implants involved coaptation of the implant and ocular prosthesis by use of magnets, with conjunctiva sandwiched in between. There were a number of variations on this premise. (Tomb & Gearhart 1954; Young 1954; Ellis & Levy 1956; Roper-Hall 1956; Gougelmann 1970). These implants had adequate movement, but if the magnet was too strong or misaligned, conjunctiva and Tenon's capsule could become compressed between the implant and the ocular prosthesis, leading to breakdown and exposure along the outer edges (Soll 1986). In 2007, magnetic coupling of implant and ocular prosthesis was reported again, but this time with porous polyethylene (Miller *et al*. 2007). It will be interesting to see, in long-term follow-up, if these new porous magnetic implants will have similar complications.

An important cause of possible tissue breakdown and late exposure (Murray *et al*. 2000) related to magnetic implants, not well described in the literature, may be ferrous toxicity and associated tissue necrosis. Over the long term the magnets rust with exposures developing over the central anterior surface, as opposed to the peripheral edges which are prone to pressure necrosis. The levels of iron in the conjunctiva have been found to be 3–5 times normal (Dr Mark A Baskin, Kaiser Permanente, Oakland, CA, personal communication, 2003).

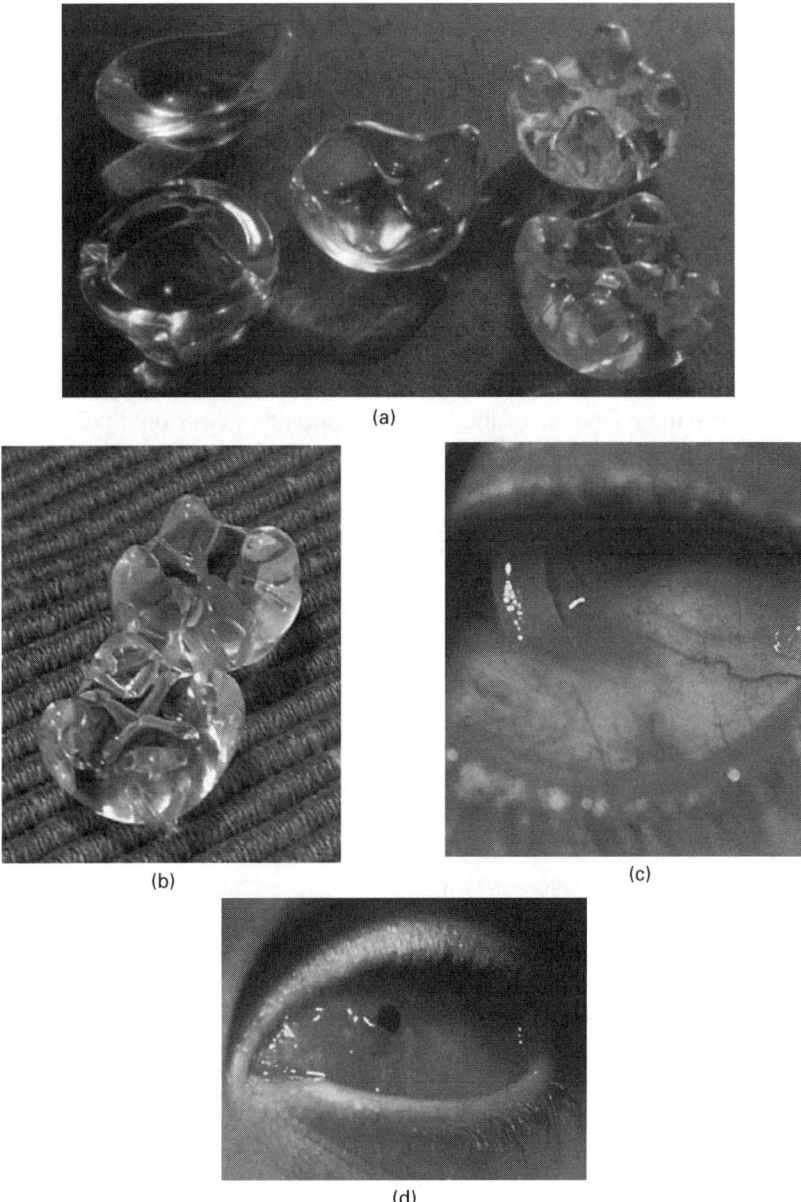

(a)

(b)

(c)

(d)

17.7 Allen, Iowa and Universal implants. (a) Allen implant, lower left corner, Iowa implant, upper right corner, Universal implant, lower right corner; upper left and middle, conformers for the Allen and Iowa implants respectively. (b) Closer view of Iowa (upper) and Universal (lower) implants (note the softer mounds on the Universal implant as compared with the Iowa implant). (c) Exposure of Allen implant (note exposure over outer ring). (d): Exposure of Iowa implant (note exposure over the mound).

17.5   Porous implants

In the absence of a vascular base, repairing or patch grafting of exposures is difficult. This led to the development of porous orbital implants using hydroxyapatite, porous polyethylene (Medpor®) and alumina. In theory, by permitting vascular ingrowth these implants should:

(a) increase the success rate of surgical repair/patch grafting when exposures develop (although porous implants appear to have a higher exposure rate overall, when compared with smooth synthetic implants) (Custer *et al.* 2003);
(b) reduce the incidence and severity of infection (since a vascular supply permits immune surveillance and defense);
(c) reduce the incidence of implant migration and extrusion. (Trichopoulos & Augsburger 2005).

17.5.1 Hydroxyapatite implants

Hydroxyapatite had been used as a bone substitute since 1975, but received US Food and Drug Administration (FDA) approval for use as an orbital implant in 1989 (Bio-Eye®: Integrated Orbital Implants, San Diego, CA) (Dutton 1991). Guist had inserted charred bone spheres into the muscle cone over 70 years earlier which produced 'considerable tissue reaction' and some reabsorption (Molteno 1980; Molteno & Elder 1991). However, hydroxyapatite implants to do not appear to absorb over time (Holmes & Hagler 1987; Sires *et al.* 1998).

Porous hydroxyapatite, $Ca_{10}(PO_4)_6(OH)_2$, is made by a specific genus of reef-building coral. The porous form has a micro-architecture similar to human cancellous (spongy) bone with interconnecting channels. Hydroxyapatite is the primary inorganic portion of human bone. The process by which hydroxyapatite implants are created from sea coral involves intense heat that denatures the proteins, to reduce immune response. When implanted next to bone, new bone growth occurs within its pores. When implanted within soft tissues, fibrovascular tissue grows into the pores (Perry 1991). Reports suggest that unwrapped hydroxyapatite does not become encapsulated as do silicone and PMMA spheres. (Holmes 1979; Dutton 1991; Perry 1991).

Hydroxyapatite incites a foreign-body giant cell reaction. (Rosner *et al.* 1992). In the animal model a foreign-body reaction may persist up to a year after implantation of a synthetic hydroxyapatite sphere (Sires *et al.* 1995; Saitoh *et al.* 1996). In addition, the rough surface of hydroxyapatite can produce exposures where implant and ocular prosthesis come into contact (Perry 1991; Buettner & Bartley 1992; Goldberg *et al.* 1992; Remulla *et al.* 1995) (Fig. 17.8). Surgeons began to wrap hydroxyapatite in banked human sclera (which adds about 1–1.5 mm to the final diameter of the implant) to decrease early exposure risk (40% exposure for unwrapped hydroxyapatite vs 7% exposure for wrapped hydroxyapatite in one study) (Remulla *et al.* 1995) and to facilitate suturing of muscles to the brittle implant (Custer *et al.* 2003). Cutting windows into the scleral wrap at the attachment site of the foure rectus muscles and associated ciliary vessels was advocated to promote faster vascularization of wrapped implants (Perry1991; Shields *et al.* 1992a; Gayre *et al.* 2002). Pore size also appears to have an effect on the rate of vascularization. Vascular ingrowth occurs more rapidly in hydroxyapatite implants with 200 mm pores than in hydroxyapatite implants with 500 mm pores (Bigham *et al.* 1999).

The scleral wrap incites a foreign-body reaction and becomes partially absorbed over time (Soll 1986; Rosner *et al.* 1992), with associated late exposure (Fig. 17.8). Thus the use of autologous grafts (e.g. temporalis fascia or fascia lata from the thigh) (Wiggs & Becker 1992; Jordan & Klapper 1999) was suggested, on the basis that a homologous graft incites less inflammation and is less likely to be absorbed. Other options for autologous wrapping materials include the rectus abdominus sheath (Kao & Chen 1999) and posterior auricular muscle (Naugle *et al.* 1999). The disadvantage is scarring, inflammation and infectious risk associated with a second surgical site. Processed wraps are also available. These include human donor fascia lata, human donor pericardium and expanded polytetrafluoroethylene (e-PTFE) (Choo *et al.* 1999; Kao 2000). The use of bovine pericardium as a wrapping material appears to be more inflammatory than scleral wrapping on histology (DeBacker *et al.* 1999) and clinically may have higher exposure rates, (Arat *et al.* 2003), although there is disagreement between authors (Gayre *et al.* 2001). Another alternative is polyglactin mesh (Jordan *et al.* 1995). A fibrovascular capsule of variable thickness forms external to the polyglactin mesh and replaces it by 12 weeks (Jordan *et al.* 2003b). Polyglactin mesh-wrapped hydroxyapatite implants must be placed deep into the orbit to prevent exposure risk (Jordan & Klapper 1999; Custer *et al.* 2003; Jordan *et al.* 2003b). More recently, the use of acellular dermis (AlloDerm – human cadaveric dermis) has been advocated as a wrapping material. Histological studies suggest that it permits vascularization of porous implants and does not incite significant inflammation. (Thakker *et al.* 2004). Although there is a theoretical risk, no case of disease transmission has been reported to date (Kadyan & Sandramouli 2008)

Polymer-coated hydroxyapatite implants became available in 2003. The coating consists of two different color-coded polymers. The anterior amber portion absorbs over 18 months and the posterior purple portion absorbs over 6 weeks. The idea is to avoid the need for a tissue wrap, with protection against anterior exposure, while promoting fibrovascular ingrowth posteriorly (Shields *et al.* 2007). Overall, the use of implant wrapping material appears to be declining among surgeons in North America (Su & Yen 2004).

A number of lower-cost versions have been developed in other countries. FCI (Issy-Les-Moulineaux, France), produces a synthetic form of hydroxyapatite. Their third-generation implant, FCI3®, has a chemical composition similar to the Bio-Eye® with minor differences in pore architecture on electron microscopy (Mawn *et al.* 1998). Drilling the FCI3® implant is easier than for the Bio-Eye® (Jordan *et al.* 1998). The Chinese hydroxyapatite implant

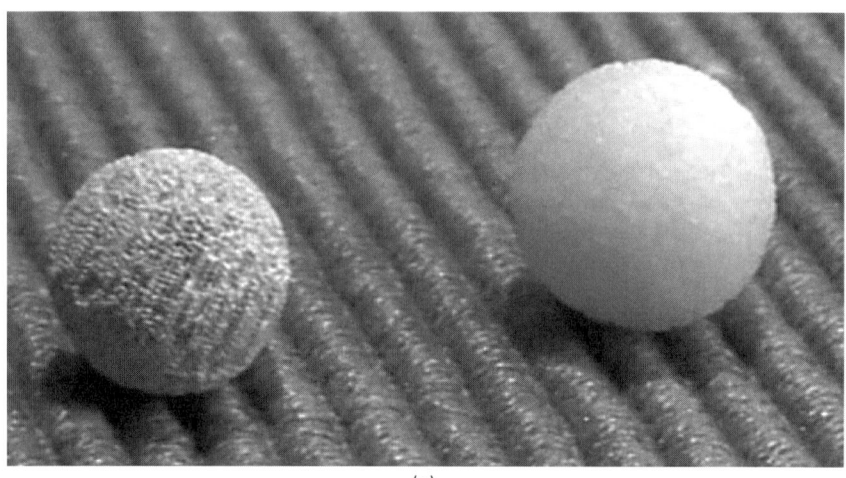

(a)

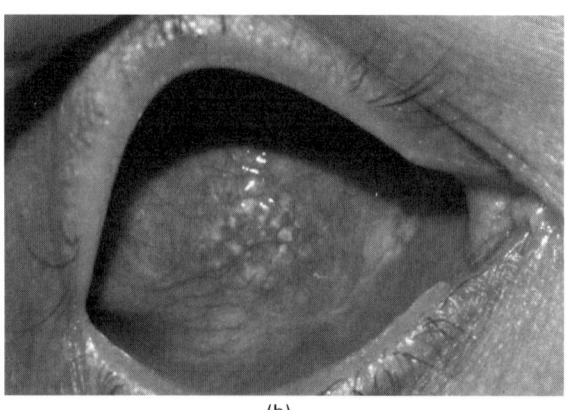

(b)

17.8 Porous implants – hydroxyapatite and porous polethylene: like hydroxyapatite, porous polyethylene permits fibrovascular ingrowth. The first generation of spherical Medpor implants had a rough surface like hydroxyapatite; subsequently, implants with a smoother anterior surface were introduced. (a) Hydroxyapatite (left) and Medpor (right) implants. (b) Early stage of exposure – hydroxyapatite implant. (c) Hydroxyapatite implant exposure. (d) Porous polyethylene implant exposure.

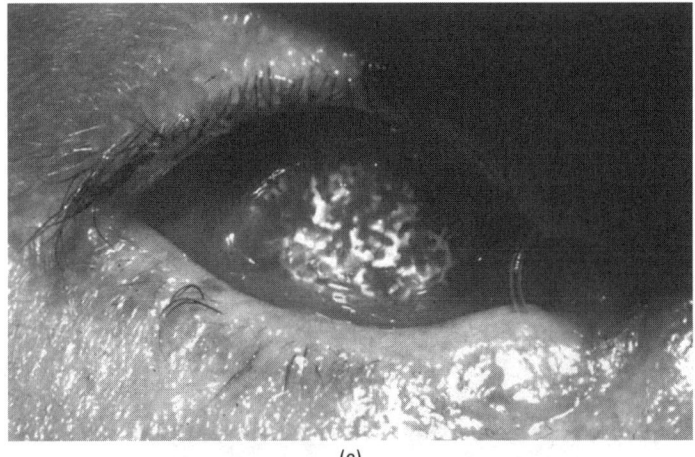

(c)

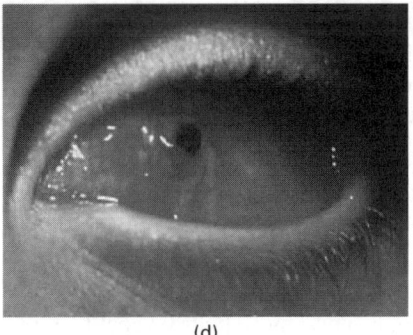

(d)

17.8 Continued

(H+Y Comprehensive Technologies, Philadelphia, PA) has been reported to contain some calcium oxide impurities. When hydrated in tissues, calcium hydroxide may form, which is caustic (Jordan *et al.* 1999c). The Brazilian hydroxyapatite implant (available in Brazil only) (Jordan *et al.* 2000b), has higher weight and lower porosity when compared with the Bio-Eye® implant (Jordan *et al.* 2000b). The Molteno M-Sphere® (IOP Inc., Costa Mesa, CA) is an antigen-free cancellous bone implant. It is comparatively fragile and may not be able to support a peg as well as the Bio-Eye® and FCI3® implants (Jordan *et al.* 2000a).

In some ways the early porous implants represented a regression in design (to the simple buried implants) in that the hydroxyapatite sphere may not translate movement to the implant as well as the irregular anterior surface of buried integrated implants (Fig. 17.9). In order to overcome this, the placement of a peg to translate movement better was advocated (Perry 1991).

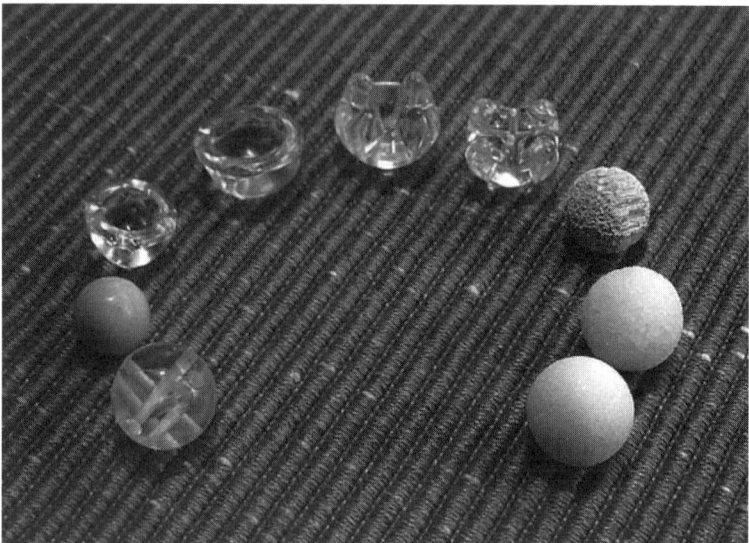

17.9 50 years of 'progress' – 1950 to 2000 (shown from left to right). In some respects, spherical porous implants represented a regression in design (to the simple buried implants) in that they may not translate movement to the implant as well as the irregular anterior surface of buried integrated implants. The irony is that after 50 years of development we returned to plastic balls with channels to permit vascular ingrowth!

Vascularization of an unwrapped hydroxyapatite implant takes approximately 6 months. However, when wrapped in sclera, the speed of vascularization is more variable. Thus it is recommended to wait at least 6 months before considering peg placement, and to confirm complete implant vascularization with gadolinium-enhanced magnetic resonance imaging (Dutton 1991; Hamilton *et al.* 1992; Spirnak *et al.* 1995; Klapper *et al.* 2003; Park *et al.* 2003). Technetium-99m bone scintillography may also be used to verify implant vascularization (Ferrone & Dutton 1992; Numerow *et al.* 1994; Leitha *et al.* 1995). Drilling 1 mm holes to the center of the implant at the time of surgery appears to accelerate implant vascularization (Perry 1991; Ferrone & Dutton 1992; Jordan *et al.* 1998).

The ocularist can assist the surgeon in drilling the implant by creating a conformer with a central opening to guide the drill. If the initial drilled tunnel is not perpendicular and central to the implant surface, re-drilling can be problematic, especially if the drill shafts need to be juxtaposed. Once adequate vascularization is confirmed, a hole (about 2–3 mm wide and 10 mm deep) is drilled into the implant and a temporary peg is placed. Follow-up with an ocularist is needed in 4–6 weeks, at which time the flat-head peg is removed (Perry 1991).

How should a pegged hydroxyapatite implant be classified: buried integrated or exposed integrated? Perry (1991) suggested that eventual vascularization of the drilled hole would allow re-epithelialization, permitting the motility advantage of exposed integrated implants with the safety profile of a buried implant. In practice, however, drilling may become complicated by exposures, chronic discharge and formation of pyogenic granulomas at the peg site. In one series the complication rate of pegging was 38% (Jordan *et al.* 1999a). The most common problems in this review ($n = 165$) included: chronic discharge, 37%; pyogenic granuloma formation, 31%; peg extrusion, 29%; poor transfer of movement, 11%; clicking with extreme gaze, 11% (the clicking appears to be related to a loose fit between the peg and ocular prosthesis, such that, when the ocular prosthesis is restricted in its motion by the fornices in extreme gaze, the peg continues to travel with the implant and knocks against the side of the drilled shaft in the implant; drilling a shaft with smaller diameter may prevent this problem). Peg complication rates as high as 67% ($n = 275$) have been reported (Shoamanesh *et al.* 2007). A study of complications associated with freestanding polycarbonate pegs found a complication rate of 71% ($n = 21$) (Fahim *et al.* 2007).

There are a number of available peg systems. In early polycarbonate pegs, used with the hydroxyapatite implant, the peg was attached to the ocular prosthesis, with the female end drilled into the implants. This made insertion and removal of the ocular prosthesis difficult and potentially traumatic to the conjunctival lining (Edelstein *et al.* 1997; Oestreicher *et al.* 1997). Thus a permanent peg was placed inside the drilled hole, with a ball at the exposed end to articulate with a corresponding indentation carved into the posterior surface of the ocular prosthesis (Perry 1991; Shields *et al.* 1994).

To decrease the high complication rate associated with non-sleeved PMMA and polycarbonate pegs, titanium peg and sleeve systems have been advocated (Jordan & Klapper 2000). Studies suggest that peg extrusion rates and pyogenic granuloma formation are reduced with sleeved peg systems (Edelstein *et al.* 1997; Jordan & Klapper 2000; Lee *et al.* 2002). In one series, sleeved peg extrusion rates were 11% ($n = 74$) compared with 27% ($n = 191$) for non-sleeved pegs (Lee *et al.* 2002). A recent large retrospective review ($n = 353$) found a significantly lower incidence of peg extrusion and granuloma formation with titanium pegged implants as compared with non-sleeved PMMA and sleeved polycarbonate pegs (Yoon *et al.* 2008).

Primary placement (i.e. at the time of enucleation) of a titanium sleeve in porous implants has been suggested to reduce the cost and complication rates (in theory) of secondary drilling and peg placement (Liao *et al.* 2005a; Liao *et al.* 2005b). In a study of 52 patients receiving a primary peg placement, a 29% complication rate was found. This complication rate is similar to reported outcomes of secondary peg insertion (Yazici *et al.* 2007). Recent surveys suggest there is a decline in placement of motility pegs by surgeons (Su & Yen 2004; Viswanathan *et al.* 2007).

17.5.2 Porous polyethylene implants

Despite the initial success of hydroxyapatite and reports of low extrusion rates when wrapped in donor sclera, a number of problems persist:

(a) a theoretical infectious risk associated with donor sclera (e.g. prion disease – although we are not aware of any reports to date);
(b) development of late exposures and pyogenic granuloma formation (Fig. 17.8);
(c) difficulty in re-drilling in cases of implant migration.

Some of these problems have been addressed by a new generation of porous polyethylene (Medpor®) implants, which can be placed safely without wrapping. An exposure rate of 1% (3/302) was reported for Medpor® implants placed without wrapping (Chen & Cui 2006). Whereas the coralline hydroxyapatite implant must be drilled with a power-tool for peg placement, porous polyethylene may be pegged by hand with a screw driver. When a hydroxyapatite sphere rotates in the orbit, re-drilling may create a large tract that does not support a peg well. With porous polyethylene, repositioning the peg is less problematic, as the tract left by the prior screw is a narrow spiral.

Like hydroxyapatite, porous polyethylene permits fibrovascular ingrowth (Karesh & Dresner 1994; Rubin *et al.* 1994). Porous polyethylene became available for orbital implantation in 1991 (Porex Surgical Inc., Newnan, GA). Animal model studies suggest that porous polyethylene incites less inflammation and fibrosis than hydroxyapatite (Goldberg *et al.* 1994; Li *et al.* 2001). Using electron microscopy, porous polyethylene implants show a smoother surface than hydroxyapatite (Bio-Eye®), synthetic hydroxyapatite (FCI3®) and aluminum oxide (alumina) implants (Jordan *et al.* 2004). The rate of vascularization of porous polyethylene appears to be slower than that for hydroxyapatite (Bio-Eye®), synthetic hydroxyapatite (FCI3®), and aluminum oxide implants (Jordan *et al.* 2004). Porous polyethylene implants with 400 um pore size vascularize more rapidly than the 200 um pore size (Goldberg *et al.* 1994; Rubin *et al.* 1994). Implant vascularization appears to be faster with the Medpor-Plus® implant, which is a combination of Medpor® and synthetic bone graft particulate (Novabone®) in a 70:30 ratio (Naik *et al.* 2007).

The first generation of spherical porous polyethylene implants had a rough surface (Li, *et al.* 2001). Subsequently, implants with a smoother anterior surface were introduced (Woog *et al.* 2004). A retrospective report of 91 enucleations suggested similar exposure rates for wrapped and unwrapped

porous polyethylene implants (<5%) (Blaydon *et al.* 2003).
Medpor® implants currently come in a number of shapes. These include but are not limited to:

(a) simple sphere;
(b) conical implants with a flat 6 mm anterior surface (Dresner);
(c) smooth surface tunnel (SST™ sphere) with suture tunnels for easier muscle attachment (Woog *et al.* 2004);
(d) conical orbital implant (Rubin *et al.* 1998) which incorporates a superior projection to reduce superior sulcus defect;
(e) 'Quad' motility implant (Anderson) – similar in design philosophy, shape and method of muscle attachment (imbrication) to the Iowa and Universal implants (Anderson *et al.* 1990; Anderson *et al.* 2002).

17.5.3 Porous aluminum oxide (Al_2O_3) implants

Implants using aluminum oxide (also known as alumina) are a recent instalment in the continuing search for better-tolerated orbital implants. Aluminum oxide has been in use for over 30 years as an implant in orthopedics and dentistry (Smith 1963). Osteoblasts and fibroblasts appear to grow faster on aluminum oxide than on hydroxyapatite in laboratory models (Mawn *et al.* 2001). Reports of aluminum encephalopathy with the use of ionocem (a biomaterial made by reacting calcium aluminum fluorosilicate with polyalkenoic acid), have raised concerns regarding aluminum-containing biomaterials. However, aluminum oxide appears to be bioinert and insoluble in tissues. Blood samples drawn from patients with alumina implants show normal aluminum levels (Christel 1992; Jordan *et al.* 2000c).

Outcomes in a review of 107 alumina implants placed over 3 years (all wrapped in polyglactin mesh) were encouraging (Jordan *et al.* 2003a). Of these, 107 implants, 76 were enucleation implants (50 as secondary implants). The overall exposure rate was 2% in 107 implants (0 in the enucleation group), as compared with 3% in 120 FCI3® implants (1995–1999), and 8% in 258 Bio-Eye® implants (1990–1995) for the same authors. However, a recent retrospective review of 108 patients found a long-term exposure rate of 7.4% for alumina implants (mean follow-up of 35.8 months) (Wang *et al.* 2009). We will have to await long-term data to make firm conclusions about the clinical efficacy of aluminum oxide as an orbital implant.

17.6   Trends in pediatric enucleation

Historically, ophthalmologists were hesitant to place orbital implants in children at the time of enucleation (De Potter *et al.* 1994). The reasons for this may have been rooted in: (a) fear of interfering with the detection of tumor recurrence (Shields *et al.* 1992b; Christmas *et al.* 2000) – since a significant portion of pediatric enucleations are done for retinoblastoma; and (b) less disfiguring appearance of acquired anophthalmia (with ocular prosthesis only) in young children as compared with adults – at least in the short term. However, animal model studies support the theory that placement of an implant is necessary for stimulation of orbital growth (Cepela *et al.* 1992). Studies on the long-term effects of pediatric enucleation in the four decades spanning 1935–1975, showed stunted orbital growth in children who did not receive implants (Taylor 1939; Pfieffer 1945; Apt & Isenberg 1973; Osborne *et al.* 1974). These observations have prompted the routine use of orbital implants after pediatric enucleation. Human follow-up studies of retinoblastoma cases suggest that childhood enucleation, when combined with a large implant, minimizes orbital growth retardation (Fountain *et al.* 1999). In addition, the role of the ocular prosthesis in stimulating orbital growth cannot be ignored (Yago & Furuta 2001).

In normal development, by 5 years of age orbital volume has reached about 80% of the volume seen at 15 years, in both sexes (Bentley *et al.* 2002). Earlier reports suggested attainment of 80% of adult size by 3 years of age (Scott 1954). Orbital volume is thought to reach adult volume by 12–14 years of age (Yago & Furuta 2001). When enucleation takes place in infancy, placement of progressively larger implants has been advocated to achieve adequate orbital growth (Vistnes 1987) In animal models, implantation of a sphere that inadequately compensates for volume loss, does not stimulate orbital growth (Sarnat & Shanedling 1970; Sarnat & Shanedling 1972; Sarnat & Shanedling 1974; Sarnat 1979; Sarnat 1981; Sarnat 1982; Reedy *et al.* 1999). In a recent study of orbital volume following childhood enucluation for retinoblastoma, 3 of 13 hydroxyapatite implants were noted to have migrated. In all 3, the orbital volume on the ipsilateral side was found to be larger than on the non-operated side. In the absence of implant migration, the operated side had a smaller volume in all cases. This argues for the significance of mechanical stimulation in orbital growth (Lyle *et al.* 2007).

Although stunted orbital growth following enucleation is well established in radiographic studies, there may not be obvious cosmetic facial asymmetry (Howard *et al.* 1965; Hintschich *et al.* 2001). More recently, orbital volume measurements using computed tomography have suggested that enucleation, in both children and adults, is associated with reduction of bony orbital volume over time (Hintschich *et al.* 2001). Other studies have found a greater impact of radiation dose (megavoltage external beam irradiation) on orbital growth than implant placement and size. In a study of irradiated orbits, secondary enucleation did not appear to have an additive growth-retarding effect (no implant placed) (Imhof *et al.* 1996). Orbital growth appears to be most affected when radiation is given in the first year (particularly in the first 6 months) of life (Imhof *et al.* 1996; Ameniya *et al.* 1977; Peylan-Ramu *et al.* 2001).

Do these studies imply that the placement of an implant after enucleation is unnecessary? No. The wealth of human clinical and experimental animal studies showing the importance of volume replacement in promoting orbital growth (Taylor 1939; Pfieffer 1945; Kennedy 1964; Apt & Isenberg 1973; Osborne *et al.* 1974; Fountain *et al.*1997; Yago & Furuta 2001; Chen & Heher 2004) cannot be discounted. Post-enucleation socket syndrome is still an important consideration and an excellent argument for placement of an implant of adequate volume in any patient. In combination with a buried integrated implant, an ocular prosthesis can show nearly life-like movements to match those of the contralateral eye, an important aspect of rehabilitation.

There has been an increasing trend to use porous implants in children (De Potter *et al.* 1992; De Potter *et al.* 2004). Fibrovascular ingrowth into these implants makes later removal difficult. (Kaltreider *et al.* 2001). One way to achieve implant motility and at the same time permit later implant exchange is to use an acrylic ball and attach the muscles to the conjunctival fornices (Soll 1972; Nunery & Hetzler 1983). A potential problem with the use of hxdroxyapatite for such an implant is that hydroxyapatite implants are radio-opaque on imaging. In theory this could interfere with detection of calcification associated with tumor recurrence in cases of retinoblastoma. However, the well-circumscribed appearance of the implant on imaging, and its intermediate signal intensity, are thought to be characteristic enough to not interfere with the radiologic features of retinoblastoma recurrence (De Potter *et al.* 1992; De Potter *et al.* 1994). In addition, coralline hydroxyapatite implants do not appear to attenuate external beam photon radiation significantly (Arora *et al.* 1992). When calcification is detected following enucleation with placement of a scleral-wrapped orbital implant, the presence of calcium may be dystrophic, and does not necessarily indicate recurrent tumor growth. (Summers 1993).

An autogenous dermis fat graft is another option (Bosniak *et al.* 1989). Graft atrophy, usually more pronounced when dermis fat grafts are placed in older patients, may also occur in children. Dermis fat graft hypertrophy may occur in growing children (Guberina *et al.* 1983; Mitchell *et al.* 2001)

In the first few months after enucleation, the rough surface of porous implants may be associated with an even higher exposure risk in children than in adults. Although there are only a handful of studies in children, scleral wrapped hydroxyapatite and polyethylene implants appear to have a reduced exposure rate compared with unwrapped implants (De Potter *et al.* 1994; Karcioglu *et al.* 1998; Christmas *et al.* 2000; Lee *et al.* 2000; Nolan *et al.* 2003; Iordanidou & De Potter 2004). The reasons for this are not well established.

17.7   Gaps in scientific knowledge and future trends

Despite the 50+ years of evolution of motility implants, our understanding about the actual motility of various implants, and the efficacy of pegging in improving motility is mostly subjective – prone to the bias of optimistic patients and surgeons. The major determinants of implant and ocular prosthesis motility are unclear. An important question is whether ocular prosthesis motility is mainly due to the retraction of conjunctival fornices by muscle contraction (De Voe 1945; Coston 1970; Soll 1982; Nunery & Hetzler 1983; Tyers & Collin 1985; Smit *et al.* 1991a), or is due to direct transmission of forces between implant and ocular prosthesis (Soll 1972; Nunery & Hetzler 1983)? In a case series of 25 patients, Nunnery and Hetzler showed that direct suturing of the rectus muscles to the conjunctival fornices can impart adequate motility to a ocular prosthesis (Nunery & Hetzler 1983).

Adequate ocular prosthesis motility does not imply movement to fully match the normal side. This would create the problems with edge show and torsion that were seen with the Allen implant (Jordan *et al.* 1987). Adequate implant motility is probably about 70–75% of the contralateral normal eye. Still, a major hurdle to social rehabilitation after enucleation continues to be poor apparent ocular prosthesis movement. Apparent, since it is unclear whether the problem is primarily an issue of inadequate implant movement, or poor translation of movement to the ocular prosthesis. Alternatively, the ocular prosthesis may be limited in motion by the conjunctival fornices, with the implant slipping underneath (Nerad *et al.* 1991). Could a large ocular prosthesis, within the confines of a small palpebral fissure and conjunctival fornices, restrict movement of the implant – especially when a peg is placed?

Studies on the relationship between implant and ocular prosthesis motility are generally lacking. A handful of investigators have attempted to assess the efficacy of various motility implants objectively; however, there are significant shortcomings. One simple approach to measuring implant motility has been to mark the conjunctival center and measure excursions in millimeters (Bosniak *et al.* 1989; Custer *et al.* 1999; Long *et al.* 2003) Custer and associates compared *implant* motility of scleral-wrapped acrylic ($n = 7$), silicone ($n = 8$) and hydroxyapatite ($n = 31$) implants. They found similar implant motility. Only age and implant size were found to be significant predictors of implant movement: vertical and horizontal movement decreased with increasing age and increased with larger implant sizes (Custer *et al.* 1999). Bosniak and associates compared *implant* motility between synthetic spherical implants ($n = 47$, all with muscle imbrication, implant sizes 14–20 mm) and autogenous dermis fat grafts ($n = 34$).(Bosniak *et al.* 1989). Overall they found better implant motility of dermis fat grafts. The diameter of spherical implants was not found to be a significant predictor of implant movement. Using the temporal and nasal limbus of the ocular prosthesis as a landmark for comparison, the difference in motility between dermis fat and synthetic implants disappeared. The authors found no correlation between ocular prosthesis motility and forniceal depth (Bosniak *et al.* 1989). Another, similar, approach is to use Kestenbaum spectacles to measure ocular prosthesis motility (Smit *et al.* 1991a). Using this approach, Smit and associates found no significant difference in ocular prosthesis motility between Allen ($n = 12$) and primary baseball (sclera-covered 18 mm acrylic, $n = 15$) implants. Motility of the ocular prosthesis was lowest in patients with no implant ($n = 11$). Patients with secondary baseball implants ($n = 11$) demonstrated ocular prosthesis motility in between the primary implantation group and patients with no implant.

Using a straight ruler to measure displacement on the curved surface of implants and ocular prostheses is inaccurate. Such measurements are subject to a significant cosine function error and are not comparable for spheres of different size, unless millimeters of movement are translated into degrees of rotation. Steven's hypothesis does not hold true for prosthetic eyes (Steven's hypothesis assumes that, for an emmetropic eye, the center of rotation and each end of the corneal diameter (12 mm) form an equilateral triangle; on this basis, linear displacement of the ocular limbus, as measured by a Wessely keratometer, can be converted into degrees of rotation) (Yamashiro 1957).

A more sophisticated approach for measuring ocular prosthesis movement is the magnetic search coil technique (Collewijn *et al.* 1975): the current generated by movement of a wire coil (placed on the ocular prosthesis) in a uniform magnetic field is used to derive the amplitude and velocity of movement (Nerad *et al.* 1991; Colen *et al.* 2000). In a series of 16 patients with Iowa and Universal implants, Nerad and associates found good initial transmission of movement to the ocular prosthesis, but final amplitudes that were on average about 50% of target movement (target = 10 degrees rotation) (Nerad *et al.* 1991). Colen and associates found similar prosthetic eye saccadic amplitudes between scleral wrapped spherical acrylic ($n = 16$) and hydroxyapatite ($n = 14$) implants (Colen *et al.* 2000). Unfortunately, the magnetic search coil technique does not give information about implant motility. It would be interesting to use this method to evaluate movement in the same patient, before and after placement of a peg. More recently, infrared oculography has been used in a prospective case series of 10 patients to quantitatively assess the effect on ocular prosthesis motility of placement of a peg. Although vertical motility was not significantly affected by peg placement, horizontal excursions did improve (Guillinta *et al.* 2003). Lucci and associates used a prism in front of the normal eye and a fixed target at 1 meter to measure ocular prosthesis movement. The prism power was increased until there was no more improvement in ocular prosthesis motility. Using this approach, a similar amplitude of movement was found in spherical and quad (Medpor®) implants (Lucci *et al.* 2007).

The development of an objective system to evaluate implant and ocular prosthesis motility is important for further development and refinement of motility implants. Such a system should permit simultaneous comparison of implant and ocular prosthesis movement, allowing investigators to better understand the dynamic relationship between the implant and ocular prosthesis movement. The surgical techniques and materials used in implantation may be culprits in limiting adequate implant motility. For example: (a) does imbrication of the rectus muscles over the surface of spherical implants produce a motility restriction by over-stretching the medial and inferior recti? (Dr A. Jampolsky, San Francisco, CA, personal communication); (b) Could the use of porous implants actually limit implant motility in the long run, in that fibrovascular ingrowth of the muscle bellies into the implant creates an adhesion-type syndrome in some patients?

To better illustrate the importance of observing ocular prosthesis and implant motility simultaneously, a simple experiment may be performed. The original impression mold of the socket may be used to produce a clear acrylic ocular prosthesis of the same shape, surface irregularities and frictional properties as the patient's own white acrylic ocular prosthesis. This allows both the socket and the implant to be observed during movement. Placement of a central conjunctival mark (with a tissue marker) allows the observer to better appreciate the relative position of implant and ocular prosthesis. This is illustrated in Fig. 17. Note that, in Fig. 17.10, poor ocular prosthesis abduction is associated with poor implant abduction, but the poor ocular prosthesis adduction is not associated with poor implant movement. The implant has slipped underneath the ocular prosthesis, suggesting that the limitation of ocular prosthesis adduction is probably related to forniceal restriction to movement. Both the implant and ocular prosthesis appear to elevate well. In depression, the ocular prosthesis appears to move well, masking the inferonasal rotation of the implant that is appreciated through the clear ocular prosthesis.

The search for more biocompatible orbital implants continues. In particular, the relationship between the microsturcture of porous implants and clinical performance requires further investigation. The ideal orbital enucleation implant would have a similar weight to the natural globe. The implant would be porous, smooth and pliable, permitting simple muscle attachment, i.e. without the need for wrapping. It should be cost effective and entirely alloplastic, eliminating potential infectious risks of donated tissue. The implant should incite no inflammation (i.e. should be inert) and be easily distinguished from surrounding tissue on imaging.

The currently available porous implants have a stiff structure (poor compliance). A more compliant implant may be more forgiving of repetitive conjuntival trauma at the implant–ocular prosthesis junction, reducing the incidence of tissue breakdown and implant exposure. Potential candidate

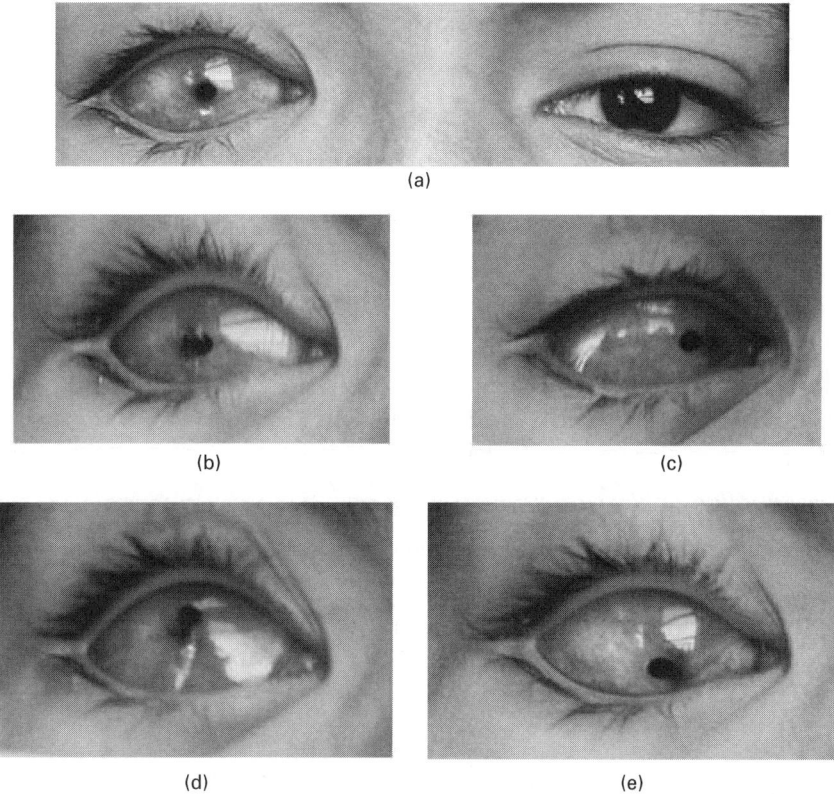

17.10 The original impression of the socket may be used to produce a clear prosthesis with the exact shape, surface irregularities and frictional properties of the patient's prosthesis. This allows both the socket and the implant to be observed during movement. The patient illustrated here is a 12-year-old boy who sustained a severe right-sided ocular injury at age 5 years. At the time of these photographs, he was 4 weeks post-enucleation, with implantation of an unwrapped 18 mm Medpor® ball. NB black mark on center of prosthesis and tissue marker on conjunctiva, placed such that in the primary position the mark on the prosthesis overlaps the tissue marker on the conjunctiva. (a) 1° position, (b) right gaze, poor implant abduction/poor prosthesis abduction, (c) left gaze, good implant adduction/poor prosthesis adduction, (d) upgaze, both implant and prosthesis elevate well, (e) downgaze, the implant extorts with infraduction, which is not apparent in the movement of the prosthesis.

materials include porous hydrogels, whose high water content allows more similar physical properties to living tissue (Chalasani *et al.* 2007). A promising design is the AlphaSphere®; this implant incorporates a spongy anterior hemisphere using poly(2-hydroxyethyl methacrylate) (PHEMA) to permit suturing of muscles, and a posterior smooth gel hemisphere, which in theory would optimize rotational movement (Hicks *et al.* 1999; Hicks *et al.* 2006).

17.8   Sources of further information and advice

Illustrations
Illustrations of the exposed integrated and buried integrated motility implants may be found in: Gougelmann H. P., The evolution of the ocular motility implant, *International Ophthalmology Clinics*, **10**, 689, 1970. Original illustrations by Lee Allen, outlining development of the Allen implant may be found in: A buried muscle cone implant – development of a tunneled hemispherical type, *Archives Ophthalmology*, **43**, 879, 1950.

Organizations and websites of interest

- Amercian Academy of Ophthalmology: www. AAO.org.
- American Society of Ocularists: www.ocularist.org.
- American Association for Pediatric Ophthalmology and Strabismus: www.AAPOS.org.

17.9   References

Allen, L. 1950, "A buried muscle cone implant – development of a tunneled hemispherical type", *Arch. Ophthalmol.*, **43**, 879–890.

Allen, L. 1970, "Fitting the ocular prosthesis: a challenge", *Trans. Am. Acad.Ophthalmol. Otolaryngol.*, vol. 74, no. 6, pp. 1318–1320.

Allen, L. 1983, "The argument against imbricating the rectus muscles over spherical orbital implants after enucleation", *Ophthalmology*, **90**, no. 9, 1116–1120.

Allen, L., Ferguson, E. C., & Braley, A. E. 1960, "A quasi-integrated buried muscle cone implant with good motility and advantages for prosthetic fitting", *Trans. Am. Acad. Ophthalmol. Otolaryngol.*, **64**, 272–286.

Allen, L. & Webster, H. E. 1969, "Modified impression method of artificial eye fitting", *Am. J. Ophthalmol.*, **67**, 189–218.

Allen. L., Spivey, B. E., & Burns, C. 1969, "A larger Iowa implant", *Am. J. Ophthalmol.*, **68**, 397–400.

Ameniya, T., Matsumura, M., & Hirose, Y. 1977, "Effects of radiation after enucleation without implantation on orbital development of patients with retinoblastoma", *Ophthalmologica*, **174**, no. 3, 137–144.

Anderson, R. L., Thiese, S. M., Nerad, J. A., Jordan, D. R., Tse, D., & Allen, L. 1990, "The universal orbital implant: indications and methods", *Adv. Ophthalmic Plast. Reconstr. Surg.*, **8**, 88–99.

Anderson, R. L., Yen, M. T., Lucci, L. M., & Caruso, R. T. 2002, "The quasi-integrated porous polyethylene orbital implant", *Ophthal. Plast. Reconstr. Surg.*, **18**, no. 1, 50–55.

Apt, L. & Isenberg, S. 1973, "Changes in orbital dimensions following enucleation", *Arch. Ophthalmol.*, **90**, 393–395.

Arat, Y. O., Shetlar, D. J., & Boniuk, M. 2003, "Bovine pericardium versus homologous sclera as a wrapping for hydroxyapatite orbital implants", *Ophthal. Plast. Reconstr. Surg.*, **19**, no. 3, 189–193.

Arora, V., Weeks, K., Halperin, E. C., & Dutton, J. J. 1992, "Influence of coralline hydroxyapatite used as an ocular implant on the dose distribution of external beam photon radiation therapy", *Ophthalmology*, **99**, no. 3, 380–382.

Bentley, R. P., Sgouros, S., Natarajan, K., Dover, M. S., & Hockley, A. D. 2002, "Normal changes in orbital volume during childhood", *J. Neurosurg.*, **96**, no. 4, 742–746.

Bigham, W. J., Stanley, P., Cahill, J. M., Jr, Curran, R. W., & Perry, A. C. 1999, "Fibrovascular ingrowth in porous ocular implants: the effect of material composition, porosity, growth factors, and coatings", *Ophthal.Plast. Reconstr. Surg.*, **15**, no. 5, 317–325.

Blaydon, S. M., Shepler, T. R., Neuhaus, R. W., White, W. L., & Shore, J. W. 2003, "The porous polyethylene (Medpor) spherical orbital implant: a retrospective study of 136 cases", *Ophthal. Plast. Reconstr. Surg.*, **19**, no. 5, 364–371.

Bosniak, S. L., Nesi, F., Smith, B. C., Schechter, B., & Cote, R. 1989, "A comparison of motility: autogenous dermis-fat vs synthetic spherical implants", *Ophthalmic Surg.*, **20**, no. 12, 889–891.

Buettner, H. & Bartley, G. B. 1992, "Tissue breakdown and exposure associated with orbital hydroxyapatite implants", *Am. J. Ophthalmol.*, **113**, no. 6, 669–673.

Cepela, M. A., Nunery, W. R., & Martin, R. T. 1992, "Stimulation of orbital growth by the use of expandable implants in the anophthalmic cat orbit", *Ophthal. Plast. Reconstr. Surg.*, **8**, no. 3, 157–167.

Chalasani, R., Poole-Warren, L., Conway, R. M., & Ben-Nissan, B. 2007, "Porous orbital implants in enucleation: a systematic review", *Surv. Ophthalmol.*, **52**, no. 2, 145–155.

Chen, D. & Heher, K. 2004, "Management of the anophthalmic socket in pediatric patients", *Curr. Opin. Ophthalmol.*, 15, no. 5, 449–453.

Chen, Y. H. & Cui, H. G. 2006, "High density porous polyethylene material (Medpor) as an unwrapped orbital implant", *J. Zhejiang. Univ Sci. B*, **7**, no. 8, 679–682.

Choo, P. H., Carter, S. R., Crawford, J. B., & Seiff, S. R. 1999, "Exposure of expanded polytetrafluoroethylene-wrapped hydroxyapatite orbital implant: a report of two patients", *Ophthal. Plast. Reconstr. Surg.*, **15**, no. 2, 77–78.

Choyce, D.P. 1952, "Orbital implants: review of results obtained at the Moorfields branch of the Moorfields, Westminster, and Central Eye Hospital, London", *Br. J. Ophthalmol.*, **36**, 123–130.

Christel, P. S. 1992, "Biocompatibility of surgical-grade dense polycrystalline alumina", *Clin. Orthop. Relat. Res.* **282**, 10–18.

Christmas, N. J., Van, Q. K., Murray, T. G., Gordon, C. D., Garonzik, S., Tse, D., Johnson, T., Schiffman, J., & O'Brien, J. M. 2000, "Evaluation of efficacy and complications: primary pediatric orbital implants after enucleation", *Arch. Ophthalmol.*, **118**, no. 4, 503–506.

Chuah, C. T., Chee, S. P., Fong, K. S., Por, Y. M., Choo, C. T., Luu, C., & Seah, L. L. 2004, "Integrated hydroxyapatite implant and non-integrated implants in enucleated Asian patients", *Ann. Acad. Med. Singapore*, **33**, no. 4, 477–483.

Colen, T. P., Paridaens, D. A., Lemij, H. G., Mourits, M. P., & van Den Bosch, W. A. 2000, "Comparison of artificial eye amplitudes with acrylic and hydroxyapatite spherical enucleation implants", *Ophthalmology*, **107**, no. 10, 1889–1894.

Collewijn, H., van der Mark, F., & Jansen, T. C. 1975, "Precise recording of human eye movements", *Vision Res.*, **15**, no. 3, 447–450.

Coston, T. O. 1970, "The spherical implant", *Trans. Am. Acad. Ophthalmol. Otolaryngol.*, **74**, no. 6, 1284–1286.

Culler, A. M. 1952, "Orbital implants after enucleation; basic principles of anatomy and physiology of the orbit and relation to implant surgery", *Trans. Am. Acad. Ophthalmol. Otolaryngol.*, **56**, no. 1, 17–20.

Custer, P. L., Kennedy, R. H., Woog, J. J., Kaltreider, S. A., & Meyer, D. R. 2003, "Orbital implants in enucleation surgery: a report by the American Academy of Ophthalmology", *Ophthalmology*, **110**, no. 10, 2054–2061.

Custer, P. L. & Trinkaus, K. M. 1999, "Volumetric determination of enucleation implant size", *Am. J. Ophthalmol.*, **128**, no. 4, 489–494.

Custer, P. L., Trinkaus, K. M., & Fornoff, J. 1999, "Comparative motility of hydroxyapatite and alloplastic enucleation implants", *Ophthalmology*, **106**, no. 3, 13–516.

Cutler, N. L. 1946, "A basket type implant for use after enucleation", *Arch. Ophthalmol.*, **35**, 71–93.

Cutler, N. L. 1947, "A positive contact ball and ring implant", *Arch. Ophthalmol.*, **37**, 73–77.

Danz, W., Sr 1990, "Mobility implants: a review", *Adv. Ophthalmic Plast. Reconstr. Surg.*, **8**, 46–52.

DeBacker, C. M., Dutton, J. J., Proia, A. D., Holck, D. E., & Stone, T. 1999, "Bovine pericardium versus homologous sclera as wrapping materials for hydroxyapatite ocular implants: an animal study", *Ophthal. Plast. Reconstr. Surg.*, **15**, no. 5, 312–316.

De Potter, P., Shields, C. L., Shields, J. A., Flanders, A. E., & Rao, V. M. 1992, "Role of magnetic resonance imaging in the evaluation of the hydroxyapatite orbital implant", *Ophthalmology*, **99**, no. 5, 824–830.

De Potter, P., Shields, C. L., Shields, J. A., & Singh, A. D. 1994, "Use of the hydroxyapatite ocular implant in the pediatric population", *Arch. Ophthalmol.*, **112**, no. 2, 208–212.

De Voe, A. G. 1945, "Experiences with the surgery of the anophthalmic orbit", *Am. J. Ophthalmol.*, **28**, 1346–1351.

Drucker, A. P. 1951, "Integrated and buried implants", *Am. J. Ophthalmol.*, **34**, 1483–1498.

Durham, D. G. 1949, "The new ocular implants", *Am.J.Ophthalmol.*, **32**, 79–89.

Dutton, J. J. 1991, "Coralline hydroxyapatite as an ocular implant", *Ophthalmology*, **98**, no. 3, 370–377.

Edelstein, C., Shields, C. L., De Potter, P., & Shields, J. A. 1997, "Complications of motility peg placement for the hydroxyapatite orbital implant", *Ophthalmology*, **104**, no. 10, 1616–1621.

Ellis, O. H. & Levy, O. R. 1956, "A new magentic orbital implant", *Arch. Ophthalmol.*, **56**, no. 352, 360.

Fahim, D. K., Frueh, B. R., Musch, D. C., & Nelson, C. C. 2007, "Complications of pegged and non-pegged hydroxyapatite orbital implants", *Ophthal. Plast. Reconstr. Surg.*, **23**, no. 3, 206–210.

Fan, J. T. & Robertson, D. M. 1995, "Long-term follow-up of the Allen implant. 1967 to 1991", *Ophthalmology*, **102**, no. 3, 510–516.

Ferrone, P. J. & Dutton, J. J. 1992, "Rate of vascularization of coralline hydroxyapatite ocular implants", *Ophthalmology*, **99**, no. 3, 376–379.

Fountain, T. R., Goldberger, S., & Murphree, A. L. 1999, "Orbital development after enucleation in early childhood", *Ophthal. Plast. Reconstr. Surg.*, **15**, no. 1, 32–36.

Frost, W. A. 1887, "On the insertion of artificial globes into Tenon's capsule after excising the eye", *Trans. Ophthalmol. Soc. UK*, **7**, 286–291.

Gale, M. E., Vincent, M. E., & Sutula, F. C. 1985, "Orbital implants and prostheses: postoperative computed tomographic appearance", *AJNR Am. J. Neuroradiol.*, **6**, no. 3, 403–407.

Gayre, G. S., DeBacker, C., Lipham, W., Tawfik, H. A., Holck, D., & Dutton, J. J. 2001, "Bovine pericardium as a wrapping for orbital implants", *Ophthal. Plast. Reconstr. Surg.*, **17**, no. 5, 381–387.

Gayre, G. S., Lipham, W., & Dutton, J. J. 2002, "A comparison of rates of fibrovascular ingrowth in wrapped versus unwrapped hydroxyapatite spheres in a rabbit model", *Ophthal. Plast. Reconstr. Surg.*, **18**, no. 4, 275–280.

Goldberg, R. A., Dresner, S. C., Braslow, R. A., Kossovsky, N., & Legmann, A. 1994, "Animal model of porous polyethylene orbital implants", *Ophthal. Plast. Reconstr. Surg.*, **10**, no. 2, 104–109.

Goldberg, R. A., Holds, J. B., & Ebrahimpour, J. 1992, "Exposed hydroxyapatite orbital implants. Report of six cases", *Ophthalmology*, **99**, no. 5, 831–836.

Gougelmann, H. P. 1970, "The evolution of the ocular motility implant", *Int. Ophthalmol. Clinics*, **10**, 689–703.

Guberina, C., Hornblass, A., Meltzer, M. A., Soarez, V., & Smith, B. 1983, "Autogenous dermis-fat orbital implantation", *Arch. Ophthalmol.*, **101**, no. 10, 1586–1590.

Guillinta, P., Vasani, S. N., Granet, D. B., & Kikkawa, D. O. 2003, "Prosthetic motility in pegged versus unpegged integrated porous orbital implants", *Ophthal. Plast. Reconstr. Surg.*, **19**, no. 2, 119–122.

Guyton, J. S. 1948, "Enucleation and allied procedures: a review and description of a new operation", *Trans. Am. Ophthalmol. Soc.*, **XLVI**, 472–527.

Hamilton, H. E., Christianson, M. D., Williams, J. P., & Thomas, R. A. 1992, "Evaluation of vascularization of coralline hydroxyapatite ocular implants by magnetic resonance imaging", *Clin. Imaging*, **16**, no. 4, 243–246.

Hicks, C. R., Clayton, A. B., Vijayasekaran, S., Crawford, G. J., Chirila, T. V., & Constable, I. J. 1999, "Development of a poly(2-hydroxyethyl methacrylate) orbital implant allowing direct muscle attachment and tissue ingrowth", *Ophthal. Plast. Reconstr. Surg.*, **15**, no. 5, 326–332.

Hicks, C. R., Morrison, D., Lou, X., Crawford, G. J., Gadjatsy, A., & Constable, I. J. 2006, "Orbital implants: potential new directions", *Expert. Rev. Med. Devices*, **3**, no. 6, 805–815.

Hintschich, C., Zonneveld, F., Baldeschi, L., Bunce, C., & Koornneef, L. 2001, "Bony orbital development after early enucleation in humans", *Br. J. Ophthalmol.*, **85**, no. 2, 205–208.

Holmes, R. E. 1979, "Bone regeneration within a coralline hydroxyapatite implant", *Plast. Reconstr. Surg.*, **63**, no. 5, 626–633.

Holmes, R. E. & Hagler, H. K. 1987, "Porous hydroxylapatite as a bone graft substitute in mandibular contour augmentation: a histometric study", *J. Oral Maxillofac. Surg.*, **45**, no. 5, 421–429.

Hornblass, A., Biesman, B. S., & Eviatar, J. A. 1995, "Current techniques of enucleation: a survey of 5,439 intraorbital implants and a review of the literature", *Ophthal. Plast. Reconstr. Surg.*, **11**, no. 2, 77–86.

Howard, G. M., Kinder, R. S., & Macmillan, A. S., Jr 1965, "Orbital growth after unilateral enucleation in childhood", *Arch. Ophthalmol.*, **73**, 80–83.

Hughes, W. L. 1948, "Integrated implants and artificial eyes for use after enucleation and evisceration", *Am. J. Ophthalmol.*, **31**, 303.

Imhof, S. M., Mourits, M. P., Hofman, P., Zonneveld, F. W., Schipper, J., Moll, A. C., & Tan, K. E. 1996, "Quantification of orbital and mid-facial growth retardation after megavoltage external beam irradiation in children with retinoblastoma", *Ophthalmology*, **103**, no. 2, 263–268.

Iordanidou, V. & De Potter, P. 2004, "Porous polyethylene orbital implant in the pediatric population", *Am. J. Ophthalmol.*, **138**, no. 3, 425–429.

Jahrling, R. C. 1979, "Statistical study of extruded implants", *Todays Ocularist*, **9**, 25–27.

Jordan, D. R. 2000, "Anophtalmic orbital implants", *Ophthalmol. Clin. N .Am.*, **13**, 587–608.

Jordan, D. R., Allen, L. H., Ells, A., Gilberg, S., Brownstein, S., Munro, S., Grahovac, S., & Raymond, F. 1995, "The use of Vicryl mesh (polyglactin 910) for implantation of hydroxyapatite orbital implants", *Ophthal. Plast. Reconstr. Surg.*, **11**, no. 2, 95–99.

Jordan, D. R., Anderson, R. L., Nerad, J. A., & Allen, L. 1987, "A preliminary report on the Universal implant", *Arch. Ophthalmol.*, **105**, no. 12, 1726–1731.

Jordan, D. R., Brownstein, S., Dorey, M., Yuen, V. H., & Gilberg, S. 2004, "Fibrovascularization of porous polyethylene (Medpor) orbital implant in a rabbit model", *Ophthal. Plast. Reconstr. Surg.*, **20**, no. 2, 136–143.

Jordan, D. R., Chan, S., Mawn, L., Gilberg, S., Dean, T., Brownstein, S., & Hill, V. E. 1999a, "Complications associated with pegging hydroxyapatite orbital implants", *Ophthalmology*, **106**, no. 3, 505–512.

Jordan, D. R., Chan, S., Mawn, L., Gilberg, S., Dean, T., Brownstein, S., & Hill, V. E. 1999b, "Complications associated with pegging hydroxyapatite orbital implants", *Ophthalmology*, **106**, no. 3, 505–512.

Jordan, D. R., Gilberg, S., & Mawn, L. A. 2003a, "The bioceramic orbital implant: experience with 107 implants", *Ophthal. Plast. Reconstr. Surg.*, **19**, no. 2, 128–135.

Jordan, D. R., Gilberg, S., Mawn, L., Brownstein, S., & Grahovac, S. Z. 1998, "The synthetic hydroxyapatite implant: a report on 65 patients", *Ophthal. Plast. Reconstr. Surg.*, **14**, no. 4, 250–255.

Jordan, D. R., Hwang, I., Brownstein, S., McEachren, T., Gilberg, S., Grahovac, S., & Mawn, L. 2000a, "The Molteno M-Sphere", *Ophthal.Plast. Reconstr. Surg.*, **16**, no. 5, 356–362.

Jordan, D. R., Hwang, I., McEachren, T., Brownstein, S., Gilberg, S., Grahovac, S., & Mawn, L. 2000b, "Brazilian hydroxyapatite implant", *Ophthal. Plast. Reconstr. Surg.*, **16**, no. 5, 363–369.

Jordan, D. R. & Klapper, S. R. 1999, "Wrapping hydroxyapatite implants", *Ophthalmic Surg. Lasers*, **30**, no. 5, 403–407.

Jordan, D. R. & Klapper, S. R. 2000, "A new titanium peg system for hydroxyapatite orbital implants", *Ophthal. Plast. Reconstr. Surg.*, **16**, no. 5, 380–387.

Jordan, D. R., Klapper, S. R., & Gilberg, S. M. 2003b, "The use of vicryl mesh in 200 porous orbital implants: a technique with few exposures", *Ophthal. Plast. Reconstr. Surg.*, **19**, no. 1, 53–61.

Jordan, D. R., Mawn, L. A., Brownstein, S., McEachren, T. M., Gilberg, S. M., Hill, V., Grahovac, S. Z., & Adenis, J. P. 2000c, "The bioceramic orbital implant: a new generation of porous implants", *Ophthal. Plast.Reconstr. Surg.*, **16**, no. 5, 347–355.

Jordan, D. R., Pelletier, C. R., Gilberg, T. S., Brownstein, S., & Grahovac, S. Z. 1999c, "A new variety of hydroxyapatite: the Chinese implant", *Ophthal. Plast. Reconstr. Surg.*, **15**, no. 6, 420–424.

Kadyan, A. & Sandramouli, S. 2008, "Porous polyethylene (Medpor) orbital implants with primary acellular dermis patch grafts", *Orbit*, **27**, no. 1, 19–23.

Kaltreider, S. A. 2000, "The ideal ocular prosthesis: analysis of prosthetic volume", *Ophthal. Plast. Reconstr. Surg.*, **16**, no. 5, 388–392.

Kaltreider, S. A., Peake, L. R., & Carter, B. T. 2001, "Pediatric enucleation: analysis of volume replacement", *Arch. Ophthalmol.*, **119**, no. 3, 379–384.

Kao, L. Y. 2000, "Polytetrafluoroethylene as a wrapping material for a hydroxyapatite orbital implant", *Ophthal. Plast. Reconstr. Surg.*, **16**, no. 4, 286–288.

Kao, S. C. & Chen, S. 1999, "The use of rectus abdominis sheath for wrapping of the hydroxyapatite orbital implants", *Ophthalmic Surg. Lasers*, **30**, no. 1, 69–71.

Karcioglu, Z. A., al-Mesfer, S. A., & Mullaney, P. B. 1998, "Porous polyethylene orbital implant in patients with retinoblastoma", *Ophthalmology*, **105**, no. 7, 1311–1316.

Karesh, J. W. & Dresner, S. C. 1994, "High-density porous polyethylene (Medpor) as a successful anophthalmic socket implant", *Ophthalmology*, **101**, no. 10, 1688–1695.

Kelley, J. J. 1970, "History of ocular prostheses", *Int.Ophthalmol.Clinics*, **10**, 713–719.

Kennedy, R. E. 1964, "The effect of early enucleation on the Oorbit in animals and humans", *Trans. Am. Ophthalmol. Soc.*, **62**, 460–509.

Kim, Y. D., Goldberg, R. A., Shorr, N., & Steinsapir, K. D. 1994, "Management of exposed hydroxyapatite orbital implants", *Ophthalmology*, **101**, no. 10, 1709–1715.

Klapper, S. R., Jordan, D. R., Ells, A., & Grahovac, S. 2003, "Hydroxyapatite orbital implant vascularization assessed by magnetic resonance imaging", *Ophthal. Plast. Reconstr. Surg.*, **19**, no. 1, 46–52.

Kronish, J. W., Gonnering, R. S., Dortzbach, R. K., Rankin, J. H., Reid, D. L., & Phernetton, T. M. 1990a, "The pathophysiology of the anophthalmic socket. Part I. Analysis of orbital blood flow", *Ophthal. Plast. Reconstr. Surg.*, **6**, no. 2, 77–87.

Kronish, J. W., Gonnering, R. S., Dortzbach, R. K., Rankin, J. H., Reid, D. L., Phernetton, T. M., Pitts, W. C., & Berry, G. J. 1990b, "The pathophysiology of the anophthalmic socket. Part II. Analysis of orbital fat", *Ophthal. Plast. Reconstr. Surg.*, **6**, no. 2, 88–95.

Langt, W. A. 1887, "On the insertion of artificial globes into Tenon's capsule after excising the eye.", *Trans. Ophthalmol. Soc. UK*, **7**, 286–291.

Lee, S. Y., Jang, J. W., Lew, H., Kim, S. J., & Kim, H. Y. 2002, "Complications in motility PEG placement for hydroxyapatite orbital implant in anophthalmic socket", *Jpn. J. Ophthalmol.*, **46**, no. 1, 103–107.

Lee, V., Subak-Sharpe, I., Hungerford, J. L., Davies, N. P., & Logani, S. 2000, "Exposure of primary orbital implants in postenucleation retinoblastoma patients", *Ophthalmology*, **107**, no. 5, 940–945.

Leitha, T., Staudenherz, A., & Scholz, U. 1995, "Three-phase bone scintigraphy of hydroxyapatite ocular implants", *Eur. J. Nucl. Med.*, **22**, no. 4, 308–314.

Li, T., Shen, J., & Duffy, M. T. 2001, "Exposure rates of wrapped and unwrapped orbital implants following enucleation", *Ophthal. Plast. Reconstr. Surg.*, **17**, no. 6, 431–435.

Liao, S. L., Chen, M. S., & Lin, L. L. 2005a, "Primary placement of a titanium sleeve in hydroxyapatite orbital implants", *Eye*, **19**, no. 4, 400–405.

Liao, S. L., Shih, M. J., & Lin, L. L. 2005b, "Primary placement of a hydroxyapatite-coated sleeve in bioceramic orbital implants", *Am. J. Ophthalmol.*, **139**, no. 2, 235–241.

Long, J. A., Tann, T. M., III, Bearden, W. H., III, & Callahan, M. A. 2003, "Enucleation: is wrapping the implant necessary for optimal motility?", *Ophthal. Plast. Reconstr. Surg.*, **19**, no. 3, 194–197.

Lucci, L. M., Hofling-Lima, A. L., Erwenne, C. M., & Toledo Cassano, E. M. 2007, "Artificial eye amplitudes and characteristics in enucleated socket with porous polyethylene spherical and quad-motility implant", *Arq Bras. Oftalmol.*, **70**, no. 5, 831–838.

Luce CM 1970, "A short history of enucleation", *Int. Ophthalmol. Clinics*, **10**, 681–687.

Lyle, C. E., Wilson, M. W., Li, C. S., & Kaste, S. C. 2007, "Comparison of orbital volumes in enucleated patients with unilateral retinoblastoma: hydroxyapatite implants versus silicone implants", *Ophthal. Plast. Reconstr. Surg.*, **23**, no. 5, 393–396.

Manson, P. N., Grivas, A., Rosenbaum, A., Vannier, M., Zinreich, J., & Iliff, N. 1986, "Studies on enophthalmos: II. The measurement of orbital injuries and their treatment by quantitative computed tomography", *Plast. Reconstr. Surg.*, **77**, no. 2, 203–214.

Mawn, L. A., Jordan, D. R., & Gilberg, S. 1998, "Scanning electron microscopic examination of porous orbital implants", *Can. J. Ophthalmol.*, **33**, no. 4, 203–209.

Mawn, L. A., Jordan, D. R., & Gilberg, S. 2001, "Proliferation of human fibroblasts in vitro after exposure to orbital implants", *Can. J. Ophthalmol.*, **36**, no. 5, 245–251.

Miller, D. M., Murray, T., Suarez, F., Cicciarelli, N. L., & Swords, G. G. 2007, "Motility assessment and clinical outcomes of a magnetically integrated microporous implant", *Ophthalmic Surg. Lasers Imaging*, **38**, no. 4, 339–341.

Mitchell, K. T., Hollsten, D. A., White, W. L., & O'Hara, M. A. 2001, "The autogenous dermis-fat orbital implant in children", *J. AAPOS.*, **5**, no. 6, 367–369.

Molteno, A. C. 1980, "Antigen-free cancellous bone implants after removal of an eye", *Trans. Ophthalmol. Soc. N. Z.*, **32**, 36–39.

Molteno, A. C. & Elder, M. J. 1991, "Bone implants after enucleation", *Aust. N. Z. J. Ophthalmol.*, **19**, no. 2, 129–136.

Mules, P. H. 1885, "Evisceration of the globe with artificial vitreous", *Trans.Ophthalmol. Soc. UK*, **5**, 200–206.

Murphey, P. J., Pitton, D. D., Schlossberg, L., & Harris, L. W. 1945, "Development of the acrylic eye ocular prosthesis at the National Naval Medical Center", *J. Am. Dent. Assoc.*, **32**, 1227–1230.

Murray, T. G., Cicciarelli, N. L., Croft, B. H., Garonzik, S., Voigt, M., & Hernandez, E. 2000, "Design of a magnetically integrated microporous implant", *Arch. Ophthalmol.*, **118**, no. 9, 1259–1262.

Naik, M. N., Murthy, R. K., & Honavar, S. G. 2007, "Comparison of vascularization of Medpor and Medpor-Plus orbital implants: a prospective, randomized study", *Ophthal. Plast. Reconstr. Surg.*, **23**, no. 6, 463–467.

Naugle, T. C., Jr, Lee, A. M., Haik, B. G., & Callahan, M. A. 1999, "Wrapping hydroxyapatite orbital implants with posterior auricular muscle complex grafts", *Am. J. Ophthalmol.*, **128**, no. 4, 495–501.

Nerad, J. A., Hurtig, R. R., Carter, K. D., Bulgarelli, D. M., & Yeager, D. C. 1991, "A system for measurement of prosthetic eye movements using a magnetic search coil technique", *Ophthal. Plast. Reconstr. Surg.*, 7, no. 1, 31–40.

Neuhaus, R. W. & Shorr, N. 1982, "The use of room temperature vulcanizing silicone in anophthalmic enophthalmos", *Am. J. Ophthalmol.*, **94**, no. 3, 408–411.

Nolan, L. M., O'Keefe, M., & Lanigan, B. 2003, "Hydroxyapatite orbital implant exposure in children", *J. AAPOS.*, **7**, no. 5, 345–348.

Numerow, L. M., Kloiber, R., Mitchell, R. J., Molnar, C. P., & Anderson, M. A. 1994, "Hydroxyapatite orbital implants. Scanning with technetium-99m MDP", *Clin. Nucl. Med.*, **19**, no. 1, 9–12.

Nunery, W. R., Cepela, M. A., Heinz, G. W., Zale, D., & Martin, R. T. 1993a, "Extrusion rate of silicone spherical anophthalmic socket implants", *Ophthal. Plast. Reconstr. Surg.*, **9**, no. 2, 90–95.

Nunery, W. R., Heinz, G. W., Bonnin, J. M., Martin, R. T., & Cepela, M. A. 1993b, "Exposure rate of hydroxyapatite spheres in the anophthalmic socket: histopathologic correlation and comparison with silicone sphere implants", *Ophthal. Plast. Reconstr. Surg.*, **9**, no. 2, 96–104.

Nunery, W. R. & Hetzler, K. J. 1983, "Improved prosthetic motility following enucleation", *Ophthalmology*, **90**, no. 9, 1110–1115.

Oestreicher, J. H., Liu, E., & Berkowitz, M. 1997, "Complications of hydroxyapatite orbital implants. A review of 100 consecutive cases and a comparison of Dexon mesh (polyglycolic acid) with scleral wrapping", *Ophthalmology*, **104**, no. 2, 324–329.

Osborne D, Hadden OB, & Deeming LW 1974, "Orbital growth after childnood enucleation", *Am. J. Ophthalmol.*, **77**, 756–759.

Park, S. W., Seol, H. Y., Hong, S. J., Kim, K. A., Choi, J. C., & Cha, I. H. 2003, "Magnetic resonance evaluation of fibrovascular ingrowth into porous polyethylene orbital implant", *Clin. Imaging*, **27**, no. 6, 377–381.

Perry, A. C. 1991, "Advances in enucleation", *Ophthalmol. Clin. N. Am.*, **4**, 173–182.

Peylan-Ramu, N., Bin-Nun, A., Skleir-Levy, M., Bibas, A., Koplewitz, B., Anteby, I., & Pe'er, J. 2001, "Orbital growth retardation in retinoblastoma survivors: work in progress", *Med. Pediatr. Oncol.*, **37**, no. 5, 465–470.

Pfieffer, R. L. 1945, "The effect of enucleation on the orbit", *Trans. Am. Acad. Ophthalmol.*, **49**, 236–239.

Reedy, B. K., Pan, F., Kim, W. S., & Bartlett, S. P. 1999, "The direct effect of intraorbital pressure on orbital growth in the anophthalmic piglet", *Plast. Reconstr. Surg.*, **104**, no. 3, 713–718.

Remulla, H. D., Rubin, P. A., Shore, J. W., Sutula, F. C., Townsend, D. J., Woog, J. J., & Jahrling, K. V. 1995, "Complications of porous spherical orbital implants", *Ophthalmology*, **102**, no. 4, 586–593.

Roper-Hall, M. J. 1956, "Magnetic orbital implant", *Br. J. Ophthalmol.*, **40**, 575.

Rosner, M., Edward, D. P., & Tso, M. O. 1992, "Foreign-body giant-cell reaction to the hydroxyapatite orbital implant", *Arch. Ophthalmol.*, **110**, no. 2, 173–174.

Rubin, P. A., Popham, J., Rumelt, S., Remulla, H., Bilyk, J. R., Holds, J., Mannor, G., Maus, M., & Patrinely, J. R. 1998, "Enhancement of the cosmetic and functional outcome of enucleation with the conical orbital implant", *Ophthalmology*, **105**, no. 5, 919–925.

Rubin, P. A., Popham, J. K., Bilyk, J. R., & Shore, J. W. 1994, "Comparison of fibrovascular ingrowth into hydroxyapatite and porous polyethylene orbital implants", *Ophthal. Plast. Reconstr. Surg.*, **10**, no. 2, 96–103.

Ruedemann, A. D. 1945, "Plastic eye implant", *Trans. Am. Ophthalmol. Soc.*, **43**, 304–307.

Saitoh, A., Tsuda, Y., Bhutto, I. A., Kitaoka, T., & Amemiya, T. 1996, "Histologic study of living response to artificially synthesized hydroxyapatite implant: 1-year follow-up", *Plast. Reconstr. Surg.*, **98**, no. 4, 706–710.

Sarnat, B. G. 1979, "Adult rabbit eye and orbital volumes after periodic intrabulbar injections of silicone", *Ophthalmologica*, **178**, no. 1–2, 43–48.

Sarnat, B. G. 1981, "The orbit and eye: experiments on volume in young and adult rabbits", *Acta Ophthalmol.* Suppl, **147**, pp. 1–44.

Sarnat, B. G. 1982, "Eye and orbital size in the young and adult. Some postnatal experimental and clinical relationships", *Ophthalmologica*, **185**, no. 2, 74–89.

Sarnat, B. G. & Shanedling, P. D. 1970, "Orbital volume following evisceration, enucleation, and exenteration in rabbits", *Am. J. Ophthalmol.*, **70**, no. 5, 787–799.

Sarnat, B. G. & Shanedling, P. D. 1972, "Orbital growth after evisceration or enucleation without and with implants", *Acta Anat. (Basel)*, **82**, no. 4, 497–511.

Sarnat, B. G. & Shanedling, P. D. 1974, "Increased orbital volume after periodic intrabulbar injections of silicone in growing rabbits", *Am. J. Anat.*, **140**, no. 4, 523–531.

Scott, J. H. 1954, "The growth of the human face", *Proc. R. Soc. Med.*, **47**, no. 2, 91–100.

Shields, C. L., Shields, J. A., & De Potter, P. 1992a, "Hydroxyapatite orbital implant after enucleation. Experience with initial 100 consecutive cases", *Arch. Ophthalmol.*, **110**, no. 3, 333–338.

Shields, C. L., Shields, J. A., De Potter, P., & Singh, A. D. 1994, "Problems with the hydroxyapatite orbital implant: experience with 250 consecutive cases", *Br. J. Ophthalmol.*, **78**, no. 9, 702–706.

Shields, C. L., Uysal, Y., Marr, B. P., Lally, S. E., Rodriques, E., Kharod, B., & Shields, J. A. 2007, "Experience with the polymer-coated hydroxyapatite implant after enucleation in 126 patients", *Ophthalmology*, **114**, no. 2, 367–373.

Shields, J. A., Shields, C. L., & De Potter, P. 1992b, "Enucleation technique for children with retinoblastoma", *J. Pediatr. Ophthalmol. Strabismus*, **29**, no. 4, 213–215.

Shoamanesh, A., Pang, N. K., & Oestreicher, J. H. 2007, "Complications of orbital implants: a review of 542 patients who have undergone orbital implantation and 275 subsequent PEG placements", *Orbit.*, **26**, no. 3, 173–182.

Sires, B. S., Holds, J. B., & Archer, C. R. 1998, "Postimplantation density changes in coralline hydroxyapatite orbital implants", *Ophthal. Plast. Reconstr. Surg.*, **14**, no. 5, 318–322.

Sires, B. S., Holds, J. B., Archer, C. R., Kincaid, M. C., & Hageman, G. S. 1995, "Histological and radiological analyses of hydroxyapatite orbital implants in rabbits", *Ophthal. Plast. Reconstr. Surg.*, **11**, no. 4, 273–277.

Smit, T. J., Koornneef, L., Groet, E., Zonneveld, F. W., & Otto, A. J. 1991a, "Ocular prosthesis motility with and without intraorbital implants in the anophthalmic socket", *Br. J. Ophthalmol.*, **75**, no. 11, 667–670.

Smit, T. J., Koornneef, L., Mourits, M. P., Groet, E., & Otto, A. J. 1990a, "Primary versus secondary intraorbital implants", *Ophthal. Plast. Reconstr. Surg.*, **6**, no. 2, 115–118.

Smit, T. J., Koornneef, L., Zonneveld, F. W., Groet, E., & Otto, A. J. 1990b, "Computed tomography in the assessment of the postenucleation socket syndrome", *Ophthalmology*, **97**, no. 10, 1347–1351.

Smit, T. J., Koornneef, L., Zonneveld, F. W., Groet, E., & Otto, A. J. 1991b, "Primary and secondary implants in the anophthalmic orbit. Preoperative and postoperative computed tomographic appearance", *Ophthalmology*, **98**, no. 1, 106–110.

Smith, L. 1963, "Ceramic-plastic material as a bone substitute", *Arch. Surg.*, **87**, 653–661.

Snyder, C. 1965, "An operation designated 'the extirpation of an eye'", *Arch. Ophthalmol.*, **74**, 429–432.

Soll, D. B. 1969, "Expandable orbital implants," in *Proc. Cent. Symp. Manhattan Eye Ear and Throat Hosp.*, 1, Turtz, A., ed., Mosby, St Louis, 197–202.

Soll, D. B. 1972, "Enucleation surgery. A new technique", *Arch. Ophthalmol.*, **87**, no. 2, 196–197.

Soll, D. B. 1982, "The anophthalmic socket", *Ophthalmology*, **89**, no. 5, 407–423.

Soll, D. B. 1986, "Evolution and current concepts in the surgical treatment of the anophthalmic orbit", *Ophthal. Plast. Reconstr. Surg.*, **2**, no. 3, 163–171.

Spirnak, J. P., Nieves, N., Hollsten, D. A., White, W. C., & Betz, T. A. 1995, "Gadolinium-enhanced magnetic resonance imaging assessment of hydroxyapatite orbital implants", *Am. J. Ophthalmol.*, **119**, no. 4, 431–440.

Spivey, B. E. 1970, "The Iowa enucleation implant", *Trans. Am. Acad.Ophthalmol. Otolaryngol.*, **74**, no. 6, 1287–1295.

Spivey, B. E., Allen, L., & Burns, C. A. 1969, "The Iowa enucleation implant. A 10-year evaluation of technique and results", *Am. J. Ophthalmol.*, **67**, no. 2, 171–188.

Su, G. W. & Yen, M. T. 2004, "Current trends in managing the anophthalmic socket after primary enucleation and evisceration", *Ophthal. Plast. Reconstr. Surg.*, **20**, no. 4, 274–280.

Summers, C. G. 1993, "Calcification of scleral-wrapped orbital implant in patients with retinoblastoma", *Pediatr. Radiol.*, **23**, no. 1, 34–36.

Taylor, W. 1939, "Effect of enucleation of one eye in childhood upon subsequent development of the face", *Trans. Ophthalm. Soc. UK*, **59**, 361–369.

Thakker, M. M., Fay, A. M., Pieroth, L., & Rubin, P. A. 2004, "Fibrovascular ingrowth into hydroxyapatite and porous polyethylene orbital implants wrapped with acellular dermis", *Ophthal. Plast. Reconstr. Surg.*, **20**, no. 5, 368–373.

Thaller, V. T. 1997, "Enucleation volume measurement", *Ophthal. Plast. Reconstr. Surg.*, **13**, no. 1, 18–20.

Tomb, E. H. & Gearhart, D. F. 1954, "A new magnetic implant", *Arch. Ophthalmol.*, **52**, 763–768.

Trichopoulos, N. & Augsburger, J. J. 2005, "Enucleation with unwrapped porous and nonporous orbital implants: a 15-year experience", *Ophthal. Plast. Reconstr. Surg.*, **21**, no. 5, 331–336.

Tyers, A. G. & Collin, J. R. 1982, "Orbital implants and post enucleation socket syndrome", *Trans. Ophthalmol. Soc. UK*, **102** (Pt 1), 90–92.

Tyers, A. G. & Collin, J. R. 1985, "Baseball orbital implants: a review of 39 patients", *Br. J. Ophthalmol.*, **69**, no. 6, 438–442.

Vistnes, L. M. 1976, "Mechanism of upper lid ptosis in the anophthalmic orbit", *Plast. Reconstr. Surg.*, **58**, no. 5, 539–545.

Vistnes, L. M. 1987, *Surgical Reconstruction in the Anophthalmic Orbit*, Aesculapius Publishing Company, Alabama.

Viswanathan, P., Sagoo, M. S., & Olver, J. M. 2007, "UK national survey of enucleation, evisceration and orbital implant trends", *Br. J. Ophthalmol.*, **91**, no. 5, 616–619.

Wang, J. K., Lai, P. C., & Liao, S. L. 2009, "Late exposure of the bioceramic orbital implant", *Am. J. Ophthalmol.*, **147**, no. 1, 162–170.

Wiggs, E. O. & Becker, B. B. 1992, "Extrusion of enucleation implants: treatment with secondary implants and autogenous temporalis fascia or fascia lata patch grafts", *Ophthalmic Surg.*, **23**, no. 7, 472–476.

Woog, J. J., Dresner, S. C., Lee, T. S., Kim, Y. D., Hartstein, M. E., Shore, J. W., Neuhaus, R. W., Kaltreider, S. A., Migliori, M. E., Mandeville, J. T., Roh, J. H., & Amato, M. M. 2004, "The smooth surface tunnel porous polyethylene enucleation implant", *Ophthalmic Surg. Lasers Imaging*, **35**, no. 5, 358–362.

Yago, K. & Furuta, M. 2001, "Orbital growth after unilateral enucleation in infancy without an orbital implant", *Jpn. J. Ophthalmol.*, **45**, no. 6, 648–652.

Yamashiro, M. 1957, "Objective measurement of the limit of uniocular movement", *Jpn. J. Ophthalmol.*, **1**, 130–136.

Yazici, B., Akova, B., & Sanli, O. 2007, "Complications of primary placement of motility post in porous polyethylene implants during enucleation", *Am. J. Ophthalmol.*, **143**, no. 5, 828–834.

Yoon, J. S., Lew, H., Kim, S. J., & Lee, S. Y. 2008, "Exposure rate of hydroxyapatite orbital implants a 15–year experience of 802 cases", *Ophthalmology*, **115**, no. 3, 566–572.

Young, J. H. 1954, "Magnetic intra-ocular implant: the magnetic artificial eye", *Br. J. Ophthalmol.*, **38**, 705–718.

18
Selected polymeric materials for orbital reconstruction

E. WENTRUP-BYRNE and K. GEORGE, QUEENSLAND
UNIVERSITY OF TECHNOLOGY, AUSTRALIA

Abstract: Despite major advances in orbital reconstruction, the orbit is still considered one of the most difficult craniofacial regions to repair. This chapter gives an historical perspective of some of the most commonly used materials including both non-biodegradable and biodegradable materials. The importance and nature of the material implant–tissue interface as well as the implant surface are discussed. Expanded polytetrafluoroethylene (ePTFE) is the example used to illustrate the role of surface modification to improve currently used materials. Finally, a short overview of current and possible future directions in bone regeneration and tissue engineering is included.

Key words: orbital reconstruction, expanded polytetrafluoroethylene (ePTFE), surface modification, non-biodegradable polymers, poly(lactide-co-glycolide) polymers.

18.1 Introduction

According to the literature and expert opinion, orbital reconstruction has advanced significantly over recent years. However, the general consensus still is that in the long term some of the most difficult craniofacial fractures and trauma damage requiring treatment are those related to the orbit. Restoration of facial defects is 'a difficult challenge for both surgeon and prosthodontist' (Beumer *et al.*, 1996). In fact, a diverse team – involving various reconstructive surgeons, neurosurgeons, ophthalmologists, prosthodontists and, indirectly, the material chemists and engineers – is required in order to achieve the optimum outcome for the patient. Of the many challenges pertaining to orbital reconstruction, selection of the most suitable repair materials is but one. It is, however, ultimately the focus of this review. In order to discuss the wide range of materials available, it is necessary to understand and appreciate the complex structure of bone as well as the facial anatomy and treatment options. For those not familiar with the surgical and treatment demands in facial reconstruction, there are excellent books, such as Beumer *et al.*'s *Maxillofacial Rehabilitation*, that cover relevant aspects. In *Maxillofacial Trauma and Esthetic Facial Reconstruction*, Cameron and Booth point out that because 'the maxillofacial region is in many ways unique – the mindless transfer of orthopaedic techniques and principles is sometimes unhelpful'

(Cameron and Booth, 2003). They recognise that the adoption of materials and fixation devices developed for orthopaedic use in the treatment of facial injuries is less than ideal, noting that it sometimes takes years for their proper evaluation in the craniofacial context to be realised. The breadth of conditions requiring surgical intervention with the use of repair materials can range from mild to serious trauma, post-traumatic deformities, defects resulting from tumour resectioning and genetic malformations. According to one recent review (Shuker, 2008) there has been 'an unprecedented increase in blast eye/orbital injuries as a result of the increased use of explosive devices, land mines, rocket-propelled grenades, thermobaric enhanced-blast explosives and explosive-forming projectiles'. A sad reflection on our society but also a confirmation that 'plastic surgery' is not just an aesthetic industry. In addition to the variety of traumas requiring intervention is the added complication of the additional issues involved when the patient is a growing child. Clearly, already several important issues have emerged that will govern the surgeon's choice of material or materials: the nature and severity of the anatomic reconstruction to be undertaken and the permanency requirements of the repair. An additional issue that at first may appear a minor one but cannot be ignored is the question of patient acceptance. According to Beumer et al. (1996), 'unrealistic patient expectations' also need to be considered since the goal of any facial reconstruction is to 'create an aesthetically pleasing and inconspicuous repair while preserving adequate function'. He ranks nasal prostheses/reconstruction at the highest satisfaction level with orbital and mid-facial prostheses/reconstruction at the lowest. Anatomic reconstruction is always demanding because of the complexity of the facial region but orbital trauma can involve not just damage to the fragile bones of the orbital rim but also damage to the bones of the floor within the orbital cavity, the eye itself, the eye lids and the lachrymal system, as well as other soft tissue damage.

The orbit comprises seven bones and all may require repair: frontal bone, maxillary bone, zygomatic bone, ethmoid bone, lacrimal bone, greater and lesser wings of the sphenoid bone and the palatine bone (Fig. 18.1). In addition, the bony orbit is divided into four compartments: superior, lateral, inferior and medial. The unique characteristics of each of these influence their response to trauma and hence each requires a strategic approach to their repair. From a materials perspective, the reconstruction team have expectations of the commercially available materials with which they are required to work. As is the case for most reconstructions – whether hips, arteries or facial – there is never one material that is ideal for all cases and situations. Since a comprehensive review of all aspects of an orbit reconstruction is beyond the scope of one chapter, we will attempt to give an overview of the choice of materials available for selected applications and a glimpse to the future as to what is expected of the next generation of repair and regeneration materials.

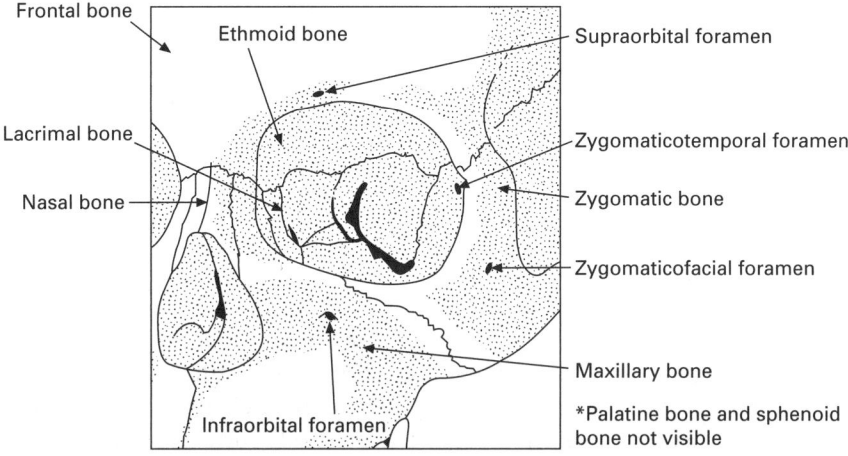

Frontal bone

Ethmoid bone

Supraorbital foramen

Lacrimal bone

Zygomaticotemporal foramen

Nasal bone

Zygomatic bone

Zygomaticofacial foramen

Maxillary bone

*Palatine bone and sphenoid bone not visible

Infraorbital foramen

18.1 Orbital bones, frontal view.

18.2   Repair strategies

When discussing a repair 'philosophy' for a particular site, it becomes clear that every repair strategy must be tailored for that particular site, and recognising the different 'environmental' demands is essential. From a materials perspective, the chemical and mechanical characteristics of the materials being used in each unique environment need to *fulfil the function for which they are intended.* Broadly speaking, an example could be the different expectations of a material being used in a load-bearing vs a non-load-bearing site: the mandible vs the eye orbit. Materials used in a mandibular reconstruction will require very different mechanical properties to ones used in a nasal or orbit repair. In addition, some general factors that need to be considered are: the age of the patient, the nature – in particular, the size – of the trauma, the permanency of the materials used and whether osseointegration of the implant is desirable. As mentioned briefly in the introduction, the age of the patient is a critical factor in developing a repair strategy. Even in more straightforward craniofacial repairs, if bones are still growing, then clearly metallic or permanent non-biodegradable polymeric materials may be unsuitable and lead to revision surgery. In this review we will not address the particular needs of such patients, although a search of the literature reveals that a review on this subject might be overdue.

Another currently much discussed aspect of tissue repair and reconstruction, the newest approach, is that of tissue engineering or regeneration. In some craniofacial applications the use of tissue-engineered biodegradable polymeric scaffolds or constructs which, with time, stimulate the growth of, and are replaced by, the body's own tissues has shown some success (Ueda, 2005). However, as far as can be ascertained, tissue regeneration is not currently an approach used in orbital repair. Since Chirila addresses this topic in Chapter 1 of this book, our emphasis in this chapter will be on repair and reconstruction. Quoting from the older but nonetheless (for the non-medical specialist) very informative *Surgery of Facial Bone Fractures* by Foster and Sherman, 'ideally fronto-naso-orbital dislocations should be totally reconstructed in one initial, well-planned surgical enterprise' (Foster and Sherman, 1987). Reading the literature, one becomes aware of the huge improvement in patient outcomes as a result of better trauma triage and surgical techniques but, although the research into improved materials is vibrant and on-going, there do not appear to be many new materials making it to commercialisation. In the words of Per-Ingvar Brånemark, one of the pioneers in the field of osseointegration of facial prostheses, 'the use of alloplastic materials in or on the body is here to stay' (Brånemark, 1997). Hence an overview of selected polymeric materials currently available and some discussion of the direction that future materials may take relative to the orbit reconstruction team may be timely.

18.3   Nature of the trauma and its influence on material choice

Size appears to be one of the critical factors by which bone and orbit defects are usually categorised (Jelks and La Trenta, 1987; Ueda, 2005). Orbital fractures can involve one or more of the following: the orbital floor cavity, the rim and surrounding facial bones, and the soft tissues. For large fractures autologous bone remains the 'gold standard' and material of choice. In practice, the amount of bone harvesting required is the limiting factor. In medium to smaller defects, especially those where other facial injuries are limited, allograft bone may be the material of choice. However, while readily available, it is associated with some risk of disease transmission. The use of alloplastic (often polymeric) materials reduces disadvantages such as cost, donor-site morbidity and increased operation time, but their use has been associated with a higher potential for infection (Firtell and Beumer, 1979). This is a significant problem in light of the fact that, of the many facial sites where restorations are routinely carried out, orbital reconstructions are the most prone to infections. In addition, in many cases more than one repair material is required. For example, when using autogenous or allograft bone, a polymer-based bone cement such as poly(methyl methacrylate) (PMMA) may also be needed.

In many orbital reconstructions the issue of orbital volume is a critical factor. After enucleation, it is essential to maintain orbital volume before an orbital implant is fitted (see Chapter 17). Again, a combination of materials may be needed in order to repair the orbital rim and floor in preparation for the actual implant (Jelks and La Trenta, 1987). Where maxillo- and craniofacial repair and reconstruction are concerned, it was generally accepted some time ago that, in the case of fixation devices, 'small is good' (Cameron and Booth, 2003). Hence, the current debate has moved on from the size of the fixation device – micro- and mini-plates are now the 'gold standard'– to whether resorbable or non-resorbable plates and screws are best. In the course of preparing this review, the fact that literature references came to light calling Teflon® an 'inorganic material' (which it is not) and Medpor® a fluoropolymer (it is not), although Teflon® is, highlights the difficulties facing writers who, although experts in their own fields, face an alarming range of terms and definitions from other specialities. In the following sections we will endeavour to present an overview of some issues relevant in orbital repair strategies with a focus on selected polymeric materials.

18.4   Choice of materials for repair

One of the earliest recorded materials used in craniofacial repair and restoration is gold, although it must be admitted that the history of facial repair and reconstruction has not been well documented. There are some discussions in the literature and even more information on the web that fascinating reading even if their historical accuracy is sometimes somewhat doubtful (Beumer *et al.*, 1996; Firtell and Beumer, 1979). One of the most interesting is the story of Tycho Brahe's artificial nose (1566) (Van Helden, 2005). After losing his nose (or part of it depending on which account one reads) in a duel he had a gold/silver prosthesis fitted using an 'adhesive balm' to keep it in place. Although renowned for his astronomical discoveries, this incident apparently kindled his keen lifelong interest in medicine. Since then many different classes of materials have been studied and trialled clinically for craniofacial repair and/or regeneration: bone autografts and allografts, ceramics (Bioglass®), metals (tantalum and titanium alloys), alloplastics and, more recently, metal/polymer composites. According to an earlier review, 'little information is available comparing the benefits, complications or selection criteria of the 20 or so alloplastic materials available for the repair of orbital blow-out fractures' (Fries, 1994). Meyer's excellent review, 'Alloplastic materials for orbital surgery' has a relevant section on *bony orbital reconstruction* (Meyer, 1995). A search of the literature, however, failed to produce more recent reviews or new critical evaluations. This may reflect both clinical and research interest in 'new' materials when they first become commercially available, as well as the need to evaluate their performance in both animal models and in clinical studies. Once their clinical efficacy, their advantages and disadvantages have been established, interest dies. In addition to this more general overview of the materials available, a selection of materials will be discussed in more depth in the following sections. Currently, micro- and mini-plates and meshes are commonly used both in orbital floor and rim repairs. These can be either permanent (titanium) (Mackenzie *et al.*, 1999; Oliver, 2000) or made from bioresorbable polymers such as polyglycolide and lactide (e.g. polyglactin 910) (see Section 18.6). Patents are currently pending for a recently developed composite material found in a series of Medpor Titan® products, which consist of a titanium mesh covered with a thin coating of high density polyethylene (HDPE). The advantage of using such composite materials is that they combine some of the advantages of both materials (in this case both materials are routinely used in a range of applications): a polymer with a metal that has good osseointegrative properties (Eppley, 2003b). They are mostly used in orbital floor and wall fracture repair. Which permanent materials are used and whether or not they should be left in place once their function has ceased are much-debated topics. For example, fixation devices (plates and screws) are often needed in conjunction with polymeric materials in order to assist healing. Cameron and Booth discuss how in Germany, for example, metal fixation devices are often removed, whereas in the UK and USA their removal is less common (Cameron and Booth, 2003). Although the use of bioreosorbable plates and screws is well established in orthopaedics, their use in craniofacial surgery is more limited but is increasingly being considered (see Section 18.6).

According to Eppley (and others too of course) (Eppley, 2003b), the concept of an alloplastic material is synonymous with the term 'synthetic' and coming from a non-biological source. The term 'alloplastic' when used in the medical literature covers manufactured materials from 'non-organic, non-human, non-animal sources', and encompasses ceramics and metals as well as plastics (which to chemists and engineers means polymers). Broadly speaking, polymeric biomaterials are divided into either permanent, non-biodegradable such as PE or polytetrafluoroethylene (PTFE), and bioresorbable polymers such as the poly(lactic acid)-based LactoSorb® (Biomet, Microfixation, FL, USA). Some of the criteria that need to be considered in choosing a repair material are summarised as follows: cost-effectiveness, biocompatibility, toxicity, antigenicity, carcinogenicity, inertness, capability to protect and provide the support that would normally be given by the defective bone; in addition, in many cases the material must be easily shaped at the operating table. It has been pointed out that 'surgeons are vulnerable to market forces from the manufacturers of fixation devices' and that 'we must always look critically at new devices since new ideas and philosophies develop' (Eppley, 2003b). Ultimately, however, it is the surgeon who must make the critical decision regarding the choice of material and it is this informed choice that will have an impact on the clinical outcomes for the patient. To summarise: while the anatomical demands of the orbital site and superb surgical expertise are major contributing factors to a positive clinical outcome, undoubtedly the judicious choice of a biocompatible and successful functioning implant material is also essential. Table 18.1 summarises the polymeric materials most commonly used in orbit repair.

18.5   Non-biodegradable polymers

18.5.1   Polytetrafluoroethylene: introduction

PTFE (Fig. 18.2) is one of a family of fluoropolymers that have been used in medical materials and devices for many years. A perusal of the literature highlights the wide range of applications using expanded PTFE (ePTFE) and its story is a good one to illustrate the long journey of a material from laboratory to industrial applications and finally its adoption in the biomedical arena (Chandler-Temple *et al.*, 2008).

Table 18.1 Polymers used in orbital reconstruction

Class	Polymer	Commercially available examples
Fluorocarbons	PTFE	Teflon®
	ePTFE*	Gore-Tex® and Proplast®
Nylon		Supramid
Polyethylenes	HDPE*	
	UHDPE	
	PHDPE*	Medpor®
	PE-coated titanium mesh*	Medpor Titan®
Polypropylene		Prolene
Polyurethane*		Bone cement and glue
Acrylic resin	Poly(methyl methacrylate)*	Bone cement
Polyesters	Polydioxanone	PDS
	Poly(ethylene terephthalate)	Marlex
	Polylactones*	Polyglactin 910 (Vicryl)
		Dexon™
		LactoSorb®
		Poliglecaprone 25 (Monocryl* Plus™ Antibacterial)
	Polyhydroxyalkanoates*	
Polyanhydrides*		
Silicones		

HDPE, high density polyethylene; UHDPE, ultra high density polyethylene; PHDPE, porous HDPE.
*Polymers discussed in this chapter.

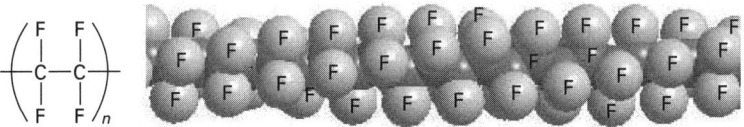

18.2 Chemical structure of polytetrafluoroethylene.

Its serendipitous discovery in 1938 led to its everyday use as Teflon®
or Gore-Tex® and finally to its use in a wide range of medical applications
such as sutures, catheters, joint coatings and vascular grafts. It has proven
to be one of the most frequently used permanent and so-called 'inert'
biomaterials. It was originally marketed in the 1980s as Proplast® for use as
a biomaterial in craniofacial applications, but proved less than successful in
mandibular applications. It was withdrawn but was reborn as a 'subcutaneous
augmentation material' (SAM) for use in plastic and reconstructive facial
applications (SAM, Gore-Tex®) as a result of Wilbert Gore's success in
developing the expanded version (ePTFE) for use in a wide range of cardiac
and vascular applications. The 1969 discovery by his son Robert Gore that
PTFE could be made in fibrillar form proved critical to this advance. The
expanded structure introduced non-interconnecting porosity while retaining
its strength and maintaining uniformity and cross-sectional shape. In addition,
this processing did not cause any significant change in its thickness. ePTFE
has a microstructure characterised by nodes interconnected by fibrils (Fig.
18.3a) and it is this fibrillar structure combined with its porosity that was a
critical factor in its adoption as a facial augmentation material. Its structure
proved conducive to microvascular in-growth but with minimal fibrous tissue
encapsulation. This offered some stabilisation but also as Eppley pointed out
'its ease of removal in subcutaneous sites due to lack of significant in-growth
offers an advantage in the event of infection or future revision procedures'
(Eppley, 2003b). Despite its widespread use, late in 2006 Gore announced
that it was 'exiting the plastic surgery market' and that SAM would no
longer be marketed as one of their products (Mercandetti, 2008, W. L. Gore
& Associates, 2006). Taking into consideration its many positive attributes
and the fact that there is fundamental research currently being published
(see section below) with a view to further improving its performance, this

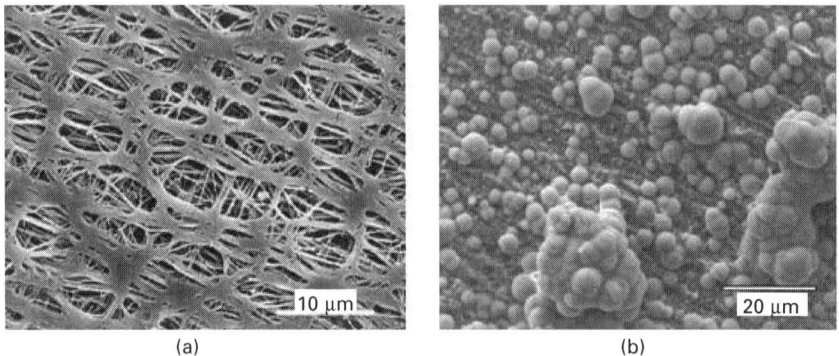

(a)   (b)

18.3 Scanning electron microscope (SEM) images of (a) untreated
membrane showing fibrillar structure and (b) mineral formation on
modified ePTFE membrane.

could present an exciting commercial opportunity for another manufacturer to enter this important market.

18.5.2 Applications

ePTFE has proven most successful in maxillofacial and periodontical applications, where it has been used as a barrier membrane for guided bone regeneration (GBR). In 1987, Karesh published the first paper specifically evaluating PTFE for 'ophthalmic plastic and reconstructive surgery' (Karesh, 1987). The paper reported both a rabbit model and a clinical study, and overall the conclusions were most positive. In a more recent review on the use of membranes for bone healing and neogenesis, Linde *et al.* state that 'virtually all investigations published on the promotion of GBR using membranes have utilised ePTFE membranes' (Linde *et al.*, 1993). Other cranial and facial applications that have benefited by the use of ePTFE membranes and ePTFE membranes reinforced with fluorinated ethylene–propylene (FEP) are at the bone interface repair sites where limited mechanical loading exists. A literature search reveals that many papers reporting their use involve the orbital floor or orbital blow-out fracture repairs (Elmazar *et al.*, 2003; Fries, 1994; Linde *et al.*, 1993; Meyer, 1995). In 1994, Hanson *et al.* evaluated the efficacy of ePTFE sheets for orbital floor reconstruction in a domestic sheep model (Hanson *et al.*, 1994). Later that year, Karesh, who had already pioneered ePTFE use in ophthalmic applications, published (in the words of Meyer) 'an erudite discussion' comparing ePTFE and HDPE for orbital repair (Karesh, 1994); Karesh analysed Hanson's study (Hanson *et al.*, 1994) and concluded that further studies were needed in order to evaluate the merits of ePTFE and HDFE, especially in the case of larger orbital defects (Karesh, 1994). In recent years many of the specialist surgeons working on the head and face have been widening their areas of operating interests. This leads to some overlapping of specialisations, as well as some confusion for the general public in knowing which specialist surgeon is best consulted for a particular reconstruction. This impression is confirmed by at least one expert in the field (Karesh, 1998). He points out that it would be necessary to 'consult journals in maxillofacial surgery, ear, nose and throat surgery, plastic surgery, ophthalmology and oculoplastic surgery to get a complete overview of all the procedures and techniques involved'. The fact that, in the hands of all these specialist surgeons, ePTFE has proven useful as a repair material at the soft–hard tissue interface merits further discussion.

18.5.3 The implant–tissue interface

From a materials point of view, a key word that can be applied to many repair and reconstruction protocols is 'interface': both the interfaces between the different tissues and the material–tissue interfaces. From both a chemical and biological perspective every interface presents a challenge in view of the fact that every 'treatment choice' will ultimately influence the final clinical and patient outcomes. The bones that make up the facial area surrounding the orbit are continuous with the orbit cavity and its walls, and they all form interfaces with the surrounding soft tissues (e.g. the eye lids) and systems such the lacrimal system. Added to Karesh's observation of the difficulty of covering the entire literature is the fact that complicated reconstructions involve more than one facial feature and hence a range of materials. In his various papers, he describes how 'PTFE implants, HDPE, polyester and polyglactin sutures, hydroxyapatite, absorbable screws and plates as well as cyanoacrylate glue' may all be required. Elmazar *et al.* are among those who point out that fixation of the PTFE implant to the orbital rim often requires a fixation device such as titanium screws or a micro-plate (Elmazar *et al.*, 2003). This creates a metallic–polymer interface which in turn means new synergies between all the different materials: biological and alloplastic.

18.5.4 Surface modification of expanded polytetrafluoroethylene

Ikada has described how the surface modification of polymeric biomaterials is a well-established method of improving commercially available products (Ikada, 1994). Over the years, much fundamental research has gone into improving the performance of various PTFE products for vascular and craniofacial applications (Colwell *et al.*, 2003; Nishibe *et al.*, 2001).

PTFE is a fully fluorinated unbranched polymer with a carbon backbone (Fig. 18.2) that contains fluorine atoms bonded to carbon to form C–F bonds. It has a helical conformation (Fig. 18.2(b)). These are the strongest chemical bonds found in polymers: this means that PTFE is extremely stable and hydrophobic. These chemical properties translate into non-adherent material surfaces with significant anti-frictional properties (excellent in vascular devices) (Kannan *et al.*, 2005). However, proteins and cells find such surfaces very unattractive. Since they play an important role in hydroxyapatite nucleation and bone growth this becomes an issue (Kasemo and Gold, 1999; Wilson Cameron *et al.*, 2005). A material surface to which proteins and cells attach is described as 'bioactive'. The bone/soft tissue–material interface requires at least some degree of attachment; yet, a fibrous tissue interface is undesirable as it can lead to micromotion and destabilisation of the implant (Maas *et al.*, 1993). Hence, a porous material with the propensity to vascularise and form a good interface with the surrounding bone and soft tissue is highly desirable from both the surgeon's and the patient's perspective. As will be discussed below, researchers have examined the custom-modification of commercially available ePTFE surfaces for specific applications, including craniofacial applications (Suzuki *et al.*, 2005).

Much of the experimental work relevant to this section aims at modifying the surface properties to increase surface bioactivity. The theory is that this will promote the cascade of events that starts with protein adhesion and eventually leads, via calcium/phosphate nucleation, to hydroxyapatite and new bone formation. In Ikada's landmark paper on surface modification he states that surface modification of biomaterials is done 'for at least two purposes; one is to render the material surface biocompatible and the other to give it physiological activity', that is, to make the surface bioactive (Ikada, 1994). Biomolecules that potentiate osseoinduction *in vivo* are well known and using such molecules to modify an implant material has the potential to improve bioactivity, biocompatibility and, most importantly, healing time. In addition, induction of hydroxyapatite growth is often achieved through the introduction of functional groups on to the surface to induce nucleation (Suzuki *et al.*, 2007; Tanahashi and Matsuda, 1997). For example, in a series of papers on the surface modification of ePTFE using phosphate-containing monomers, Grøndahl *et al.* demonstrated that modified ePTFE surfaces promoted nucleation of a range of calcium phosphate phases (including in some cases hydroxyapatite) (Grøndahl *et al.*, 2003). Figure 18.3(b) clearly shows the calcium/phosphate mineral growth on the 'activated' surface, whereas there is zero mineral observed on the untreated membrane. Later, Suzuki *et al.* demonstrated that, in addition to calcium/phosphate mineral growth in simulated body fluid, protein and cell adhesion also improved on phosphate-modified surfaces. Figure 18.4 shows how both the morphology and extent of the attached osteoblasts were significantly enhanced after surface modification of the ePTFE surface (Suzuki *et al.*, 2005). As has been emphasised throughout this overview, there is no ideal repair material and

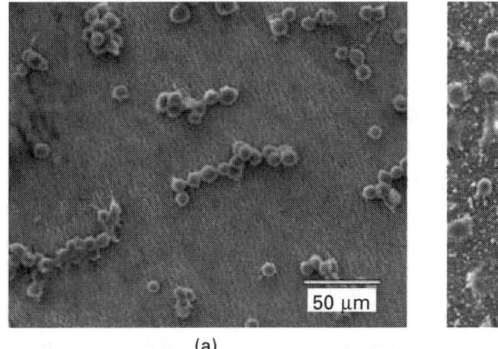
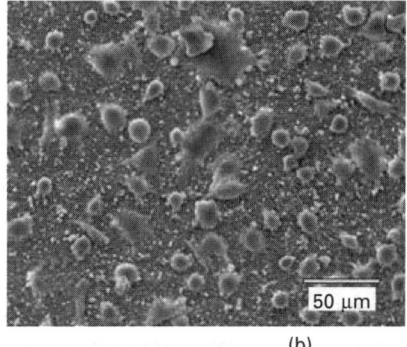

(a)   (b)

18.4 Osteoblast-like SaOS-2 cells on unmodified (a) and modified (b) ePTFE membranes.

ePTFE is no exception. There have been cases of secondary complications and infections are not unknown (Daniel, 1994; Mercandetti, 2008). It is not always obvious why products are withdrawn from the market and clearly clinical efficacy based on sound scientific principle and research is the priority; however, it is a long and winding road from laboratory-based research to the development of new biomaterials to commercial realisation. Modification of successful and approved materials makes sense both from a research and a commercial point of view, so hopefully the final chapter in the ePTFE story is yet to be written (Mercandetti, 2008).

18.5.5 High density polyethylene

PE is another polymer that has made a very successful transition from the laboratory to industrially oriented applications to biomedical applications. Different medical applications require one of the typically commercially available grades: low density PE (LDPE), HDPE and ultra high molecular weight PE (UHMWPE). Each grade has different properties (e.g. mechanical), which render them more or less suitable for different applications; for example, load-bearing orthopaedic applications use UHMWPE, craniofacial repairs use HDPE and porous HDPE (PHDPE). The higher tensile strength of HDPE compared with LDPE is advantageous in facial reconstruction (Bikhazi and Van Antwerp, 1991; Wellisz, 1993). HDPE is somewhat more difficult to sculpt than SAM and tends to form a thin fibrous in-growth layer which stabilises the implant; the downside is that, in the event of revision surgery, subsequent removal becomes more difficult. Importantly, the drilling and fixation techniques, which are mandatory in so many orbit reconstructions, do not fracture HDPE (Eppley, 2003a). The extremely useful and well-tested porous form, PHDPE, is found in the MedPor® range of products (Porex Surgical Inc., GA, USA). Incidentally, this manufacturer has a most informative and helpful website for their products (Porex Corporation, 2008). In a recent review, Lee *et al.* report on a retrospective analysis of 170 patients 'to determine the safety and efficacy of using PHDPE in the repair of orbital defects'. They concluded that it was so successful, and overall outcomes were so positive, that it has now been adopted as part of their clinical practice. This also eliminates potential problems associated with donor site morbitity (Lee *et al.*, 2005). According to Eski *et al.*, the best clinical outcomes using PHDPE are found for mild to moderate zygomatico-orbital fractures (Eski *et al.*, 2007). However, revision surgery cannot be ruled out in cases requiring complex repair and restoration procedures, and Antonopoulous *et al.* report the successful use of Medpor® in revision surgery of an 'enormous composite defect' after an initial reconstruction using cement had failed (Antonopoulous *et al.*, 2006). After a 2-year follow-up, no infection was observed and the cosmetic outcome was described as 'satisfactory'. This is just one case that highlights some of the challenges and choices (discussed in the Introduction) in the selection of suitable materials. PE in its various forms is one of the most successful and oft-cited biomaterials used in orbital reconstruction: its future appears secure.

18.5.6 Bone cements

It is difficult to discuss bone cements without reference to orthopaedic and, to a lesser extent, dental applications. However, despite the warning in the Introduction that care must be taken not to 'mindlessly adopt' orthopaedic materials and methods, it is for applications in these areas that bone cements have been largely developed. In craniofacial applications bone cements are generally used in conjunction with a variety of other repair materials. Hence, Donkerwolcke's general review on 'Tissue and bone adhesives – historical aspects' is a useful introduction (Donkerwolcke et al., 1998). In his 'State of the art review', Lewis points out that the success of the two-part self-polymerising PMMA system is such that it is now generally known as 'bone cement'. Although primarily focused on orthopaedic applications, this system is included because of its probable general interest (Lewis, 1997).

Acrylic and methacrylic-based polymeric materials are made from either acrylic or methacrylic acids or their esters. The best-known example, PMMA, was developed for use in dentistry in the 1930s and soon became popular in orthopaedic applications. In 1944, Blum reported the use of 'acrylic dough' in spinal fixations and for the repair of skull defects in animals (Blum, 1944). In the 1950s cold-curing acrylic cements became available. The pioneering English orthopaedic surgeon Sir John Charnley, who developed and gave his name to the hip replacement device, worked in collaboration with industry to develop bone cement in 1958 (Charnley, 1960). However, 'cranioplasty' applications soon became just as frequent (Prolo, 1985). Eppley gives a useful discussion on the advantages and limitations of PMMA (Eppley, 2003a). The latest generation of bone cements are more custom-designed to be used for specific applications. Generally, they are antibiotic-loaded to reduce the risk of infection in both primary and revision operations.

In a review in 1999, the degradable calcium phosphate cements were predicted to be the 'new technology' in craniofacial surgery and maxillofacial reconstruction in the new century (Schmitz et al., 1999). A carbonated apatite cement was used in a series of cranio-maxillofacial cases including 'post-traumatic bone defects in the orbital, periorbital and malar regions' (Wolff et al., 2004). No adverse effects were found after a mean follow-up period of 29 months, no inflammation was reported and the conclusion was that this was a suitable material for treating moderate-sized defects. Adverse effects, however, have been reported in other applications. Burstein et al. have compared the use of two forms of hydroxyapatite cements in craniofacial (including orbit) reconstruction. In their first study they used a granular form and described how most of the complications manifested themselves after the first 18 months (Burstein *et al.*, 1997). In a subsequent pioneering study of 61 patients (56 of whom were children) they used a powdered form of the hydroxyapatite cement and reported greatly improved clinical handling and results. This paper is impressive in its honesty in so far that the authors report that some of the complications subsequently observed were due to their 'inexperience during their early use of [hydroxyapatite] HAP cements'. This paper illustrates clearly the learning curve facing surgeons when first using materials that are new to the market (Burstein *et al.*, 1999).

18.5.7 Polyurethanes

Polyurethane-based materials have a long history of use as biomaterials. Their good biocompatibility as well as excellent strength have seen them used in a wide variety of biomedical implants and devices such as cardiac pacemakers and vascular grafts. Like many biomaterials, however, their development involved some less than successful products. As described in a review by Donkerwolke *et al.*, their use as bone glues, particularly in orthopaedic applications, dates back to the 1950s and 1960s (Donkerwolcke *et al.*, 1998). In 1958, Manderino and Salvatore (1959) announced the use of a polyurethane polymer as a bone glue or cement. It was described in *Time* magazine in 1959 as 'the realisation of a dream' but unfortunately with time the reality did not live up to that dream. Later, both animal and human studies showed a plethora of infections and the formation of a fibrotic, non-adhesive layer. However, the overall good biocompatibility as well as the excellent strength of polyurethane polymers has seen them used in a wide variety of biomedical implants, including cardiac pacemaker leads and catheters (Gunatillake and Adhikari, 2003).

This later success of polyurethane-based devices has sparked some interest in producing biodegradable polyurethanes. This is usually achieved through the coupling of degradable prepolymers with urethane linkages. A diisocyanate can be used to create a urethane linkage with a degradable hydroxy-terminated polyester to create a poly(ester-urethane) (Fig. 18.5). This approach enables chain-extended and cross-linked materials (if a triisocyanate is used) to be easily synthesised. Using such procedures makes it possible to control and modify the degradation rate and hence control the reduction in mechanical strength (Seppälä *et al.*, 2004). These advances in the control of properties that are critical in facial repair and reconstruction may open up the possibility of future commercial development of polyurethanes for a wider range of applications.

HO—$\left(\text{R}\right)_m$—OH + O=C=N—R'—N=C=O

$$+O-\left(R\right)_m-O-\overset{\displaystyle O}{\overset{\|}{C}}-NH-R'-NH-\overset{\displaystyle O}{\overset{\|}{C}}\rightarrow_n$$

18.5 Synthesis of poly(ester-urethane) where R = polyester.

18.6   Biodegradable and bioresorbable polymers

18.6.1 Introduction

There is some confusion in the literature because different disciplines – such as tissue engineersing and materials chemistry – use different definitions of the terms biodegradable, bioresorbable, bioabsorbable and bioerodible. Therefore, although the term biodegradable is the one most frequently used in its broadest sense, it is pertinent to define these terms because they can be important when discussing the chemical and physical properties of the kinds of polymers used in the materials and devices discussed in this review. Vert *et al.*'s definitions given below for solid polymeric materials and devices are generally accepted by the materials and tissue engineering communities (Albertsson and Varma, 2003; Vert *et al.*, 1992).

- Biodegradables break down due to macromolecular degradation. There is *in vivo* dispersion of the fragments/by-products but no proof of elimination from the body.
- Bioresorbables show bulk degradation and further resorb *in vivo*: i.e. the original foreign material and its breakdown products can be shown to be eliminated through the body's natural pathways.
- Bioerodibles show surface degradation and further resorb *in vivo*. Total elimination of low molecular weight by-products is inherent.
- Bioabsorbables can dissolve in body fluids in the absence of polymer chain cleavage or molecular mass loss, such as in the slow dissolution of water-soluble materials.

18.6.2 Natural biodegradable polymers

The rationale for the use of 'natural biodegradable' polymers such as the hydrogels gelatine and collagen, particularly when they are present in the patient's own system, i.e. collagen, appears to be logical. These polymers usually degrade *in vivo* enzymatically but many are also susceptible to hydrolysis. The degradation by-products are usually disposed of, or recycled, by the body through normal metabolic pathways. Furthermore, because of the chemical similarity between these polymers and extracellular matrix

18.6 Structures of (a) PHB, (b) PHV and (c) PHHx.

components already present in tissues, biocompatibility and integration would be expected to be enhanced. Unfortunately, the polymers of natural origin generally do not perform as well as expected. In order to produce enough material for the scaffold, the crude polymer is usually sourced from a different species to the patient. As a result, there is concern regarding not only disease transmission, but also the variable quality of these polymers, which often differs between batches. Furthermore, for many of these natural polymers, the mechanical properties of the processed products are less than ideal.

Natural polymers obtained from non-animal sources may overcome some of the disadvantages discussed above. Polyhydroxyalkanoates (PHAs) are polyesters that are produced by micro-organisms and degrade via hydrolysis of the ester linkages. The most commonly studied PHAs for biomedical applications are poly(3-hydroxybutyrate) (PHB), poly(3-hydroxyvalerate) (PHV) and poly(3-hydroxyhexanoate) (PHHx), and their copolymers. A drawback of the use of PHAs in biomedical devices is their limited availability and the often time-consuming extraction techniques necessary. Undesirable endotoxins are sometimes incorporated by the polymer-synthesising bacteria colonies, hence there is some concern over their use as implant materials. The structures of these homopolymers are shown in Fig. 18.6.

18.6.3 Polylactones: introduction

Due to their good biocompatibility and ability to bioresorb, polylactones – such as polylactide (PLA), polyglycolide (PGA), poly(ε-caprolactone) (PCL) (Fig. 18.7) – and their copolymers have been studied for biomedical purposes since the 1960s (Albertsson and Varma, 2003). The first commercially available product, launched in 1962, was a polyglycolide suture, Dexon™ (Tyco Healthcare Group, CT, USA) (Albertsson and Varma, 2003). Poly(lactide-co-glycolide) (PLGA) sutures became available a few years later. The latest generation of sutures uses other polylactones acids) and incorporates factors such as antibacterials. Commercially available products such as Monocryl™ Plus Antibacterial is a glycolide/ε-caprolactone copolymer (poliglecaprone 25)

18.7 Structures of (a) PLA, (b) PGA and (c) PCL.

(Johnson & Johnson Gateway). The advantage of such composite polymers is that they not only combine some of the advantages of each component, but they also often make it possible to tailor the various properties (mechanical and/or degradative).

18.6.4 Poly(lactide-*co*-glycolide) polymers

Lactosorb SE®, one of the most successful materials used in maxillo and craniofacial applications, became available commercially in 1996. It is a copolymer of L-lactic acid (82%) and glycolic acid (18%) and, although it has a specific strength comparable with titanium, it degrades *in vivo* within 12 months. LactoSorb SE® overcame many of the limitations encountered with earlier bone substitutes such as with the permanent PTFE-based Proplast® series (mouldability, delamination, fragmentation and trans-cranial migration) discussed earlier. With respect to orbit repair, the most common LactoSorb SE® devices used are bone fixation devices such as sutures, micro- and mini-plates, and screws.

In 1996, Eppley reviewed the obstacles and 'potential role' of resorbable plates and screws in cranio-maxillofacial trauma (Eppley *et al.*, 1996). In 1997, he observed that 'favourable clinical experiences have been very limited', although that same year Kumar *et al.* reviewed their use in 22 paediatric cases (Eppley and Prevel, 1997; Kumar *et al.*, 1997). However, Kumar recognised that 'further experience using this technology' would be required before it could be adopted as 'the standard of care' in infants. In 2005, Eppley again reviewed the use of resorbable plates and screws in paediatric fractures (Eppley, 2005). Although a pilot study using them in large orbital wall repairs appeared in 1996, it was not until 2007 that a specific reference to an orbital rim repair using a resorbable plate appeared. 'An excellent cosmetic and functional outcome' was reported by Curtis *et al.* in a complicated case involving both a corticocancellous bone graft and the biosorbable plate to treat a rare intraosseous hemangioma (Al-Sukhun *et al.*, 2006; Curtis and Zoellner, 2007).

Polymeric materials, including PLA–PGA copolymers, with tailored properties are feasible in the laboratory at least. For biomedical applications, such polyesters are usually synthesised by ring opening polymerisation reactions. Unlike the condensation polymerisation of monomeric lactic acid, the ring opening approach can produce polymers of high molecular weight. Under certain conditions the polymerisation is living and proceeds in a controlled fashion yielding a narrow molecular weight distribution. In such systems, the molecular weight and, consequently, the physical properties of the polymer can be controlled easily by the ratio of monomer to initiator. Block copolymers can be synthesised by the addition of a second monomer after the polymerisation of the first monomer is complete. Molecular weight is related to bioresorption and biodegradation, hence – in theory at least – devices could be produced for very specific applications, such as orbital rim repair. In practice, such a finely tailored range of products is seldom commercially available. Since these synthetic polymers have had US Food and Drug Administration (FDA) and Therapeutic Goods Administration (TGA) (Australia) approval for nearly 50 years, as well as being already used in a range of craniofacial applications, they clearly lend themselves to further laboratory-based research with a view to extending commercial interest and development of new products.

As mentioned previously, there is no perfect polymeric repair material and in this case there is some concern regarding the release of acidic degradation products and the negative effect this can have at the implant site. It is argued that, although the degradation products can be eliminated from the body via well-understood metabolic pathways, since the PLLA undergoes bulk degradation there is a burst release of a high concentration of acidic by-products that can be entrapped inside the polymer material. This lowers the local pH and can trigger an inflammatory response. The surface of these polymers is generally considered to be less than ideal for interacting with the biological environment because of a lack of suitable functional groups (Suh *et al.*, 2001). Consequently, many studies have been directed towards overcoming this through surface modification of the polyesters. Attachment of biologically active molecules, such as silk fibroin and type I atelocollagen has been shown to have a favourable effect on osteoblast cell behaviour *in vitro* (Cai *et al.*, 2002; Suh *et al.*, 2001).

If polylactones and other polymers are to be made more attractive clinically, then the ability to tailor their properties is essential, not only for promoting initial bone formation, but also for controlling the degradation rate and subsequent loss in mechanical properties. This is important not only for device stability but for the remodelling of the new and surrounding bone needed to ensure full restoration of bone function at the defect site.

18.7   The future: composite materials, bone regeneration and tissue engineering

New materials are constantly being developed. Although their immediate application may be in areas far removed from the medical arena, as discussed in this chapter, they do often eventually find use as biomaterials. Fundamental research on the surface modification of materials will continue to make an important contribution. Another trend is the merging of material science with biology and pharmacology to introduce antibacterials, antibiotics and growth factors in order to produce 'activated' biomaterials. Although this chapter is limited to polymeric materials and did not cover ceramics or metals, it should be mentioned that there are some interesting reports on the development of composite materials that combine polymers with other alloplastic compounds. Of particular relevance for craniofacial reconstruction is that of a polymer and a bioactive ceramic such as hydroxyapatite or tricalcium phosphate (TCP). This approach is not new, of course, but in spite of some major challenges, one of which is achieving the right chemical or physical binding between the two materials, a range of bone repair composite materials has reached both the commercialisation and clinical stages. These materials were developed by an interdisciplinary group at the National University of Singapore (Hutmacher *et al.*, 2007). Both polycaprolactone/hydroxyapatite and poly(ε-caprolactone/TCP scaffolds were used in orbital floor reconstruction with good clinical outcomes after 12 months.

Hopefully, some of the fundamental research advances being made in developing new materials, hybrid/composite materials and tissue-engineered constructs will translate into some exciting new biomaterials for use in complex and demanding orbital repair and reconstruction applications.

18.8   References

Albertsson A-C and Varma I K (2003), 'Recent Developments in Ring Opening Polymerization of Lactones for Biomedical Applications'. *Biomacromolecules*, **4**, 1466–1486.

Al-Sukhun J, Tornwall J, Lindqvist C and Kontio R (2006), 'Bioresorbable Poly-L/Dl-Lactide (P[L/DL]LA 70/30) Plates Are Reliable for Repairing Large Inferior Orbital Wall Bony Defects: A Pilot Study'. *J. Oral Maxillofac. Surg.*, **64**, 47–55.

Antonopoulous D, Tsiliboti D, Skarpetas D and Masmanidis A (2006), 'Complete Orbit and Forehead Reconstruction Using a Free Latissimus Dorsi Flap and Medpor Implants'. *Head Neck*, **28**, 559–563.

Beumer J, III, Ma T, Marunick M T, Roumanas E and Nishimura R (1996) 'Restoration of Facial Defects: Etiology, Disability and Rehabilitation', in Beumer J, III, Curtis TA and Marunick MT (Eds), *Maxillofacial Rehabilitation: Prosthodontics and Surgical Considerations* St Louis, Ishiyaku EuroAmerica, pp. 377–438.

Bikhazi H B and Van Antwerp R (1991) 'The Use of Medpor in Cosmetic and Reconstructive Surgery: Experimental and Clinical Evidence', in Stucher F, *Plastic and Reconstructive*

Surgery of the Head and Neck: Proceedings of the Fifth International Symposium/ American Academy of Facial Plastic and Reconstructive Surgery, Mosby, St Louis, B.C. Decker.

Blum G (1944), 'Phosphatase and Repair of Fractures'. *Lancet*, **II**, 75–78.

Brånemark P-I (1997) 'Osseointegration: Anchorage of Craniofacial Prostheses', in Brånemark P-I and De Oliveira M F (Eds), *Craniofacial Prostheses*, Chicago, Quintessence Books, p. 85.

Burstein F, Cohen S, Hudgins R and Boydston W (1997), 'The Use of Porous Granular Hydroxyapatite in Secondary Orbitocranial Reconstruction'. *Plast. Reconstr. Surg.*, **100**, 869–873.

Burstein F, Cohen S, Hudgins R and Boydston W (1999), 'The Use of Hydroxyapatite Cement in Secondary Craniofacial Reconstruction'. *Plast. Reconstr. Surg.*, **104**, 1270–1275.

Cai K, Yao K, Cui Y, Yang Z, Li X, Xie H, Qing T and Gao L (2002), 'Influence of Different Surface Modification Treatments on Poly(D,L-Lactide) with Silk Fibroin and their Effects on the Culture of Osteoblast in Vitro'. *Biomaterials*, **23**, 1603–1611.

Cameron M and Booth P W (2003) 'Principles of Reduction of Fractures and Methods of Fixation', in Booth P W., Eppley B L and Schmelzeisen R (Eds), *Maxillofacial Trauma and Esthetic Facial Reconstruction*, Edinburgh; New York, Churchill Livingstone.

Chandler-Temple A, Wentrup-Byrne E and Grøndahl L (2008), 'Expanded Poly (Tetrafluoroethylene): From Conception to Biomedical Device'. *Chem. Aust.*, **75**, 3–6.

Charnley J (1960), 'Anchorage of the Femoral Head Prosthesis to the Shaft of the Femur'. *J. Bone Jt Surg.*, **42–B**, 28–30.

Colwell J M, Wentrup-Byrne E, Bell J M and Wielunski L S (2003), 'A Study of the Chemical and Physical Effects of Ion Implantation of Microporous and Nonporous PTFE'. *Surf. Coat. Technol.*, **168**, 216–222.

Curtis N and Zoellner H (2007), 'Resection of an Orbital Rim Intraosseous Cavernous Hemangioma and Reconstruction by Chin Graft and Resorbable Fixation Plate'. *Ophthal. Plast. Reconstr. Surg.*, **23**, 232–234.

Daniel R K (1994), 'The Use of Gore-Tex for Nasal Augmentation: A Retrospective Analysis of 106 Patients, Discussion'. *Plast. Reconstr. Surg.*, **94**, 249–250.

Donkerwolcke M, Burny F and Muster D (1998), 'Tissues and Bone Adhesives – Historical Aspects'. *Biomaterials*, **19**, 1461–1466.

Elmazar H, Jackson I T, Degner D, Miyawaki T, Barakat K, Andrus L and Bradford M (2003), 'The Efficiency of Gore-Tex Vs Hydroxyapatite and Bone Graft in Reconstruction of Orbital Floor Defects'. *Eur. J. Plast. Surg.*, **25**, 362–368.

Eppley B L (2003a) 'Alloplastic Biomaterials for Facial Reconstruction', in Booth P W, Eppley B L and Schmelzeisen R (Eds), *Maxillofacial Trauma and Esthetic Facial Reconstruction*, Edinburgh; New York, Churchill Livingstone, pp. 144–145.

Eppley B L (2003b) 'Alloplastic Biomaterials for Facial Reconstruction', in Booth P W, Eppley, B L and Schmelzeisen R (Eds), *Maxillofacial Trauma and Esthetic Facial Reconstruction*, Edinburgh; New York, Churchill Livingstone, pp. 139–150.

Eppley B L (2005), 'Use of Resorbable Plates and Screws in Pediatric Facial Fractures'. *J. Oral Maxillofac. Surg.*, **63**, 385–391.

Eppley B L and Prevel C D (1997), 'Nonmetallic Fixation in Traumatic Midfacial Fractures'. *J. Craniofac. Surg.*, **8**, 103–109.

Eppley B L, Prevel C D, Sadove A M and Sarver D (1996), 'Resorbable Bone Fixation: Its Potential Role in Cranio-Maxillofacial Trauma'. *J. Craniomaxillofac. Trauma*, **2**, 56–60.

Eski M, Sengezer M, Turegun M, Deveci M and Isik S (2007), 'Contour Restoration of the Secondary Deformities of Zygomatico-orbital Fractures with Porous Polyethylene Implant'. *J. Craniofac. Surg.*, **18**, 520–525.

Firtell D N and Beumer J, III (1979) 'Cranial and Facial Implants', in Beumer J, III, Curtis, T A and Firtell D N (Eds), *Maxillofacial Rehabilitation: Prosthodontic and Surgical Considerations*, St Louis, C.V. Mosby, pp. 372–397.

Foster C A and Sherman J E (1987) 'Maso-Orbital Fractures', in Foster C A and Sherman, J E (Eds), *Surgery of Facial Bone Fractures*, New York, Churchill Livingston, pp. 39–65.

Fries P D (1994), 'Autogenous, Alloplastic, Integrated and Resorbable Implants for Orbital Blow-out Fracture Repair; A Review'. *Orbit*, **13**, 135–145.

Grøndahl L, Cardona F, Chiem K, Wentrup-Byrne E and Bostrom T (2003), 'Calcium Phosphate Nucleation on Surface-Modified PTFE Membranes'. *J. Mater. Sc. Mater. Med.*, **14**, 503–510.

Gunatillake P A and Adhikari R (2003), 'Biodegradable Synthetic Polymers for Tissue Engineering'. *Euro. Cell Mater.*, **5**, 1–16.

Hanson L J, Donovan M G, Hellstein J W and Dickerson N C (1994), 'Experimental Evaluation of Expanded Polytetrafluoroethylene for Reconstruction of Orbital Floor Defects'. *J. Oral Maxillofac. Surg.*, **52**, 1050–1055; discussion 1056–1057.

Hutmacher D W, Schantz J T, Lam C X F, Tan K C and Lim T C (2007), 'State of the Art and Future Directions of Scaffold-Based Bone Engineering from a Biomaterials Perspective: Review Article'. *J. Tissue Eng. Regen. Med.*, **1**, 245–260.

Ikada Y (1994), 'Surface Modification of Polymers for Medical Applications'. *Biomaterials*, **15**, 725–736.

Jelks G W and La Trenta G (1987) 'Orbital Fracture', in Foster C A and Sherman, J E (Eds), *Surgery of Facial Bone Fractures*, New York, Churchill Livingston, pp. 67–91.

Johnson & Johnson Gateway Features and Benefits, http://www.jnjgateway.com/home.jhtml?loc=USENG&page=viewContent&contentId=edea000100002187&parentId=fc0de00100000345.

Kannan R Y, Salacinski H J, Butler P E, Hamilton G and Seifalian A M (2005), 'Current Status of Prosthetic Bypass Grafts: A Review'. *J. Biomed. Mater. Res. B. Appl. Biomater.*, **74B**, 570–581.

Karesh J W (1987), 'Polytetrafluoroethylene as a Graft Material in Ophthalmic Plastic and Reconstructive Surgery. An Experimental and Clinical Study'. *Ophthal. Plast. Reconstr. Surg.*, **3**, 179–185.

Karesh J W (1994), 'Experimental Evaluation of ePTFE for Reconstruction of Orbital Floor Defects'. *J. Oral Maxillofac. Surg.*, **52**, 1056–1057.

Karesh J W (1998), 'Biomaterials in Ophthalmic Plastic and Reconstructive Surgery'. *Curr. Opin. Ophthalmol.*, **9**, 66–74.

Kasemo B and Gold J (1999), 'Implant Surfaces and Interface Processes'. *Adv. Dent. Res.*, **13**, 8–20.

Kumar A V, Staffenberg D A, Petronio J A and Wood R J (1997), 'Bioabsorbable Plates and Screws in Pediatric Craniofacial Surgery: A Review of 22 Cases'. *J. Craniofac. Surg.*, **8**, 97–99.

Lee S, Maronian N, Most S P, Whipple M E, Mcculloch T M, Stanley B and Farwell D G (2005), 'Porous High-Density Polyethylene for Orbital Reconstruction'. *Arch. Otolaryngol. Head Neck Surg.*, **131**, 446–50.

Lewis G (1997), 'Properties of Acrylic Bone Cement: State of the Art Review'. *J. Biomed. Mater. Res. B. Appl. Biomater.*, **38**, 155–182.

Linde A, Alberius P, Dahlin C, Bjurstam K and Sundin Y (1993), 'Osteopromotion: A Soft-Tissue Exclusion Principle Using a Membrane for Bone Healing and Bone Neogenesis'. *J. Periodontol.*, **64**, 1116–1128.

Maas C S, Gnepp D R and Bumpous J (1993), 'Expanded Polytetrafluoroethylene (Gore-Tex Soft-Tissue Patch) in Facial Augmentation'. *Arch. Otolaryngol. Head Neck Surg.*, **119**, 1008–1014.

Mackenzie D J, Arora B and Hansen J (1999), 'Orbital Floor Repair with Titanium Mesh Screen'. *J. Cranio Maxill. Trauma*, **5**, 9–18.

Mandarino M P and Salvatore J E (1959), 'Polyurethane Polymer; Its Use in Fractured and Diseased Bones'. *Am. J. Surg.*, **97**, 442–446.

Mercandetti M (2008) Implants, Soft Tissue, Gore-Tex, http://www.emedicine.com/ent/fulltopic/topic376.htm, accessed 19 August 2008.

Meyer D R (1995), 'Alloplastic Materials for Orbital Surgery'. *Curr. Opin. Ophthalmol.*, **6**, 43–52.

Nishibe T, O'Donnel S, Pikoulis E, Rich N, Okuda Y, Kumada T, Kudo F, Tanabe T and Yasuda K (2001), 'Effects of Fibronectin Bonding on Healing of High Porosity Expanded Polytetrafluoroethylene Grafts in Pigs'. *J. Cardiovasc. Surg.*, **42**, 667–73.

Oliver A J (2000), 'The Use of Titanium Mesh in the Management of Orbital Trauma – a Retrospective Study'. *Ann. R. Australas. Coll. Dent. Surg.*, **15**, 193–198.

Porex Corporation (2008) Options: Medpor Biomaterial and Surgical Implants, http://www.porexsurgical.com/english/surgical/smedpor.asp, accessed 20 August 2008.

Prolo D (1985) 'Cranial Defects and Cranioplasty', in *Neurosurgery*, Wilkins R H and Rengachary S S (Eds), New York, McGraw-Hill, pp. 646–851.

Schmitz J P, Hollinger J O and Milam S B (1999), 'Reconstruction of Bone Using Calcium Phosphate Bone Cements: A Critical Review'. *J. Oral Maxillofac. Surg.*, **57**, 1122–1126.

Seppälä J V, Helminen A O and Korhonen H (2004), 'Degradable Polyesters through Chain Linking for Packaging and Biomedical Applications'. *Macromolecular Bioscience*, **4**, 208–217.

Shuker S T (2008), 'Mechanism and Emergency Management of Blast Eye/Orbit Injuries'. *Expert Rev. Ophthalmol.*, **3**, 229–246.

Suh H, Hwang Y-S, Lee J-E, Han C D and Park J-C (2001), 'Behaviour of Osteoblasts on a Type I Atelocollagen Grafted Ozone Oxidized Poly L-Lactic Acid Membrane'. *Biomaterials*, **22**, 219–230.

Suzuki S, Grøndahl L, Leavesley D and Wentrup-Byrne E (2005), 'In Vitro Bioactivity of Methacryloyloxyethyl Phosphate Grafted Polytetrafluoroethylene Membranes for Craniofacial Applications'. *Biomaterials*, **26**, 5303–5312.

Suzuki S, Rintoul L, Monteiro M J, Wentrup-Byrne E and Grøndahl L (2007), '*In Vitro* Mineralization of Phosphate-Containing Polymer Ad-Layers'. *Poly. Prepr.*, **48**, 430–431.

Tanahashi M and Matsuda T (1997), 'Surface Functional Group Dependence on Apatite Formation on Self-Assembled Monolayers in a Simulated Body Fluid'. *J. Biomed. Mater. Res.*, **34**, 305–315.

Ueda M (2005) 'Maxillofacial Bone Regeneration Using Tissue Engineering Concepts', in *Engineered Bone*, Petite H and Quarto R (Eds), Austin, Landes Bioscience, pp. 183–194.

Van Helden A (2005), 'Tycho Brahe'. The Galileo Project, http://galileo.rice.edu/sci/brahe.html, accesed 24 July 2009.

Vert M, Li S M, Spenlehauer G and Guerin P (1992), 'Bioresorbability and Biocompatibility of Aliphatic Polyesters'. *J. Mater. Sci.: – Mater. M ed.*, **3**, 432–446.

W. L. Gore & Associates (2006) Gore & Associates to Exit the Plastic Surgery Market, http://www.goremedical.com/press/news/sam-03nov2006, accessed 25 August 2008.

Wellisz T (1993), 'Clinical Experience with the Medpor Porous Polyethylene Implant'. *Aesthetic Plast. Surg.*, **17**, 339–344.

Wilson C J, Clegg R E, Leavesley D I and Pearcy M J (2005), 'Mediation of Biomaterial-Cell Interactions by Adsorbed Proteins: A Review'. *Tissue Eng.*, **11**, 1–18.

Wolff K-D, Swaid S, Nolte D, Bockmann Roland A, Holzle F and Muller-Mai C (2004), 'Degradable Injectable Bone Cement in Maxillofacial Surgery: Indications and Clinical Experience in 27 Patients'. *J. Craniomaxillofac. Surg.*, **32**, 71–79.

19

Physicochemical properties of hydrogels for use in ophthalmology

B. J. TIGHE, Aston University, UK

Abstract: This chapter deals with the physicochemical aspects of structure–property relationships in hydrogels, with particular reference to their application in optometry and ophthalmology. It demonstrates the ways in which the amount of water contained in the hydrogel network can be manipulated by changes in copolymer composition, and illustrates the advantages and limitations imposed by use of water as a means of influencing surface, transport and mechanical properties of the gel. The chapter then proceeds to show how interpenetrating networks and macroporous materials, in which behaviour is not so centrally dominated by the equilibrium water content as is the case with homogeneous hydrogels, provide advantageous ways of extending the properties of these interesting materials.

Key words: hydrogels, equilibrium water content, oxygen permeability, surface energy, macroporous hydrogels, interpenetrating networks.

19.1   Introduction

The treatment presented here deals with the physicochemical aspects of structure-property relationships in hydrogels and aims to indicate what is achievable in terms of those properties that are particularly important in ophthalmic applications, dealing with both advantages and limitations. The chapter outlines the principles involved in the formation of those forms of hydrogels, such as interpenetrating networks and macroporous materials, in which the properties are not so centrally dominated by the equilibrium water content as is the case with homogeneous hydrogels. The question of so-called silicone hydrogels is touched upon, but is dealt with in more detail in Chapter 12. It is inevitable that homogeneous hydrogels will assume a position of central importance in any treatment that deals with those properties of hydrogels that are of relevance in ophthalmic applications. In this context it is important to show that poly(2-hydroxyethyl methacrylate) or PHEMA is only one material in a synthetically diverse field, and to appreciate the possibilities and limitations in the design of hydrogels that possess appropriate properties for a given application.

The special position that hydrogels occupy in the biomedical field can be illustrated by comparing their properties with more established biomaterials and with natural tissue. The feature that characterises non-hydrogel polymers such as polyethylene, polypropylene, silicone rubber and poly(vinyl chloride) – all of which have important biomaterials applications – is their relative hydrophobicity. Even the more polar materials, such as poly(methyl methacrylate) (PMMA) and poly(ethylene terephthalate), have polar components of surface energy that are much lower in magnitude than the dispersive, or non-polar, component of the polymer; in contrast to water which has a surface energy dominated by its polar component. The behaviour of water at the surfaces of these relatively non-polar polymers is necessarily dominated by hydrophobic interactions and this is a feature that contributes to their success in the biomedical fields for which they were developed. In contrast, the cell surface is greatly influenced by more hydrophilic groups such as oligosaccharide units, and the wide variety of soft tissue interfaces in the body interact with water in a quite different way from conventional synthetic hydrophobic polymers.

It is this aspect of behaviour that sets the class of polymeric materials known collectively as hydrogels apart from conventional synthetic polymers. There is no precise and limiting definition of the term hydrogel, and problems always arise when attempts are made to apply such definitions to the range of materials that may be encompassed by the term. Perhaps the most useful description that may be given is that hydrogels are water-swollen polymer networks, of either natural or synthetic origin. Of these, it is the crosslinked, covalently bonded, synthetic hydrogels whose biomedical use has grown most dramatically in recent years, including composite structures involving both natural and synthetic hydrophilic materials. This aspect points to the central problem in the design of polymeric biomaterials. Whereas the biological structure to be replaced, or with which an interface is required, is invariably structurally complex, the historic tendency has been to choose biomaterials from a range of simple homogeneous synthetic polymers. As a result, the single synthetic material is required to produce a combination of surface and mechanical properties that is achieved by a combination of elements in the natural host. The obvious requirement for the development of more effective synthetic biologically compatible composites can only be achieved by reaching a better understanding of the behaviour of homogeneous hydrogels in biological environments, and by optimising their synthetic versatility. This chapter is not a review of current hydrogel literature, which is extremely extensive; it aims, rather, to summarise the well-established physicochemical principles that provide the necessary basis for the optimisation of hydrogel design for specific applications.

19.2   Water in hydrogels: effects of monomer structure

The vast majority of work in this field can be traced back to the pioneering work of Otto Wichterle, who was not only the 'father' of hydrogels, but also an early advocate of the principles of biomimesis. He recognised quite clearly the importance of attempting to match mechanical properties of the host tissue, allow diffusion of metabolites and achieve a compatible interface with biological fluids. In order to achieve these ends he attempted to harness water as a component of the biomaterial and together with his coworker Drahoslav Lim he demonstrated the usefulness, for biological applications, of lightly crosslinked polymers of 2-hydroxyethyl methacrylate (usually referred to simply as HEMA) (Wichterle and Lim, 1960). The great advantages of this material over most other hydrophilic gels (such as the synthetic acrylamide gels that have been known for many years) are its stability to varying conditions of pH, temperature and osmolarity, such as are commonly encountered in biomedical use. The foundations of the subject were laid in a range of reviews, edited symposia and reference works (Wichterle, 1971; Andrade, 1976; Peppas, 1986, 1987a, 1987b).

Hydrogels are normally prepared by free radical addition polymerisation of unsaturated monomers that contain functional groups capable of interacting with water. The single most commonly used monomer is still HEMA – which is a tribute to the enduring nature of Wicherle's work. Indeed, one of the problems associated with the development of hydrogels for biomedical applications has been the assumption, by those unfamiliar with the synthetic versatility of this class of materials, that the properties attainable with hydrogel devices are limited to those associated with lightly crosslinked, homogeneous, polymers of HEMA. Because of the central position occupied by HEMA, both as a monomer and polymer, it is convenient to use this as a starting point in developing a consideration of structure–property relationships in hydrogels. When HEMA is polymerised in the absence of water, it is glassy and similar in many ways to PMMA. The difference between PHEMA and PMMA becomes quite apparent, however, when the materials are immersed in water. Whereas PMMA is relatively little affected by water, PHEMA absorbs some two-thirds of its own weight to form an elastic gel that contains around 40% by weight of water and is remarkably stable to changes in its aqueous environment.

The amount of water held by the hydrogel is described by the equilibrium water content (EWC):

EWC = (weight of water in the gel/total weight of hydrated gel) × 100%

[19.1]

The EWC is undoubtedly the single most important property of a hydrogel because this, in turn, influences several other properties. The water in a hydrogel acts as:

• a transport medium for dissolved species;
• a surface energy 'bridge' between the hydrogel and the external environment;

- a plasticiser, giving the material flexibility;
- a lubricant, influencing the coefficient of friction.

The underlying role of water in acting as a plasticiser, a transport medium in the polymer matrix for dissolved species (such as oxygen) and a 'bridge' between the very different surface energies of synthetic polymers and body fluids, is responsible for the unique position that hydrogels occupy in the field of biomaterials. Thus, the permeability of the membranes, their mechanical properties, their surface properties and resultant behaviour at biological interfaces are all a direct consequence of the amount and nature of water held in this way.

The EWCs of hydrogels are governed by a range of factors. These include the nature of the hydrophilic monomer used in preparing the gel, the nature and density of the crosslinking agent (the most common crosslinking agent being ethylene glycol dimethacrylate) and external factors such as the temperature, osmolarity (and nature of the constituent ions) and pH of the hydrating medium. Although PHEMA is relatively stable to these external factors, this is not the case for hydrogels derived from other hydrophilic monomers; especially responsive to these factors are hydrogels that contain anionic or cationic monomers.

There is a great deal of evidence that has been accumulated to suggest that water in polymers can exist at any one time in more than one state and that these states of water in the hydrogel will also affect its properties. Various descriptions have been applied to the nature of water held in the hydrogel network, although these are not usually regarded as thermodynamically stable states. Rather, the water present in a polymer network can be envisaged to exist in a continuum of states between two extremes. These are, water strongly associated with the polymer network through hydrogen bonding, and water with a much greater degree of mobility, unaffected by the polymeric environment. Several techniques, such as differential scanning calorimetry (DSC) and nuclear magnetic resonance (NMR) have been applied to the study of water binding in natural and synthetic polymers and the ratio of the various states of water obtained will depend on the experimental technique used. The technique used to study water binding in hydrogels has to some extent determined both the number of states into which the water is classified and the terms used to describe those states. When water binding is studied by DSC, it is convenient and unambiguous to refer directly to the experimentally determined states (i.e. non-freezing and freezing water) rather than to imply any particular molecular interpretation. The properties of a hydrogel are therefore strongly influenced both by the EWC of the hydrogel and by the ratio of freezing to non-freezing water. This difference becomes less important as the EWC of the hydrogel rises but, as will become apparent, it affects behaviour quite markedly at values of EWC below that of PHEMA (Pedley and Tighe, 1979; Corkhill *et al.*, 1987; Roorda, 1990; Wang and Gunasekaran, 2006; Kishi *et al.*, 2008).

19.2.1 Hydroxyalkyl acrylates and methacrylates

Because of the influence that water exerts on such a range of properties, it is important to understand the ways in which both the total amount of water and the nature of water binding are influenced by the constituent monomers in a hydrogel. A useful starting point is the hydroxyalkyl acrylate and methacrylate family. Figure 19.1 shows the structure of the parent acrylic acid (AA) and methacrylic acid (MA) monomers and three important hydroxyalkyl methacrylates. Figure 19.2 compares the EWCs of homopolymers of: 2-hydroxyethyl acrylate (HEA), 2-hydroxypropyl acrylate (HPA), 2-hydroxyethyl methacrylate (HEMA), 2-hydroxypropyl methacrylate (HPMA) and 2,3-dihydroxypropyl methacrylate (DHPMA) – more commonly known as glyceryl methacrylate (GMA). Each is copolymerised with 1% (w/w) ethylene glycol dimethacrylate as a crosslinking agent.

The EWC increases as the hydrophilicity of the monomer increases, which in turn depends upon the balance of contributing steric and polar effects. The polar contribution arises predominantly from the hydroxyl group and to a lesser extent from the ester group; whereas the steric effect arises from the combined contribution of the α-methyl group and alkyl side chain component of the hydrophilic monomer. It can be seen that the hydrophilicities of

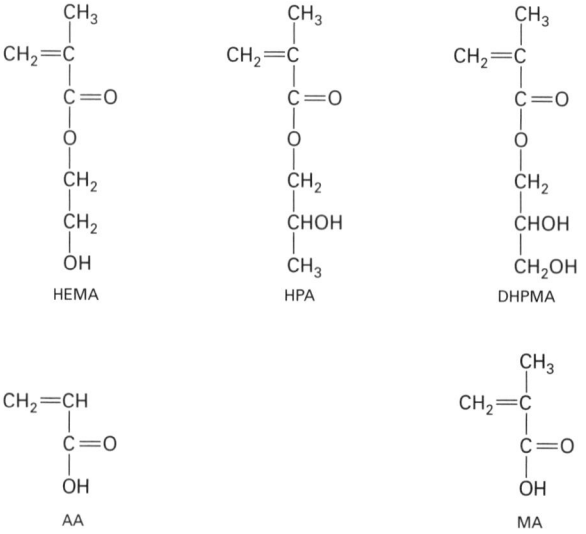

19.1 Structures of monomers containing hydroxyl and carboxyl groups

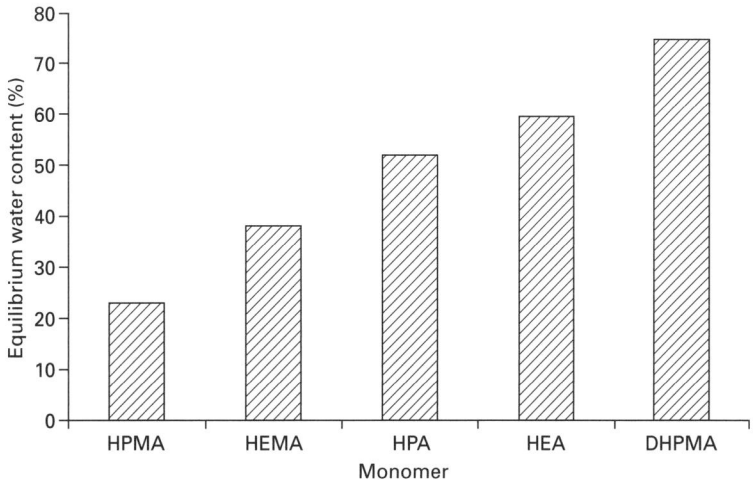

19.2 Equilibrium water contents of homopolymers of monomers containing hydroxyl groups.

the monomers decrease in the order: DHPMA > HEA > HPA > HEMA > HPMA. As expected, the additional steric hindrance of the α-methyl group on the methacrylate polymer backbone means that the homopolymers of HEA and HPA are more hydrophilic, respectively, than those of HEMA and HPMA, respectively Similarly, the EWCs of the homopolymers derived from HPA and HPMA are more hydrophobic than those derived from HEA and HEMA, respectively, because of the extra CH_2 group in the side chain. It is interesting to compare the isomeric monomers HPA and HEMA. The higher water content of the homopolymer (and copolymers) derived from HPA compared with those based on HEMA illustrates that a greater reduction in water content is obtained by inserting the methylene group on to the backbone, than introducing it in the side chain. This principle applies extensively in hydrogel copolymer systems.

A great deal of interest in the field of synthetics has focused on the synthesis of hydrogels that have higher EWCs than those attainable by hydroxyalkyl acrylates alone. One of the major driving forces has been the desire to produce contact lens materials with higher oxygen permeability than that achievable with PHEMA. In the 30 years following Wichterle's original disclosure, well over 100 patent specifications described conventional (non-silicone-containing) hydrogel copolymers for contact lens uses, many of them claiming oxygen permeabilities of a sufficiently high level for extended wear. The validity of this claim is considered in Chapter 12. The hydrogel chemistry disclosed in these patent specifications and the compositions currently used in commercial contact lens materials have been previously reviewed (Tighe, 1987, 2007).

19.2.2 Vinyl amides and substituted acrylamides

One of the most widely used methods of producing hydrogels with enhanced water contents for contact lens use depends upon the incorporation of N-vinylpyrrolidone (NVP). The structures of this and other nitrogen-containing monomers are shown in Fig. 19.3.

The range of EWCs obtained by copolymerising HEMA with both the more hydrophilic monomer NVP and with methyl methacrylate (MMA), which has no independent hydrophilic characteristics, is exemplified in Fig. 19.4. This figure illustrates a general principle that is applicable to other monomers that are either more, or less, hydrophilic than HEMA. This provides an effective way of preparing copolymers of any desired water content from approaching zero to greater than 80%. The 60:40 NVP–HEMA copolymer, which is seen to have an EWC in excess of 70%, is still commonly used as a material for the manufacture of so-called high-water-content conventional hydrogel contact lenses.

Two further figures serve to extend these points and conclude this section. Figure 19.5 shows how the EWC of the HEMA–MMA copolymers contained in Fig. 19.4 relates to the experimentally determined freezing water content. This illustrates the point previously made that water binding effects of this type become more markedly differentiated at lower water contents. The relevance of this effect to hydrogel behaviour will become apparent when the relationships between EWC and surface, mechanical and transport properties are discussed in the next section.

Figure 19.6 shows how variations in the structure of monomers that contain the hydrophilic —N—CO— grouping influence the EWCs of HEMA copolymers. The series shown in Fig. 19.6 is based on monomer ratios of

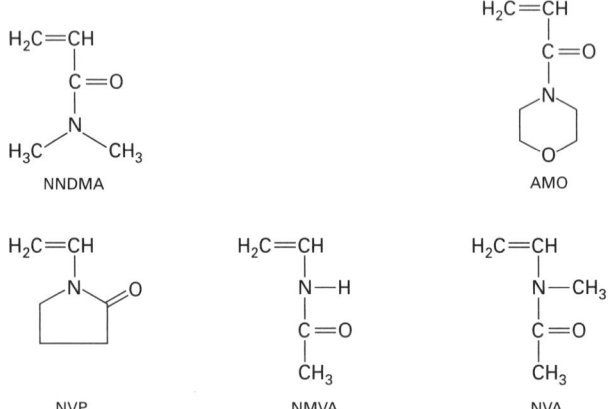

19.3 Structures of nitrogen-containing monomers: N, N-dimethyl acrylamide (NNDMA), acryloyl morpholine (AMO), N-vinyl pyrrolidone (NVP), N-methyl vinyl acetamide (NMVA) and N-vinyl acetamide (NVA).

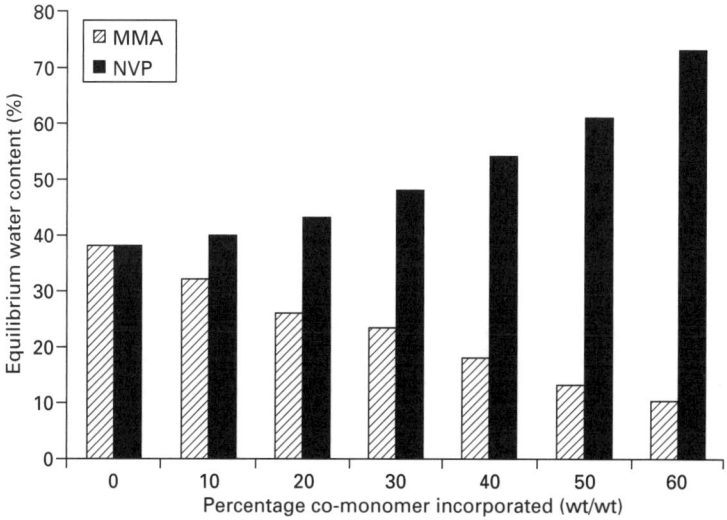

19.4 Equilibrium water contents of copolymers of HEMA–MMA and HEMA–NVP.

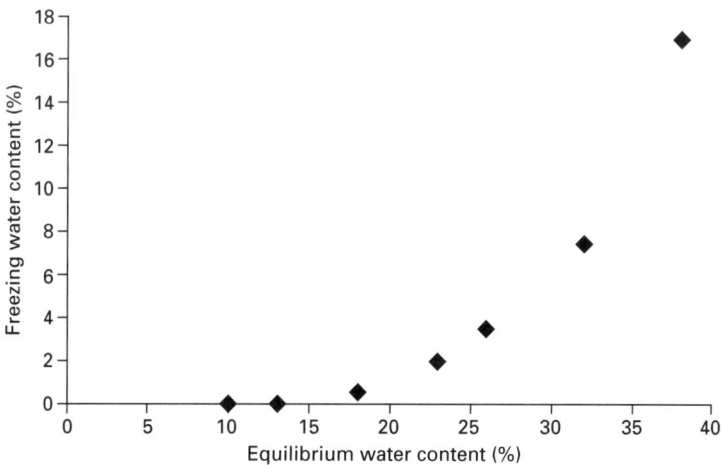

19.5 Comparison of equilibrium water contents and freezing water contents of HEMA–MMA copolymers.

30:70 (wt:wt) of the N—CO— monomer with HEMA. It is important to note that this is not a universally applicable 'hydrophilicity series' because intramolecular hydrogen bonding competes with water binding in hydrogel polymers and the balance of these two effects varies with particular monomer pairs. Nonetheless, inspection of the monomer structures shows a similar balance of polar and steric effects to that seen with the hydroxyalkyl acrylates.

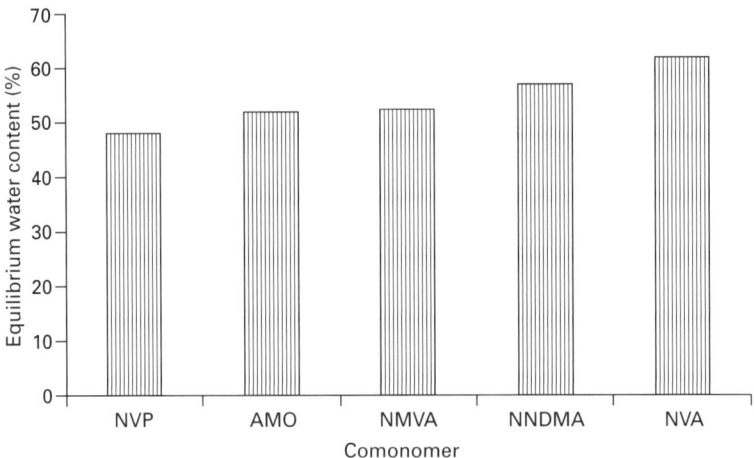

19.6 Equilibrium water contents of 70:30 (wt:wt) copolymers of HEMA and monomers containing the N—C— group.
$$\underset{O}{\overset{\parallel}{}}$$

The closeness of the nitrogen atom to the polymer backbone in the *N*-vinyl amides (NVP, NMVA and NVA) gives somewhat lower EWCs – for a given level of hydrophobic methyl or methylene substitution – than in the substituted acrylamides (AMO, NNDMA). Differences in reactivity ratios of the two families in copolymerisation provide useful versatility in influencing sequence distribution in hydrogels of similar water content.

The nitrogen-containing monomers represent the most widely used family of neutral hydrophilic monomers employed in the preparation of hydrogels that have EWCs greater than that of HEMA. Anionic monomers, such as sulphonates and carboxylates, are much more hydrophilic but are extremely susceptible to variations (e.g. pH, osmolarity) in their aqueous environment. For that reason, their greater hydrophilicity is more difficult to exploit in applications where dimensional stability is important. The one monomer of this group that has found significant use in the contact lens field, particularly in disposable lenses, is methacrylic acid. Although the unionised carboxyl group is only modestly hydrophilic, at physiological pH the monomer exists in the form of the carboxylate anion. The level of hydrophilicity that this brings to hydrogels is illustrated by the fact that the range of EWCs shown (Fig. 19.6) by the incorporation into HEMA copolymers of 30 wt% of the nitrogen-containing monomers is achieved with only 3–4% by weight of methacrylic acid.

19.3   Effect of hydrogel water content on properties

We now turn to the effect of EWC, monomer structure and water binding characteristics on the surface, mechanical, and transport properties of hydrogels. The central importance of transport phenomena, particularly oxygen permeability, to the contact lens field (see Chapter 12) led to the establishment of sound experimental methodologies. Standardisation of techniques for measurement of surface and mechanical properties of hydrogels in a reproducible and unambiguous manner has been more difficult to achieve. This is in part becouse of the inherent properties that the materials possess, but to a large extent is related to the difficulties associated with the loss of water from the gel, when held in a non-aqueous environment. A variety of techniques has been used to probe the surface properties of hydrogels including sessile drop methods, inverted droplet techniques, the Wilhelmy plate method and predictive methods. All these methods have previously been described in detail and the many problems associated with the surface analysis of hydrogels have also been discussed. A similar level of attention has been paid to methodologies for the measurement of mechanical properties and useful summaries and descriptions of novel techniques have been presented (Yang *et al.*, 2007; Ahearne *et al.*, 2008; Lee *et al.*, 2008).

19.3.1 Surface properties

Surface and interfacial properties are extremely important in the general biomaterials field and no less so in the area of ophthalmic biomaterials. One key aspect of this subject is the question of surface energy and, in order to deal with this, some definitions and concepts need to be addressed, starting with surface energy and surface tension. Surface tension has the dimension of force per unit length (mN/m), which is equivalent to the older erg/cm^2 unit (i.e. energy per unit area). The term surface tension is synonymous with surface energy – which is a more useful descriptor since it applies equally to both solids and liquids. In surface chemistry the total surface energy (γ_t) of a covalently bonded liquid or solid is commonly and conveniently separated into polar (γ_p) and dispersive (γ_d) components. These are treated additively, i.e. $\gamma_t = \gamma_d + \gamma_p$. It is useful to summarise briefly the molecular implications as they relate to the particular features of hydrogels and biological interfaces. In covalently bonded molecules there are two weaker forms of intermolecular attractions – dispersion forces and dipole–dipole attractions. In addition, we have hydrogen bonding which is a stronger and much more specific form of intermolecular force. In surface energy considerations dipole–dipole and related forces taken together with hydrogen bonding are drawn together under the heading of 'polar forces' and are designated γ_p.

Dispersion forces are also known as van der Waals dispersion forces or London forces (named after Fritz London who first suggested how they might arise). The origin of van der Waals dispersion forces lies in temporary fluctuating dipoles. These arise because electrons are mobile, and are repeatedly asymmetrically located in a molecule. This constant mobility of the electrons in the molecule causes rapidly fluctuating dipoles. This sets up an induced dipole in adjacent molecules. The polarities continue to fluctuate synchronously in adjacent molecules so that attraction is maintained. As the number of electrons and the area over which they operate increases, so does the magnitude of the dispersion forces. Longer linear molecules can develop bigger temporary dipoles and can also pack more closely, as the contribution of rotational freedom at chain ends diminishes. As a result, dispersion forces (and the surface energies arising from them) increase as molecular weight increases – thus surface energy increases with molecular weight.

It is important to realise that all molecules experience dispersion forces. Dipole–dipole interactions are not an alternative to dispersion forces – they occur in addition to dispersion forces. Additionally, and perhaps surprisingly, dipole–dipole attractions (as distinct from hydrogen bonding) are fairly minor compared with dispersion forces. The consequence is that the additional effect of any dipolar contribution in polymers is usually relatively small. The increase in the dispersion forces as chain length increases from low molecular weight monomers and oligomers to polymers more than outweighs the usually insignificant contribution of dipole–dipole interactions.

The uniquely hydrogen-bonded structure of water and its ubiquitous presence in biological systems alter these considerations, however. Water has a total surface energy (or surface tension) of 72.8 mN/m. Of this total, the dispersive component is unexceptional (21.8 mN/m) and of similar magnitude to that of many covalently bonded liquids, whereas the polar component makes by far the dominant contribution (51.0 mN/m).

The significance of the magnitude of polar and dispersive components of surface energy becomes clearer when we consider the interfacial tension or interfacial energy between two phases. For the interface to be stable, the interfacial tension should be low. If there is an imbalance, a thermodynamic driving force will exist tending to reduce it. For a synthetic material in a biological environment, deposition processes usually achieve this. The interfacial tension ($\gamma_{1,2}$) between a solid (phase 1) and a liquid (phase 2) can be described in terms of the polar (γ_p) and dispersive (γ_d) components of surface energy of the two phases:

$$\gamma_{1,2} = \gamma_1 + \gamma_2 - 2(\gamma_{1d}\gamma_{2d})^{1/2} - 2(\gamma_{1p}\gamma_{2p})^{1/2} \qquad [19.2]$$

It can be seen by inspection that, for the interfacial tension to reach zero, the polar and dispersive components on both sides of the interface must match. Similarly, if a solid substrate has a polar component of zero, the interfacial tension between water and that substrate is going to be significant. Oils, fats and waxes, for example, have polar components that are very small and as a result show interfacial tensions with water of around 50 mN/m.

Hydrogels, as might be expected, show very low interfacial tensions with water but, in order to understand interfacial behaviour and the complexities of hydrogel design for particular environments, we need to know more precisely how structural factors and EWC affect the surface energy components of hydrogels. Figure 19.7 shows changes in polar (γ_p) and dispersive (γ_d) components of hydrogel surface energy as a function of changing water content in the gel. These results are based on literature and in-house measurements of copolymers based on a wide range of hydroxyalkyl acrylates and methacrylates (Andrade, 1976; Andrade *et al.*, 1976; Ratner, 1986; Baker *et al.*, 1988; Barnes *et al.*, 1988).

Values for the interfacial tensions between water and the hydrogels derived from this copolymer series can be derived from equation [19.2] in conjunction with the information contained in Fig. 19.7. The greatest change in the polar component (γ_p) occurs during the incorporation of the first 20% of water by weight and the interfacial tension has already become very low at this point. Based on Fig. 19.7 and equation [19.2] the interfacial tension is calculated to fall very little thereafter – from around 1.6 mN/m at 20% EWC to around 0.8 mN/m at 60% EWC.

Two important observations need to be made at this point. The first is that the surface energy changes dramatically in a region where very little freezing water is available. As subsequent results will show, the introduction of water in the sub-20% region does little to enhance transport properties or to enhance flexibility. The water in this region appears to be strongly associated with the polymer and is effectively behaving as an extension of the monomer structure. In that role it contributes dramatically to the enhancement of the polar component of surface energy. The second observation is simply that

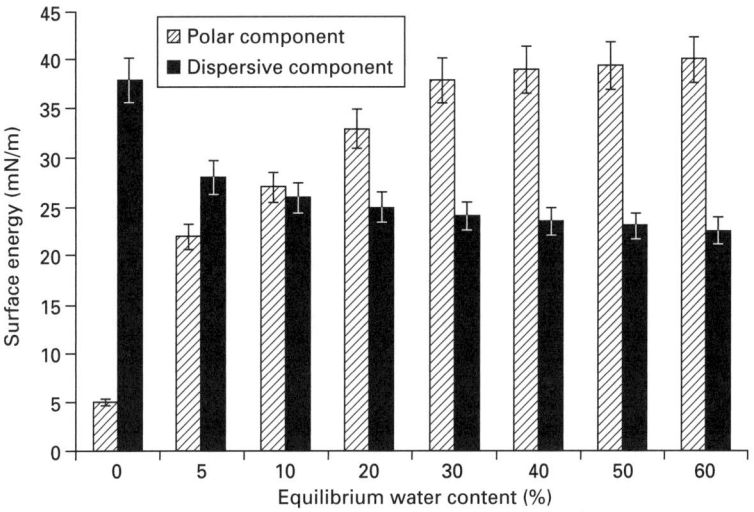

19.7 Changes in polar and dispersive components of hydrogel surface energy as a function of EWC.

biological fluids such as blood and tears contain naturally occurring surface active molecules whose size generally precludes them from entering the hydrogel matrix. The consequence of the presence of these surface active species is that biological fluids show surface tensions appreciably lower than that of water (typically around 50 mN/m or below), which is achieved solely by reduction in the polar component. The consequence is that polar component values fall to around the level of the dispersive component (c. 20–25 mN/m), which is both lower than that of water and, initially at least, lower than that of the water-swollen matrix. This presents a paradox that will become increasingly apparent. In order to match both the polar and the dispersive component of tears, the EWC of the hydrogel would need to be reduced to a level such that water would make virtually no contribution to the desired transport and mechanical properties.

It is apparent that the types of synthetic hydrogels under consideration here do not suffer deficiencies in terms of inherent wettability, provided that they are fully hydrated. Two further factors influence their behaviour in the anterior eye, however. The first is the fact that the anterior surface of the lens will progressively lose water, especially in adverse environmental conditions. The second is that the polymer chains are able to rotate rapidly in response to a changed interface. In contact with aqueous fluids the hydrophilic groups rotate to the surface, whereas in contact with more hydrophobic interfaces, such as air or lipids during tear film break-up, the hydrophilic groups 'bury' themselves within the gel and a more hydrophobic surface is exposed. Chain rotation is a dynamic process, whereas evaporative water loss is a progressive process. Molecular processes such as protein deposition and denaturation are well able to respond to the dynamic processes, which is why the eye presents such a challenging environment. The progressive dehydration has a more influential effect on the gross surface properties of the hydrogel and is part of the complex process that produces end of day discomfort for many hydrogel contact lens wearers.

19.3.2 Transport properties

Oxygen permeability

The transport of the gas through a polymer membrane is expressed in the following terms:

$$P = DS \qquad\qquad [19.3]$$

In this expression, P is the permeability coefficient for a given combination of polymer and permeant (i.e. gas), D is the diffusion coefficient of the gas through the polymer, and S is the solubility of the gas in the polymer. Much of the standardisation work on oxygen permeability measurements with hydrogels has been related to contact lens materials and was carried out by Irving Fatt, who chose to use the alternative term k to represent gas solubility (e.g. Weissman and Fatt, 1991). For this reason, the contact lens literature favours the use of the term Dk, whereas in membrane science, DS or more commonly, simply P is used. Thus Dk (or P) is the permeability coefficient for a given material, whereas DK/t or P/t refers specifically to the permeability (transmissibility) of a sample (such as a contact lens) of that material of a given thickness, t. The symbol L is also used to represent lens thickness, hence the term Dk/L is also found in the hydrogel literature. In order to determine the permeability coefficient (P or Dk) of a material at a given temperature, it is necessary to measure the rate (volume per unit time) at which the chosen gas passes through a sample of membrane of given dimensions (area and thickness) for a given gas pressure. The units of Dk take these variables into account and are quite complex. It is common therefore to quote the value in barrers (1 barrer $= 1 \times 10^{-11} cm^3 O_2$ (STP) cm/s cm^2 mmHg).

Since the oxygen passing through a contact lens is consumed by the cornea, it is apparent that, in principle, it should be possible to balance this consumption requirement with the oxygen flux through a contact lens of given dimensions and given conditions, and to define the required lens behaviour in terms of a permeability (Dk value). It is important to recognise, however, that the measured and quoted Dk values for contact lenses will only serve as a guide to their relative ability to deliver oxygen to the cornea. It is a very good guide, but not a precise indication. The question is much more critical in the case of extended (overnight) wear. For this reason it is important to identify carefully between the factors that affect the oxygen permeability of conventional hydrogels and to examine the principles involved in the development of so-called silicone hydrogels. This is the substance of Chapter 12, whereas this chapter will deal solely with factors affecting the permeability of homogeneous hydrogels.

In order to understand the permeability of hydrogel polymers, we have to look separately at the two terms that are involved: D and k, diffusion and solubility. While the diffusion term is related to the mobility of the polymer chains and the ease with which the oxygen molecule can meander through them, the solubility term is governed by the amount of oxygen that the material can dissolve. Incorporating water into a glassy polymer that resembles PMMA not only increases the ease of diffusion but also provides a medium that very effectively dissolves oxygen. Not surprisingly, then, the more water that the polymer contains, the greater amount of oxygen that it will dissolve and the higher the resultant permeability. Additionally, the water acts as a plasticiser and progressively increases the ease of diffusion. Because of this combined effect, the product of diffusion and solubility (i.e. permeability or Dk) in a conventional hydrogel will always be significantly below the value for water itself, which at 34 °C is around 100 barrers.

The precise way in which the oxygen permeability varies with water content at a given temperature was established in the mid 1970s. The relationship is an empirical one in which permeability (Dk) is seen to increase exponentially with EWC (W (in %)). That is:

$$Dk = A\,e^{-BW} \tag{19.4}$$

where A and B are experimentally determined constants for a given temperature. This means that, if the water content and the constants A and B are known at a given temperature (say $34\,^\circ C$), a reasonably exact value of the oxygen permeability can be calculated.

There is a clear pitfall here, however. Because of the ways in which water content varies with temperature, it is not possible to make comparative predictions of the permeabilities at $34\,^\circ C$ for different materials from their water contents at room temperature. As previously explained, PHEMA is atypically well-behaved in respect of the stability of its water content with temperature and can not be taken as a model for the behaviour of other polymers. If the water content of hydrogels were to remain unchanged between $20\,^\circ C$ and $34\,^\circ C$, the oxygen permeability would almost double over that temperature range. Since water contents usually fall with this temperature rise, however, the gain in oxygen permeability between room temperature and eye temperature is significantly less for most contact lens materials. These points are illustrated in Fig. 19.8, which collects quoted Dk values

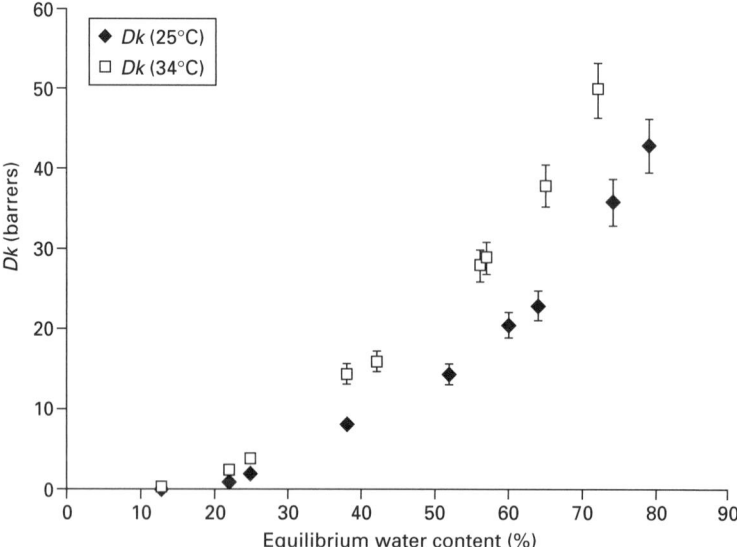

19.8 Effect of EWC on the oxygen permeability (Dk) of hydrogels at $25\,^\circ C$ and $34\,^\circ C$.

for a series of hydrogel membranes and commercial lenses as a function of water content. The figure contains data measured at both 25 °C and 34 °C.

Comparison of Fig. 19.8 with Figs. 19.7 and 19.5 illustrates the constraining factor in hydrogel design already referred to. Whereas the polar component of surface energy rises dramatically as water is introduced into the hydrogel, oxygen permeability – and indeed the permeability of all water-borne species – rises only as freezing water becomes available. This latter fact has been well recognised by various workers and is indeed an important element of the design of reverse osmosis (salt rejection) membranes that allow molecular passage of water but not that of hydrated ions (Yasuda and Lamaze, 1971; Frommer and Lancet, 1972; Pedley and Tighe, 1979; Uragami *et al.*, 1984; Hamilton *et al.*, 1988; Murphy *et al.*, 1988; McConville *et al.*, 2002).

Permeation models and polymer–solute interaction

In addition to work on ionic inorganic species, the first two decades following Wichterle's disclosures saw a range of studies into the fundamental nature of permeation through hydrogels of a range of additional species including steroids, sugars and water itself (Yasuda *et al.*, 1972; Zentner *et al.*, 1979; Kim *et al.*, 1980; Wisniewski and Kim, 1980). Because an understanding of the transport processes involved, and thus an ability to influence permeability and permselectivity, is important in applications such as reverse osmosis, kidney dialysis, sensors and drug delivery, there have been many attempts to rationalise available data in the form of a universally applicable transport model. Most of these seek to link permeability or diffusivity to the overall amount of water in the gel matrix. The free-volume model proposed by Yasuda is, perhaps, the one that has been most successful. This model applies to homogeneous water-swollen polymer matrices, where it is assumed that there is neither macroscopic phase separation of the polymer and non-polymer components nor any heterogeneity in these components. The free-volume model takes a partly thermodynamic, partly statistical approach in which the transported species is associated only with the water phase, with its diffusion being dependent upon the probability of it being located next to a suitable hole that is both unobstructed and large enough to accept the permeant. In the free-volume model the flux from high to low concentrations reflects the fact that fewer holes are occupied in the less concentrated regions and the penetrant has a higher probability of jumping to an unoccupied hole in the low concentration regions. The model predicts a linear relationship between $\ln P$ and $1/H$, where P is the permeability coefficient in the hydrogel and H is the degree of hydration. It also predicts that permeability decreases exponentially with increasing solute size and that the permselectivity of solutes increases as the degree of membrane hydration decreases. Other models have explored the applicability of the linear relationship between

$1/H$ and the logarithm of P or D, which gives the best fit for some sets of experimental data. More sophisticated models relate diffusion coefficient to an array of factors, including the degree of swelling, the radius of the solute, the number averaged molecular weight between crosslinks and function related to the mesh size, taking into account the effects of barriers such as those due to crosslinks and entanglements (Yasuda *et al.*, 1968, 1969; Kojima *et al.*, 1984; Peppas and Moynihan, 1985; Moynihan *et al.*, 1986; Amsden, 1998; Hamilton *et al.*, 1988; Murphy *et al.*, 1988).

It is clear that the transport of small, water-soluble molecules through hydrogels with moderate to high EWCs is relatively well understood and predictable. The range of applications previously mentioned includes those in which permselectivity and controlled release characteristics are required. Here the chemical composition of the polymer, its water content, and the nature of the solute to be transported interact together to enable transport behaviour to be manipulated in such a way that a degree of specificity and control is achieved. In some applications it is desirable to circumvent the overriding influence of water content on the transport process. Two examples are silicone hydrogels, dealt with in Chapter 12, and macroporous hydrogels, which are described in Section 19.4.

19.3.3 Mechanical properties

In its dehydrated state, PHEMA (and indeed most other hydrogel-forming polymers) is hard and brittle. In this, it resembles PMMA. When swollen in water, however, it becomes soft and rubber-like with a very low tear and tensile strength. This lack of mechanical strength can have a profound effect on the usefulness of hydrogels as biomaterials. Even with a supported structure such as a contact lens, the lack of durability had a marked effect on the lifetime of the lens, which caused significant problems before the advent of disposability and frequent replacement. Although the water content has a marked effect on mechanical strength within a given family of materials, the chemical structure of the polymer also plays a large part. This is not surprising, since mechanical properties are markedly influenced by chain rotation and even at an EWC of 50% the interchain distance is little more than 0.5 nm. By choosing co-monomers with bulky substituents (both cyclohexyl methacrylate and tetrahydrofurfuryl methacrylate have been used in this way) the energy barrier to rotation of the hydrogel polymer backbone can be raised considerably. In consequence, it is not difficult to increase the initial modulus – or stiffness – of a hydrogel. This approach does, however, reduce elasticity and achievable elongation of the hydrogel under tension. Increasing stiffness and reducing elasticity in this way often increases brittle failure and leads to a net reduction in tensile strength. It is generally true that homogeneous hydrogels compete poorly with natural tissue in terms of mechanical properties. This point is illustrated by comparing the strength of synthetic hydrogels such as PHEMA with that of natural composite hydrophilic gels, such as articular cartilage, intervertebral disc and the cornea. Cartilage has a modulus and tensile strength more than ten times greater than that of PHEMA, despite having double the water content (around 80%). Illustrative data are included in Table 19.1.

In summary, the elastic behaviour and rigidity of hydrogels are closely governed by monomer structure and effective crosslink density, which includes not only covalent crosslinks but also ionic, polar and steric interchain forces. To achieve good strength, network perfection, rather than the chain rotational behaviour of individual segments alone is a key factor. By use of modified monomer combinations and crosslinking agents and reducing impurity levels, high-EWC copolymer networks with improved stability and elasticity can be prepared. The currently available commercial high-water-content lenses illustrate this attention to detail and are vastly superior in strength to the first generation of fragile gels of similar water content based on HEMA–NVP. As a general rule of thumb, however, it is still true to say that increased water content reduces durability, particularly resistance to tearing, and this still presents a major limitation to the widespread use of hydrogels in more demanding applications. The logical biomimetic approach is to try to use nature's composite tissue structures as models, and the logical way to approach this is with interpenetrant technology, described in Section 19.4.

It is important to examine the way in which increases in EWC influence mechanical properties – progressively and linearly or resembling either oxygen permeability on the one hand or surface properties on the other. Figure 19.9

Table 19.1 Mechanical properties under tension (modulus, Emod; tensile strength, Ts; and elongation at break, Eb) of hydrogel interpenetrating networks and reference materials based on: cellulose acetate butyrate (CAB), polyurethane (PU), tetrahydrofurfuryl methacrylate (THFMA), *N,N*-dimethyl acrylamide (NNDMA), acryloyl morpholine (AMO), *N*-vinyl pyrrolidone (NVP) and methyl methacrylate MMA).

Monomer 1–monomer 2–interpenetrant (%, wt:wt:wt)	EWC (%)	E Mod (MPa)	Ts (MPa)	Eb (%)
NVP-MMA-CAB (48:32:20)	41*	89.0	10.9	122
NVP-MMA-CAB (54:36:10)	42*	34.2	7.4	133
NVP-THFMA-PU (42:36:22)	45	21.9	4.6	67
NVP-THFMA-PU (50:30:20)	51	13.0	4.0	70
AMO-THFMA-PU (50:30:20)	41	9.2	1.3	139
NNDMA-THFMA-PU (50:30:20)	59	5.0	0.8	79
NVP-MMA (80:20)	75	0.2	0.2	90
NVP-MMA (70:30)	65	0.5	1.1	264
PolyHEMA	38	0.5	0.5	180
Articular cartilage	75	10–100	10–30	80

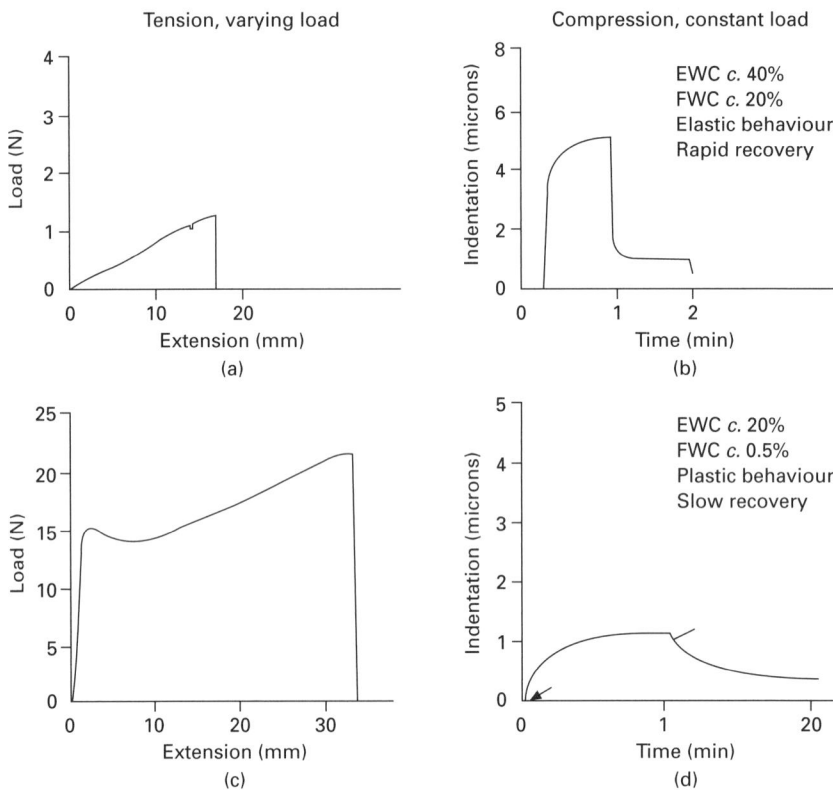

19.9 Deformational behaviour of two hydrogels under tension (left hand panels) and compression (right hand panels): comparative effect of equilibrium water content (EWC) and freezing water content (FWC).

provides the answer. It illustrates the effect of water content, and freezing water content on the behaviour of HEMA-based hydrogels in tension and compression. Tensile testing involves the application of a steadily increasing load and monitors the strain (elongation) of the sample. The absence of freezing water conveys on the sample plastic rather than elastic deformation. The behaviour is reflected in the behaviour under compression. A static load is applied and the compressive deformation of the sample monitored. The load is removed and the sample recovery curve recorded. In both tensile and compressive deformation the PHEMA sample behaves elastically and the HEMA copolymer, although containing around 20% water, shows typical thermoplastic behaviour. The results show clearly the plasticising effect of freezing water in contrast to the absence of a plasticising effect in the absence of freezing water. This behaviour is analogous to that observed with oxygen permeability and contrasts markedly with the effect of water on surface energy.

19.3.4 Density and refractive index

These properties are inter-related and both (unlike surface, transport and mechanical properties) vary progressively and substantially linearly with water content. Both depend upon the combined effect of water content and monomer composition. For conventional hydrogels based on hydroxyl and amido/acrylamido groups, densities at 20 °C decrease progressively from around 1.16 at 38% water content to around 1.05 at 75% water content.

Refractive index is a particularly important property in intraocular lens (IOL) design and manufacture. For conventional hydrogels the refractive index decreases progressively with increasing water content with values lying within a fairly narrow, almost rectilinear band, decreasing (at 34 °C) from 1.46–1.47 at 20% water content to 1.37–1.38 at 75% water content. It is for this reason that refractive index is sometimes used (with a hand-held refractometer) as a rapid method of determining the approximate water content of an unknown gel. Although the method is convenient, it suffers from inherent inaccuracies, including the erroneous assumption that dehydrated hydrogels all have the same refractive index. The extensive series of patents on new IOL materials illustrate this. The disclosures seek to demonstrate combinations of monomers with high refractive index (typically containing aromatic or heterocyclic groups) and sufficient water content to endow a degree of flexibility. The magnitude of the increase achievable by monomer structure can be seen by comparing the refractive index of PMMA (1.489) with that of poly(N-vinylphthalimide) (1.620) and poly(vinylnaphthalene) (1.681). The necessary incorporation of both hydrophilic monomer and water markedly reduces the apparent margin of improvement to a maximum net gain of around 0.05 over the refractive index of conventional methacrylate hydrogels in the 25–30% EWC region. This means that achievable refractive indices for usable hydrogel IOLs lie in the region of 1.52.

19.4   Modified hydrogels

These limitations in the ability to control independently the mechanical, surface and transport properties of homogeneous hydrogels have led to the development of modified hydrogels. Three important examples are relevant here since they have led to commercial products that would not otherwise have been achieved:

- interpenetrating networks;
- macroporous hydrogels;
- silicone hydrogels (dealt with in Chapter 12).

19.4.1 Semi-interpenetrating polymer networks

In the past two decades there has been a growing interest in applying polymer blend, composite technology, and interpenetrating network technology to hydrogels, principally because of the enhanced mechanical properties that these systems often possess. Expectation exists that this approach may enable the design of synthetic hydrogels that mimic some aspects of the behaviour of biological composites. There is sometimes confusion about the precise distinction between blends and composites when applied to polymers. Blends have been defined as 'a mix of components which are inseparable and indistinguishable' in contrast to the definition of composites as 'a material made of constituents which remain recognizable'. Problems arise, however, when trying to apply these terms on a molecular level. Interpenetrating polymer networks (IPNs) have been more specifically defined as a combination of two polymers, each in network form, at least one of which has been synthesised and/or crosslinked in the presence of the other. Varying methods are used to synthesise IPNs and this, in turn, determines the class of IPN produced. These methods may be described as follows.

1. Monomer I is polymerised and crosslinked to give a polymer which is then swollen with monomer II plus its own crosslinker and initiator. Polymerisation of monomer II *in situ* produces a *sequential IPN*.
2. If only one polymer in the system is crosslinked, the network formed is called a *semi-IPN* (SIPN). With sequential polymerisation four such *semi-IPNs* may be produced.
3. Simultaneous polymerisation, of a solution of both monomers with their crosslinkers and initiators, by two different, non-interfering methods produces a *simultaneous-IPN* or SIN.

Although these materials are known as IPNs, it is only if there is total mutual solubility that full intermolecular interpenetration occurs. In most IPNs there is, therefore, some phase separation but this may be reduced by chain entanglement between the polymers. IPNs have been used in a wide range of applications and several reviews are available describing both these applications and the fundamental theory of IPNs (Frisch *et al.*, 1981; Sperling, 1981; Klempner and Berkowski, 1987).

Hydrogel IPNs usually consist of a linear reinforcing polymer and an entwined crosslinked hydrogel copolymer. A similar principle describes the function of collagen, which reinforces the hydrophilic matrix of natural hydrogels such as articular cartilage. This technology allows hydrogels to be synthesised that have water contents similar to conventional hydrogels but which are mechanically tougher and stronger. Using this approach several examples of semi-interpenetrating hydrogel polymer networks (SIPNs) have been prepared in which preformed polymers are dissolved in hydrophilic monomer and crosslinking agent mixtures, which are subsequently polymerised. In this way a synthetic hydrogel network is formed around a primary polymer chain with the primary polymer modifying the behaviour of the hydrogel. The most obviously beneficial effects of interpenetration techniques used in this way relate to mechanical behaviour, but water binding, surface and optical properties are also affected. Optical properties are most strongly influenced by compatibility phenomena, which occur at two levels. The initial solubility of the 'filler' polymer and matrix monomer governs the first essential step in SIPN formation. This dissolution process can be assisted by use of non-reactive solvents that are subsequently removed but this has no beneficial effect on the compatibility of matrix polymer and 'filler' polymer in the dehydrated state. In hydrogel-based IPNs, additional and separate compatibility considerations in the hydrated state are involved because of the necessary presence of water as the essential third component. Translucence in the hydrated systems is generally a result of preferential water clustering around the more hydrophilic moieties creating a degree of phase segregation of hydrophobic blocks. Although high-water-content, optically clear SIPNs have considerable potential utility in ocular applications, translucent or opaque materials are of potential value both in non-ophthalmic biomaterials such as wound dressings and synthetic articular cartilage and in ocular implants and devices that do not demand optical clarity (Corkhill and Tighe, 1990, 1992; Corkhill et al., 1993).

Table 19.1 illustrates the use of interpenetrating network technology with two different types of interpenetrant in the synthesis of both translucent and optically clear systems exhibiting a range of mechanical properties. The properties of typical conventional homogeneous hydrogels are shown for comparison, together with articular cartilage. The marked effect that SIPN formation has in increasing initial modulus and tensile strength at the expense of elasticity is of considerable interest, since these are the characteristic ways in which biological composite hydrogels differ from their homogeneous synthetic counterparts.

Practical use has been made of hydrogel IPN technology in two quite different types of ocular device: the hydrogel keratoprosthesis (Chirila, 2001) and the contact lens (Hu et al., 2000; Maiden et al., 2002; Broad, 2008). Whereas the purpose of the IPN in the keratoprosthesis is to promote mechanical integration, the contact lens applications quoted have a different purpose. They make use of the observation that surface properties of SIPN materials are influenced by the nature of the interpenetrant. It was pointed out at the beginning of this section that interpretation of the molecular nature of polymer composites is difficult, but it appears that the materials described by Hu's and Maiden's groups are conventional SIPNs in which poly(ethylene glycol) and poly(N-vinylpyrrolidone), respectively, are used to enhance the hydrophilicity of the contact lens surface. The materials described by Broad, however, appear to involve sequential IPNs formed *in situ* from NVP for the same ultimate purpose. Commercial silicone hydrogel contact lenses that make use of the different technologies described in Maiden's and Broad's patents are described in Chapter 12.

19.4.2 Macroporous hydrogels

The versatility of hydrogel polymers and their numerous potential applications in the field of biomedicine stem from the extensive range of hydrophilic monomers available for their formation and from the ability to control the extent and nature of water binding within the polymer matrices. One feature of the materials is that in homogeneous hydrogels the transport properties are limited by effective mean pore, or mesh, diameters within the polymer. Although this feature may be employed to advantage in the design of permselective membranes, it limits the utilisation of hydrogels for the transport of high molecular weight species. This limitation is of prime importance in the design of hydrogels for use as sorbents in haemoperfusion and in macromolecular drug-delivery systems. An additional aspect of the application of hydrogels in bodily repair and regeneration is their use in implants requiring cellular integration, such as articular cartilage repair and keratoprosthesis.

Three different approaches to the preparation of macroporous hydrogels illustrate the fact that both pore size and detailed morphology can be manipulated in response to the requirements of different applications. These approaches are:

- freeze–thaw polymerisation;
- incorporation of water-extractable porosigens;
- phase-separation polymerisation.

The first two of these methods of increasing the effective pore size of polymers involve polymerising monomers around a crystalline matrix that is subsequently dispersed or dissolved to leave an interconnected meshwork. The significance of the freeze–thaw technique for hydrophilic monomers lies in the fact that aqueous systems can be induced to form ice-based crystalline matrices by rapid cooling of homogeneous solutions of these monomers. Crosslinking monomers are necessary to control the integrity of the resultant macroporous polymers and the solubility of the non-aqueous components must be maintained during cooling to avoid phase separation before ice crystal formation. The formation of macroporous hydrophilic matrices by the freeze–thaw technique consists, in principle, of freezing a monomer/crosslinker/solvent mixture on to a cold plate, or by dropping the mixture into a cold non-solvent, to create a system that consists of a solid monomer matrix around and between solvent crystals. This monomer matrix is then

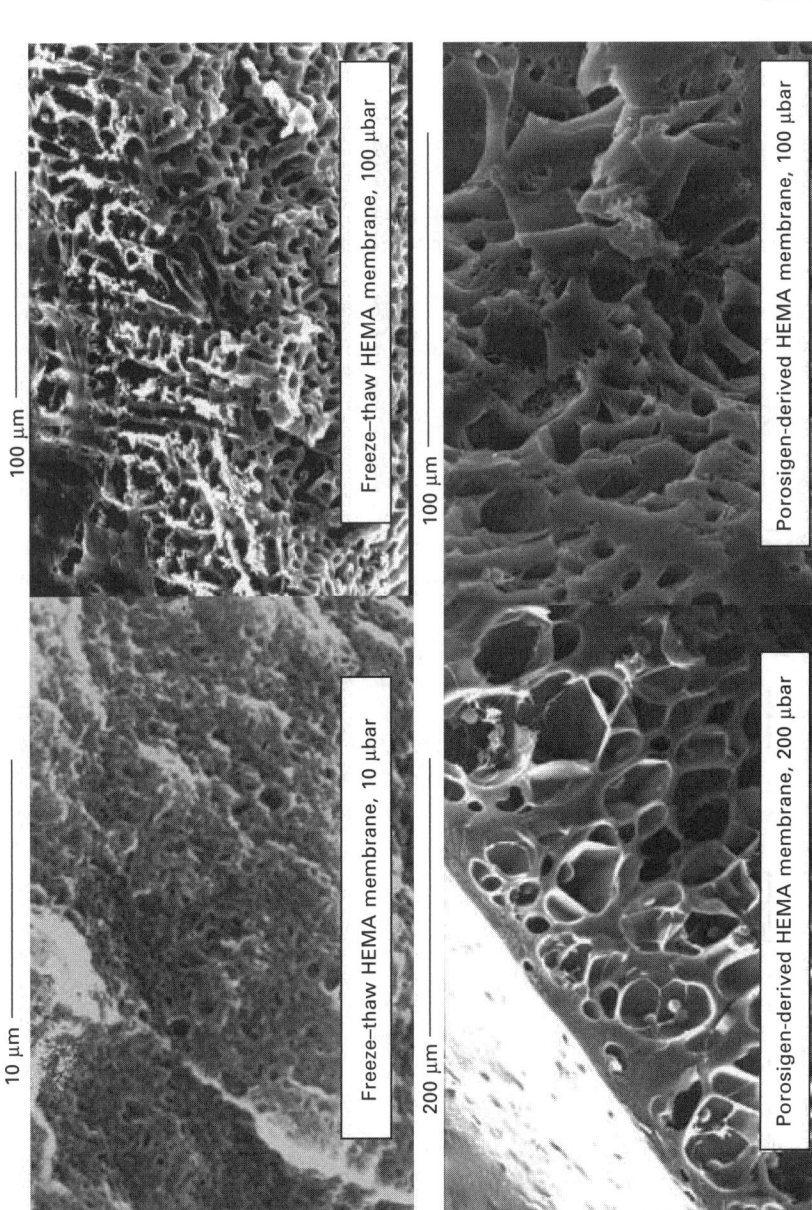

100 μm

Freeze–thaw HEMA membrane, 100 μbar

10 μm

Freeze–thaw HEMA membrane, 10 μbar

100 μm

Porosigen-derived HEMA membrane, 100 μbar

200 μm

Porosigen-derived HEMA membrane, 200 μbar

19.10 Examples of macroporous hydrogel structures.

polymerised by photopolymerisation, utilising a water-soluble photocatalyst, such as uranyl nitrate. After polymerization, the aqueous solvent is removed by thawing and a macroporous polymer results. The principle can be employed to prepare membranes or particulates with morphologies based on interconnected pores with diameters in the range 1–20 μm (Krauch and Sanner, 1968; Haldon and Lee, 1972; Skelly and Tighe, 1979; Murphy et al., 1992; Oxley et al., 1993).

Polymerisation around pre-formed porosigens, although less elegant than freeze–thaw polymerisation, does allow a wider range of hydrogel compositions, including IPNs, to be prepared in macroporous form. Additionally, hydrogels with larger pores and asymmetric pore distributions can be prepared. These features are illustrated in Fig. 19.10.

The most dramatic success in the practical use of macroporous hydrogel technology in ophthalmic applications is found in phase separation technology and its application to the AlphaCor™ keratoprosthesis. The principle of phase-separation polymerisation lies in the selection of a solvent in which the monomer system but not the resultant polymer is soluble. Above a particular concentration of, in this case, water, phase-separation develops during polymerisation (Chirila et al., 1993; Chirila, 2001).

19.4.3 Silicone hydrogels

Macroporosity provides a means of overcoming the limitations imposed by the presence of the polymer structure on transport through the aqueous phase of the hydrogel. Silicone hydrogels seek to make use of the polymer to enhance transport through the gel. The principle is simple: since silicone rubber has an oxygen permeability at least ten times greater that that of water, why not make use of that in preparing 'super-permeable' hydrogels? As is often the case, the principle is simple but translating it into practice is not. The last decade has seen the principle harnessed so successfully that it now forms the basis of a multi-billion dollar industry – the silicone hydrogel contact lens. This is such a large and important subject that it requires separate treatment, and is discussed in Chapter 12.

19.5   References

Ahearne M, Yang Y and Liu K K (2008), 'Mechanical characterisation of hydrogels for tissue engineering applications', in Ashammakhi N, Reis R and Chiellini F, Eds, *Topics in Tissue Engineering*, Vol. 4. Available from: http://www.oulu.fi/spareparts/ebook_topics_in_t_e_vol4/published_chapters.html [Accessed 15th March 2009].

Amsden B (1998), 'Solute diffusion within hydrogels. Mechanisms and models', *Macromolecules*, **31**, 8382–8395.

Andrade, J D, Ed. (1976), *Hydrogels for Medical and Related Applications,* ACS Symposium Series No. 31, American Chemical Society, Washington DC.

Andrade J D, King R N, Gregonis D E and Coleman D L (1976), 'Surface characterization of poly (HEMA) and related polymers. I. Contact angle methods in water', *J Polym Sci Polym Symp*, **66**, 313–336.

Baker D A, Corkhill P H, Ng C O, Skelly P J and Tighe B J (1988), 'Synthetic hydrogels. II. Copolymers of carboxyl-, lactam and amide-containing monomers – structure property relationships', *Polymer*, **29**, 691–700.

Barnes A, Corkhill, P H and Tighe B J (1988), 'Synthetic hydrogels. III. Hydroxyalkyl acrylate and methacrylate copolymers: surface and mechanical properties', *Polymer*, **29**, 2191–2202.

Broad R A (2008), 'Contact lens', WO/2008/061992, 29.05.2008.

Chirila T V, Chen Y-C, Griffin B J and Constable I (1993), 'Hydrophilic sponges based on 2-hydroxyethyl methacrylate I, Effect of monomer mixture composition on pore size', *Polym Int*, **32**, 221–232.

Chirila T V (2001), 'An overview of the development of artificial corneas with porous skirts and the use of PHEMA for such an application', *Biomaterials*, **22**, 3311–3317.

Corkhill P H and Tighe B J (1990), 'Synthetic hydrogels 7. High EWC semi-interpenetrating polymer networks based on cellulose esters and *N*-containing hydrophilic monomers', *Polymer*, **31**, 1526–1537.

Corkhill P H and Tighe B J (1992), 'Synthetic hydrogels 8. Physicochemical properties of *N,N*-dimethylacrylamide semi-interpenetrating polymer network hydrogels', *J Mater Chem*, **2**, 491–496.

Corkhill P H, Fitton J H and Tighe B J (1993), 'Towards a synthetic articular cartilage', *J Biomater Sci Polym Edn*, **4**, 615–630.

Frisch H L, Frisch K C and Klempner D (1981), 'Advances in interpenetrating polymer networks', *Pure Appl Chem*, **53**, 1557–1566.

Frommer M and Lancet D (1972), 'Freezing and non-freezing water in cellulose acetate membranes', *J Appl Polym Sci*, **16**, 1295–1303.

Haldon R A and Lee B E (1972), 'Structure and permeability of porous films of poly(hydroxyethyl methacrylate)', *Br Polym J*, **4**, 491–501.

Hamilton C J, Murphy S M, Atherton N D and Tighe B J (1988), 'Synthetic hydrogels 4. The permeability of poly(2-hydroxyethyl methacrylate) to cations – an overview of solute–water interactions and transport processes', *Polymer*, **29**, 1879–1886.

Hu H, Briggs C R, Nguyen T, Tran H and Rossberg E. (2000), 'Interpenetrating polymer network hydrophilic hydrogels for contact lens', WO/2000/002937, 20.01.2000.

Kim S W, Cardinal J R, Wisniewski S and Zentner G M (1980), 'Solute permeation through hydrogel membranes', in Rowland S P, Ed., *Water in Polymers*, ACS Symposium Series, Vol. 127, American Chemical Society, Washington DC, pp. 347–359.

Kishi A, Tanaka M and Mochizuki A (2008), 'Comparative study on water structures in polyHEMA and polyMEA by XRD-DSC simultaneous measurement', *J Appl Polym Sci,* **111**, 476–481.

Klempner D and Berkowski L (1987), 'Interpenetrating polymer networks', in Kroschwitz J I, Ed., *Encyclopedia of Polymer Science and Engineering*, Vol. 8, Wiley-Interscience, New York, pp. 279–341.

Kojima Y, Furuhata, K and Miyasaka, K (1984) 'Diffusive permeability of solutes in poly(vinylalcohol) membranes as a function of the degree of hydration', *J Appl Polym Sci*, **29**, 533–546.

Krauch C H and Sanner A (1968), 'Polymerisation auf kristalliner matrix', *Naturwissenschaft*, **55**, 539–540.

Lee S J, Bourne G R, Chen X, Sawyer G and Sarntinoranont M (2008), 'Mechanical characterization of contact lenses by microindentation: Constant velocity and relaxation testing', *Acta Biomater*, **4**, 1560–1568.

Maiden A C, Vanderlaan D G, Turner D C, Love R N, Ford J D, Molock F F, Steffen R B, Hill G A, Alli A and McCabe K P (2002), 'Hydrogel with internal wetting agent', United States Patent 6367929, 04.09.2002.

McConville P, Whittaker M K and Pope J M (2002), 'Water and polymer mobility in hydrogel biomaterials quantified by 1H NMR: A simple model describing both T1 and T2 relaxation', *Macromolecules*, **35**, 6961–6969.

Moynihan H J, Honey M S and Peppas N A (1986), 'Solute diffusion in swollen membranes V. Solute diffusion in poly(2-hydroxyethyl methacrylate)', *Polym Eng Sci*, **26**, 1180–1185.

Murphy S M, Hamilton C J and Tighe B J (1988), 'Synthetic hydrogels 5. Transport processes in 2-hydroxyethyl methacrylate copolymers', *Polymer*, **29**, 1887–1893.

Murphy S M, Skelly P J and Tighe B J (1992), 'Synthetic hydrogels 9. Preparation and characterisation of macroporous hydrophilic matrices', *J Mater Chem*, **2**, 1007–1013.

Oxley H R, Corkhill P H, Fitton J H and Tighe B J (1993), 'Macroporous hydrogels for biomedical applications: methodology and morphology', *Biomaterials*, **14**, 1064–1072.

Pedley D G and Tighe B J (1979), 'Water binding properties of hydrogel polymers for reverse osmosis and related applications', *Br Polym J*, **11**, 130–136.

Peppas N A and Moynihan H J (1985), 'Solute diffusion in swollen membranes. IV. Theories for moderately swollen networks', *J Appl Polym Sci*, **30**, 2859–2606.

Peppas N A, Ed. (1986), *Hydrogels in Medicine and Pharmacy*, Vol. 1, *Fundamentals*, CRC Press, Boca Raton, Florida.

Peppas N A, Ed. (1987a), *Hydrogels in Medicine and Pharmacy*, Vol. 2, *Polymers*, CRC Press, Boca Raton, Florida.

Peppas N A, Ed. (1987b), *Hydrogels in Medicine and Pharmacy,* Vol. 3, *Properties and Applications*, CRC Press, Boca Raton, Florida.

Ratner B D (1986), 'Hydrogel surfaces', in Peppas N A, Ed., *Hydrogels in Medicine and Pharmacy*, Vol. 1, *Fundamentals*, CRC Press, Boca Raton, Florida, pp. 85–94.

Roorda W E, de Bleyser J, Junginger H E and Leyte J C (1990), 'Nuclear magnetic relaxation of water in hydrogels', *Biomaterials*, **11**, 17–23.

Skelly P J and Tighe B J (1979), 'Novel macroporous hydrogel adsorbents for artificial liver support perfusion systems', *Polymer*, **20**, 1051–1052.

Sperling L H (1981), *Interpenetrating Polymer Networks and Related Materials*, Plenum Press, New York.

Tighe B J (1987), 'Hydrogels as contact lens materials', in Peppas N A, Ed., Chapter 3, *Hydrogels in Medicine and Pharmacy,* Vol. 3, *Properties and Applications*, CRC Press, Boca Raton, Florida, pp. 53–82.

Tighe B J (2007), 'Contact lens materials', in Phillips A J and Speedwell L, Eds, *Contact Lenses,* 5th Edition, Butterworths, London, pp. 59–78.

Uragami T, Furukawa T and Sugihara M.(1984), 'Studies on syntheses and permeabilities of special polymer membranes. VII. Permeability of solute through polymer membranes and state of water in their membranes', *Polym Commun,* **25**, 30–33.

Wang T and Gunasekaran S (2006), 'State of water in chitosan–PVA hydrogel', *J Appl Polym Sci*, **101**, 3227–3232.

Weissman B A and Fatt, I (1991) 'Contact-lens wear and oxygen permeability measurements', *Current Opinion in Ophthalmology* **2**: (1) 88–94.

Wichterle O and Lim D (1960), 'Hydrophilic gels for biological use', *Nature*, **185**, 117–118.

Wichterle O (1971), 'Hydrogels', in Mark H and Gaylord N, Eds, *Encyclopedia of Polymer Science and Technology*, Vol. 15, Wiley-Interscience, New York, pp. 273–290.

Wisniewski S and Kim S W (1980), 'Permeation of water through poly(2-hydroxyethyl methacrylate) and related polymers: temperature effects', *J Membrane Sci*, **6**, 309–318.

Yang Y, Bagnaninchi P O, Ahearne M, Wang R K and Liu K K (2007), 'A novel optical coherence tomography-based micro-indentation technique for mechanical characterization of hydrogels', *J Roy Soc Interface*, **4**, 1169–1173.

Yasuda H and Lamaze G E (1971), 'Permselectivity of solutes in homogeneous water-swollen polymer membranes', in Rogers C E, Ed., *Permselective Membranes*, Marcel Dekker, New York, pp. 111–134.

Yasuda H, Lamaze G E and Ikenberry L D (1968), 'Permeability of solutes through hydrated polymer membranes I. Diffusion of sodium chloride', *Makromol Chem*, **118**, 19–35.

Yasuda H, Ikenberry L D and Lamaze G E (1969), 'Permeability of solutes through hydrated polymer membranes II. Permeability of water soluble organic solutes', *Makromol Chem*, **125**, 108–118.

Yasuda H, Olf H G, Crist B, Lamaze G E and Peterlin A (1972), 'Movement of water in homogeneous water-swollen polymers', in Jellinek H H G, Ed., *Water Structure at the Water–Polymer Interface*, Plenum Press, New York, pp. 39–45.

Zentner G M, Cardinal J R, Feijen J and Song S Z (1979), 'Progestin permeation through polymer membranes IV. Mechanism of steroid permeation and functional group contributions to diffusion through hydrogel films', *J Pharm Sci*, **68**, 970–975.

Index